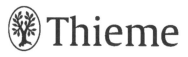

Fundamental Topics in Plastic Surgery

Diego Marré, MD
Consultant
Department of Plastic and Reconstructive Surgery and Burns
Clínica Las Condes
Emergency Public Hospital
Santiago, Chile

457 illustrations

Thieme
Stuttgart • New York • Delhi • Rio de Janeiro

Library of Congress Cataloging-in-Publication Data

Names: Marre, Diego, editor.
Title: Fundamental topics in plastic surgery / [edited by]
Diego Marré.
Description: Stuttgart ; New York : Thieme, [2018] |
Includes bibliographical
   references and index. |
Identifiers: LCCN 2018007646 (print) | LCCN
2018008885 (ebook) | ISBN
   9783132059214 () | ISBN 9783132059115
   (hardcover : alk. paper)
Subjects: | MESH: Reconstructive Surgical
Procedures--methods
Classification: LCC RD118 (ebook) | LCC RD118 (print) |
NLM WO 600 | DDC
   617.9/52--dc23
LC record available at https://lccn.loc.gov/2018007646

© 2018 by Georg Thieme Verlag KG

Thieme Publishers Stuttgart
Rüdigerstrasse 14, 70469 Stuttgart, Germany
+49 [0]711 8931 421, customerservice@thieme.de

Thieme Publishers New York
333 Seventh Avenue, New York, NY 10001 USA
+1 800 782 3488, customerservice@thieme.com

Thieme Publishers Delhi
A-12, Second Floor, Sector-2, Noida-201301
Uttar Pradesh, India
+91 120 45 566 00, customerservice@thieme.in

Thieme Publishers Rio, Thieme Publicações Ltda.
Edifício Rodolpho de Paoli, 25º andar
Av. Nilo Peçanha, 50 - Sala 2508
Rio de Janeiro 20020-906 Brasil
+55 21 3172 2297 / +55 21 3172 1896

Cover design: Thieme Publishing Group
Typesetting by DiTech Process Solutions Pvt. Ltd., India

Printed in Germany by CPI Books   5 4 3 2 1

ISBN 978-3-13-205911-5

Also available as an e-book:
eISBN 978-3-13-205921-4

Important note: Medicine is an ever-changing science undergoing continual development. Research and clinical experience are continually expanding our knowledge, in particular our knowledge of proper treatment and drug therapy. Insofar as this book mentions any dosage or application, readers may rest assured that the authors, editors, and publishers have made every effort to ensure that such references are in accordance with **the state of knowledge at the time of production of the book.**

Nevertheless, this does not involve, imply, or express any guarantee or responsibility on the part of the publishers in respect to any dosage instructions and forms of applications stated in the book. **Every user is requested to examine carefully** the manufacturers' leaflets accompanying each drug and to check, if necessary in consultation with a physician or specialist, whether the dosage schedules mentioned therein or the contraindications stated by the manufacturers differ from the statements made in the present book. Such examination is particularly important with drugs that are either rarely used or havebeen newly released on the market. Every dosage schedule or every form of application used is entirely at the user's ownrisk and responsibility. The authors and publishers request every user to report to the publishers any discrepancies or inaccuracies noticed. If errors in this work are found after publication, errata will be posted at www.thieme.com on the product description page.

Some of the product names, patents, and registered designs referred to in this book are in fact registered trademarks or proprietary names even though specific reference to this fact is not always made in the text. Therefore, the appearance of a name without designation as proprietary is not to be construed as a representation by the publisher that it is in the public domain.

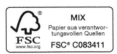

Contents

Contents

Contents

Foreword

The plastic surgeon is both an artisan and an artist and aims to re-create what is lost following injury, disease, or the aging process. The medium is the living tissue, with its own fickle intrinsic power of repair and memory. At its best, the surgeon's repair will be a replica of what was lost in form and function, with the almost invisible mending of primary healing; at its worst, it will be the scarred horror of secondary healing with contraction and deformity. How does the surgeon ensure that the pendulum is always weighted toward the former? Like all artistic pursuits, although plastic surgeons will likely boast an element of innate talent, they cannot perfect their craft until they have mastered its underlying fundamental principles. Very often in life and in our jobs, we assume we understand core principles and proceed directly to the specifics of a task. But these fundamentals may never have been learned, and instead were subliminally assumed and accreted piecemeal, often from disparate contexts, and, when challenged, we realize that our understanding is superficial and often erroneous. In plastic surgery, without a thorough grounding in these fundamentals, we are destined to flounder because they are the key to design concepts, technical mastery, and the avoidance of complications.

This book, edited by Dr. Diego Marré, is the one we all wish we had read before our entrenched habits took hold. It teaches us principles we did not even know we did not know. It is targeted at the plastic surgery trainee/resident level, but it is an excellent source for those who are not trainees as well as those who are specialists. It aims to cover all the fundamentals so that the reader, once grounded in the conceptual roots, can confidently move on to the specifics of plastic surgery. It deliberately excludes detailed surgical techniques. The authors are a balanced mix of those of the younger generation and senior specialists. The former bring new talent, their own perspective and insights as to what is important and what is not, and a refreshing contemporary feel to the work. The latter bring invaluable experience and expertise unique to senior specialists.

The book is of a digestible size, has a limited but targeted scope, avoids repetition, and is engaging and a joy to read. It collates and distills the latest information, which is not readily accessible in standard texts. The format and style are uniform and pleasing. The text is presented in two sections: Principles and Techniques. The principles presented in section 1 are interesting and eclectic. The chapters provide detailed discussion of topics that are often taken for granted or are not presented in easy format elsewhere and hence are never fully learned or understood. Examples include safety in the operating theater, antibiotics in plastic surgery, biomaterials, osteosynthesis, and statistics for plastic surgery. Section 1 also impresses on us the collaborative and interdisciplinary role that plastic surgeons play and the need to understand the fundamentals of other disciplines, as highlighted by chapters on dermatology, infections, and osteosynthesis. Section 2, Techniques, gives us the core requirements for success: blood supply, wound healing and suture techniques, and flaps and grafts, among many others.

This book offers something quite different from its contemporaries and others before it, and I very much appreciate the honor to be asked to write this Foreword. I congratulate the editor for his insight to discern the need for such a volume amid the myriad existing texts on plastic surgery, and to the multiple authors who have contributed to bring this superb book to fruition. Those who have the privilege to read it will long savor its merits.

Wayne Morrison, MBBS, FRACS

Plastic and Hand Surgeon
Department of Plastic Reconstructive and Hand Surgery
St. Vincent's Hospital
Melbourne, Australia

Preface

Plastic surgery is one of the surgical disciplines with most presence in the media and, paradoxically, one of the most misunderstood too. Although the majority of lay public (and of course medical staff) have a very good idea of what an orthopaedic or cardiothoracic surgeon does, their knowledge about the daily practice of a plastic surgeon is generally limited to the aesthetic branch of our specialty, which, despite its great value, does not represent the whole scope of plastic surgery. In addition, the prototype of the plastic surgeon presented in advertising, television series, and movies in most cases makes the gap between illusion and reality even bigger. Furthermore, it is both surprising and demoralizing to realize every now and then how our own colleagues from other medical or surgical fields still do not understand the breadth of plastic surgery outside its cosmetic realms, a phenomenon that is highly contradictory as the roots of plastic surgery actually derive from its reconstructive legacy.

So what is plastic surgery? The name comes from the Greek word *plastikos*, meaning "to mold or to shape," which, although etymologically correct, and seemingly a good and intelligent answer to give our friends or patients when they ask the question, tells us little about what we actually do as plastic surgeons. Without a system or anatomical region of its own, it is hard to box plastic surgery into one specific definition or scope of practice. For example, how is a complex craniofacial reconstruction related to the tangential excision and grafting of a burn or to a flexor tendon repair in the hand? In the very broad sense, plastic surgery could be thought of as the surgical specialty in charge of repairing what is wounded, replacing what is missing, restoring what is altered, and reshaping what is deformed.

At the start of our training, most of us had an idea of what we were getting ourselves into, though probably for most, it was rather vaguely so, with very little interconnection between these fascinating things we started seeing every day, a lot of them for the very first time. And so, in this whirlwind of new concepts and techniques, we started digging into specific flaps for specific needs or reading on specific procedures and classifications, in an effort to prepare ourselves in the best possible way for the next case, studying on a case-by-case basis rather than on a principles-based approach. Not surprisingly then, trainees may sometimes know all about the anatomy and the technical aspects of the deep inferior epigastric perforator (DIEP) flap, but have a hard time describing the different ways in which flaps can be classified. And so the obvious becomes clear: in order to build our knowledge we need to start from the basics. But then comes the issue of where to begin the study from. Where do I find a good chapter on flaps? Where is tissue expansion described in detail? And again we start diving through pages of numerous textbooks, one with a good chapter on a specific topic but falling short on another one that is equally important, all of which renders difficult the study of these essential issues. This is especially the case during the early years of training, in which time is limited and thus going through different textbooks becomes frustrating and ineffective. In this context, *Fundamental Topics in Plastic Surgery* would help the reader as it has been designed and written to provide trainees with a solid foundation and a detailed description of the basic principles of our specialty.

The book is divided in two sections: Principles and Techniques. The first section, Principles, comprises 11 chapters, including topics such as patient safety, wound healing, dressings, and negative pressure wound therapy, among others. In addition, this section incorporates topics such as infections and antibiotics in plastic surgery and principles of osteosynthesis, which despite being part of our everyday practice, are sometimes hard to find in reference books. The second section, Techniques, describes the theoretical and technical aspects of procedures that are common to virtually the whole scope of plastic surgery, starting with basic techniques and local flaps and then navigating through grafts, flaps, tissue expansion, and microsurgery, the latter including a detailed description on the necessary elements for a successful laboratory training as well as the physiological and clinical features of microsurgical tissue transfer. In addition, chapters on burns, facial trauma, and hand trauma have been included in this second section to provide the basic theory and principles of treatment of these conditions, commonly seen by trainees in the emergency department.

In all, *Fundamental Topics in Plastic Surgery* has been devised as the starting point for anyone interested in pursuing this fascinating specialty. In addition, senior trainees, fellows, and consultants might also find it useful as a reference resource and as a teaching resource as well. The concepts and information provided throughout the following pages should help the reader build a solid foundation of the core topics of plastic surgery, and then be able to move confidently forward into more specialized reading.

Diego Marré, MD

Consultant
Department of Plastic and Reconstructive Surgery and Burns
Clínica Las Condes
Emergency Public Hospital
Santiago, Chile

Acknowledgments

First and foremost I want to thank my beloved wife, Isabel, and our children, Juan Diego and Agustin. Not only has Isabel been the pillar of our family throughout my years of residency and fellowship, but she has managed to do so while being a resident and fellow herself, which has led her to become the accomplished dermatologist she is today. Her help and sage advice have been vital for this book to come to fruition, by making me see things in different ways at times of frustration and despair, by bringing new and fresh ideas that have really enhanced the work, and by contributing with a fabulous chapter. But above all, I thank her for being a wonderful wife and a loving mother.

I would like to thank my parents for encouraging me to study medicine and supporting me in every step of the way. My mother, who always managed to find time away to come and visit and stay with us no matter how far we were, and my father, for his example of hard work. And, very especially to Juan and Maribel, without whom our life overseas would not have been possible.

This book represents the culmination of the generous contributions from several authors. I am indebted to each of them for their participation in this wonderful project.

I offer sincere thanks to my mentors and friends in plastic surgery. A special recognition goes to Dr. Wilfredo Calderon and the whole Burns and Plastic Surgery Unit at Hospital del Trabajador during my stay there many years ago. Many thanks to Alex Eulufi, Patricio Léniz, and Álvaro Cuadra for their friendship and support, and Dr. Hector Roco, who became my role model very early in my career and with whom I took my first steps in reconstructive surgery and microsurgery. I am deeply grateful to Bernardo Hontanilla and Cristina Aubá, my tutors in Spain, for being my teachers and surgical mentors and for showing me the value of and passion for research. I thank all my colleague residents—we shared such wonderful moments throughout our training. A special thanks to my colleague and close friend Alvaro Cabello, a skillful surgeon and one of the most virtuous people I know. My deepest gratitude to Professor Wayne Morrison, a true master, a person whose door and mind are always open to new ideas, and with whom I had the privilege to share thoughts, projects, and countless hours in theater during my 2 years in Melbourne. To everyone at O'Brien Institute, I really enjoyed my research time there! Thanks to Mr. Tim Bennet, Eldon Mah, and the whole Plastic Surgery Unit at St. Vincent's Hospital Melbourne for an amazing year as your reconstructive surgery fellow; that period has left an indelible mark in my career and my life. To my new colleagues and team members at Hospital de Urgencia de Asistencia Pública and Clinica Las Condes, I really enjoy working with you.

I want to thank all the people at Thieme for their invaluable support. It has been a true honor to publish this book with you and become a Thieme author.

Lastly, I would like to pay tribute to and honor the memory of two very special people, Dr. Ernesto Medina Lois and Dr. Ana María Kaempffer, two outstanding physicians, leaders in their respective fields, but more than that, my two loving grandparents. Their contributions to Chilean medicine and the World Health Organization are countless, as are the number of students that had the privilege to attend their lessons. They were the first couple to ever receive the Professor Emeritus distinction from Universidad de Chile, and my grandmother was one of the few women to be honored with such a remarkable recognition. Every memory I have of them is a joyful one, and I am sure they would have been proud to see this book published.

Contributors

Cristina Aubá, MD, PhD
Consultant
Department of Plastic, Reconstructive and
Aesthetic Surgery
University Clinic of Navarra
Pamplona, Spain

Patricio Andrades, MD
Consultant
Department of Surgery
University of Chile Clinical Hospital
Hospital del Trabajador
Santiago, Chile

Pedro Bolado, MD
Resident
Division of Plastic and Reconstructive Surgery
La Paz University Hospital
Madrid, Spain

Jorge Bonastre, MD, PhD
Consultant
Division of Plastic and Reconstructive Surgery
La Paz University Hospital
Madrid, Spain

Edward P. Buchanan, MD
Assistant Professor
Division of Plastic Surgery
Texas Children's Hospital
Michael E. Debakey Department of Surgery
Baylor College of Medicine
Houston, Texas, USA

Javier Buendia, MD
Consultant
Department of Plastic and Reconstructive Surgery
San Carlos Clinical Hospital
Madrid, Spain

Álvaro Cabello, MD, PhD
Consultant
Department of Plastic and Reconstructive Surgery
University Clinic of Navarra
Pamplona, Spain

Daniel Calderón, MD
Instructor
Department of Surgery
University of Chile
Santiago, Chile

Wilfredo Calderón, MD
Professor of Plastic Surgery
Chief of Plastic and Reconstructive Surgery
Salvador Hospital
Santiago, Chile

Marcus Castro Ferreira, MD, PhD
Full Professor of Plastic Surgery
University of São Paulo
School of Medicine
Coordinator of the Complex Wound Center
Syrian-Lebanese Hospital
São Paulo, Brazil

Alejandro Conejero, MD, FACS
Faculty
Department of Plastic and Reconstructive Surgery
Assistant Professor of Surgery
Albert Einstein College of Medicine
Montefiore Medical Center
New York, New York, USA

Álvaro Cuadra, MD
Faculty
Department of Plastic and Reconstructive Surgery
University Hospital
Pontifical Catholic University of Chile
Santiago, Chile

Bruno Dagnino, MD
Assistant Professor
Head of Plastic Surgery Division
Department of Surgery
University Hospital
Pontifical Catholic University of Chile
Santiago, Chile

Stefan Danilla, MD, MSc
Consultant
Plastic Surgery Unit
Department of Surgery
Clinical Hospital
University of Chile
Santiago, Chile

José Manuel Collado Delfa, MD
Chief of Burn Unit
Department of Plastic and Reconstructive Surgery
and Burns
Vall d'Hebron University Hospital
Barcelona, Spain

Sandhya Deo, MD
Plastic and Reconstructive Surgeon
Wellington Regional Plastic, Maxillofacial and
Burns Unit
Hutt Hospital
Lower Hutt, New Zealand

Chiara Distefano, MD
Plastic Surgeon
Private practice
Catania, Italy

Alex Eulufí, MD
Consultant
Department of Plastic and Reconstructive Surgery
Clinica Alemana
Santiago, Chile

Tomas Gantz, MD
Consultant
Department of Surgery
Padre Hurtado Hospital
Santiago, Chile

Ismael González, MD
Consultant
Ibermutuamur
Madrid, Spain

Bernardo Hontanilla, MD, PhD
Professor of Plastic Surgery
Chief of Plastic and Reconstructive Surgery
University Clinic of Navarra
Pamplona, Spain

Isabel Irarrazaval, MD
Consultant
Dermatology Department
University Clinic of Los Andes
Exequiel Gonzalez Cortes Hospital
Santiago, Chile

Leigh Jansen, MD, MSc, FRCSC
Plastic Surgeon
Vancouver, British Columbia, Canada

Matthew G. Kaufman, MD
Resident
Division of Plastic Surgery
Baylor College of Medicine
Houston, Texas, USA

Luis Landin, MD, PhD
Consultant
Division of Plastic and Reconstructive Surgery
La Paz University Hospital
Madrid, Spain

Matthew R. Louis, MD
Resident
Division of Plastic Surgery
Michael E. DeBakey Department of Surgery
Baylor College of Medicine
Houston, Texas, USA

Diego Marré, MD
Consultant
Department of Plastic and Reconstructive Surgery
and Burns
Clínica Las Condes
Emergency Public Hospital
Santiago, Chile

Aránzazu Menéndez, MD
Consultant
Department of Plastic and Reconstructive Surgery
University Clinic of Navarra
Pamplona, Spain

Pablo Monedero, MD, PhD
Consultant
Department of Anesthesiology and Critical Care
University Clinic of Navarra
Pamplona, Spain

Ester Moreno-Artero, MD
Dermatologist
Dermatology Department
University Clinic of Navarra
Pamplona, Spain

Jesús Olivas, MD
Resident
Department of Plastic and Reconstructive
Surgery
University Clinic of Navarra
Pamplona, Spain

Nicolás Pereira, MD, MSc
Assistant Professor in Plastic Surgery
Department of Plastic and Reconstructive Surgery
Hospital del Trabajador
Clínica Las Condes
Santiago, Chile

Gustavo Perez-Abadía, MD
Assistant Professor of Physiology and Biophysics
Director and Instructor of Microsurgery Teaching
Course
University of Louisville
Louisville, Kentucky, USA

Brent B. Pickrell, MD
Resident
Harvard Plastic Surgery Residency Program
Boston, Massachusetts, USA

José L. del Pozo, MD, PhD
Consultant
Division of Infectious Diseases
University Clinic of Navarra
Pamplona, Spain

Maider Pretel, MD, PhD
Consultant
Dermatology Department
University Clinic of Navarra
Pamplona, Spain

Shan Shan Qiu, MD
Consultant
Department of Plastic and Reconstructive Surgery
Maastricht University Medical Center
Maastricht, The Netherlands

Pedro Redondo, MD, PhD
Professor of Dermatology
University of Navarra
Consultant Dermatology Department
University Clinic of Navarra
Pamplona, Spain

Ricardo Roa, MD
Chief
Department of Plastic and Reconstructive Surgery
and Burns
Hospital del Trabajador
Santiago, Chile

Héctor Roco, MD
Chief
Department of Plastic and Reconstructive Surgery
Chilean Air Force Hospital
Santiago, Chile

Marco Romeo, MD, PhD
Consultant
Department of Plastic and Reconstructive Surgery
Jiménez Díaz Foundation University Hospital
Madrid, Spain

S. Raja Sabapathy, MS, MCh, DNB, FRCS(Ed), MAMS
Chairman
Division of Plastic Surgery, Hand and
Reconstructive Microsurgery and Burns
Ganga Hospital
Coimbatore, India

R. Raja Shanmugakrishnan, MD
Senior Fellow
Department of Plastic Surgery, Hand and
Reconstructive Microsurgery and Burns
Ganga Hospital
Coimbatore, India

Cristián Taladriz, MD, MSc
Consultant
Department of Plastic and Reconstructive Surgery
and Burns
Hospital del Trabajador
Santiago, Chile

Michael Tecce, MD
Clinical Research Fellow
Division of Plastic Surgery
University of Pennsylvania
Philadelphia, Pennsylvania, USA

Ekaterina Troncoso Olchevskaia, MD, MSc
Plastic Surgery Resident
Department of Plastic and Reconstructive Surgery
University of Chile
Santiago, Chile

Andrew P. Trussler, MD
Plastic Surgeon
Private practice
Austin, Texas, USA

Pablo Zancolli, MD
Microsurgery Fellow
Kleinert Kutz Institute
Louisville, Kentucky, USA

To our god-daughter, Maria, our angel looking after us every day from above

Section I
Principles

I

1 Patient Safety in Plastic Surgery

Brent B. Pickrell, Andrew P. Trussler

Abstract

This chapter provides a brief overview of the topics most pertinent to patient safety for the busy practicing surgeon and advanced trainees. It is organized to provide a longitudinal account of the patient encounter, beginning in the clinic ("Practice-Based Safety"), where patients are often first evaluated and their consent is sought for the recommended procedure. The discussion moves to a discussion of risk factors ("Risk Stratification"), with particular emphasis on smoking and patient safety. Finally, safety topics are outlined, with current supporting evidence from the literature ("Intraoperative Patient Safety").

Keywords: informed consent, intraoperative risks, preoperative risk assessment, venous thromboembolism

1.1 Introduction

Patient safety has become a national focus in recent years, since the Institute of Medicine published *To Err Is Human* (2000), alerting the public to the serious and potentially deadly dangers posed by medical errors occurring in the health care setting. The authors estimated that approximately 44,000–98,000 Americans die annually secondary to preventable medical errors costing approximately US $79 billion. Thereafter, initiatives and guidelines have evolved to define, measure, and improve patient safety practices and culture.

Despite perceptions of the lay public, even in the elective office-based setting, plastic surgery is not without risk to the patient. Although plastic surgery often poses less risk than procedures of other surgical subspecialties, the risk of surgical complications should not be minimized. Even though the majority of complications from plastic surgery include scarring, infection, and bleeding, more serious complications, such as venous thromboembolism, do occur and can have devastating consequences.

1.2 Practice-Based Safety

1.2.1 Informed Consent

Opportunities to obtain patient consent abound in clinical practice, and physicians are required to obtain the informed consent of their patients before initiating treatment. That is, valid informed consent is premised on educating competent patients with the appropriate information so that they may make a conscious, voluntary choice. When patients lack the competence to make a decision about treatment, substitute decision makers must be sought if the scenario is nonemergent. If a surrogate decision maker must be sought, it is the physician's responsibility to follow the given state's statutes and contact family members in the correct order of priority.

Patient education begins preoperatively with a clear explanation of the procedure, along with the risks, benefits, and alternatives, if available. This necessary counseling can help avoid surprise and confusion if a complication arises postoperatively. Indeed, failure to inform patients is a common secondary claim in malpractice lawsuits. For specific procedures, the surgeon should consider providing standardized preoperative and postoperative patient education.

Informed consent should include the type of surgery and its potential risks, including anticipated outcomes, benefits, and possible consequences and side effects. When discussing risks with patients, one should avoid a recitation of statistics because they are frequently misunderstood or misinterpreted. Documentation of the informed consent should be noted in the medical record and revisited by the surgeon on the day of the operation.

> **Note**
>
> Spending time informing patients in the preoperative period can increase patient satisfaction and potentially lead to fewer claims in malpractice suits.

1.2.2 Reporting Adverse Events

It is important that a medical system has a standardized process for reporting adverse events that is valid, reliable, and actionable. Historically, many physicians have abstained from reporting their errors for fear of liability. To this end, the protocol should encourage honest reporting without fear of ramifications; an in-depth, comprehensive review of adverse events is key to improving the culture of patient safety. In 2002, the American Society of Plastic Surgeons/Plastic Surgery Educational Foundation and the American Board of Plastic Surgery collaborated to create the "Tracking Operations and Outcomes for Plastic Surgeons," a web-based database that compiles plastic surgery procedures and outcomes information. This database, which is compliant with the Health Insurance Portability and Accountability Act, serves as an internal quality control mechanism for the sole purpose of reducing morbidity and mortality and improving patient care. Because this information is not discoverable or admissible as evidence in a court of law, physicians need not fear liability for reporting their adverse events.

1.3 Patient Risk Stratification

Identification of preoperative patient risk factors is essential during initial consultation. It is appropriate for plastic surgeons to maintain a low threshold for primary care referrals for medical evaluation if a patient is over the age of 40 and wishes to undergo an elective procedure. Screening should be evidence based to avoid unnecessary use of patient and health care resources.

1.3.1 Smoking Cessation

The risks associated with smoking in the surgical patient are well documented. In particular, perioperative pulmonary complications have been shown to be four times more frequent in current smokers than in people who have never smoked. In a multicenter, randomized, controlled trial, patients who were randomized to receive preoperative smoking intervention (i.e., counseling, nicotine replacement, and either cessation or reduction of smoking) 6 to 8 weeks before surgery had fewer complications than control patients who did not receive the intervention.

A number of studies have linked tobacco use with complications following plastic surgery operations, most frequently in the context of the deleterious effects on wound healing. Chang et al. found an increased risk of mastectomy flap and abdominal wall necrosis following free transverse rectus abdominal myocutaneous flap reconstruction. Rees et al reported that smokers undergoing face-lifts were more likely to suffer skin slough. Coon et al. reported significantly higher overall complication rates, tissue necrosis rates, and the likelihood of reoperation. In a retrospective review of 1,881 patients, smoking was found to correlate with decreased skin graft survival.

Deciding whether to operate on a smoking patient is ultimately up to the surgeon, but the current literature supports an increased risk of complications that may be unacceptable for elective operations. Even so, a large survey by Rohrich et al. in 2002 suggests that many plastic surgeons elect to operate on patients who are known smokers, but the majority refused to offer skin flaps or procedures with extensive undermining.

Caution
Smokers will often misrepresent their tobacco status in the doctor's office. Use of preoperative cotinine levels may help avoid tobacco-associated complications in these patients.

1.4 Intraoperative Risk

1.4.1 Patient Positioning

Complications arising from patient positioning are an underappreciated source of intraoperative morbidity. The risks of improper patient positioning include peripheral neuropathies, brachial plexopathies, myopathies, compartment syndromes, and pressure ulcers (▶ Fig. 1.1). Given that plastic surgeons will often require unusual positioning in the operating room (OR) for adequate exposure, it is extremely important that the surgeon takes the appropriate precautions to prevent these complications.

Eighty percent of operations take place in the supine position. The two most common postoperative neuropathies, brachial and ulnar plexopathy, result from improper positioning and padding. These complications may be avoided by abducting the arms < 90 degrees to avoid traction on the brachial plexus. Additionally, the arms should remain supinated while abducted to avoid pressure on the

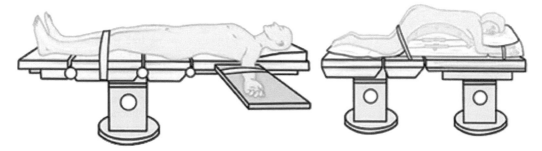

Fig. 1.1 Common patient positions and safety considerations.

ulnar nerve as it passes posterior to the medial epicondyle. Members of the surgical team should also be discouraged from leaning on extremities during the case. Similarly, cachexia may produce bony prominences and predispose the patient to compressive neuropathies or pressure ulcers.

Prone positioning is the second most common position in plastic surgery. Aside from respiratory and cardiovascular concerns, complications related to prone positioning include vertebral artery occlusion causing stroke, brachioplexopathy, and pain from shoulder impingement. Most complications are related to excessive pressure on the head and neck, including blindness secondary to ischemic optic neuropathy. As such, a well-padded headrest should be used for every prone case. The neck should be stabilized in a neutral, non-extended position, avoiding neck rotation and accelerated movements. Bilateral chest rolls placed lengthwise should support the patient's weight on the clavicles and iliac crests to lessen compressive forces that have the potential to negatively impact cardiopulmonary status. Lastly, female breasts and male genitals should be free from pressure and torsion.

> **Note**
>
> Postoperative neuropathies are a common source of malpractice claims and can be avoided through proper patient positioning and arm board padding.

1.4.2 Hypothermia

Hypothermia, defined as a body temperature lower than 36°C, is a risk factor for coagulopathy, cardiac events, and wound infection. A meta-analysis that pooled the results of 14 randomized trials found that even mild hypothermia (35–36°C) was associated with a 16% increase in blood loss and a 22% increase in the relative risk of transfusion. In another study, hypothermic patients undergoing plastic surgery were found to have an 8.3% prolongation of activated partial thromboplastin time as compared with those patients with mild intraoperative hypothermia. Additionally, Coon et al. found that lower OR temperatures were associated with an increased risk of seroma formation following postbariatric body contouring procedures.

Hypothermia is most frequently caused by cold OR temperatures, infusion or irrigation with temperate fluids, and anesthesia-induced impairments of thermoregulatory mechanisms. Procedures with a large surface area exposed, such as multisite or large body-contouring cases, large-volume liposuction, and cases lasting longer than 2 hours, are associated with an increased risk of hypothermia.

Proactive methods to decrease the risk of intraoperative hypothermia include using only warm infiltration/irrigation fluids and applying cutaneous warming devices or forced-air warming blankets. The surgeon, anesthesiologist, and OR staff should ensure that the temperature of the OR remains at a level that allows the patient to remain normothermic throughout the case.

1.4.3 Malignant Hyperthermia

Malignant hyperthermia is an inherited myopathy that presents as a hypermetabolic reaction to certain anesthetic gases, including halothane, enflurane, sevoflurane, desflurane, and isoflurane, and the depolarizing muscle relaxant succinylcholine.

Desflurane and sevoflurane are less potent triggers, producing a more gradual onset of clinical signs. The onset may be dramatic if succinylcholine is used in genetically susceptible patients.

A variety of unusual conditions (e.g., sepsis, thyroid storm, pheochromocytoma) may resemble malignant hyperthermia during anesthesia and eclipse the initial diagnosis. Classically, an impending episode is heralded by a rising end tidal carbon dioxide level in the anesthetized patient. Hyperthermia is most often a late sign.

Given its autosomal dominant inheritance pattern with variable penetrance, careful preoperative screening can identify susceptible individuals, who should then undergo the caffeine halothane contracture test. Even then, susceptible patients may actually undergo anesthesia several times before a clinical event occurs.

Initial management of malignant hyperthermia should include immediate discontinuation of all volatile anesthetic agents and succinylcholine, followed by administration of dantrolene, given as a 2.5 mg/kg rapid bolus through a large-bore IV, with repeated administration every 10 minutes until the initial signs of the episode have ceased. Pediatric dosing is the same as for adults. Stopping all surgery, hyperventilating with 100% oxygen, volume resuscitation, and correcting hyperkalemia are also important. In the acute scenario, rapid dantrolene administration is of the highest priority; thus it is critical that perioperative staff are aware of its treatment role in this disease process. A continuous administration of 10 mg/kg/d should then be started for at least 24 hours, during which the patient should be transferred and observed in an acute care facility due to the risk of recrudescence (▶Table 1.1). It is important to ensure that all surgical suites be ready and able to handle a malignant hyperthermia emergency.

Remember	M!
Rising end-tidal CO_2 is often the first sign of a malignant hyperthermia episode.	

1.4.4 Duration of Procedure

Increased surgery length has been correlated with increased rates of hypothermia, wound infection, postoperative nausea and vomiting, and hospital admission in the outpatient surgery setting. In a study that examined 35 different procedures, long-duration procedures (> 95% upper confidence limit of expected operative time) had significantly greater risk of mortality, acute renal failure, cardiac arrest requiring cardiopulmonary resuscitation (CPR), superficial/deep surgical site infection, deep vein thrombosis, prolonged intubation, pneumonia, progressive renal insufficiency,

Table 1.1 Management of malignant hyperthermia in the operating room

- Discontinue volatile anesthetic agents and triggers.
- Halt procedure as soon as possible.
- Administer 100% O_2, high flow 10L/min.
- Increase minute ventilation (hyperventilate).
- Administer dantrolene 2.5 mg/kg intravenous (IV) bolus, then give 1–2.5 mg/kg every 10 minutes until signs of episode have resolved and the patient is stable.
- Actively cool the patient with ice packs, cooling blankets, and cool nasogastric lavage.
- Treat hyperkalemia: calcium chloride 1 g IV; D_{50} 1 Ampule IV (25 g dextrose) + regular insulin 10 units IV; sodium bicarbonate 1 Ampule.
- Treat cardiac arrhythmias (most often from hyperkalemia). Consult Advanced Cardiac Life Support (ACLS) guidelines as needed.
- Send labs for arterial blood gas, myoglobin, creatine kinase, prothrombin time/partial thromboplastin time, and lactic acid.
- Place a Foley catheter for monitoring urine output.
- Admit the patient to the intensive care unit for postoperative care and monitoring.
- Continue dantrolene 1 mg/kg every 4–6 hours for 24–36 hours.
- Call Malignant Hyperthermia Hotline with questions: 1–800-MH-HYPER (1–800–644–9737).

sepsis/septic shock, unplanned intubation, urinary tract infection, and wound disruption.

Plastic surgery operations lasting longer than 6 hours should be evaluated critically for close postoperative monitoring and an overnight stay for observation, depending on the time of day at which the operation ends and any confounding patient risk factors.

1.4.5 Venous Thromboembolism

Venous thromboembolism (VTE) has a varying range of incidence within the field of plastic surgery. The literature states that incidence ranges from 1 to 2% of all patients undergoing plastic surgery, although there is significant variance among the breadth of procedures. Among plastic surgical procedures, the risk of symptomatic pulmonary embolism is highest in liposuction, with a reported maximum incidence of 23%. Breast reconstruction is second, with a maximum incidence of 6%, followed by thermal injuries (4.4%), abdominoplasty (0.3–3.4%), and oncological head and neck reconstruction (0.1–0.4%).

Patients most at risk for VTE include those undergoing combined procedures, belt lipectomy, and abdominoplasty. Keyes et al found that 13 of the 23 deaths in the outpatient setting were caused by pulmonary embolism, and 12 of the deaths were associated with abdominoplasty alone or in association with one or more surgical procedures. Similarly, Grazer and Goldwyn reported a deep vein thrombosis incidence of 1.1% and a pulmonary embolism incidence of 0.8% in abdominoplasty patients.

Despite the severe consequences of VTE, a 2007 survey of members of the American Society of Plastic Surgeons found that only 43.7% of surgeons performing liposuction, 48.7% performing face-lifts, and 60.8% performing a combined procedure used VTE prophylaxis all the time. Until recently, there had been no data that addressed either risk stratification or thromboprophylaxis in plastic surgery patients. Recognizing the void of plastic surgery–specific literature, Seruya et al devised a VTE prophylaxis algorithm tailored specifically to plastic surgery patients. The authors provide an overall score for patients to stratify them into one of four risk groups (▶Fig. 1.2): low, moderate, high, or highest. For each group, the authors recommend a VTE regimen, including early ambulation, positioning, intermittent pneumatic

compression stockings, and/or low-molecular-weight heparin (LMWH). Importantly, Seruya et al demonstrated that the appropriate use of chemoprophylaxis did not result in statistically significant increased rates of hematoma among the highest-risk patients. Similarly, Pannucci et al showed that postoperative enoxaparin does not produce a clinically relevant increase in observed rates of reoperative hematoma.

There are certain preoperative factors known to increase the risk of VTE (▶Table 1.2); these should be explored on initial consultation for risk category assignment. Ideally, patients with an inherited bleeding disorder are identified preoperatively; however, some patients may not know their family history or may not think to disclose this information to the surgeon. As such, a thorough history and exam, including familial history, is imperative to gaining key information to identify potentially high-risk patients.

> **Caution** ⚠
>
> Patients most at risk for venous thromboembolism include those undergoing combined procedures, belt lipectomy, and abdominoplasty.

1.4.6 Surgical Site Infections

It is estimated that as much as 40–60% of surgical site infections may be preventable. The indications for the administration of prophylactic antibiotics are limited to clean-contaminated and contaminated procedures, although the significant morbidity that ensues from the infection of implants should warrant their use in clean procedures. Choice antibiotics include a first-generation cephalosporin (e.g., cefazolin), typically 1 g given intravenously (IV), or 2 g in the patient who weighs at least 160 pounds. Patients with a β-lactam allergy can be given clindamycin (600–900 mg IV) or vancomycin (1–1.5 g IV).

Antibiotic administration should be completed at least 30–60 minutes before incision. Additional administration should be performed every 3 to 5 hours until the wound has closed or if a significant amount of blood loss has occurred. Numerous studies have shown that continued administration of antibiotics after the completion of surgery is not indicated, and current Surgical Infection Prevention Project panel recommendations dictate the discontinuation of antimicrobial prophylaxis within 24 hours from the completion of surgery.

Step I.   Total = _____

Exposing Risk Factors

Check the box corresponding to each condition

1 Factor		2 Factors		3 Factors		5 Factors	
Minor surgery	☐	*Minor surgery	☐	Previous myocardial infarction	☐	Hip, pelvis, or leg fracture	☐
		Immobilizing plaster cast	☐	Congestive heart failure	☐	Stroke	☐
		Patient confined to bed for > 72 hrs	☐	Severe sepsis	☐	Multiple trauma	☐
		Central venous access	☐	Free flap	☐	Acute spinal cord injury	☐

*Major surgery is defined by the use of general anesthesia or any procedure lasting longer than 1 hour.

Step II.   Total = _____

Predisposing Risk Factors

Check the box corresponding to each condition

Clinical Setting		Inherited		Acquired	
Age 40 to 60 (1 Factor)	☐	Any genetic hypercoaguable disorder (3 Factors)	☐	Lupus anticoagulant (3 Factors)	☐
Age > 60 (2 Factors)	☐			Antiphospholipid antibodies (3 Factors)	☐
History of DVT/PE (3 Factors)	☐			Myeloproliferative disorders (3 Factors)	☐
Pregnancy or < 1 month postpartum (1 Factor)	☐			Heparin-induced thrombocytopenia (3 Factors)	☐
Malignancy (2 Factors)	☐			Hyperviscosity (3 Factors)	☐
Obesity > 20% IBW (1 Factor)	☐			Homocystinemia (3 Factors)	☐
Oral contraceptive / hormone replacement therapy (1 Factor)	☐				

Step III.   Total Step I and Step II = _____   Factors

Step IV. Orders

1 Factor	Low risk	Ambulate patient TID	☐
2 Factors	Moderate risk	Intermittent pneumatic compression stocking with elastic compression stocking at all times when not ambulating	☐
3-4 Factors	High risk	Intermittent pneumatic compression stockings with elastic compression stockings on at all times when not ambulating	☐
> 4 Factors	Highest risk	Intermittent pneumatic compression stockings with elastic compression stockings on at all times when not ambulating + 1. Enoxaparin (Lovenox) 40mg SQ once daily post op ☐ **For1 : Give first dose 12 hours Post Op**	

Signature _____   Date/Time _____
Print Name   Pager #

Fig. 1.2 Venous prophylaxis form for plastic surgery patients devised by Seruya et al.

Table 1.2 Factors that increase risk of venous thromboembolism

- Older age
- Underlying malignancy
- History of spontaneous miscarriage
- Pregnancy
- Oral contraceptive use
- Previous venous thromboembolism
- Heart failure
- Obesity
- Paralysis
- Presence of thrombophilic abnormality[a]

[a] Factor V Leiden, prothrombin variant 20210A, antiphospholipid antibodies, protein C or protein S deficiency, antithrombin deficiency or dysfunction, hyperhomocysteinemia, heparin-induced thrombocytopenia, dysfibrinogenemia, and polycythemia vera.

1.4.7 Hypertension

Management of perioperative blood pressure control is largely unstandardized in the field of plastic surgery, even though hypertension is known to correlate significantly with hematoma rate and bleeding. It is well known that perioperative hypertension is the most significant risk factor in the development of hematoma after face-lift. To date, several studies have shown that the incidence of hematoma formation after face-lift can be reduced with close blood pressure control. Specifically, Ramanadham et al. use a transdermal clonidine patch on every patient undergoing rhytidectomy at their institution, and they report a postoperative hematoma rate of 0.9%. Although there is still a lack of consensus regarding treatment thresholds, perioperative hypertension requires consideration and careful management by the surgeon.

1.4.8 Liposuction

Liposuction is considered to be one of the most frequently performed plastic surgery procedures in the United States. Infiltration solutions containing up to 35 mg/kg of lidocaine are considered safe, provided that they are injected into the subcutaneous fat and contain epinephrine. Epinephrine doses between 1:100,000 and 1:1,000,000 are generally administered, with maximal doses not to exceed 0.07 mg/kg. Epinephrine is a critical additive in infiltrate solutions because it provides hemostasis and delays the rate of local anesthetic absorption from infiltrated tissue (▶ Table 1.3).

In 1990, the dermatologist Klein demonstrated that the systemic absorption of lidocaine after tissue tumescence is equivalent to a slow, continuous infusion of the drug. Through this, he established a conservative maximum dose of lidocaine for tissue tumescence at 35 mg/kg. Klein also demonstrated that, when the total dose of lidocaine and infiltration time were held constant, the more-dilute solutions delay systemic absorption. By effectively slowing down the rate of absorption by using dilute lidocaine, rapid absorption from highly vascularized tissue or inadvertent intravascular injection is less likely to result in toxicity.

As a more potent local anesthetic, the toxic dose of bupivacaine (2.5 mg/kg) is far less than the toxic dose of lidocaine. Additionally, bupivacaine has a much longer duration of action (up to 10 hours) compared to that of lidocaine (up to 3 hours) due to higher protein binding. Toxicity of bupivacaine

Table 1.3 Commonly used local anesthetics

Agent	Recommended dosage (mg/kg)	Duration of action (min)
Lidocaine	Without epinephrine: 4.5 With epinephrine: 7	30–60 120–360
Procaine	7	15–60
Prilocaine	8	30–90
Bupivacaine	Without epinephrine: 2.5 With epinephrine: 2.5–4	120–240 180–420

was originally noted to cause a therapy-resistant and nearly universally fatal cardiovascular collapse due to irreversible heart block. The first case of successful human rescue from refractory cardiac toxicity from bupivacaine was published in 2006. Intravenous 20% lipid emulsion (Intralipid, Baxter) has been shown to reduce mortality and should be stocked in facilities using bupivacaine.

> **Caution** ⚠️
>
> Intralipid is used to treat bupivacaine toxicity and should be stocked appropriately.

1.4.9 Lidocaine Toxicity

Toxic effects of local anesthetics result from inappropriately high dosages or accidental intravascular injection. Signs and symptoms of lidocaine toxicity include light-headedness, restlessness, drowsiness, tinnitus, metallic taste in the mouth, slurred speech, and numbness of the lips and tongue. Plasma lidocaine levels peak 10–14 hours after infiltration into most fatty body areas when epinephrine is present in the wetting solution. Levels peak more quickly when the working area is highly vascularized, such as in the neck (6 hours). As such, the surgeon must be aware that tumescent anesthesia in the head and neck and other well vascularized tissues may show signs of toxicity sooner and at lower doses compared to the trunk (12 hours).

Cessation of administration, ensuring adequate oxygenation, and close electrocardiogram monitoring should be prompt, with supportive care in the form of IV fluids and vasopressors as needed, usually in the form of small doses of epinephrine. Seizure control is most appropriately managed with benzodiazepines (e.g., diazepam, midazolam).

> **Caution** ⚠️
>
> Different anatomical sites have different rates of local anesthetic absorption.

1.4.10 Operative Room Fires

There are approximately 100 OR fires per year in the United States, responsible for an average of two deaths annually. The vast majority of all fires occur during facial, neck, and tonsil surgery. Aside from fiberoptic lights, lasers, and electrocautery devices, supplemental oxygen has traditionally been a lesser-known risk for surgical fires among OR personnel.

For surgical fires to occur, the classic triad must be present: a spark, flame, or heat source to cause ignition; a fuel source (a flammable item); and an oxidative material (e.g., oxygen). Further, the likelihood of fire depends on (1) the oxygen flow rate, (2) the power of the heat source (e.g., Bovie device), and (3) the distance between the heat source and the supplemental oxygen.

To mitigate the risk of surgical fires, some have advocated for techniques that reduce facial oxygen concentrations to ambient levels through use of a nasopharyngeal tube in lieu of a nasal cannula. Under this design, the two cut ends of the nasal cannula are placed down the nasopharyngeal tube. Others use an 8-French feeding tube to ensure oxygen delivery to the posterior pharynx. Indeed, one of the most critical elements in preventing OR fires involves communication between the surgeon and the anesthesiologist in cases where electrocautery is used in the head/neck or oropharynx in the presence of supplemental oxygen.

1.5 Conclusions

The culture of patient safety has undergone significant change in recent years and continues to make strides to improve the safety of health care delivery. Given the astounding breadth of plastic and reconstructive surgery, the surgeon must remain current on not only the expanding technology and surgical techniques but also the processes that make these procedures safe for our patients.

1.6 Key Points

- Patient safety begins preoperatively with patient education and proper consent.
- Active smoking can limit surgical options and should be addressed on initial consultation.
- Improper patient positioning in the OR can seriously harm patients.
- Close intraoperative monitoring can limit the risk of hypothermia.
- All surgical suites should be equipped to handle an episode of malignant hyperthermia.
- VTE prophylaxis should be considered in all procedures, especially combined operations.
- Surgical site infections can be limited by proper antibiotic administration 30–60 minutes before the operation.

- Reducing facial oxygen concentrations can limit the risk of OR fires.

Recommended Readings

Allen GC, Brubaker CL. Human malignant hyperthermia associated with desflurane anesthesia. Anesth Analg. 1998; 86(6):1328–1331

Aly AS, Cram AE, Chao M, Pang J, McKeon M. Belt lipectomy for circumferential truncal excess: the University of Iowa experience. Plast Reconstr Surg. 2003; 111(1):398–413

American Society of Plastic Surgeons. Cosmetic and reconstructive plastic surgery trends. 2007. http://www.plasticsurgery.org/media/statistics/loader.cfm?url=/commonspot/security/getfile.cfm&pageID=29285

Baudendistel L, Goudsouzian N, Cote' C, Strafford M. End-tidal CO_2 monitoring. Its use in the diagnosis and management of malignant hyperthermia. Anaesthesia. 1984; 39(10):1000–1003

Beale EW, Rasko Y, Rohrich RJ. A 20-year experience with secondary rhytidectomy: a review of technique, longevity, and outcomes. Plast Reconstr Surg. 2013; 131(3):625–634

Beer GM, Goldscheider E, Weber A, Lehmann K. Prevention of acute hematoma after face-lifts. Aesthetic Plast Surg. 2010; 34(4):502–507

Bluman LG, Mosca L, Newman N, Simon DG. Preoperative smoking habits and postoperative pulmonary complications. Chest. 1998; 113(4):883–889

Bratzler DW, Houck PM; Surgical Infection Prevention Guideline Writers Workgroup. Antimicrobial prophylaxis for surgery: an advisory statement from the National Surgical Infection Prevention Project. Am J Surg. 2005; 189 (4):395–404

Brechtelsbauer PB, Carroll WR, Baker S. Intraoperative fire with electrocautery. Otolaryngol Head Neck Surg. 1996; 114(2):328–331

Broughton G II, Rios JL, Rohrich RJ, Brown SA. Deep venous thrombosis prophylaxis practice and treatment strategies among plastic surgeons: survey results. Plast Reconstr Surg. 2007; 119(1):157–174

Burk RW III, Guzman-Stein G, Vasconez LO. Lidocaine and epinephrine levels in tumescent technique liposuction. Plast Reconstr Surg. 1996; 97(7):1379–1384

Cavallini M, Baruffaldi Preis FW, Casati A. Effects of mild hypothermia on blood coagulation in patients undergoing elective plastic surgery. Plast Reconstr Surg. 2005; 116(1):316–321, discussion 322–323

Chang DW, Reece GP, Wang B, et al. Effect of smoking on complications in patients undergoing free TRAM flap breast reconstruction. Plast Reconstr Surg. 2000; 105(7):2374–2380

Chen CM, Disa JJ, Mehrara BJ. The incidence of venous thromboembolism in head and neck reconstruction. Paper presented at: 24th Annual Meeting of the Northeastern Society of Plastic Surgeons; October 3–6, 2007; Southampton, Bermuda

Coon D, Michaels J V, Gusenoff JA, Chong T, Purnell C, Rubin JP. Hypothermia and complications in postbariatric body contouring. Plast Reconstr Surg. 2012; 130(2):443–448

Coon D, Tuffaha S, Christensen J, Bonawitz SC. Plastic surgery and smoking: a prospective analysis of incidence, compliance, and complications. Plast Reconstr Surg. 2013; 131(2):385–391

Daane SP, Toth BA. Fire in the operating room: principles and prevention. Plast Reconstr Surg. 2005; 115(5):73e–75e

Daley BJ, Cecil W, Clarke PC, Cofer JB, Guillamondegui OD. How slow is too slow? Correlation of operative time to complications: an analysis from the Tennessee Surgical Quality Collaborative. J Am Coll Surg. 2015; 220(4): 550–558

Davison SP, Venturi ML, Attinger CE, Baker SB, Spear SL. Prevention of venous thromboembolism in the plastic surgery patient [published correction appears in Plast Reconstr Surg 2004;114(5):1366. Dosage error in article text]. Plast Reconstr Surg. 2004; 114(3):43E–51E

Geerts WH, Heit JA, Clagett GP, et al. Prevention of venous thromboembolism. Chest. 2001; 119(1), Suppl:132S–175S

Grant GP, Szirth BC, Bennett HL, et al. Effects of prone and reverse trendelenburg positioning on ocular parameters. Anesthesiology. 2010; 112(1):57–65

Grazer FM, Goldwyn RM. Abdominoplasty assessed by survey, with emphasis on complications. Plast Reconstr Surg. 1977; 59(4):513–517

Greco RJ, Gonzalez R, Johnson P, Scolieri M, Rekhopf PG, Heckler F. Potential dangers of oxygen supplementation during facial surgery. Plast Reconstr Surg. 1995; 95(6):978–984

Gronert GA. Malignant hyperthermia. Anesthesiology. 1980; 53(5):395–423

Gurunluoglu R, Swanson JA, Haeck PC; ASPS Patient Safety Committee. Evidence-based patient safety advisory: malignant hyperthermia. Plast Reconstr Surg. 2009; 124(4), Suppl:68S–81S

Haeck PC, Swanson JA, Gutowski KA, et al. ASPS Patient Safety Committee. Evidence-based patient safety advisory: liposuction. Plast Reconstr Surg. 2009; 124(4), Suppl:28S–44S

Hatef DA, Trussler AP, Kenkel JM. Procedural risk for venous thromboembolism in abdominal contouring surgery: a systematic review of the literature. Plast Reconstr Surg. 2010; 125(1):352–362

Hester TR, Jr, Baird W, Bostwick J, III, Nahai F, Cukic J. Abdominoplasty combined with other major surgical procedures: safe or sorry? Plast Reconstr Surg. 1989; 83(6):997–1004

Horton JB, Janis JE, Rohrich RJ. MOC-PS(SM) CME article: patient safety in the office-based setting. Plast Reconstr Surg. 2008; 122(3), Suppl:1–21

Institute for Healthcare Improvement. 5 Million Lives Campaign. Getting Started Kit: Prevent Surgical Site Infections How-to Guide. Cambridge, MA: Institute for Healthcare Improvement; 2008

Iverson RE, Lynch DJ, ASPS Task Force on Patient Safety in Office-Based Surgery Facilities. Patient safety in office-based surgery facilities: II. Patient selection. Plast Reconstr Surg. 2002; 110(7):1785–1790, discussion 1791–1792

Keyes GR, Singer R, Iverson RE, et al. Mortality in outpatient surgery. Plast Reconstr Surg. 2008; 122(1):245–250, discussion 251–253

Klein JA. Tumescent technique for regional anesthesia permits lidocaine doses of 35 mg/kg for liposuction. J Dermatol Surg Oncol. 1990; 16(3):248–263

Klein JA. Tumescent technique for local anesthesia improves safety in large-volume liposuction. Plast Reconstr Surg. 1993; 92(6):1085–1098, discussion 1099–1100

Kohn LT, Corrigan JM, Donaldson MS, eds. To Err Is Human: Building a Safer Health System. Committee on Quality of Health Care in America. Institute of Medicine. Washington. D.C.: National Academy Press; 2000

Laffan M. Genetics and pulmonary medicine. 4. Pulmonary-embolism. Thorax. 1998; 53(8):698–702

Levine JM, Goldstein AB, Kelly AB, Pribitkin EA. Informed consent for rhytidectomy: a survey of AAFPRS fellowship programs. Arch Facial Plast Surg. 2004; 6(1):61

Mattucci KF, Militana CJ. The prevention of fire during oropharyngeal electrosurgery. Ear Nose Throat J. 2003; 82(2): 107–109

Meneghetti SC, Morgan MM, Fritz J, Borkowski RG, Djohan R, Zins JE. Operating room fires: optimizing safety. Plast Reconstr Surg. 2007; 120(6):1701–1708

Millsaps CC. Pay attention to patient positioning! RN. 2006; 69(1):59–63

Miszkiewicz K, Perreault I, Landes G, et al. Venous thromboembolism in plastic surgery: incidence, current practice and recommendations. J Plast Reconstr Aesthet Surg. 2009; 62(5):580–588

Møller AM, Villebro N, Pedersen T, Tønnesen H. Effect of preoperative smoking intervention on postoperative complications: a randomised clinical trial. Lancet. 2002; 359(9301):114–117

Motykie GD, Zebala LP, Caprini JA, et al. A guide to venous thromboembolism risk factor assessment. J Thromb Thrombolysis. 2000; 9(3):253–262

Pannucci CJ, Wachtman CF, Dreszer G, et al. The effect of postoperative enoxaparin on risk for reoperative hematoma. Plast Reconstr Surg. 2012; 129(1):160–168

Pérez-Guisado J, Gaston KL, Benítez-Goma JR, et al. Smoking and diabetes mellitus type 2 reduce skin graft take; the use of fibrin glue might restore graft take to optimal levels. Eur J Dermatol. 2011; 21(6):895–898

Podnos YD, Williams RA. Fires in the operating room. American College of Surgeons, Committee of Perioperative Care. Bull Am Coll Surg. 1997; 82:14–17

Poore SO, Sillah NM, Mahajan AY, Gutowski KA. Patient safety in the operating room: I. Preoperative. Plast Reconstr Surg. 2012; 130(5):1038–1047

Rajagopalan S, Mascha E, Na J, Sessler DI. The effects of mild perioperative hypothermia on blood loss and transfusion requirement. Anesthesiology. 2008; 108(1):71–77

Ramanadham SR, Mapula S, Costa C, et al. Evolution of hypertension management in face lifting in 1089 patients: optimizing safety and outcomes. Plast Reconstr Surg. 2015; 135(4):1037–1043

Rees TD, Liverett DM, Guy CL. The effect of cigarette smoking on skin-flap survival in the face lift patient. Plast Reconstr Surg. 1984; 73(6):911–915

Reyes RJ, Smith AA, Mascaro JR, Windle BH. Supplemental oxygen: ensuring its safe delivery during facial surgery. Plast Reconstr Surg. 1995; 95(5):924–928

Rohrich RJ, Coberly DM, Krueger JK, Brown SA. Planning elective operations on patients who smoke: survey of North American plastic surgeons. Plast Reconstr Surg. 2002; 109(1):350–355, discussion 356–357

Rohrich RJ, White PF. Safety of outpatient surgery: is mandatory accreditation of outpatient surgery centers enough? Plast Reconstr Surg. 2001; 107(1):189–192

Rosenblatt MA, Abel M, Fischer GW, Itzkovich CJ, Eisenkraft JB. Successful use of a 20% lipid emulsion to resuscitate a patient after a presumed bupivacaine-related cardiac arrest. Anesthesiology. 2006; 105(1):217–218

Rosenfield LK, Chang DS. Flash fires during facial surgery: recommendations for the safe delivery of oxygen. Plast Reconstr Surg. 2007; 119(6):1982–1983

Seruya M, Venturi ML, Iorio ML, Davison SP. Efficacy and safety of venous thromboembolism prophylaxis in highest risk plastic surgery patients. Plast Reconstr Surg. 2008; 122(6):1701–1708

Shermak M, Shoo B, Deune EG. Prone positioning precautions in plastic surgery. Plast Reconstr Surg. 2006; 117(5):1584–1588, discussion 1589

Shulman M, Braverman B, Ivankovich AD, Gronert G. Sevoflurane triggers malignant hyperthermia in swine. Anesthesiology. 1981; 54(3):259–260

Souba WW. ACS Surgery: Principles and Practice. New York, NY: WebMD Professional; 2006

Sys J, Michielsen J, Mertens E, Verstreken J, Tassignon MJ. Central retinal artery occlusion after spinal surgery. Eur Spine J. 1996; 5(1):74–75

Tucker GT. Pharmacokinetics of local anaesthetics. Br J Anaesth. 1986; 58(7):717–731

Wahl WL, Brandt MM. Potential risk factors for deep venous thrombosis in burn patients. J Burn Care Rehabil. 2001; 22(2):128–131

Wolfe SW, Lospinuso MF, Burke SW. Unilateral blindness as a complication of patient positioning for spinal surgery. A case report. Spine. 1992; 17(5):600–605

2 Wound Healing

Matthew G. Kaufman, Matthew R. Louis, Shan Shan Qiu, Edward P. Buchanan

Abstract
Complete understanding of wound healing mechanisms is fundamental knowledge for the plastic surgeon, as management decisions and the development of new therapeutics rely on optimizing these processes. In order to provide a thorough background on wound healing, we will address the intrinsic processes that drive normal wound healing, discuss local and systemic factors that can affect the normal healing process, and provide an overview of wound management options. Physiologic wound healing includes hemostasis, an inflammatory phase, a proliferative phase, and a remodeling phase. Factors affecting wound healing include oxygen delivery, smoking, chronic disease states, immunosuppressive therapy, nutrition, age, infection, and radiation exposure. Special attention should be paid to new wound care modalities, which should be employed to suit patient-specific needs, with an eye toward possible side effects and supportive evidence. In some populations, the healed wound may transform into either a hypertrophic scar or a keloid. Silicone gel sheeting (SGS) has been found to be the most effective method to treat and prevent these pathological scars.

Keywords: wound healing, chronic wounds, wound care, hypertrophic scars, keloids

2.1 Introduction

Plastic surgeons' expertise lies in the management of all wounds, whether they are traumatic, surgical, or secondary to another etiology. Complete understanding of wound healing mechanisms is fundamental knowledge for the plastic surgeon, because management decisions and the development of new therapeutics rely on optimizing these processes. In order to provide a thorough background on wound healing, we will address the intrinsic processes that drive normal wound healing, discuss local and systemic factors that can affect the normal healing process, and provide an overview of wound management options.

2.2 Basic Science

2.2.1 Physiologic Wound Healing

In order to explain wound healing, one must start with the normal physiologic mechanisms that occur following a traumatic cutaneous injury. Classically, wound healing has been described in terms of three discrete phases: the hemostatic and inflammatory phase, the proliferative phase, and the remodeling phase. Although this model has been used to describe healing in a more understandable fashion, the actual healing process is a dynamic interplay of the local wound environment and biochemical signals. Following tissue injury, hemostasis is achieved and the inflammatory phase begins, representing the acute phase of inflammation that occurs within the first week after injury. The proliferative phase involves the processes of fibroblast growth, production of granulation tissue, wound contraction, and epithelialization. Finally, the maturation/remodeling phase describes the changes healed scars undergo as they mature.

Hemostasis

Immediately following a vascular injury, the body's response is to initiate hemostasis to curb further blood loss. Hemostasis requires the coordination between the blood's coagulation pathways and the local vasculature (▶ Fig. 2.1). A sympathetic nervous response to injury leads to release of norepinephrine, which drives vasoconstriction. The violation of the vascular endothelium results in exposure of subendothelial collagen and tissue factor, which in turn activates the intrinsic and extrinsic blood-clotting cascades, respectively. The extrinsic pathway acts to initiate the formation of a platelet plug while the intrinsic pathway amplifies the process. Simultaneously, circulating platelets begin to adhere and aggregate at the site of injury.

The formation of a platelet plug and the resultant clot bridges hemostasis and the inflammatory phase. The clot, composed of cross-linked fibrin,

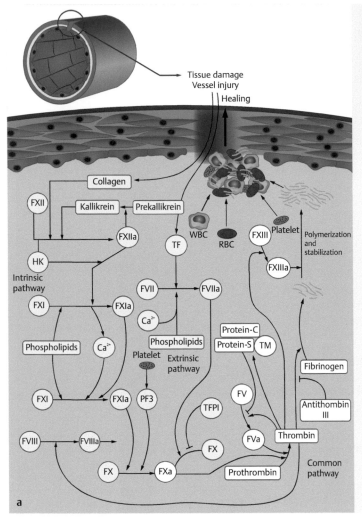

Fig. 2.1 Wound healing through time. (a) Hemostasis. Demonstrate clot formation through fibrin, platelets, the intrinsic and extrinsic pathway along white blood cells (WBCs) and red blood cells (RBCs).

(Continued)

platelets, erythrocytes, and other extracellular matrix (ECM) proteins, serves many purposes; it aids in hemostasis, provides a barrier against infiltrating bacteria, attracts inflammatory and stem cells, and establishes scaffolding for future repair.

Thrombin is a protease that cleaves inactivated fibrinogen to produce fibrin. Fibrin functions as a latticework through which various hemostatic cells are woven together to create an insoluble clot. Not only does thrombin drive the cleavage of fibrinogen, but it is also a powerful proinflammatory agent. After the initial protective vasoconstriction, thrombin induces vasodilation, leading to edema and expression of adhesion molecules on endothelial cells, which in turn provide binding sites for inflammatory cell extravasation. In

the presence of thrombin, endothelial cells will then release cytokines (CCL2, interleukin [IL]-6 and IL-8) that are used to attract monocytes to the wound. As the monocytes arrive, thrombin induces them to release IL-6, interferon-γ, IL-1β, and tumor necrosis factor-α (TNF-α) leading to the transformation of these monocytes into wound macrophages (▶Table 2.1).

Cross-linked fibrin is an integral molecule in initiating wound healing via its various binding capabilities. Through its interaction with integrins CD11b and CD18 on monocytes and neutrophils, fibrin draws key inflammatory cells into the damaged area to initiate healing. Stromal cell propagation is guided by fibrin's binding to insulin-like growth factor-1 (IGF-1). Angiogenesis is promoted by fibrin's

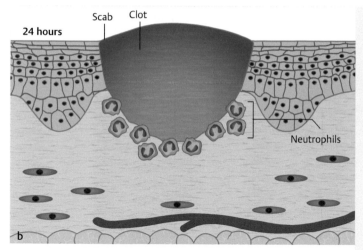

24 hours

Scab · Clot

Neutrophils

b

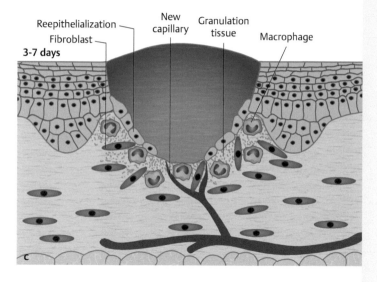

Reepithelialization
Fibroblast
3-7 days

New capillary · Granulation tissue

Macrophage

c

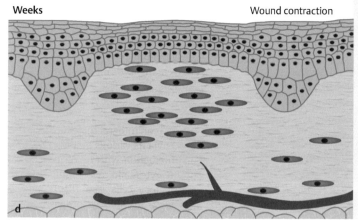

Weeks

Wound contraction

d

Fig 2.1 *(Continued)* **(b)** The inflammatory phase. Neutrophils predominate and use the respiratory burst to kill both local tissue and invading microbes. **(c)** The proliferative phase follows 48 hours after injury and will last for approximately 3 weeks. In this phase, there is significant deposition of collagen, the formation of granulation tissue, angiogenesis, and reepithelialization. **(d)** The maturation and remodeling phase begins 3 weeks after injury and is marked by collagen remodeling from type III to type I collagen, with wound strength reaching 80% after 2–3 months.

Table 2.1 Inflammatory cytokines and their effects.

Cytokine	Source	Inflammatory effect
EGF	Platelets	Reepithelialization, angiogenesis
FGF	Macrophages, mast cells, T lymphocytes, endothelial cells	Fibroblast recruitment, angiogenesis
IFN-α	Monocytes, macrophages	Inhibit collagen production
PDGF	Platelets, macrophages, fibroblasts, keratinocytes	Fibroblast chemotaxis, myofibroblast stimulation, and ECM production
TNF-α	Neutrophils, macrophages, T lymphocytes, keratinocytes	Leukocyte chemotaxis, wound fibroplasia
TGF-β	Platelets, fibroblasts, macrophages	Reepithelialization
IL-1	Keratinocytes, macrophages, neutrophils	Leukocyte chemotaxis, wound fibroplasia
IL-8	Endothelial cells, macrophages	Angiogenesis, Reepithelialization
IL-10	Lymphocytes, monocytes	Limit fibroblast proliferation and downregulation of inflammation

Abbreviations: ECM, extracellular matrix; EGF, epithelial growth factor; FGF, fibroblast growth factor; IFN, interferon; IL, interleukin; PDGF, platelet-derived growth factor; TGF, transforming growth factor; TNF, tumor necrosis factor.
Source: Modified from Henry and Garner.

connection with fibroblast growth factor-2 (FGF-2) and vascular endothelial growth factor (VEGF).

Inflammatory Phase

Once injured, tissue immediately enters an acute-phase inflammatory state, which sets the stage for later tissue repair (▶ Fig. 2.1). The inflammatory phase is classically characterized by *calor, dolor, tumor,* and *rubor* (heat, pain, swelling, and redness, respectively).

On a cellular level, platelet cells, mast cells, neutrophils, and macrophages coordinate the release of cytokines and other biologically active agents that influence the molecular processes of the inflammatory phases. Bridging the gap between hemostasis and inflammation, platelets in the clot release significant amounts of chemotaxic agents, such as thrombin, serotonin, transforming growth factor-β (TGF-β), platelet-derived growth factor (PDGF), and VEGF. These cytokines, along with monocyte chemoattractant protein-1 (MCP-1) (CCL2), macrophage inflammatory protein (MIP-1α) (CCL3), TGF-α, fibronectin, elastin, C5a, C3a, nerve growth factor, and ECM components, initiate the process of chemotaxis of inflammatory cells to the wound from the peripheral circulatory system.

Neutrophils are drawn to the site of injury and constitute the predominant cell type 24–48 hours after the inciting event. These cells use the respiratory burst to generate reactive oxygen species thereby killing both infectious cells and local tissues. Interestingly, although neutrophils are the first inflammatory cells to arrive at the wound, there is some question as to how significant a role they play in the wound healing process. Studies have demonstrated that neither the absence of neutrophils themselves nor the absence of the cytokines they produce has any bearing on the wound's ability to heal, and some have even postulated that the free radicals produced by neutrophils during the myeloperoxidase system may contribute to chronic wounds. However, other studies insist that neutrophils are necessary for their ability to modify and orchestrate macrophage function. What is certain is that, after a few days, the neutrophils present in the wound begin to undergo apoptosis and are ultimately phagocytized by macrophages.

As the neutrophil population dwindles, macrophages become the dominant inflammatory cell in the acute wound. Circulating monocytes are signaled to the wound by the interplay of a series of growth factors, cytokines, chemokines, and other biologically active factors, enabling the monocytes to extravasate from the circulation, enter the wound, and transform into macrophages. Once in the wound, these cells are responsible for the debridement of dead neutrophils and fibrin. Macrophages are also responsible for the production of growth factors (TGF-β, TGF-α, basic FGF [bFGF], VEGF, and PDGF) that drive the proliferative phase of healing. Whereas the presence of neutrophils may or may not be critical to wound healing, macrophages are without question vital to normal physiologic healing and are responsible for the resolution of the inflammatory state.

Proliferative Phase

Taking place 2 days after the inciting injury and lasting for 3 weeks postinjury, the proliferative phase is characterized by the processes of collagen deposition, formation of granulation tissue, angiogenesis, and finally epithelialization (▶ Fig. 2.1). Fibroblasts, the dominant cell of this phase, are responsible for producing the collagen, elastin, and glycosaminoglycans that produce a well-vascularized fibrous connective tissue known as granulation tissue. This tissue is the framework upon which wound healing occurs and contains an abundance of type III collagen.

Revascularization of the wound itself is a very important aspect of this phase of healing because it is essential to deliver oxygen and nutrients to the wound to meet the high metabolic demands of the wound repair process. Vascularization occurs either by angiogenesis (branching of preexisting microvasculature in the wound periphery) or vasculogenesis (formation of new blood vessels by stem cells). Angiogenesis is initiated by local hypoxia and driven by FGF, PDGF, VEGF, and IL-8.

Once the granulation tissue is appropriately vascularized, unopposed wound edges must undergo closure via contraction. Epidermal cells at the wound margins arrange themselves circumferentially and produce a contractile "purse-string" force that helps contract the wound. This occurs as myofibroblasts (specialized fibroblast cells that express alpha-smooth muscle actin and intercellular adhesion factors in response to TGF-β1) initiate the process of wound contraction.

Finally, reepithelialization must occur for the wound to be considered fully closed. Keratinocytes present at the wound edges and adnexal structures (e.g., hair follicles, sebaceous glands) are signaled to multiply by epidermal growth factor, FGF, and TGF-β. This process requires the loss of contact inhibition, allowing cells to travel across the wound. Contact inhibition is reestablished after successful migration. Evidence suggests that chronic wounds may develop secondary to the failure of keratinocyte migration. Reepithelialization is accelerated by a moist healing environment as well as the presence of matrix metalloproteinase-1 (MMP-1).

Maturation/Remodeling Phase

The final phase of healing is an ongoing process that can extend up to a year after the initial insult. Approximately 3 weeks postinjury, the inflammatory and proliferative phases have transformed the acute wound into a healing bed composed of immature type III collagen, providing approximately 20% of the strength of uninjured skin. Collagen remodeling continues to take place with no net change in collagen production. Slowly, the wound fibroblasts begin shifting the ratio of type III to type I collagen, and with this the wound will strengthen proportionately. The wound will achieve 80% of its premorbid strength after 2–3 months, but will never reach 100%. Over time, the wound will continue to contract, with the amount of wound contraction being inversely proportional to the thickness of the wound dermis.

2.3 Factors Affecting Wound Healing

Using knowledge of the intrinsic physiologic healing mechanism as a foundation, the plastic surgeon must also be able to incorporate these concepts into clinical scenarios and understand how various systemic conditions of each patient will impact wound healing. Knowledge of the healing capacity of a 70-year-old smoker as compared to an infant, for example, will provide prognostic value and drive therapeutic decision making.

2.3.1 Oxygen Delivery

The rapid turnover of cells in the acute wound is a highly catabolic, energy-intensive process; therefore sufficient delivery of oxygen to the wound is critical. In patients where the local microvasculature has been compromised, local tissue hypoxia will adversely impact wound healing. The arterial oxygen partial pressure (PaO_2) is representative of the amount of oxygen arriving to the wound. The normal range of PaO_2 is 75–100 mm Hg at sea level, but this can be variable based on the anatomical location tested. The vasoconstrictive effects of cold temperature, increased sympathetic tone secondary to pain, nicotine, vasopressive medications, and hypovolemic shock decrease tissue perfusion and thus inhibit wound healing. These factors must be optimized in the context of the patient's overall health. It is also important to consider the anatomical location of the wound; the head and neck region are inherently better perfused than the lower extremity. Adjunctive wound healing modalities, such as hyperbaric oxygen therapy, aim to augment oxygen delivery if perfusion is adequate.

2.3.2 Smoking

Smoking is a major inhibitor of wound healing, and its effects are multifactorial. It has frequently been cited that smoking one cigarette leads to an average reduction in digital blood-flow velocity of 42%. Nicotine is also prothrombotic through is effects on platelet adhesion, further producing tissue hypoxia. Smoking decreases the amount of inflammatory cells that are able to infiltrate the wound. As if the effects of nicotine were not enough, carbon monoxide and hydrogen cyanide, just 2 of the over 4,000 components of cigarette smoke, decrease the amount of oxygen transported to the wound. Cigarette smoking has been shown to decrease prostacyclin production, leading to increased platelet aggregation, decreased collagen production, increased fibrinogen production, and decreased leukocyte function. Carbon monoxide competitively inhibits oxygen binding to hemoglobin, shifting the oxygen–hemoglobin saturation curve to the left, in essence making the wound more hypoxic. There have been multiple studies demonstrating the negative effects of smoking on wound healing, with all data showing higher rates of wound complication, wound necrosis, and surgical site infection.

For elective cases, it is generally recommended that smoking be discontinued beginning at least 4 weeks prior to the operation until 4 weeks following the operation. In patients where compliance may be an issue, levels of cotinine, a tobacco metabolite, may be checked to ensure the patient has truly abstained from nicotine exposure. The role of nicotine replacement therapy has not been clearly delineated, but it stands to reason that these products should also be avoided.

2.3.3 Chronic Disease States

The overall health of the patient must be taken into consideration when managing wounds. As such, it is vital to identify medical comorbidities that may negatively impact wound healing. Some of these comorbidities include, but are not limited to, peripheral artery disease, diabetes mellitus, and chronic venous insufficiency.

In patients with diabetes, three factors converge to negatively impact wound healing: (1) vasculopathy, (2) neuropathy, and (3) immunopathy.

Adding to this complexity, diabetic patients also frequently have associated comorbidities, such as peripheral artery disease and atherosclerosis. These elements not only impair wound healing but also predispose the diabetic patient to various wounds, such as foot ulcers. It is estimated that 25% of diabetic patients will develop a foot ulcer.

Diabetic neuropathy affects sensory, motor, and autonomic nerves. With decreased sensation, patients have altered perception of pain, which may negatively impact healing by removing this protective mechanism. The diabetic patient may have motor neuropathy in the foot leading to the classic claw foot deformity and development of pressure points over the plantar metatarsal heads. Autonomic neuropathy negatively impacts healing by preventing the normal secretion of sweat and oils, which prevents the skin from drying out.

The immunopathy of diabetic patients ultimately leads to an unfavorable local environment for wound healing. Macrophage function is impaired, keratinocyte migration is inhibited, fibroblasts experience a phenotypic change, and the accumulation of ECM components is impaired. Remodeling of the wound bed by MMPs is decreased, and collagen accumulation is abnormal.

Patients with peripheral artery disease have by definition impaired arterial blood flow. This leads to decreased delivery of vital nutrients and oxygen to tissue while simultaneously decreasing the removal of metabolic waste products. These features combine to impair wound healing and predispose to ulceration in distal blood flow sites.

Chronic venous insufficiency leads to incompetent venous valves and venous stasis. The areas affected are essentially experiencing chronic inflammation without resolution of wound healing. White blood cells are activated by the increased stress experienced by the endothelial blood cells and enter the interstitial space. Inflammatory cytokines and cells are recruited, and wound healing is impaired.

2.3.4 Nutrition

The wound healing process by definition is an anabolic state, with increased production of substances such as collagen and other proteins in the ECM in an attempt to restore the body to its premorbid state. It stands to reason that nutritional status can significantly impact the patient's ability to heal. Caloric energy, amino acids, fatty acids, vitamins, and cofactors are all required for the healing process to succeed. When initially assessing a patient's nutritional status, a thorough history and physical exam are crucial. Previous work by Molnar et al stated, "all geriatric wound patients are malnourished until proven otherwise." If malnutrition is suspected, laboratory studies can be performed to provide a quantitative assessment (▶Table 2.2), though these values may not always directly correlate with nutritional status in cases of inflammation or trauma.

A dietary treatment plan should be provided to address deficiencies and allow for systemic optimization. Protein is recommended to be 1–2 g/kg/d. Addition of arginine has been shown to aid in collagen production. Vitamin C supplementation can also be given to healing patients because it is a critical substrate in the hydroxylation reactions that take place during collagen cross-linking. In patients who are receiving systemic corticosteroid therapy, vitamin A can be supplemented to offset the epithelialization-inhibiting effects of steroids while maintaining their immunosuppressant properties. Cofactors such as zinc are necessary for proper proliferation of epithelial cells and fibroblasts.

Tight glucose control has been increasingly recognized as paramount in various outcomes in surgery. Proper blood glucose control is extremely important perioperatively to avoid a wide variety of complications. Ramos et al demonstrated a 30% increase in the postoperative infection rate for each 40 mg/dL over 110 mg/dL. Latham et al found that surgical site infection rates of diabetic patients with a hemoglobin A1c > 8% was more than two times that of the group with an A1c < 8%. Some experts recommend that blood glucose measurements should be < 200 mg/dL and hemoglobin A1c < 6.5% in high-risk wound closure populations for lower rates of dehiscence. Delay of operation should be considered in patients with an A1c > 9%, and perioperative blood glucose levels should be maintained between 140 and 180 mg/dL. The surgeon should have a low threshold for involving endocrinology and a multidisciplinary approach to the diabetic patient.

2.3.5 Age

As people age, significant changes in skin can make the elderly more susceptible to trauma. The epidermis, basement membrane, and dermis all significantly thin, leading to impaired barrier function and thinner appearance of skin. Water loss and susceptibility to infection increase. Blood vessels become more friable and fragile, as seen in senile purpura. Age has often been viewed as an independent risk factor for impaired wound healing; however, evidence in the literature suggests that not age but rather the concomitant risk factors in the elderly may be to blame.

One large study by Karamanos et al found no difference in wound dehiscence rates between patients younger than 30 years and older than 30 years but identified postoperative abscess development, paraplegia, quadriplegia, steroid and tobacco use, deep surgical-site infection development, increased body mass index (BMI), and wound classification at the end of surgery as independent risk factors for wound dehiscence.

On the other hand, when comparing breast reduction surgery outcomes between women younger and older than 40, Shermak et al found older women have increased likelihood of experiencing postoperative infection and wound healing problems, and they require subsequent wound debridement. Once again, BMI was found to significantly correlate with infection risk (each point rise in BMI increased infection risk by 7%). This group suggested that declines in estrogen levels were the cause of wound healing problems because patents on hormone replacement therapy and oral contraceptive therapy had a reduced risk of postoperative infection.

Commonly underappreciated, older patients cosmetically heal better and have less significant scarring. This can be attributed to a curbed inflammatory reaction during wound healing. Fewer lymphocytes infiltrate the wound but at the same time have enhanced cytokine release while macrophages

Table 2.2 Albumin and prealbumin as markers for nutritional status

Albumin	Prealbumin
Mild deficiency: 2.8–3.5 g/dL	Mild deficiency: < 15 mg/dL
Moderate deficiency: 2.1–2.7 g/dL	Moderate deficiency: < 10 mg/dL
Severe deficiency: < 2.1 g/dL	Severe deficiency: < 5 mg/dL
Half-life: 20 days	Half-life: 3 days

Note: The relationship between these values and nutritional status may be unreliable in cases with an associated inflammatory state.

have decreased phagocytic ability. Although age has been associated with delayed time to epithelialization, the relative amount of collagen deposition remains unchanged with age. This has been posited to be caused by the decreased proliferative response by keratinocytes, fibroblasts, and endothelial cells.

On the opposite end of the spectrum, fetal wounds have been found to undergo scarless healing until 24 weeks' gestation. When fetal tissue is injured, the dermis can reconstitute a nondisrupted collagen matrix identical to the premorbid tissue. Additionally, dermal structures such as sebaceous glands and hair follicles are regenerated.

Scarless healing in fetuses can be attributed to differences across all phases of wound healing. The inflammatory phase of wound healing in the fetus is relatively blunted, with decreased platelet degranulation and aggregation to initiate the inflammatory cycle. Fewer neutrophils are recruited into the wound. In the proliferative phase, fibroblasts of the fetus secrete more type III and IV collagen in addition to increased proliferation of fibroblasts and collagen. There are no myofibroblasts. Cell signaling is decreased with less TGF-β IL-6, and IL-8, which decreases chemotaxis and inflammatory cell mediator recruitment. The content of hyaluronic acid in the fetal skin increases faster than in adult wounds. Hyaluronic acid has a negative charge and effectively impedes water molecule movement into the wound. Compared to adults, there is an increased ratio of type I to III collagen in wounds. In the remodeling phase, there is rapid upregulation of genes involved in cell growth and proliferation leading to rapid wound closure in the fetus. Further research into these topics may yield significant advances in scarless healing.

2.3.6 Infection

A significant impediment to proper wound healing is local and systemic infection. When considering infected wounds, it is useful to group them as acute and chronic infections because the treatment strategy varies significantly. Although acute and chronic infectious are usually treated similarly, their biology dictates alternative approaches.

Acute infections generally involve a single microbe, whereas chronic infections are polymicrobial and often consist of a biofilm. A biofilm is a group of microorganisms living within a matrix of extracellular polymeric substance that is resistant to conventional wound care therapy. The differences between these two infections lie in the survival strategies employed by the microbe rather than the host immune response, location, or type of microbe. In acute infections, the bacteria rapidly damage tissue until either the infection is quelled or the host dies. Biofilm bacteria are more patient and employ a parasitic-like strategy. The microbes will evoke a persistent hyperinflammatory response from the host and will feed on plasma exudate. Unlike acute infections, these chronic infections respond only partially to antibiotics and will make a quick resurgence once the antibiotics are removed.

The biofilm phenotype is becoming more widely appreciated in morbidity of chronic wounds. It is estimated by some sources that 65% of all human infectious disease is caused by the biofilm phenotype, whereas the National Institutes of Health (NIH) estimates as much as 80%. The biology of biofilms begins with attachment to the wound bed. The growth state of the biofilm is guided by quorum sensing, which directs gene expression for the various microbes living in the biofilm environment. Substances are then secreted to protect the biofilm from bacteriophages, light, and desiccation. This substance is usually a polysaccharide but may consist of host DNA from neutrophils, bacterial DNA, bacterial proteins, or plasma components, such as fibrin and albumin. The composition of this protective substance may change in order to adapt to environmental stressors and make culturing biofilms difficult.

Therapeutics should be targeted as a biofilm-based strategy, including multimodality debridement (sharp, energy transfer, ultrasound, biological); anti-biofilm agents, such as lactoferrin (which disrupts attachment at the wound base), xylitol (for degrading the biofilm matrix), and hamamelitannin (which disrupts quorum sensing); as well as bactericidal agents.

2.3.7 Radiation

As radiation therapy has become a commonly employed cancer treatment modality, wounds in irradiated fields have also become a frequently encountered problem for plastic surgeons. Soon after the implementation of radiation therapy, it was noted that irradiated tissues experience delayed wound healing. Significant advances have been achieved since that time, and high-energy megavolt therapy is being used with increased accuracy for tumor-laden tissue while sparing more superficial structures. Radiation causes direct DNA damage and cellular damage, which lead to both immediate and long-term effects. The acute effects include erythema, dry desquamation, and wet desquamation. The delayed effects include changes in pigmentation, fibrosis of the skin and subcutaneous tissues, changes in sweat gland function, as well as necrosis and tumorigenesis.

Nearly every aspect of wound healing is affected by radiation therapy. The immediate damage to the basement membrane leads to the release of serotonin and histamines, inducing an erythematous response. As vessels are damaged, the permeability of the capillaries increases, leading to local inflammation. The acute inflammatory stage is often prolonged and leads to fibrosis.

Radiation-induced fibrosis can occur in nearly any tissue. It progresses over 4–12 months and is clinically noted by skin thickening, induration, and ulceration in the skin. The pathogenesis extends from the acute inflammatory phase and involves direct DNA damage as well as the production of reactive oxygen species and reactive nitrogen species. The inflammatory state leads to increased differentiation of fibroblasts into myofibroblasts. Although these myofibroblasts are creating excess collagen, leading to a bulky ECM, there are decreased ECM remodeling enzymes due to free radical damage. The end result is an edematous ECM with decreased tissue compliance and lower breaking strength.

Direct damage to blood vessels in the wound bed, so-called obliterative endarteritis, produces decreased oxygen tension. Radiated wounds are unable to respond with angiogenesis, leading to a suboptimal wound bed in radiated tissues. Radiated wounds have hyperkeratotic edges, which impair both contraction and keratinocyte migration. Because cells with the highest mitotic rate are most affected by radiation, keratinocyte production is significantly altered, leading to slower reepithelialization.

Strategies to mitigate the sequelae of radiation exposure are aimed at decreasing inflammation and subsequent fibrosis. Topical agents and systemic agents have little evidence to support their use. Calendula ointment has been found to decrease dermatitis in patients with breast cancer.

2.3.8 Biomarkers for Wound Healing

As evidenced by the foregoing discussion of various systemic and local factors, evaluation of chronic and abnormally healing wounds is challenging and fraught with confounding factors. In order to properly assess and manage wounds in the future, it is important to identify local and systemic biomarkers that will help tailor management of complex wounds. Biomarkers in chronic wounds can be split into tissue biomarkers, wound fluid biomarkers, and systemic biomarkers. Development and research of biomarkers are cumbersome, but greater use of large datasets may yield promising patient-specific patterns that can direct wound care.

2.4 Wound Care Management

Wound care management is a cornerstone of the practice of a plastic surgeon. Many new therapies have emerged in recent years with equivocal supporting evidence. The surgeon should be judicious in employing new therapies and should tailor treatment strategies to patients based on their overall state of health and etiology of tissue injury.

General treatment strategies for wound healing often involve antiseptic agents and wound irrigating agents. Some options include povidone-iodine solutions, octenidine, polyhexamethylene biguanide derivatives, and Dakin's solution. In a Cochrane Review, povidone-iodine solutions had acceptable antimicrobial activity in 64% of combinations, octenidine had 54% of combinations with appropriate antibacterial activity, and polyhexamethylene had only 32.5% sufficient antimicrobial activity. Studies evaluating antibiotics and antiseptics for surgical wound healing by secondary intention have not demonstrated robust evidence to support the use of any antiseptic/antibiotic/antibacterial preparation.

In a Cochrane Review assessing dressings for foot ulcers in diabetic patients, there was no significant evidence suggesting one dressing improves outcomes compared to another. Wound dressings assessed included absorbent dressings, alginate dressings, hydrogel dressings, films, soft polymer dressings, hydrocolloid dressings, foam dressings, capillary action dressings, iodine-impregnated dressings, silver-impregnated dressings, and chlorhexidine gauze.

Topical silver, with its antimicrobial effects and favorable toxicity profile, is an effective treatment for infected wounds that has been used since the times of the ancient Greeks and Romans. Although the use of silver in treating infected wounds was less pervasive following the introduction of antibiotics, a renewed interest was taken in silver-containing topical treatments as antibiotic resistance emerged. However, a review demonstrated no significant difference in silver-containing foam dressings compared to standard practices and wound dressings.

Much like silver, honey has been used since ancient times in wound care. Numerous trials have evaluated the use of honey in various clinical settings. There is high-quality evidence that honey dressings heal partial-thickness burns more quickly than conventional dressings. There is low-quality evidence that burns treated with honey heal more quickly than those treated with silver sulfadiazine and high-quality evidence that there is no difference in overall risk of healing within 6 weeks in honey compared to silver sulfadiazine. In postoperative infected wounds, those dressed with honey were shown to heal more quickly than those treated with antiseptic washes followed by gauze and were additionally associated with fewer adverse events.

Dakin's solution was developed by Henry Dakin and Alexis Carrel around the time of the First World War. The solution was composed by buffering 0.05% sodium hypochlorite with boric acid. When used properly, Dakin's solution is bactericidal to commonly encountered organisms in open wounds. Like other antiseptics, Dakin's solution is indicated for use in the inflammatory phase of wound repair in the face of contaminated and dirty wounds. One must be careful when using the solution because it has been found to be cytotoxic and may inflict significant cellular damage. Typically it is used for 3 days to sterilize a dirty wound bed.

An emerging wound treatment modality is platelet-rich plasma (PRP). PRP is composed of the patient's own plasma that has a high concentration of platelets and associated growth factors. To date, there have been 10 randomized controlled trials evaluating the use of PRP. Overall, the data suggest that PRP may help with the healing of foot ulcers associated with diabetes mellitus (low-quality evidence), but other indications have not yet been validated.

Complement C5 has been described in a topical form in a rat skin model to increase maximum wound breaking strength as well as collagen and fibronectin via the chemotactic cytokine properties of C5 and may be a promising compound for future study in human models.

Ultrasound has been suggested for use in wound healing and is thought to work via cavitation (creation of micrometer-sized bubbles) and microstreaming (fluid movement along acoustic boundaries). Mechanical vibration created by these devices induces changes at the cellular level leading to favorable effects at all stages of wound healing. Randomized controlled trials have not demonstrated any changes in wound healing but have shown reduction in pain.

Electrical stimulation has been suggested for use in wound healing since 1980. The theory behind the application of this technology is based on the direct current electrical gradient that exists within 1 mm of the wound. It is theorized that manipulation of this current could potentiate wound healing. Some authors have found that using electrical stimulation causes enhanced cellular migration, whereas other authors argue against it. Electrical stimulation increases angiogenesis via enhanced release of VEGF. Robust clinical trials in human are lacking, but some suggest there may be positive wound healing and pain effects. Further study is required.

Negative pressure wound therapy was first introduced in 1997 and was quickly touted as a useful adjuvant to complicated wound healing. Open-cell foam dressing is packed into the wound cavity, a seal is created with impermeable drapes, and negative pressure is then applied to the system. The purported mechanism is fourfold: increasing blood flow, causing cellular deformation leading to increased mitotic rate, removing exudate and reducing bacterial load, and increasing the rate of granulation tissue formation. Increased mitotic rate and subsequent cell proliferation are the products of the tensile forces that are exerted on the tissues by the vacuum devices. In the initial study, 296 of 300 wounds treated responded favorably with increased granulation tissue formation.

Negative pressure wound vacuums are contraindicated in exposed vessels, malignancy, necrotic tissue, untreated osteomyelitis, or nonenteric and unexplored fistulas. Care must be taken when combined with anticoagulation. Although widely hailed as critical to current wound care management, significant questions have been raised as to the mechanism of action and purported benefits. In one study using different methods to assess for blood flow, the authors found that negative wound therapy actually decreased local blood flow. This suggests that negative pressure wound therapy should be used cautiously in wounds in which the tissue perfusion may be compromised.

In a Cochrane Review evaluating nine clinical trials, mixed evidence was found as to whether negative pressure wound therapy reduces surgical site infections, decreases wound dehiscence, and decreases healing time. It is suggested that hospitals use "home-made" systems as opposed to commercial products because the cost is significantly lower and pain may be lower as well. A comprehensive review by Anghel and Kim found that negative pressure wound therapy is effective in complicated wounds in patients with diabetes, provides enhanced outcomes in acute injury and burn patients, and reduces inflammation and edema after skin-grafted free muscle flaps.

Stem cells are a promising area of research for application in wound healing. These undifferentiated cells are divided into pluripotent (able to transform into any cell of the three germ cell layers) or multipotent (only able to transform into cells of one germ cell layer). Because there is hot debate on the ethical use of pluripotent embryonic stem cells, research has focused on the use of multipotent stem cells (MSCs). In animal studies assessing MSC use in wound healing, the data are promising. The most common source of MSCs is placental tissue. EpiFix (MiMedx Group) is a dehydrated human amnion/chorion membrane and has been found to induce MSC recruitment, migration, and proliferation. When compared to standard therapy, evidence suggests it has higher wound closure rates. Grafix (Osiris Therapeutics), which contains fibroblasts, MSCs, and epithelial cells, has been compared to standard therapy and demonstrated higher wound closure rates, reduction in wound size, and decreased wound infections. In their review of available literature, Sorice et al posit that stem cell therapies will be the standard of wound care in the future.

Hyperbaric oxygen therapy is an effective modality used in the treatment of difficult wounds to increase tissue oxygenation. This therapy consists of delivering 100% oxygen above atmospheric pressure for weeks to months. Sessions typically last 1–2 hours. Hyperbaric oxygen therapy is thought to improve wound healing by increasing blood perfusion, thereby delivering more growth factors into the wound bed while decreasing inflammatory cytokines and increasing fibroblast activity in the proliferative phase. In a review evaluating the use of hyperbaric oxygen therapy for treatment of surgical and traumatic wounds, there was found to be increased graft survival in one trial, no difference in a second, decreased necrosis and better wound healing in a third, and no difference in graft survival compared to dexamethasone or heparin in the fourth. In the treatment of chronic wounds, hyperbaric oxygen therapy has been found to increase ulcer healing in the short term without significant effects in the long term.

2.5 Scar Management

Patients frequently seek out a plastic surgeon for cosmetic concerns over their scars. These may be poorly healed surgical scars, burn scars, hypertrophic scars, or keloids. Keloids and hypertrophic scars are significant problems faced by the plastic surgeon and affect up to 5 to 15% of wounds. Although the terms are commonly used interchangeably, keloids and hypertrophic scars are physiologically different. Varying pathological mechanisms at different stages of wound healing are responsible for the development of abnormal scars, including increased response to growth factors and excess collagen deposition after tissue injury (▶Table 2.3). Hypertrophic scars will respect the injury boundaries, whereas keloids invade into normal surrounding tissue. Moreover, the etiology differs as well, with keloids developing after minimal tissue insults (e.g., vaccinations and piercings), whereas hypertrophic scars commonly arise following significant lesions caused by surgery and burns. Additionally, certain areas of the body are more prone than others to scar abnormally: the lower face, pectoral areas of the chest, upper back, ears, neck, and lateral aspect of the arm. ▶Table 2.4 summarizes the main differences between keloids and hypertrophic scars.

Tensile forces and movement acting at the site of a scar often lead to a poor scar appearance for a number of reasons. Tension has been found to prolong the inflammatory phase of wound healing and may increase the risk of hypertrophic or keloid scar formation. Other factors that may contribute to the likelihood of hypertrophic and keloid scar formation include genetics, age, method of injury, and healing by secondary intention.

Unfortunately, there remains to be a single compound to treat and improve hypertrophic scars and keloids. The plastic surgeon must use a cocktail of various topical agents with dubious efficacy. There are numerous topical therapies available for use,

Table 2.3 Pathological mechanisms leading to excessive scarring

	Normal healing	Excessive scarring
Inflammatory phase	Immediately after injury	Prolonged response to proinflammatory cytokines
	Homeostasis	
	Induction of cell proliferation	
	PDGF, TGF-β, FGF	
Proliferative phase	2–3 days after injury	Increase the response of fibroblasts toward TGF-β1 and TGF-β2
	Angiogenesis/vasculogenesis	Increase deposition of collagen
	Formation of granulation tissue Myofibroblasts	Increase the differentiation of fibroblasts to myofibroblasts
Remodeling phase	Reepithelialization	Inhibition of matrix metalloproteinases
	Proteolytic enzymes	
	Matrix metalloproteinases	Keloids collagen I:III ratio = 17:1
	Collagen I:III ratio = 3:1 Normalization of cell density	Overexpression of proliferative cytokines

Abbreviations: FGF, fibroblast growth factor; PDGF, platelet-derived growth factor; TGF, transforming growth factor.

Table 2.4 Main characteristics of keloids and hypertrophic scars

	Keloid	Hypertrophic scar
Location	Dermis	Dermis
Extension	Beyond the original scar	Confined to the original scar
Histological features	Fibroproliferative tumor	Excessive collagen deposition
α-SMA	Protomyofibroblast (-)	Myofibroblast (+)
Predisposing factors	Genetic predisposition	Genetic predisposition
	Ethnic (Asian, African)	Ethnic (Asian, African)
	Hormone	Suture material
	Surgical site Age (10–30 years old)	Surgical site Depth of injury
Progression	Does not regress	May regress

Abbreviation: SMA, smooth muscle actin.

both over the counter and by prescription. Notable therapies include vitamin E derivatives, SGS, moist exposed burn ointment, onion extract–based gel, retinoids, botulinum toxin A, intradermal injections of human mesenchymal stem cells and human TGF-β3, as well as numerous laser modalities.

SGS has been found to be effective in scars and keloids and is widely accepted as the most efficacious modality in treating these scar types. Although the exact mechanism of action remains unknown, the prevailing theory is the increased static charge of silicone sheeting leads to increased occlusion and hydration of wounds while decreasing capillary activity and collagen production and potential modulation of growth factors. This modality is most effective in patients who have had a scar revision and in patients who are apt to develop hypertrophic and keloid scars. In a Cochrane Review of 20 trials involving 873 patients, the efficacy of SGS for prevention and treatment of hypertrophic and keloid scarring was evaluated. SGS was found to be most useful in the treatment of scar reduction thickness and color amelioration, whereas SGS for prevention was not found to be more beneficial than no treatment.

Intralesional injection of steroids has been found to be effective in the treatment of hypertrophic scars and keloids. Triamcinolone is usually administered at concentrations of 10 mg/mL for moderate scars and 40 mg/mL for thick keloids using a fine needle. The recommended dose is 0.1 - 0.2 mL/cm² of the involved skin with the total dose not exceeding 1 or 2 mL per application. The solution can be injected in full strength or diluted to half strength with saline or local anesthetic. It is important to note that the injection must be done within the scar avoiding deep subcutaneous delivery of the steroid as this can lead to atrophy of the underlying fat.

Vitamin E derivatives are the most prevalent antioxidant in the skin. For this reason, it has been hypothesized that using topical vitamin E during the inflammatory phase of wound healing can lessen scar development by scavenging excess free radicals and inhibiting fibroblast and keratinocyte proliferation. There have been case reports of vitamin E helping improve scar appearance, but larger, more elegantly designed studies have not shown any benefit. In fact, vitamin E has been found to cause significant contact dermatitis in individuals.

Onion extract–based gel is a compound that contains *Allium cepa* as the active ingredient and has been touted as improving scar appearance. However, no method of action has been elucidated, and there are no data supporting its ability to improve scarring compared to standard petrolatum emollients.

Botulinum toxin A has been used in numerous applications in not only plastic surgery but also other fields. The neuromodulating effects of this toxin may also help in scar management. In facial surgery, injection of the muscles surrounding the surgical site will reduce tension on wound closure and may allow the surgeon to use finer suture, thus creating a less noticeable scar.

Human mesenchymal stem cells may become a more prominent tool for the plastic surgeon in scar revision. These multipotent cells may be injected into the closure site and function to decrease scar formation while increasing the tensile strength of the scar after healing.

Fat grafting has been used extensively in plastic surgery, and there is increased interest in its utilization in wound healing and scarring via optimization of angiogenesis, curbing the inflammatory response, and ameliorating pain. Although subjective measures are promising, increased investigation is required to determine the extent of the effects of autologous fat grafting on scarring.

Different phototherapy modalities, including laser-assisted healing, pulsed dye laser for vascular lesions, nonablative laser resurfacing, and ablative laser resurfacing, have been used to decrease scar appearance and improve wound healing. The exact mechanism accounting for improvement in scar appearance has not yet been determined. In a prospective cohort study evaluating lasers in the treatment of hypertrophic burn scars, significant improvement was noted compared to controls in both subjective and objective analysis. In a review evaluating seven randomized controlled trials with 403 participants evaluating the effects of phototherapy on the healing of pressure ulcers, there is insufficient evidence to recommend its utilization until more convincing evidence arises.

Pressure dressings have become an integral tool in the treatment of burn scars and hypertrophic scars. Burn wounds heal with a large amount of collagen at the site of injury. The initial scar is red, raised, and often rigid. During this phase of scar maturation, pressure therapy is thought to be best equipped to prevent scar hypertrophy. It is thought that pressure therapy modulates scar appearance during this phase by decreasing blood flow to the pressurized site. The decreased blood flow ultimately curbs collagen deposition at the site. Initially, low pressures are used (15–17 mm Hg), then custom-made garments are used to deliver more pressure (24–28 mm Hg). Pressure therapy is to be maintained on a continuous basis and may be initiated as soon as the burn site can tolerate the application of these devices. The ultimate goal of therapy is to decrease scar height while maintaining scar pliability. Efficacy is most notable in the treatment of ear keloids via pressure earrings. Evidence of efficacy is otherwise paltry to support the widespread use in scar management because it can be uncomfortable and can cause ulceration and skin maceration. Considering the possible side effects and lack of significant evidence, pressure therapy is not the standard of care in all scar treatment regimens, but it is more useful in burn patients. Similar to pressure dressings, adhesive paper tape may improve scar appearance by minimizing tension across the healing wound.

Semiocclusive dressings and ointments promote moist wound healing and timely reepithelialization, thereby decreasing hypertrophic scar formation. Growth factors that are within the wound bed are kept within the wound by these dressings. Symptoms of pain and itching have been found to decrease with these dressings, but data are lacking as to whether the scar appearance is improved.

Aloe vera has long been used as an adjuvant compound in wound healing. In a rat model in which wound surface, contraction, and epithelialization were monitored there was a dose-dependent relationship between strength and modulus of elasticity compared to the control. Aloe vera was found to decrease inflammation and improve wound epithelialization while decreasing scar tissue size and improving organization of scar tissue.

Various devices have been invented to improve not only surgical wound closure but also scarification. The DERMABOND PRINEO Skin Closure System (Ethicon) was found to be equivalent to intradermal suturing in breast procedures and was 6.3 times faster for wound closure with comparable wound healing and scar cosmesis. The Embrace (Neodyne) device was recently used in scar revision surgery in a randomized controlled trial involving 12 patients as self controls. The 6-month assessment found significant improvement in scar appearance. The device functions via force offloading on the incision and mechanomodulation to reduce scarring.

In the multidisciplinary treatment of burn patients, massage therapy has been used as a potential therapy to decrease scarring; however, there is little evidence to suggest that it has any benefits in this parameter.

As opioid use has increased in recent years, with more focus on addiction and overdose, it is important to evaluate alternative sources of pain management. Pulsed electromagnetic fields have been found to decrease pain in bone and wound repair as well as reduce edema. Mean IL-1 β concentration in wound exudate was found to be significantly lower in addition. In the patients evaluated, there was a two-fold reduction in narcotic use.

In summary, therapies validated by evidence-based studies include pressure therapy, SGS and intralesional corticosteroid injection. Therapies lacking consensus and significant evidence include various creams, massage therapy, laser therapy, radiotherapy, intralesional injection of products other than corticosteroids, splinting, and antihistamines.

2.5.1 Emergent Therapies

Over the past decades new promising therapies have been developed for scar treatment including inhibitors of collagen synthesis and blockers of TGF-β1. However, to date, neither the traditional nor the new emergent modalities have been fully effective in achieving significant clinical improvement and thus the ideal treatment remains elusive.

Inhibitors of Collagen Synthesis

These agents ameliorate the fibrotic process by inhibition of collagen synthesis. They include anti-Co1 antisense oligodeoxynucleotide, basic FGF, and histone deacetylase inhibitor.

Decorin is a natural antagonist of TGF-β fibrotic activity, and its effectiveness has been tested in renal fibrosis. Indoleamine 2.3 dioxygenase is available for topical application and can increase MMP-1 and -3 activity, enhancing collagen fiber breakdown.

Some agents can inhibit cell proliferation, such as tacrolimus and angiotensin, whereas others can induce cell apoptosis, such as 5 aminolevulinic acid photodynamic laser and high-dose ultraviolet light.

The results shown in animal models or in vitro have been promising for many of these emergent agents; however, further studies are needed to confirm their safety and efficacy in the clinical setting.

TGF-β 1 Blockers

Among the cytokines participating in the wound healing process, some of them show a TGF-β1 antagonist effect, with most of them blocking its effector receptors or its effect in the different targets. Smad 7 belongs to Smad proteins responsible for the intracellular effect of TGF-β1 signaling. Smad 7 is the unique negative feedback regulator of TGF-β1. Interferon-α2b (IFN-α2b) downregulates the expression of TGF-β1, promoting myofibroblast apoptosis and decreasing VEGF-mediated angiogenesis. A trial in burned patients showed its effectiveness when administered subcutaneously. Epidermal growth factor (EGF) decreases the collagen type III synthesis and the levels of α -smooth muscle actin (SMA) regulated by TGF-β1. In addition, an increased expression of decorin, a small, leucine-rich proteoglycan, may decrease TGF-β1 fibrotic activity. TNF-α inhibits ECM synthesis, activates MMPs, and inhibits the α -SMA expression and subsequent myofibroblast differentiation in human dermal fibroblast.

Botulinum toxin A reduces the TGF-β1 secretion and can inhibit fibroblast growth in human hypertrophic scars. Putrescine or 1,4 diaminobutane induces fibroblast apoptosis and decreases the fibrotic effect of TGF-β1 by inhibition of tissue transglutaminase. Tetrandrine produces an upregulation of Smad7 and consequently inhibits the effect of TGF-β1 as it is described above.

Regarding the inhibition of TGF-β1 receptor, several peptide inhibitors have been described. Quercetin can inhibit TGF-β1 receptor types I and II, as well as the Smad2/3 system, in keloids' fibroblasts. Several studies have shown the effect of an inhibitor of TGF-β1 (P144; Digna Biotech) in reducing fibrosis in different tissues. Intraperitoneal administration reduced myocardial and liver fibrosis in rats, whereas topical administration improved scleroderma in mice with implanted human skin samples. Additionally, topical application of this peptide improved scar maturation and morphological features of hypertrophic scars implanted on the back of nude mice. Given its key role in the development of abnormal scarring, modulation of TGF-β1 may hold promise in the treatment of hypertrophic scars and keloids.

2.6 Conclusion

Mastery of wound healing is important in any plastic surgeon's practice. When approaching challenging wounds, it is helpful to think of wounds in their various phases: hemostasis, inflammation, proliferation, and remodeling. Basic science research elucidating roles of various cells, growth factors, and signaling molecules may bring revolutionary techniques to the field of wound healing and regenerative medicine. Consideration of patient factors is vital to understand why various wounds are more difficult to heal. As more products come to market touting wound healing benefits, a critical appraisal of the evidence is paramount before application of these products.

2.7 Key Points

- Physiologic wound healing includes hemostasis, an inflammatory phase, a proliferative phase, and a remodeling phase.
- Factors affecting wound healing include oxygen delivery, smoking, chronic disease states, immunosuppressive therapy, nutrition, age, infection, and radiation exposure. Oxygen delivery

to tissue should be optimized. Smoking should be avoided. Chronic disease states should be considered in difficult-to-heal wounds. Aging confers the benefit of more cosmetic scars, but epithelialization is delayed. Acute and chronic infections should be thoughtfully treated for resolution of a wound. Irradiated tissues often undergo fibrosis and heal poorly.
- Wound care management is critical in the practice of a plastic surgeon. Various solutions are available to aid wound healing with variable efficacy. In lieu of fad solutions, evidenced based wound care solutions should be employed which are tailored to the patient while avoiding possible side effects.
- Plastic surgeons are often sought after for scar management. Commonly encountered but difficult to treat are keloids and hypertrophic scars. Silicone gel sheeting has been found to be the most effective method to treat and prevent these pathologic scars.

Recommended Readings

Anghel EL, Kim PJ. Negative-Pressure Wound Therapy: A Comprehensive Review of the Evidence. Plast Reconstr Surg. 2016; 138(3), Suppl:129S–137S

Armour A, Scott PG, Tredget EE. Cellular and molecular pathology of HTS: basis for treatment. Wound Repair Regen. 2007; 15 Suppl 1:S6–S17

Baumann LS, Spencer J. The effects of topical vitamin E on the cosmetic appearance of scars. Dermatol Surg. 1999; 25(4):311–315

Baur PS Jr, Parks DH, Hudson JD. Epithelial mediated wound contraction in experimental wounds—the purse-string effect. J Trauma. 1984; 24(8):713–720

Blondeel PN, Richter D, Stoff A, Exner K, Jernbeck J, Ramakrishnan V. Evaluation of a new skin closure device in surgical incisions associated with breast procedures. Ann Plast Surg. 2014; 73(6):631–637

Boulton AJM, Armstrong DG, Albert SF, et al; American Diabetes Association. American Association of Clinical Endocrinologists. Comprehensive foot examination and risk assessment: a report of the task force of the foot care interest group of the American Diabetes Association, with endorsement by the American Association of Clinical Endocrinologists. Diabetes Care. 2008; 31(8):1679–1685

Bowering CK. Diabetic foot ulcers. Pathophysiology, assessment, and therapy. Can Fam Physician. 2001; 47:1007–1016

Brem H, Tomic-Canic M. Cellular and molecular basis of wound healing in diabetes. J Clin Invest. 2007; 117(5):1219–1222

Brown RJ, Lee MJ, Sisco M, Kim JYS, Roy N, Mustoe TA. High-dose ultraviolet light exposure reduces scar hypertrophy in a rabbit ear model. Plast Reconstr Surg. 2008; 121(4):1165–1172

Burns JL, Mancoll JS, Phillips LG. Impairments to wound healing. Clin Plast Surg. 2003; 30(1):47–56

Chen C, Hou W-H, Chan ES, Yeh M-L, Lo H-LD. Phototherapy for treating pressure ulcers. In: Cochrane Database of Systematic Reviews. John Wiley & Sons, Ltd; 2014. http://onlinelibrary.wiley.com.ezproxyhost.library.tmc.edu/doi/10.1002/14651858.CD009224.pub2/abstract. Accessed July 11, 2016

Chen MA, Davidson TM. Scar management: prevention and treatment strategies. Curr Opin Otolaryngol Head Neck Surg. 2005; 13(4):242–247

Condé-Green A, Marano AA, Lee ES, et al. Fat Grafting and Adipose-Derived Regenerative Cells in Burn Wound Healing and Scarring: A Systematic Review of the Literature. Plast Reconstr Surg. 2016; 137(1):302–312

Cullum N, Al-Kurdi D, Bell-Syer SE. Therapeutic ultrasound for venous leg ulcers. In: Cochrane Database of Systematic Reviews. John Wiley & Sons, Ltd; 2010. http://onlinelibrary.wiley.com.ezproxyhost.library.tmc.edu/doi/10.1002/14651858.CD001180.pub3/abstract. Accessed June 24, 2016

Daley JM, Reichner JS, Mahoney EJ, et al. Modulation of macrophage phenotype by soluble product(s) released from neutrophils. J Immunol. 2005; 174(4):2265–2272

Dauwe PB, Pulikkottil BJ, Lavery L, Stuzin JM, Rohrich RJ. Does hyperbaric oxygen therapy work in facilitating acute wound healing: a systematic review. Plast Reconstr Surg. 2014; 133(2):208e–215e

Davis JC, Hunt TK, eds. Problem Wounds: The Role of Oxygen. New York, NY: Elsevier; 1988

Desai KK, Hahn E, Pulikkottil B, Lee E, Lee E. Negative pressure wound therapy: an algorithm. Clin Plast Surg. 2012; 39(3):311–324

Diao J-S, Xia W-S, Yi C-G, et al. Histone deacetylase inhibitor reduces hypertrophic scarring in a rabbit ear model. Plast Reconstr Surg. 2013; 132(1):61e–69e

Dolynchuk KN, Ziesmann M, Serletti JM. Topical putrescine (Fibrostat) in treatment of hypertrophic scars: phase II study. Plast Reconstr Surg. 1996; 97(1):117–123, discussion 124–125

Dumville JC, Owens GL, Crosbie EJ, Peinemann F, Liu Z. Negative pressure wound therapy for treating surgical wounds healing by secondary intention. In: Cochrane Database of Systematic Reviews. John Wiley & Sons, Ltd; 2015. http://onlinelibrary.wiley.com.ezproxyhost.library.tmc.edu/doi/10.1002/14651858.CD011278.pub2/abstract. Accessed June 24, 2016

Endara M, Masden D, Goldstein J, Gondek S, Steinberg J, Attinger C. The role of chronic and perioperative glucose management in high-risk surgical closures: a case for tighter glycemic control. Plast Reconstr Surg. 2013; 132(4):996–1004

Ennis WJ, Lee C, Gellada K, Corbiere TF, Koh TJ. Advanced Technologies to Improve Wound Healing: Electrical Stimulation, Vibration Therapy, and Ultrasound-What Is the Evidence? Plast Reconstr Surg. 2016; 138(3), Suppl:94S–104S

Eskes A, Vermeulen H, Lucas C, Ubbink DT. Hyperbaric oxygen therapy for treating acute surgical and traumatic wounds. In: Cochrane Database of Systematic Reviews. John Wiley & Sons, Ltd; 2013. http://onlinelibrary.wiley.com.ezproxyhost.library.tmc.edu/doi/10.1002/14651858.CD008059.pub3/abstract. Accessed July 11, 2016

Ezquerro I-J, Lasarte J-J, Dotor J, et al. A synthetic peptide from transforming growth factor beta type III receptor inhibits liver fibrogenesis in rats with carbon tetrachloride liver injury. Cytokine. 2003; 22(1–2):12–20

Field FK, Kerstein MD. Overview of wound healing in a moist environment. Am J Surg. 1994; 167(1A):2S–6S

Foo CW, Tristani-Firouzi P. Topical modalities for treatment and prevention of postsurgical hypertrophic scars. Facial Plast Surg Clin North Am. 2011; 19(3):551–557

Gisquet H, Liu H, Blondel WCPM, et al. Intradermal tacrolimus prevent scar hypertrophy in a rabbit ear model: a clinical, histological and spectroscopical analysis. Skin Res Technol. 2011; 17(2):160–166

Henry G, Garner WL. Inflammatory mediators in wound healing. Surg Clin North Am. 2003; 83(3):483–507

Hermida N, López B, González A, et al. A synthetic peptide from transforming growth factor-beta1 type III receptor prevents myocardial fibrosis in spontaneously hypertensive rats. Cardiovasc Res. 2009; 81(3):601–609

Hirsch T, Limoochi-Deli S, Lahmer A, et al. Antimicrobial activity of clinically used antiseptics and wound irrigating agents in combination with wound dressings. Plast Reconstr Surg. 2011; 127(4):1539–1545

Holt DR, Kirk SJ, Regan MC, Hurson M, Lindblad WJ, Barbul A. Effect of age on wound healing in healthy human beings. Surgery. 1992; 112(2):293–297, discussion 297–298

Honardoust D, Varkey M, Marcoux Y, Shankowsky HA, Tredget EE. Reduced decorin, fibromodulin, and transforming growth factor- ß 3 in deep dermis leads to hypertrophic scarring. J Burn Care Res. 2012; 33(2):218–227

Hultman CS, Friedstat JS, Edkins RE, Cairns BA, Meyer AA. Laser resurfacing and remodeling of hypertrophic burn scars: the results of a large, prospective, before-after cohort study, with long-term follow-up. Ann Surg. 2014; 260(3):519–529, discussion 529–532

Huntington JA, Williams LV, Schwarzbauer JE. Molecular recognition mechanisms of thrombin. J Thromb Haemost. 2005; 3(8):1861–1872

Ingber DE, Folkman J. Mechanochemical switching between growth and differentiation during fibroblast growth factor-stimulated angiogenesis in vitro: role of extracellular matrix. J Cell Biol. 1989; 109(1):317–330

Janis JE, Harrison B. Wound healing: part I. Basic science. Plast Reconstr Surg. 2014; 133(2):199e–207e

Janis JE, Harrison B. Wound Healing: Part I. Basic Science. Plast Reconstr Surg. 2016; 138(3), Suppl:9S–17S

Jull AB, Cullum N, Dumville JC, Westby MJ, Deshpande S, Walker N. Honey as a topical treatment for wounds. In: Cochrane Database of Systematic Reviews. John Wiley & Sons, Ltd; 2015. http://onlinelibrary.wiley.com.ezproxyhost.library.tmc.edu/doi/10.1002/14651858.CD005083.pub4/abstract. Accessed June 24, 2016

Kairinos N, Voogd AM, Botha PH, et al. Negative-pressure wound therapy II: negative-pressure wound therapy and increased perfusion. Just an illusion? Plast Reconstr Surg. 2009; 123(2):601–612

Karamanos E, Osgood G, Siddiqui A, Rubinfeld I. Wound healing in plastic surgery: does age matter? An American College of Surgeons National Surgical Quality Improvement Program study. Plast Reconstr Surg. 2015; 135(3):876–881

Kavalukas SL, Barbul A. Nutrition and wound healing: an update. Plast Reconstr Surg. 2011; 127 Suppl 1:38S–43S

Klebanoff SJ. Myeloperoxidase: friend and foe. J Leukoc Biol. 2005; 77(5):598–625

Kranke P, Bennett MH, Martyn-St James M, Schnabel A, Debus SE, Weibel S. Hyperbaric oxygen therapy for chronic wounds. In: Cochrane Database of Systematic Reviews. John Wiley & Sons, Ltd; 2015. http://onlinelibrary.wiley.

com.ezproxyhost.library.tmc.edu/doi/10.1002/14651858. CD004123.pub4/abstract. Accessed July 11, 2016

Kreymerman PA, Andres LA, Lucas HD, Silverman AL, Smith AA. Reconstruction of the burned hand. Plast Reconstr Surg. 2011; 127(2):752–759

Krueger JK, Rohrich RJ. Clearing the smoke: the scientific rationale for tobacco abstention with plastic surgery. Plast Reconstr Surg. 2001; 108(4):1063–1073, discussion 1074–1077

Larson BJ, Longaker MT, Lorenz HP. Scarless fetal wound healing: a basic science review. Plast Reconstr Surg. 2010; 126(4):1172–1180

Latham R, Lancaster AD, Covington JF, Pirolo JS, Thomas CS Jr. The association of diabetes and glucose control with surgical-site infections among cardiothoracic surgery patients. Infect Control Hosp Epidemiol. 2001; 22(10):607–612

Leibovich SJ, Ross R. The role of the macrophage in wound repair. A study with hydrocortisone and antimacrophage serum. Am J Pathol. 1975; 78(1):71–100

Li X, Zhou ZP, Hu L, Zhang WJ, Li W. Apoptotic cell death induced by 5-aminolaevulinic acid-mediated photodynamic therapy of hypertrophic scar-derived fibroblasts. J Dermatolog Treat. 2014; 25(5):428–433

Lim AF, Weintraub J, Kaplan EN, et al. The embrace device significantly decreases scarring following scar revision surgery in a randomized controlled trial. Plast Reconstr Surg. 2014; 133(2):398–405

Lindley LE, Stojadinovic O, Pastar I, Tomic-Canic M. Biology and Biomarkers for Wound Healing. Plast Reconstr Surg. 2016; 138(3), Suppl:18S–28S

Liu A, Moy RL, Ozog DM. Current methods employed in the prevention and minimization of surgical scars. Dermatol Surg. 2011; 37(12):1740–1746

Madden JW, Peacock EE Jr. Studies on the biology of collagen during wound healing. I. Rate of collagen synthesis and deposition in cutaneous wounds of the rat. Surgery. 1968; 64(1):288–294

Martinez-Zapata MJ, Martí-Carvajal AJ, Solà I, et al. Autologous platelet-rich plasma for treating chronic wounds. In: Cochrane Database of Systematic Reviews. John Wiley & Sons, Ltd; 2016. http://onlinelibrary.wiley.com.ezproxy-host.library.tmc.edu/doi/10.1002/14651858.CD006899. pub3/abstract. Accessed June 24, 2016

Mahdavian Delavary B, van der Veer WM, van Egmond M, Niessen FB, Beelen RHJ. Macrophages in skin injury and repair. Immunobiology. 2011; 216(7):753–762

Marfella R, Sasso FC, Cacciapuoti F, et al. Tight glycemic control may increase regenerative potential of myocardium during acute infarction. J Clin Endocrinol Metab. 2012; 97(3):933–942

Martin P, Leibovich SJ. Inflammatory cells during wound repair: the good, the bad and the ugly. Trends Cell Biol. 2005; 15(11):599–607

McCullough M, Carlson GW. Dakin's solution: historical perspective and current practice. Ann Plast Surg. 2014; 73(3):254–256

Midwood KS, Williams LV, Schwarzbauer JE. Tissue repair and the dynamics of the extracellular matrix. Int J Biochem Cell Biol. 2004; 36(6):1031–1037

Mills JL Sr, Conte MS, Armstrong DG, et al; Society for Vascular Surgery Lower Extremity Guidelines Committee. The Society for Vascular Surgery Lower Extremity Threatened Limb Classification System: risk stratification based on wound, ischemia, and foot infection (WIfI). J Vasc Surg. 2014; 59(1):220–34.e1, 2

Molnar JA, Vlad LG, Gumus T. Nutrition and chronic wounds: improving clinical outcomes. Plast Reconstr Surg. 2016; 138(3), Suppl:71S–81S

Monaco JL, Lawrence WT. Acute wound healing an overview. Clin Plast Surg. 2003; 30(1):1–12

Monstrey S, Middelkoop E, Vranckx JJ, et al. Updated scar management practical guidelines: non-invasive and invasive measures. J Plast Reconstr Aesthet Surg. 2014; 67(8):1017–1025

Morykwas MJ, Argenta LC, Shelton-Brown EI, McGuirt W. Vacuum-assisted closure: a new method for wound control and treatment: animal studies and basic foundation. Ann Plast Surg. 1997; 38(6):553–562

Negenborn VL, Groen J-W, Smit JM, Niessen FB, Mullender MG. The Use of Autologous Fat Grafting for Treatment of Scar Tissue and Scar-Related Conditions: A Systematic Review. Plast Reconstr Surg. 2016; 137(1):31e–43e

Neligan P, ed. Plastic Surgery. 3rd ed. London; New York: Elsevier Saunders; 2013

Norman G, Dumville JC, Mohapatra DP, Owens GL, Crosbie EJ. Antibiotics and antiseptics for surgical wounds healing by secondary intention. In: Cochrane Database of Systematic Reviews. John Wiley & Sons, Ltd; 2016. http://onlinelibrary.wiley.com.ezproxyhost.library.tmc.edu/doi/10.1002/14651858. CD011712.pub2/abstract. Accessed June 24, 2016

O'Brien L, Jones DJ. Silicone gel sheeting for preventing and treating hypertrophic and keloid scars. In: Cochrane Database of Systematic Reviews. John Wiley & Sons, Ltd; 2013. http://onlinelibrary.wiley.com.ezproxyhost.library.tmc.edu/doi/10.1002/14651858.CD003826.pub3/abstract. Accessed July 9, 2016

O'Sullivan ST, O'Shaughnessy M, O'Connor TP. Aetiology and management of hypertrophic scars and keloids. Ann R Coll Surg Engl. 1996; 78(3 (Pt 1)):168–175

Olascoaga A, Vilar-Compte D, Poitevin-Chacón A, Contreras-Ruiz J. Wound healing in radiated skin: pathophysiology and treatment options. Int Wound J. 2008; 5(2):246–257

Oryan A, Mohammadalipour A, Moshiri A, Tabandeh MR. Topical Application of Aloe vera Accelerated Wound Healing, Modeling, and Remodeling: An Experimental Study. Ann Plast Surg. 2016; 77(1):37–46

Peters T, Sindrilaru A, Hinz B, et al. Wound-healing defect of CD18(-/-) mice due to a decrease in TGF-beta1 and myofibroblast differentiation. EMBO J. 2005; 24(19):3400–3410

Pietramaggiori G, Liu P, Scherer SS, et al. Tensile forces stimulate vascular remodeling and epidermal cell proliferation in living skin. Ann Surg. 2007; 246(5):896–902

Pilcher BK, Dumin JA, Sudbeck BD, Krane SM, Welgus HG, Parks WC. The activity of collagenase-1 is required for keratinocyte migration on a type I collagen matrix. J Cell Biol. 1997; 137(6):1445–1457

Poormasjedi-Meibod M-S, Hartwell R, Kilani RT, Ghahary A. Anti-scarring properties of different tryptophan derivatives. PLoS One. 2014; 9(3):e91955

Qiu SS, Dotor J, Hontanilla B. Effect of P144® (Anti-TGF-ß) in an "In Vivo" Human Hypertrophic Scar Model in Nude Mice. PLoS One. 2015; 10(12):e0144489

Raffetto JD. Pathophysiology of wound healing and alterations in venous leg ulcers-review. Phlebology. 2016; 31(1), Suppl:56–62

Raja SK, Sivamani K, Garcia MS, Isseroff RR. Wound re-epithelialization: modulating keratinocyte migration in wound healing. Front Biosci. 2007; 12:2849–2868

Ramos M, Khalpey Z, Lipsitz S, et al. Relationship of perioperative hyperglycemia and postoperative infections in patients who undergo general and vascular surgery. Ann Surg. 2008; 248(4):585–591

Reddy M. Skin and wound care: important considerations in the older adult. Adv Skin Wound Care. 2008; 21(9):424–436, quiz 437–438

Rinker B. The evils of nicotine: an evidence-based guide to smoking and plastic surgery. Ann Plast Surg. 2013; 70(5):599–605

Roeckl-Wiedmann I, Bennett M, Kranke P. Systematic review of hyperbaric oxygen in the management of chronic wounds. Br J Surg. 2005; 92(1):24–32

Rohde C, Chiang A, Adipoju O, Casper D, Pilla AA. Effects of pulsed electromagnetic fields on interleukin-1 beta and postoperative pain: a double-blind, placebo-controlled, pilot study in breast reduction patients. Plast Reconstr Surg. 2010; 125(6):1620–1629

Römling U, Balsalobre C. Biofilm infections, their resilience to therapy and innovative treatment strategies. J Intern Med. 2012; 272(6):541–561

Sahni A, Odrljin T, Francis CW. Binding of basic fibroblast growth factor to fibrinogen and fibrin. J Biol Chem. 1998; 273(13):7554–7559

Santiago B, Gutierrez-Cañas I, Dotor J, et al. Topical application of a peptide inhibitor of transforming growth factor-beta1 ameliorates bleomycin-induced skin fibrosis. J Invest Dermatol. 2005; 125(3):450–455

Sarin CL, Austin JC, Nickel WO. Effects of smoking on digital blood-flow velocity. JAMA. 1974; 229(10):1327–1328

Sen CK, Roy S. Oxygenation state as a driver of myofibroblast differentiation and wound contraction: hypoxia impairs wound closure. J Invest Dermatol. 2010; 130(12):2701–2703

Serghiou M, Cowan A, Whitehead C. Rehabilitation after a burn injury. Clin Plast Surg 2009; 36(4):675–686

Seth AK, Geringer MR, Nguyen KT, et al. Bacteriophage therapy for Staphylococcus aureus biofilm-infected wounds: a new approach to chronic wound care. Plast Reconstr Surg. 2013; 131(2):225–234

Shermak MA, Chang D, Buretta K, Mithani S, Mallalieu J, Manahan M. Increasing age impairs outcomes in breast reduction surgery. Plast Reconstr Surg. 2011; 128(6):1182–1187

Shi H-X, Lin C, Lin B-B, et al. The anti-scar effects of basic fibroblast growth factor on the wound repair in vitro and in vivo. PLoS One 2013; 8(4):e59966

Shih R, Waltzman J, Evans GRD; Plastic Surgery Educational Foundation Technology Assessment Committee. Review of over-the-counter topical scar treatment products. Plast Reconstr Surg. 2007; 119(3):1091–1095

Simpson DM, Ross R. The neutrophilic leukocyte in wound repair a study with antineutrophil serum. J Clin Invest. 1972; 51(8):2009–2023

Sinno H, Malhotra M, Lutfy J, et al. Accelerated wound healing with topical application of complement C5. Plast Reconstr Surg. 2012; 130(3):523–529

Sorice S, Rustad KC, Li AY, Gurtner GC. The Role of Stem Cell Therapeutics in Wound Healing: Current Understanding and Future Directions. Plast Reconstr Surg. 2016; 138(3), Suppl:31S–41S

Straub JM, New J, Hamilton CD, Lominska C, Shnayder Y, Thomas SM. Radiation-induced fibrosis: mechanisms and implications for therapy. J Cancer Res Clin Oncol. 2015; 141(11):1985–1994

Uzun H, Bitik O, Hekimoglu R, Atilla P, Kayikçioglu AU. Angiotensin-converting enzyme inhibitor enalapril reduces formation of hypertrophic scars in a rabbit ear wounding model. Plast Reconstr Surg. 2013; 132(3):361e–371e

Vermeulen H, van Hattem JM, Storm-Versloot MN, Ubbink DT, Westerbos SJ. Topical silver for treating infected wounds. In: Cochrane Database of Systematic Reviews. John Wiley & Sons, Ltd; 2007. http://onlinelibrary.wiley.com.ezproxyhost.library.tmc.edu/doi/10.1002/14651858.CD005486.pub2/abstract. Accessed July 9, 2016

Wittenberg GP, Fabian BG, Bogomilsky JL, et al. Prospective, single-blind, randomized, controlled study to assess the efficacy of the 585-nm flashlamp-pumped pulsed-dye laser and silicone gel sheeting in hypertrophic scar treatment. Arch Dermatol. 1999; 135(9):1049–1055

Wolcott R, Dowd S. The role of biofilms: are we hitting the right target? Plast Reconstr Surg. 2011; 127 Suppl 1:28S–35S

Wong VW, Martindale RG, Longaker MT, Gurtner GC. From germ theory to germ therapy: skin microbiota, chronic wounds, and probiotics. Plast Reconstr Surg. 2013; 132(5):854e–861e

Wu L, Norman G, Dumville JC, O'Meara S, Bell-Syer SE. Dressings for treating foot ulcers in people with diabetes: an overview of systematic reviews. In: Cochrane Database of Systematic Reviews. John Wiley & Sons, Ltd; 2015. http://onlinelibrary.wiley.com.ezproxyhost.library.tmc.edu/doi/10.1002/14651858.CD010471.pub2/abstract. Accessed July 9, 2016

Xiao Z, Zhang F, Lin W, Zhang M, Liu Y. Effect of botulinum toxin type A on transforming growth factor beta1 in fibroblasts derived from hypertrophic scar: a preliminary report. Aesthetic Plast Surg. 2010; 34(4):424–427

Xie J, Qi S, Yuan J, et al. Effects of antisense oligodeoxynucleotide to type I collagen gene on hypertrophic scars in the transplanted nude mouse model. J Cutan Pathol. 2009; 36(11):1146–1150

Yuan J, Li T, Qi S. [Effect of Col I A1 antisense oligodeoxynucleotide on collagen synthesis in human hypertrophic scar transplanted nude mouse model] Zhongguo Xiu Fu Chong Jian Wai Ke Za Zhi. 2011; 25(6):718–723

Zhang Z, Garron TM, Li X-J, et al. Recombinant human decorin inhibits TGF-beta1-induced contraction of collagen lattice by hypertrophic scar fibroblasts. Burns. 2009; 35(4):527–537

Zunwen L, Shizhen Z, Dewu L, Yungui M, Pu N. Effect of tetrandrine on the TGF-ß-induced smad signal transduction pathway in human hypertrophic scar fibroblasts in vitro. Burns. 2012; 38(3):404–413

3 Wound Management and Pressure Sores

Ricardo Roa, Cristián Taladriz, Daniel Calderón, Wilfredo Calderón

Abstract

This chapter focuses on wound dressings and skin substitutes, their history, evolution, and current indications. It provides summarized information about the basic science of wounds and their physiopathology. It is important to know how to treat wounds according to their stage of evolution. It is also important to know the different types of wound dressings to ensure proper treatment. The chapter describes wound management and the management of pressure sores. The latter are caused by multiple factors, all of which need to be addressed and corrected to achieve healing. Surgical treatment is reserved for ulcers in advanced stages and should be performed only after all factors have been addressed.

Keywords: chronic wounds, dermal substitutes, pressure sores, wound dressings, wound management

3.1 Introduction

Complex wounds can be defined as lesions that do not heal after at least 3 months of proper treatment. These types of wounds usually carry a significant financial burden for every health care system, with some reports predicting that the global wound care market will reach more than US$22 billion annually by 2020. According to Gottrup (2004) at least 1% of the population of developed countries will have a complex wound during their lifetime. In North America alone more than 6.5 million people have a type of complex wound, and this number increases annually. In addition, complex wounds are a major health care problem, not only from an economical standpoint but also because of their significant impact on patients' quality of life. Therefore it is important to find cost-effective treatments that allow us to improve our results without overly increasing costs.

Complex wounds can be divided into three categories:

1. Wounds resulting from a chronic disease (diabetes, venous ulcers)
2. Pressure ulcers
3. Nonhealing surgical wounds

The treatment of complex wounds must be targeted according to the type of wound. For example, management of complex wounds associated with chronic diseases usually involves treating the underlying condition. On the other hand, patients with pressure ulcers associated with neurological or mobility disability require special care before any improvement can be expected. Finally, nonhealing surgical wounds need other considerations, such as immune response or previous antibiotic treatments.

3.2 Basic Science

3.2.1 Physiopathology of Chronic Wounds

As we have already mentioned, chronic wounds are associated with increased health care costs that affect millions of patients every year worldwide.

Chronic wounds are difficult to study because they do not occur in animals, so most studies involve humans, which unfortunately leaves inevitable gaps in understanding the etiology and pathogenesis of chronic wounds.

The hypothesis is that chronic wounds do not have a single causative factor but rather represent a combination of factors that affect the healing process, including the following:

1. **Hypoxia** Local tissue hypoxia impairs healing. Levels of partial oxygen pressure < 30 mm Hg are related to an 80% reduction in wound-healing rate at 7 days. However, many chronic wounds develop without any measurable ischemia.
2. **Edema** Edema is another factor that hinders wound healing by increasing the distance between cells and capillaries, which in turn affects the distance for oxygen diffusion, resulting in cellular hypoxia. Although the magnitude of this factor is unclear, chronic venous ulcers in edematous limbs improve following standard management involving the use of compression garments.
3. **Bioburden** The presence of bacteria is also related to impaired wound healing. Within 48 hours, an open wound becomes contaminated by bacteria from the surrounding skin.

Depending on the presence of bacteria and the host's reaction, wounds are usually described as *contaminated*, when microorganisms have reached the wound but are not expanding; *colonized*, when there is active replication of bacteria but no clinically evident host response; and *infected*, when bacteria proliferation is accompanied by clinical signs of infection, with or without systemic manifestations. Clinically, it is not possible to distinguish between contaminated and colonized wounds. According to Robson, bacterial levels > 100,000/g of tissue are associated with skin graft failure. Biofilm also promotes chronic wound perpetuation by reducing the way the host can interact with bacteria.

4. **Chronic inflammation and local environment** Some authors have demonstrated major differences between acute and chronic wounds. The latter have increased protease and proinflammatory levels and reduced growth factor levels. Acute wounds normally heal in a sequenced and timely manner, characterized by four major phases (hemostasis, inflammation, proliferation, and remodeling). On the contrary, chronic wounds remain in one particular stage of healing (usually the inflammation phase). This alters the balance between deposition and degradation of extracellular matrix components. The degradation and remodeling of extracellular matrix by proteases, particularly by matrix metalloproteinases (MMPs), is a key element of tissue repair and plays a role in various wound-healing mechanisms.

5. **Ischemia–reperfusion injury** Cycles of ischemia and reperfusion have recently been associated with chronic wound pathogenesis. Although at the molecular level, ischemia–reperfusion is equivalent to that in other organs, the main difference in chronic wounds is that it occurs in a repetitive fashion, with the degree of injury increasing with each cycle. This mechanism can be seen in pressure ulcers in patients with paraplegia, in whom postural changes, despite being a well-intentioned preventive measure, produce cycles of ischemia and reperfusion in the wound, which may have detrimental clinical effects.

6. **Aging and impaired stress response** Most chronic wounds occur in elderly patients, usually over the age of 60. Aging cells have an impaired response to stress. Aged human fibroblasts fail to proliferate under hypoxic conditions. This limited ability to respond to stress in aged patients contributes a great deal to the impaired healing response.

7. **Nutrition** According to a Cochrane systematic review there is currently no clear evidence that nutritional interventions reduce the development of pressure ulcers. However, another recently published systematic review and meta-analysis of nutritional supplementation in chronic lower-extremity wounds shows that nutritional supplementation in populations who are receiving health care and who are malnourished or at risk of malnutrition show benefits in the healing of chronic lower-extremity venous, diabetic, and sickle cell ulcers. In any case, good nutritional support is an important pillar in wound management, aiming for enteral nutrition whenever possible and normal values of albumin (e.g., > 3.5 g/dL). In some cases, because albumin's half-life is 20 days and has a large serum pool, it may be a late indicator of malnutrition, in which case prealbumin, which has a half-life of 48 hours, is a better parameter.

3.3 Wound Assessment

Proper wound assessment prior to the implementation of any therapy is important, not only to decide on the best available treatment but also to facilitate communication among wound care personnel. Some definitions are as follows:

1. Wound bed
   a) *Granulation* This is a healthy red tissue, formed by collagen, elastin, and capillary networks. It is usually well vascularized and can bleed very easily.
   b) *Epithelializing* Once the granulation process is complete, a new epithelium will grow on top of healthy granulation tissue and cover the wound surface.
   c) *Slough* This is a yellowish, devitalized tissue. It is not pus; it is formed by an accumulation of dead cells.
   d) *Necrotic tissue* This is dead tissue, which is usually seen as a dark, hard, dry plaque. It prevents the wound from healing properly.
   e) *Hypergranulation* This is seen when granulation tissue grows above the wound margins and is associated with an extended proliferative phase.

2. Wound measurements

Every wound must be measured so that the healing rate can be evaluated. Flat lesions are usually measured in two dimensions (e.g., length and width in millimeters), whereas wounds with a cavity also need to include depth as a measurement.

3. Wound edges

a) Healthy wound edges are usually seen as a pink epithelium growing over healthy granulation tissue.

b) Erythema surrounding the wound can be associated with an inflammatory response or cellulitis.

c) Raised edges may indicate pressure, trauma, or malignant changes.

d) Rolled edges indicate chronicity or stagnation.

4. Exudate

Exudate is fluid produced by all acute and chronic wounds and is part of the natural healing process. It contains nutrients and growth factors as well as high levels of white blood cells. Exudate aids wound healing by cleansing the wound, promoting epithelialization, and maintaining a moist environment.

Excessive exudate can lead to skin maceration, whereas too little can result in a dry wound bed. It is important to differentiate between different types of exudate because it can indicate an infection. An exudate can be serous, hemoserous, sanguinous, or purulent.

5. Infection

Described as the presence of bacteria or other microorganisms in the wound accompanied by a response from the host. Local clinical indicators of wound infection include pain, swelling, erythema, increased temperature, malodor, purulent drainage, and a delayed or abnormal healing process. Systemic signs comprise fever, general malaise, lymphangitis, and elevated C-reactive protein and white blood cell count. If any of these indicators is present, then a culture biopsy, wound swab, or both should be done.

3.4 Wound Debridement

Once a correct assessment of the wound has been made, the wound bed can be prepared.

There are four basic components to wound preparation:

1. Tissue debridement
2. Inflammation and infection control
3. Moisture balance (optimal dressing selection)
4. Epithelial edge advancement

3.4.1 Tissue Debridement

There are different methods of wound debridement, including surgical (sharp), biosurgical (maggots), autolytic, hydrosurgical, and ultrasonic.

Usually considered the gold standard method of debridement, sharp debridement allows complete removal of devitalized tissue and necrotic plaques as well as drainage of collections and alleviation of pressure, all of which eventually maximize the effectiveness of topical preparations (▶ Fig. 3.1). It is an invasive procedure and should be performed only by trained physicians.

The use of larvae (biosurgical debridement) is a safe and effective debridement technique. Its ease allows it to be performed by any practitioner, with good results in a relatively rapid and atraumatic way. Some reviews suggest that the use of larvae may improve outcomes when compared to autolytic debridement with hydrogel.

Hydrosurgical debridement is another type of wound debridement that uses water to create a high-energy cutting beam, allowing visualization and removal of devitalized tissue in the wound bed.

Autolytic debridement uses a moist wound dressing to soften and remove devitalized tissue. It is painless, selective, and very comfortable for the patient. However, care must be taken to avoid maceration of the surrounding skin. Autolytic debridement is not recommended in the presence of infection, ischemia, or dry gangrene.

Enzymatic debridement is a topical treatment that uses naturally occurring proteolytic enzymes or proteinases, which are critical to the wound repair process. Proteinase activity in chronic wounds is useful not only for the purpose of debridement but also for more fundamental aspects of cell migration necessary for epithelialization. The two most commonly enzymatic agents used for chronic wounds are papain–urea combinations in a cream base and collagenase in a petrolatum base.

Ultrasonic debridement delivers low-frequency ultrasound waves via a saline solution either by contact or noncontact means. This method is selective and immediate. Although the initial equipment cost is high, cost per treatment is lower

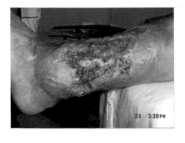
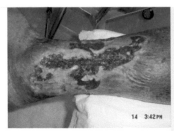
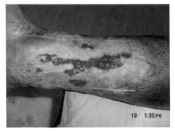
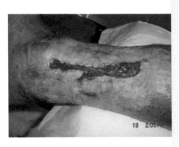
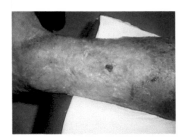
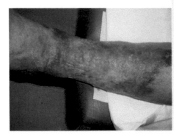

Fig. 3.1 Healing process of a venous ulcer.

than that of surgical and hydrosurgical debridement. This method, however, is not suitable for all wound types.

3.4.2 Infection Control

Infections are associated with increased rates of morbidity and mortality and should therefore be treated early and aggressively. Although there is no indication for systemic antibacterial therapy in clinically uninfected wounds, virtually all those infected will require antibiotics. In the presence of mild infections in patients without previous antibiotic therapy, swabs or tissue biopsies should be obtained to determine flora and antimicrobial resistance that will guide optimal therapy. In the meantime, empirical oral treatment should be started targeting *Staphylococcus aureus* and β-hemolytic streptococcus.

Topical antimicrobials do not drive any resistance. They provide high local concentrations but do not penetrate deeper soft tissue or intact skin, which makes them useful for patients with poor vascular supply or in cases of nonhealing wounds without signs of infection but with suspicion of increased bacterial bioburden.

In cases of deep tissue infection, intravenous broad-spectrum antibiotics should be initiated promptly. Tissue and/or exudate samples must be obtained to identify specific microorganisms in the wound and adjust antibiotic treatment according to antibiogram. Antibiotic therapy should be continued until resolution of infection, with optimal duration depending on the severity of infection and response to treatment.

Biofilm is a matrix produced by bacteria, which acts as a protective barrier that reduces antimicrobial action. Repeated debridement and wound cleansing disrupt the biofilm, whereas antimicrobial dressings prevent its reformation and attachment.

3.4.3 Moisture Balance: Optimal Dressing Selection

Dressings are usually designed to create a moist environment to support wound healing but are not substitutes for debridement or infection control. Dressings that can help to manage wound exudate optimally and promote a balanced environment are key to improving outcomes. There is a great range of dressings available, with no single one specifically designed for any type of wound; therefore health care professionals should use the one that best applies to the clinical appearance and site of the wound.

Factors to consider when choosing a wound dressing are location and extent of the wound, amount and type of exudate, type of tissue on the wound surface, condition of the surrounding skin, risk of infection, and pain and trauma at dressing changes.

▶Table 3.1 and ▶Table 3.2 provide a summary of the type of recommended dressings and wound management.

Table 3.1 Types of wound dressings available

Type	Actions/advantages	Indications/use	Precautions/contraindications
Alginates/CMC*	Absorb fluid Promote autolytic debridement Moisture control Adapt well to wound bed	Moderate- to high-exuding wounds Special rope or ribbon presentations for wounds with cavities Combined presentation with silver for antimicrobial activity	Do not use on dry/necrotic wounds Use with caution on friable tissue (may cause bleeding) Do not pack cavity wounds tightly
Foams	Absorb fluid Moisture control Adapt well to wound bed	Moderate- to high-exuding wounds Special rope or ribbon presentations for wounds with cavities Low-adherent versions available for patients with fragile skin Combined presentation with silver or polyhexamethylene biguanide (PHMB) for antimicrobial activity	Do not use on dry/necrotic wounds or those with minimal exudate
Honey	Rehydrate wound bed Promote autolytic debridement Antimicrobial action	Sloughy wounds with low to moderate exudate Critically colonized or infected wounds	May cause "drawing" pain (osmotic effect) Known sensitivity
Hydrocolloids	Absorb fluid Promote autolytic debridement	Clean wounds with low to moderate exudate Combined presentation with silver for antimicrobial activity	Do not use on dry/necrotic wounds or high-exuding wounds May encourage overgranulation May cause maceration
Hydrogels	Rehydrate wound bed Moisture control Promote autolytic debridement Cooling	Dry wounds or those with low to moderate exudate Combined presentation with silver for antimicrobial activity	Do not use on highly exuding wounds or where anaerobic infection is suspected May cause maceration
Iodine	Antimicrobial action	Critically colonized or infected wounds Wounds with low to high exudate	Do not use on dry necrotic tissue Known sensitivity to iodine Short-term use recommended (risk of systemic absorption)
Low-adherent wound contact layer (silicone)	Protect new tissue growth Atraumatic to periwound skin Adapts well to anatomical contours	Wounds with low to high exudate Used as contact layer on superficial wounds with low exudate	May dry out if left in place for too long Known sensitivity to silicone

(Continued)

Table 3.1 *(Continued)* Types of wound dressings available

Type	Actions/advantages	Indications/use	Precautions/contraindications
PHMB	Antimicrobial actions	Wounds with low to high exudate Critically colonized or infected wounds May require secondary dressing	Do not use on dry/necrotic wounds Known sensitivity
Odor control (activated charcoal)	Odor absorption	Malodorous wounds (due to excess exudate) May require antimicrobial if due to increased bioburden	Do not use on dry wounds
Protease modulating	Active or passive control of wound's protease levels	Clean wounds that are not progressing despite correction of underlying causes, exclusion of infection, and optimal wound care	Do not use on dry wounds or those with leathery eschar
Silver	Antimicrobial action	Critically colonized or infected wounds Wounds with low to high exudate Combined presentation with foam and alginates/CMC for increased absorbance Also in paste form	Some may cause discoloration Known sensitivity Discontinue after 2 weeks if no improvement and reevaluate
Polyurethane film	Moisture control Breathable bacterial barrier Transparent	Primary dressing over superficial low-exuding wounds Secondary dressing over alginate or hydrogel for rehydration of wound bed	Do not use on patients with fragile/ compromised periwound skin Do not use on moderate- to high-exuding wounds

* Wound dressings may contain alginates or CMC only; alginates may also be combined with CMC.
Abbreviation: CMC, carboxymethyl cellulose.
Source: Data from International Best Practice Guidelines: Wound Management in Diabetic Foot Ulcers. London: Wounds International; 2013.

Table 3.2 Wound management

Type of tissue in the wound	Therapeutic goal	Role of dressing	Treatment options		
			Wound bed preparation	Primary dressing	Secondary dressing
Necrotic, black, dry	Remove devitalized tissue Do not attempt debridement if vascular insufficiency suspected Keep dry and refer for vascular assessment	Hydration of wound bed Promote autolytic debridement	Surgical or mechanical debridement	Hydrogel Honey	Polyurethane film dressing

Table 3.2 *(Continued)* Wound management

Type of tissue in the wound	Therapeutic goal	Role of dressing	Treatment options		
Sloughy, yellow, brown, black, or gray Dry to low exudate	Remove slough Provide clean wound bed for granulation tissue	Rehydrate wound bed Control moisture balance Promote autolytic debridement	Surgical or mechanical debridement If appropriate Wound cleansing (consider antiseptic wound cleansing solution)	Hydrogel Honey	Polyurethane film dressing Low adherent (silicone) dressing
Sloughy, yellow, brown, black, or gray Moderate to high exudate	Remove slough Provide clean wound bed for granulation tissue Exudate management	Absorb excess fluid Protect periwound skin to prevent maceration Promote autolytic debridement	Surgical or mechanical debridement if appropriate Wound cleansing (consider antiseptic wound cleansing solution) Consider barrier products	Absorbent dressing (alginate/CMC/foam) For deep wounds, use cavity strips, rope, or ribbon versions	Retention bandage or polyurethane film dressing
Granulating, clean, red Dry to low exudate	Promote granulation Provide healthy wound bed for epithelialization	Maintain moisture balance Protect new tissue growth	Wound cleansing	Hydrogel Low-adherent (silicone) dressing For deep wounds use cavity strips, rope, or ribbon versions	Pad and/ or retention bandage Avoid bandages that may cause occlusion and maceration Tapes should be used with caution due to allergy potential and secondary complications
Granulating, clean, red Moderate to high exudate	Exudate management Provide healthy wound bed for epithelialization	Maintain moisture balance Protect new tissue growth	Wound cleansing Consider barrier products	Absorbent dressing (alginate/CMC/foam) Low adherent (silicone) dressing For deep wounds, use cavity strips, rope, or ribbon versions	
Epithelializing, red, pink No to low exudate	Promote epithelialization and wound maturation (contraction)	Protect new tissue growth	Hydrocolloid (thin) Polyurethane film dressing Low-adherent (silicone) dressing		
Infected Low to high exudate	Reduce bacterial load Exudate management Odor control	Antimicrobial action Moist wound healing Odor absorption	Wound cleansing (consider antiseptic wound cleansing solution) Consider barrier products	Antimicrobial dressing	

Source: Data from International Best Practice Guidelines: Wound Management in Diabetic Foot Ulcers. London: Wounds International; 2013.

3.5 Skin Substitutes

It is known that skin substitutes have been used for a long time. According to historical reviews, skin grafts were used to treat mutilated extremities in India as early as 2500 BC. In 1874, Karl Thiersch reported for the first time the use of partial-thickness skin grafts, which allowed the development of the first commercially available dermatomes. Prior to World War II the use of allografts became popularized by Brown and McDowell, who used skin from fresh cadavers to cover and stabilize acute wounds. Unfortunately they were unable to maintain the viability of these grafts for more than 3 to 4 weeks. The first skin bank was created in 1949, setting the stage for the birth and evolution of skin substitutes.

The main objective of treatment of skin injuries is to achieve early cover of the lesion. This allows the body to generate a functional and stable barrier that will evolve into a scar, followed by an aesthetically pleasing unit. Usually the first option for cover is the autologous graft, which offers rapid, permanent, and satisfactory results. However, in some situations it is not possible to do a partial-thickness skin graft, or the chances of failure are too high, especially in cases of an inappropriate wound bed or severe infection. The use of temporary substitutes will improve viability of the wound, reduce the risk of infection, and minimize pain and metabolic stress.

The depth of the wound will indicate the type of skin substitute to use. Temporary skin substitutes can be employed to treat superficial and intermediate burns. Deep burns will probably require autologous grafts.

Although great effort has gone into the development of skin substitutes, to date nothing exists that completely replaces native skin. Sheridan and Tompkins in 1999 proposed a list of characteristics of the ideal skin substitute, such as low antigenicity, durability, affordable price, and easy handling (▶Table 3.3).

Benefits of skin substitutes include reducing fluid loss from evaporation, ameliorating pain, and decreasing metabolic stress.

Table 3.3 The ideal skin substitute

Characteristics of the ideal skin substitute
Cost-effective
Easy handling
Long lasting
Low antigenicity
Durable
Flexible
Avoid loss of water
Protective barrier/reduced pain
Adaptable to irregular surfaces
Easy fixation
Grows with the patient
Applicable in one surgery
No hypertrophy

Source: Adapted from Sheridan RL, Tompkins RG. Skin substitutes in burns. Burns 1999;25(2):97–103.

3.5.1 Surgical Technique

There must be a differentiation between chronic and acute patients for surgical technique.

Acute wounds require a clean and healthy wound bed, without devitalized tissue, free of infection, and ideally noncontaminated. This can be confirmed by negative cultures. Before starting, antibiotic prophylaxis is administered according to institutional protocols. A surgical cleansing is performed, and the skin substitute applied to the wound, which is then dressed with moisturized gauze or a negative pressure system. Dressing changes will depend on the characteristics of the skin substitute employed and the institution's protocol.

For chronic wounds in cases of contractured or unstable scars, it is important that, prior to applying a dermal substitute, all fibrous tissue is removed and a healthy, well-vascularized bed is generated. When used for coverage of chronic ulcers, negative cultures are mandatory before application of any dermal substitute to reduce the chances of failure due to local infection.

3.5.2 Synthetic Bioengineered Dermal Substitutes

The main objective of dermal substitutes is to provide cover to the wound while a functional barrier is formed that will be the base of a future scar. Technological advances have allowed the development of multiple skin substitutes of different origins (▶Table 3.4). There is a wide range of skin cover products and there are many ways of classifying them, according to their origins or indications of use.

Acellular Dermal Substitutes

Bilayer Dermal Substitutes

These substitutes are composed of a porous matrix that contains collagen, hyaluronic acid, fibronectin, and other extracellular matrix proteins, covered by a thin silicone layer that helps protect the wound from fluid evaporation and infection.

Biobrane

Biobrane (Smith & Nephew) is a bilayer dermal substitute that was approved by the U.S. Food and Drug Administration (FDA) in 1979. It is composed of a nylon mesh to which porcine type I collagen is added in a covalent manner to improve the product's adherence. On top of this nylon layer lies a silicone sheet that reduces loss of evaporation and at the same time acts as an epidermic layer. Biobrane's transparency permits continuous evaluation of the wound bed, while its elasticity allows a good range of movement. It must be applied to clean, noninfected wounds that are free of nonviable tissue. Hematomas developing under Biobrane must be drained due to their risk of becoming infected. Additionally, any zones not adhered to the wound bed must be removed. To ensure good

Table 3.4 Bioengineered skin substitutes

Tissue of origin	Product	Structure
Xenograft	Permacol (Medtronic)	Porcine dermis
	EZ Derm (Mölnlycke Health Care)	Porcine dermis + collagen
	Matriderm (Ideal Medical Solutions)	Bovine collagen covered with elastin
	Oasis (Cook Biotech)	Porcine intestinal submucosa
Synthetic	Biobrane (Smith & Nephew)	Bilayer of silicone mesh and nylon + porcine collagen
	Integra (Integra LifeSciences)	Bilayer of silicone and bovine collagen + chondroitin 6-sulfate
	Advanced Wounds Bioengineered Alternative Tissue (AWBAT)	Porous bilayer of nylon and silicone + porcine collagen
	Hyalomatrix (Medline Industries)	Bilayer of silicone and esterified hyaluronan
Allogenic		
Acellular	Cadaveric	Fresh allogeneic processed dermis
	Alloderm (Biohorizons)	Allogeneic processed dermis
	GraftJacket (Wright Medical Group)	Frozen decellularized allogeneic dermis
	GammaGraft (Promethean Life Sciences)	Gamma-irradiated allogeneic dermis
Epidermis	Stratagraft (Stratatech Corp.)	Allogeneic dermis + stratified keratinocytes
Dermis	Dermagraft (Organogenesis)	Bioabsorbable polyglactin mesh + neonatal fibroblast
	TransCyte (BioCentury)	Silicone bilayer + nylon/collagen with neonatal fibroblasts
	ICX-SKN (BioCentury)	Allogeneic extracellular matrix + fibroblasts
Composed	Apligraf (Organogenesis)	Neonatal keratinocytes + collagen matrix with neonatal fibroblasts
	OrCel (Ortec International Inc.)	Neonatal keratinocytes + bovine collagen with neonatal fibroblasts

Source: Adapted from Markéta Límová. Active Wound Coverings: Bioengineered Skin and Dermal Substitutes. Surg Clin N Am 2010;(90):1237–1255.

adherence, Biobrane is covered with compressive gauze for 24–48 hours. Finally, the shift from the transparent to an opaque appearance indicates reepithelialization of the skin and means the substitute can be removed.

Integra

Integra (Integra LifeSciences) is a bilayer matrix which creates a mesh that allows dermal regeneration and temporary wound cover. It is formed by an internal layer of known porosity and degradation rate composed of bovine collagen fibers cross-linked with chondroitin 6-sulfate. The external layer is made of a synthetic polymer that retains humidity and at the same time protects the wound against infections. During the healing process, the collagen matrix is infiltrated by fibroblasts and other cells to eventually disappear and become completely replaced by the host's tissue, forming a neodermis. After 2–3 weeks, the silicone layer is removed, and a partial-thickness skin graft is placed. Integra is usually employed for partial- or full-thickness wounds or burns. Among its uses are retracted scars, extensive acute burns, and chronic ulcers. The main advantage of Integra is that it provides dermal regeneration with good aesthetic and functional results, similar to native skin (▶Fig. 3.2). The main disadvantage of dual-layer Integra is that it requires two surgeries: one to place it and another one 3 weeks after for skin grafting. However, this shortcoming can be avoided by using single-layer

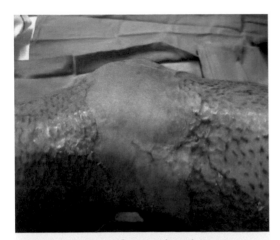

Fig. 3.2 Comparison of scar results with Integra + split-thickness skin graft in the center versus meshed split-thickness skin graft on the sides.

Integra. Another disadvantage is that it does not tolerate any infections or bleeding of the wound bed.

Hyalomatrix

Hyalomatrix (Anika Therapeutics) is a bilayer dermal substitute composed of hyaluronic acid and a semipermeable silicone membrane that controls evaporation and at the same time provides a flexible and resistant wound cover. It can be used in partial- or full-thickness skin wounds. Its biodegradable matrix acts as a base for cellular growth and development of new capillaries.

EZ Derm

EZ Derm (Mölnlycke Health Care) consists of a porcine dermal patch that has been shown to be useful in partial-thickness burns, allowing reduced hospitalization times. Porcine skin does not support capillary growth and dehydrates when exposed. This generates a less elastic cover, which limits the range of motion during cicatrization and the healing process. However, it provides good epidermal protection that favors epithelialization and management of pain. Importantly, patients with certain religious beliefs do have some issues with using porcine products. EZ Derm can also be employed as a transitory skin substitute.

3.6 Clinical Applications

Wound dressings are part of the everyday practice of every plastic surgeon. As said earlier, selection of a particular dressing will depend on a number of factors, including wound characteristics and institutions' infrastructure. In this sense, it is impossible to illustrate the clinical use of each dressing in a single chapter; thus the focus here is on the use of dermal substitutes, which currently have an important role in reconstructive surgery.

3.6.1 Case 1

A 28-year-old active, working man presented with a severe contracture of his right axilla following deep burns treated with early debridement and split-thickness skin grafting. On examination he had marked contracture of his right axillary scars, which limited his shoulder abduction to just above 90 degrees. He underwent debridement and release of his scars and application of Integra to cover the defect. Three weeks later, once the Integra had "taken" and become revascularized, the second stage was performed, which consisted of removal of the silicone layer and coverage with a split-thickness skin graft. No complications were observed, and the patient recovered uneventfully. Six months after the surgery, the patient was able to fully abduct his arm (▶Fig. 3.3).

3.6.2 Case 2

A 32-year-old man suffered a deep second-degree burn on the dorsum of his left hand. After tangential excision, the wound was covered with Integra. Three weeks later, once the matrix had become revascularized, the silicone layer was removed and replaced with a split-thickness skin graft. The graft survived in its entirety, and a stable, pliable coverage was achieved (▶Fig. 3.4).

3.7 Pressure Sores

Pressure sores are soft tissue injuries resulting from prolonged pressure of skin over a bony prominence. A number of factors contribute to the development of a pressure sore, including reduced mobility, local inflammation, altered sensation, spasticity, shear, malnutrition, and poor hygiene. Patients at risk of developing pressure sores include bed- or wheelchair-bound patients, such as paraplegic or tetraplegic patients, nursing home residents, patients with altered sensation, and those with a long hospital stay.

It is estimated that approximately 10% of hospitalized patients develop a pressure sore, with prevalence rates ranging from 3.5 to 29.5% for acute and long-term care facilities. According to the National Pressure Ulcer Advisory Panel, in the United States 60,000 patients die each year as a result of a pressure sore. From an economic point of view, the costs of treatment of each individual patient with a

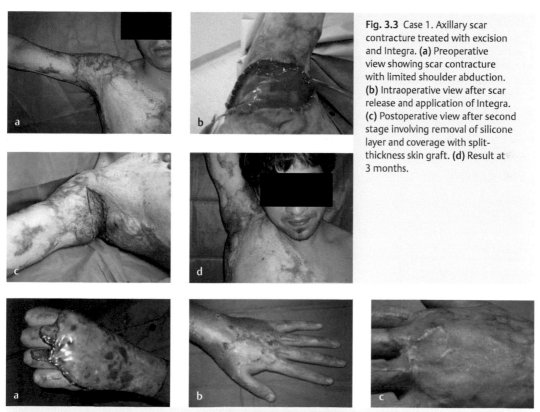

Fig. 3.3 Case 1. Axillary scar contracture treated with excision and Integra. (a) Preoperative view showing scar contracture with limited shoulder abduction. (b) Intraoperative view after scar release and application of Integra. (c) Postoperative view after second stage involving removal of silicone layer and coverage with split-thickness skin graft. (d) Result at 3 months.

Fig. 3.4 Case 2. Deep second-degree burn on the dorsum of the hand treated with tangential excision and Integra. (a) After tangential excision, the wound was covered with Integra. View prior to skin grafting. (b) Postoperative result at 1 month after second stage. (c) Postoperative result at 4 months showing stable cover.

pressure ulcer ranges from $US20,900 to $151,700 per ulcer.

3.8 Basic Science

The common underlying etiology for all pressure sores is pressure over a bony prominence. Compression results in ischemia, which, if prolonged, subsequently leads to necrosis and ulceration. In addition, other factors may contribute to the development, perpetuation, and aggravation of a pressure ulcer, all of which should be considered and addressed when managing a patient at risk or with an established ulcer.

3.8.1 Pressure

When external pressure exceeds the capillary pressure, blood flow is interrupted. Capillary pressure has been found to be 12 mm Hg on the venous side and 32 mm Hg on the arterial side; therefore, any pressure greater than the latter will produce ischemia. It is important to note that pressure does not distribute evenly within the lesion, with the highest values (and hence the greatest injury) seen on the deep tissues, and the skin wound being only the "tip of the iceberg." In addition, pressure is distributed unevenly throughout the body in the supine, prone, and sitting positions, with the sacrum and ischial tuberosities being the most affected areas in supine and seated positions,

respectively (▶ Fig. 3.5). Time is also an important factor when it comes to pressure loading; it has been demonstrated that pressure of 70 mm Hg for 2 hours or longer produces irreversible changes, whereas no injury develops if pressure is relieved for as little as 5 minutes, even with pressure over 400 mm Hg. Lastly, it is important to note that the greater the pressure applied, the less time needed to develop an ulcer.

3.8.2 Friction and Shear

Friction and shear can contribute to the development or worsening of a pressure ulcer in a susceptible patient. Although they are different phenomena, they usually occur in conjunction. *Shear* refers to forces acting in opposite directions over an area of skin, for example when a patient is seated up in bed and slides down but the skin does not slide (▶ Fig. 3.6). Shear is then dependent on the coefficient of friction between the surfaces and the degree of contact between them. When shear occurs, perforators to the skin are stretched or compressed, resulting in decreased blood flow. *Friction* results from the dragging of skin across a surface, for example, when a patient is mobilized in bed or the bed linens are pulled under him. While the insult resulting from shear occurs in the deep tissues, friction causes injury to the skin, usually in the form of an abrasion or superficial laceration.

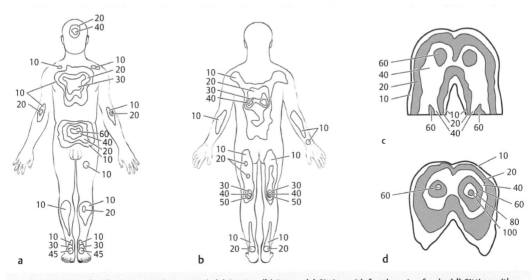

Fig. 3.5 Pressure-distribution maps (in mm Hg). **(a)** Supine. **(b)** Prone. **(c)** Sitting with feet hanging freely. **(d)** Sitting with feet supported. (Reproduced from Janis, Essentials of Plastic Surgery, 2nd edition, © 2014, Thieme Publishers, New York.)

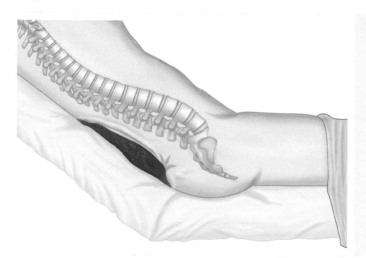

Fig. 3.6 Diagram showing shear phenomenon at the sacral area.

3.8.3 Local Conditions

Unfavorable local conditions can predispose to the development of an ulcer in a high-risk area of a susceptible patient. Extravasation of fluid to the interstitial space may hinder proper oxygen delivery and accentuate the ischemic insult of pressure. Likewise, healing of an established ulcer may be affected by edema of the surrounding tissues. Inflammation also contributes to the development and perpetuation of a pressure sore as these are often chronic wounds with low grade, long-term perilesional inflammation that reduces the healing capacity of the wound. Pressure sores are often chronic wounds with low-grade, long-term perilesional inflammation that reduces the healing capacity of the wound. Contamination is frequent in these types of wounds; therefore efforts must be taken to keep contamination a strict minimum. The skin should be cleaned from urine or fecal material and kept adequately hydrated, always avoiding maceration. In some cases a urine or rectal catheter or even a colostomy may be considered to minimize the risk of contamination and subsequent infection. Infected pressure sores need prompt treatment with a combination of broad-spectrum antibiotics, which should be narrowed once culture results are back, antiseptic dressings, and surgical debridement and washout depending on the extent of infection. Negative tissue cultures should be obtained before proceeding with reconstruction. Osteomyelitis is not infrequent and should be suspected in lesions with exposed bone. Magnetic resonance imaging is the most sensitive test to detect osteomyelitis, and a definitive diagnosis is made with bone biopsies (see Chapter 6). In cases of osteomyelitis, debridement down to healthy bleeding bone should be performed at the time of closure.

3.8.4 Spasticity

As mentioned earlier, neurologic patients are among the population at risk of developing pressure sores. Apart from the fact that these patients are bed or wheelchair bound, a unique feature that puts them at higher risk is spasticity, which is characterized by hyperreflexia, clonus, and increased muscle tone. Spasticity is common in patients with spinal cord injury and represents a risk factor because it causes shear and friction. In addition, spasticity increases mechanical stress, alters weight distribution, and complicates patient positioning, skin inspection, and hygiene. The higher the level of spinal injury, the greater the incidence of spasticity and therefore the risk of developing a pressure sore. Spasticity should therefore be addressed early in the process, prior to any surgical reconstruction of the wound. Medical therapy includes baclofen, diazepam, and dantrolene. Botulinum toxin injection is also an effective and safe strategy to treat spasticity. Patients who fail to respond to these therapies may benefit from more invasive procedures, such as peripheral nerve blocks, epidural stimulators, baclofen pumps, and rhizotomy.

3.8.5 Systemic Conditions

Medical comorbidities that affect wound healing should be addressed in patients with pressure sores. Smokers must be strongly encouraged to reduce, or better yet suspend, their habit. Diabetes should be well controlled and monitored with hemoglobin A1c, which should ideally be under 6%. Peripheral vascular disease may delay wound healing in patients with pressure sores of the heel or ankle; therefore, consultation with vascular specialists should be sought if needed. Nutrition plays a major role in both the development and the healing of pressure sores. Given the profile of patients at higher risk of developing pressure sores, they often present with varying degrees of malnutrition, which needs prompt correction. Protein intake should be 1.5–3 g/kg/d, aiming for an albumin of 3 g/dL or higher. However, because the half-life of albumin is 3 weeks, it is not a valuable marker to assess progress of nutritional status over short periods of time. Prealbumin instead has a half-life of 2 days, which makes it a good indicator of visceral protein status because it is affected earlier by acute variations in protein balance. Prealbumin levels should ideally be > 18 mg/dL. Carbohydrate intake should be approximately 25–35 kcal/kg/d and vitamin and iron supplements should be given as necessary. Consultation with a nutritional specialist is valuable in these cases.

3.9 Classification

Pressure sores are classified into four stages according to their depth (▶ Fig. 3.7).
- Stage 1: intact skin with nonblanchable erythema
- Stage 2: superficial ulcer involving the epidermis and partial thickness of the dermis, presenting as an abrasion, blister, or very shallow ulcer
- Stage 3: full-thickness skin ulceration down to the subcutaneous fat, without extending beyond the deep fascia
- Stage 4: full-thickness ulceration with involvement of muscle, bone, tendon, ligament, or joint capsule
- Unstageable: full-thickness skin or soft tissue loss in which depth is obscured by slough or eschar (after surgical debridement, these ulcers are commonly stage 3 or 4)

3.10 Treatment

Management of pressure sores involves a spectrum of measures and therapies, aimed first at correcting precipitating factors and second at promoting wound healing. When managing a patient at risk of ulcerating or with an established pressure sore, the importance of preventive measures cannot be overemphasized to either prevent the development of an ulcer or stop its progression. Relief

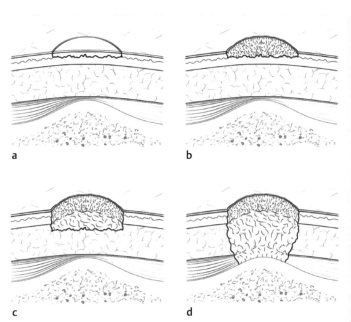

Fig. 3.7 Classification of pressure sores. **(a)** Stage 1. **(b)** Stage 2. **(c)** Stage 3. **(d)** Stage 4. (Reproduced from Janis, Essentials of Plastic Surgery, 2nd edition, © 2014, Thieme Publishers, New York.)

a

b

c

d

of pressure is a pillar and includes frequent postural changes (every 2 hours or less), and the use of adequate devices, such as air fluid mattresses, foams, and specialized wheelchair cushions. Donut cushions, once thought to be useful, may actually produce more harm because they relieve pressure over the area at risk but create a halo of pressure around it, which reduces blood flow; therefore, their use should be discouraged. Keeping the skin clean and well hydrated and avoiding maceration are important aspects as well. Any preexisting comorbidities and the patient's nutritional status should be optimized.

For established ulcers, treatment will depend on the characteristics of the wound and its stage. In general terms, stage 1 and 2 pressure sores should be treated conservatively with local wound care and relief of pressure, whereas patients with stage 3 and 4 lesions should be managed surgically.

3.10.1 Surgical Management

Even though the principles of surgical management of pressure sores follow those of every chronic wound, there are some aspects unique to these types of wounds that must be considered to optimize the outcome of surgical therapy in these patients. First, debridement of all devitalized, contaminated, and infected tissue and obtaining negative cultures are essential steps to convert a chronic wound into an acute clean one. Total excision of the ulcer's bursa is paramount. Applying diluted methylene blue to the wound just before resection is a useful aid to determine the extent of devitalized tissue. Removal of the underlying bony prominence, particularly in cases of osteomyelitis, is crucial to avoid recurrence; nevertheless, it should be done mindfully because too much resection may create an imbalance, with redistribution of pressure points to other areas. Following thorough hemostasis, dead

space should be obliterated with well vascularized tissue and the wound closed with flaps, preferably muscle or musculocutaneous flaps. When planning flap reconstruction of pressure sores, the patient's ambulatory status should be considered because sacrifice of muscles, such as the gluteus maximus, can have serious consequences for hip stability and gait. Furthermore, the planned flap should be large enough so as to keep suture lines away from zones of pressure, and, because recurrence is not uncommon in these patients, the flap should be designed in a way that other potential donors are not violated or that allows reuse of the same flap, for example, rerotation or readvancement. Finally, after surgery, no pressure is allowed over the flap and suture lines for at least 3 weeks.

With respect to flap selection, a number of factors influence the decision, such as ambulatory status, availability of local/regional tissue, previous operations, and scars. Nevertheless, common options for the most common sites include the following:

- **Sacral ulcers**
  ○ Unilateral or bilateral gluteal fasciocutaneous or myocutaneous V-Y advancement flaps (▶Fig. 3.8)
  ○ Fasciocutaneous or myocutaneous gluteal rotation flaps (▶Fig. 3.9)
  ○ Fasciocutaneous lumbosacral flap
- **Ischial ulcers**
  ○ Posterior hamstring myocutaneous V-Y advancement flap (▶Fig. 3.10)
  ○ Posterior thigh fasciocutaneous V-Y advancement flap
  ○ Gluteal fasciocutaneous or myocutaneous rotation or V-Y advancement flaps (▶Fig. 3.11)
  ○ Tensor fascia lata flap
- **Trochanteric ulcers**
  ○ Tensor fascia lata flap
  ○ Pedicled anterolateral thigh ± vastus lateralis flap

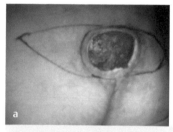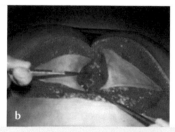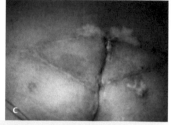

Fig. 3.8 Sacral pressure sore treated with bilateral V-Y advancement myocutaneous flaps. (a) Design of flaps. (b) Flaps raised and advanced onto sacral wound. (c) Six months postoperative view.

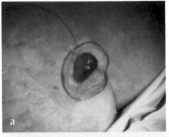
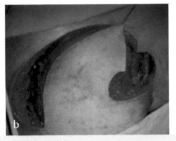
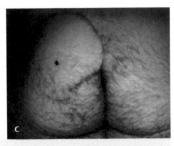

Fig. 3.9 Sacral pressure sore treated with gluteus maximus myocutaneous rotation flap. (a) Design of flap. (b) Flap raised and rotated onto sacral wound. (c) Six months postoperative view.

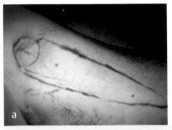
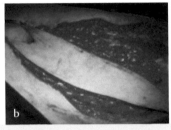
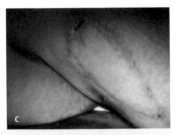

Fig. 3.10 Ischial pressure sore treated with hamstring V-Y myocutaneous advancement flap. (a) Design of flap. (b) Flap raised and rotated onto sacral wound. (c) Six months postoperative view.

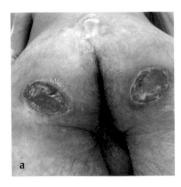
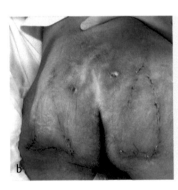

Fig. 3.11 Bilateral ischial ulcers treated with V-Y gluteus maximus myocutaneous advancement flaps. (a) Bilateral ischial ulcers. (b) Postoperative view at 4 weeks.

Negative pressure therapy (discussed in detail in Chapter 4) is currently an established tool in the armamentarium of possible therapies for pressure sores. Through its ability to remove exudate, reduce bacterial load, and stimulate angiogenesis leading to the formation of granulation tissue, negative pressure wound therapy has proven useful, either as first-line treatment of a number of pressure ulcers, particularly stage 3 ulcers, or as a bridge prior to surgical intervention of stage 4 wounds. Because these ulcers often present with varying degrees of contamination/infection, proper follow-up by nursing and medical staff is mandatory to prevent

complications. In addition, pressure sores in the buttock region are sometimes difficult to seal with negative pressure wound therapy, and the presence of feces is at times hard to manage as well.

Lastly, as mentioned earlier, recurrence of pressure sores is not infrequent and should be considered in the initial surgical plan. Sameem et al. conducted a meta-analysis to study the complication and recurrence rates of fasciocutaneous, myocutaneous, and perforator flaps for pressure sores. These authors found that myocutaneous flaps had a complication rate of 18.6% and a recurrence rate of 8.9%, whereas fasciocutaneous flaps had 11.7% and 11.2%, respectively. Perforator flaps had the highest rate of complications, 19.6%, but also the lowest recurrence rate, 5.6%.

3.11 Conclusions

Technological advances searching for the ideal skin substitute proposed by Sheridan and Tompkins have led to a new, wide range of synthetic bioengineered products that are currently used as temporary skin substitutes. Unfortunately, as these authors mentioned, the ideal substitute has not yet become available. The same applies to the treatment of complex wounds, where a vast array of alternatives are offered with which to provide our patients with better chances of recovery, although none of them is the perfect solution.

Many authors have demonstrated the versatility of the different skin substitutes for treatment of trauma and partial- or full-thickness burns. Most of these skin substitutes and wound dressings have been employed in our department, and each has its advantages and disadvantages. Therefore, it is important to use them and create your own experience according to the economic, clinical, and professional conditions of each particular plastic surgery unit.

It is also important to have a long-term vision so that your main goals aim to provide your patients with better functional and aesthetic results while improving cost-effectiveness and reduced hospitalization times.

3.12 Key Points

- A wide variety of wound dressings are available today, although there is little robust evidence to support the use of one over another.
- Selection of the dressing should be based on wound characteristics, which should be assessed periodically as the wound gradually changes during the healing process.
- Proper wound assessment prior to the implementation of any therapy includes the characteristics of the wound bed, the dimensions of the wound, the edges of the wound, the type and amount of exudate, and the presence of infection.
- The four basic components of wound preparation include tissue debridement, inflammation and infection control, moisture balance (optimal dressing selection), and epithelial edge advancement.

- There are different methods of wound debridement, including surgical (sharp), biosurgical (maggots), autolytic, hydrosurgery, and ultrasonic debridement.
- Skin substitutes provide a valuable replacement of the dermal component of the skin, leading to better-quality scars and more pliable skin than compared with traditional split-thickness skin grafts.
- Resistance and elasticity of the skin depend on the amount of dermis remaining on the generated scar.
- Pressure sores represent an important economic burden for any health system.
- Continuous pressure and subsequent ischemia of skin and soft tissues over a bony prominence form the basic physiopathological mechanisms of pressure sores.
- Prevention is key in the management of pressure sores, and the importance of frequent postural changes cannot be overemphasized.
- Medical comorbidities, nutrition, spasticity, and other factors need to be addressed and optimized prior to surgical intervention for a pressure sore.
- Surgical management is often reserved for stage 3 and 4 ulcers, although with the advent of negative pressure wound therapy, many stage 3 ulcers are amenable to treatment with this modality alone.
- The patient's ambulatory status and specific aspects of flap design should be considered during the preoperative planning.
- Recurrence of pressure sores is common, although different rates have been reported for different kinds of flaps, with perforator flaps having the lowest rate of recurrence.

Recommended Readings

Bishop JF, Demling RH, Hansbrough JF. Indications for use of Biobrane in wound management. Proceedings of a conference held in Houston, Texas. J Burn Care Rehabil. 1995; 16:341–342

Bishop S, Walker M, Rogers AA, Chen WY. Importance of moisture balance at the wound-dressing interface. J Wound Care. 2003; 12(4):125–128

Bolgiani A, Lima E, Do Valle Freitas M. Matrices de Regeneración Dérmica. En: Bolgiani A, ed. Quemaduras: Conductas clínicas y Quirúrgicas. São Paulo, Brazil: Editora Atheneu; 2013:151–157

Bowler PG. Wound pathophysiology, infection and therapeutic options. Ann Med. 2002; 34(6):419–427

Brown JB, McDowell F. Massive repairs of burns with thick split-skin grafts: emergency"dressings" with homografts. Ann Surg. 1942;115(4):658–674

Buck BW, Galiano RD. Wound care. In: Thorne CH, Chung KC, Gosain AK et al., eds. Grabb and Smith's Plastic Surgery. 7th ed. Philadelphia, PA: Elsevier; 2014:20–28

Butcher G, Pinnuck L. Wound bed preparation: ultrasonic-assisted debridement. Br J Nurs. 2013; 22(6):S36 S38–S43

Canadian Association of Wound Care. Best practicearticles. https://www.woundscanada.ca/health-care-profession-al/education-health-care-professional/advanced-educa-tion/12-healthcare-professional/110-supplements. Accessed November 11, 2017

Calderón W, Andrades P, Leniz P, et al. The cone flap: a new and versatile fasciocutaneous flap. Plast Reconstr Surg. 2004; 114(6):1539–1542

Calderón W, Oyarse E, Calderón D, et al. Hatchet-shaped tensor fascia lata flap for the treatment of trochanteric pressure sores. Cir plast.iberolatinoamer. 2010; 36(4):355–358

Can pressure ulcers be prevented using differents support sur-faces? Cochrane database of systematic reviews. 2015

Chadwick P. International Case Series: Using Askina® Calgitrol® Paste in the Treatment of Diabetic Foot Infection: Case Studies. London: Wounds International; 2013

Cuadra A, Piñeros JL, Roa R. Quemaduras faciales: Manejo inicial y tratamiento. Rev Med Clin Las Condes. 2010; 21:41–45

Davis SC, Martinez L, Kirsner R. The diabetic foot: the impor-tance of biofilms and wound bed preparation. Curr Diab Rep. 2006; 6(6):439–445

Edwards R, Harding KG. Bacteria and wound healing. Curr Opin Infect Dis. 2004; 17(2):91–96

Edwards J, Stapley S. Debridement of diabetic foot ulcers. Co-chrane Database Syst Rev. 2010; 1(1):CD003556

European Wound Management Association (EWMA). Position document: Wound bed preparation in practice. London: MEP Ltd; 2004

Game F. The advantages and disadvantages of non-surgical management of the diabetic foot. Diabetes Metab Res Rev. 2008; 24(Suppl 1):S72–S75

Girdner J. Skin grafting with grafts taken from dead subjects. Med Rec. 1881; 20:119–120

Global Industry Analysts. Advanced wound care: a global stra-tegic business report. http://www.marketresearch.com/ Global-Industry-Analysts-v1039/Advanced-Wound-Care-8102385/. Accessed August 4, 2017

Gottrup F. A specialized wound-healing center concept: impor-tance of a multidisciplinary department structure and surgical treatment facilities in the treatment of chronic wounds. Am J Surg 2004; 187(5A):38S–43S

Grab WC. Grabb and Smith's Plastic Surgery book: Lippincot-Raven; 1997:1086–1097

Haycocks S, Chadwick P. Debridement of diabetic foot wounds. Nurs Stand. 2012; 26(24):51–52, 54, 56 passim

Haycocks S, Chadwick P. Sharp debridement of diabetic foot ul-cers and the importance of meaningful informed consent. Wounds UK. 2008; 4(1):51–56

Heimbach D, Luterman A, Burke J, et al. Artificial dermis for major burns. A multi-center randomized clinical trial. Ann Surg. 1988; 208(3):313–320

Hosseini SN, Mousavinasab SN, Fallahnezhat M. Xenoderm dressing in the treatment of second degree burns. Burns. 2007;33(6):776–781

Jull AB, Rodgers A, Walker N. Honey as a topical treatment for wounds. Cochrane Database Syst Rev. 2008(4):CD005083

Llanos S, Calderón W. Colgajo miocutáneo de gluteo mayor en isla con cierre en V-Y para la cobertura de úlcera isquiática. Cir Plast iberolatinoamer. 2006; 32(1):41–48

Lipsky BA, Berendt AR, Cornia PB, et al; Infectious Diseases Society of America. 2012 Infectious Diseases Society of America clinical practice guideline for the diagnosis and treatment of diabetic foot infections. Clin Infect Dis. 2012; 54(12):e132–e173

Lipsky BA, Hoey C, Zasloff M. Topical antimicrobial thera-py for treating chronic wounds. Clin Infect Dis. 2009; 49(10):1541–1549

McCallon SK, Weir D, Lantis JC II. Optimizing Wound Bed Prepa-ration With Collagenase Enzymatic Debridement. J Am Coll Clin Wound Spec. 2015; 6(1–2):14–23

McCarty SM, Percival SL. Proteases and Delayed Wound Healing. Adv Wound Care (New Rochelle). 2013; 2(8):438–447

Medina A, Scott PG, Ghahary A, Tredget EE. Pathophysiology of chronic nonhealing wounds. J Burn Care Rehabil. 2005; 26(4):306–319

Mogford JE, Sisco M, Bonomo SR, Robinson AM, Mustoe TA. Impact of aging on gene expression in a rat model of ischemic cutaneous wound healing. J Surg Res. 2004; 118(2):190–196

Moore ZE, Cowman S. Risk assessment tools for the preven-tion of pressure ulcers. Cochrane Database Syst Rev. 2014(2):CD006471

Mustoe TA, O'Shaughnessy K, Kloeters O. Chronic wound patho-genesis and current treatment strategies: a unifying hy-pothesis. Plast Reconstr Surg. 2006; 117(7, Suppl):35S–41S

Mustoe T. Understanding chronic wounds: a unifying hypothesis on their pathogenesis and implications for therapy. Am J Surg. 2004; 187(5A):65S–70S

National Institute for Health and Clinical Excellence. Diabetic Foot Problems: Inpatient Management of Diabetic Foot Problems. Clinical Guideline no. 119. London: NICE; 2011

Pereira C, Gold W, Herndon D. Review paper: burn coverage technologies: current concepts and future directions. J Bio-mater Appl. 2007; 22(2):101–121

Phillips PL, Wolcott RD, Fletcher J, Schultz GS. et al; Biofilms Made Easy. Wounds International 2010; 1(3): Available from http://www.woundsinternational.com

Richard JL, Sotto A, Lavigne JP. New insights in diabetic foot in-fection. World J Diabetes. 2011; 2(2):24–32

Roa R, Las Heras R, Piñeros JL, Correa G, Norambuena H, Marré D. Contractura axilar por quemadura tratada con Integra®. Rev Chil Cir. 2011; 63(3):276–279

Robson MC. Wound infection. A failure of wound healing caused by an imbalance of bacteria. Surg Clin North Am. 1997; 77(3):637–650

Saffle JR. Closure of the excised burn wound: temporary skin substitutes. Clin Plast Surg. 2009; 36(4):627–641

Sameem M, Au M, Wood T, Farrokhyar F, Mahoney J. A systematic review of complication and recurrence rates of musculo-cutaneous, fasciocutaneous, and perforator-based flaps for treatment of pressure sores. Plast Reconstr Surg. 2012; 130(1):67e–77e

Scottish Intercollegiate Guidelines Network. Management of Diabetes. A National Clinical Guideline. Guideline no. 116. Edinburgh: SIGN; 2010

Sen CK, Gordillo GM, Roy S, et al. Human skin wounds: a major and snowballing threat to public health and the economy. Wound Repair Regen. 2009; 17(6):763–771

Sisco M, Mustoe TA. Animal models of ischemic wound healing. Toward an approximation of human chronic cutaneous ul-cers in rabbit and rat. Methods Mol Med. 2003; 78:55–65

Smith DJ Jr. Use of Biobrane in wound management. J Burn Care Rehabil. 1995; 16:317–319

Steed DL, Donohoe D, Webster MW, Lindsley L; Diabetic Ulcer Study Group. Effect of extensive debridement and treatment on the healing of diabetic foot ulcers. J Am Coll Surg. 1996; 183(1):61–64

Stern R, McPherson M, Longaker MT. Histologic study of artificial skin used in the treatment of full-thickness thermal injury. J Burn Care Rehabil. 1990; 11(1):7–13

Still J, Donker K, Law E, Thiruvaiyaru D. A program to decrease hospital stay in acute burn patients. Burns. 1997; 23(6):498–500

Thompson D. A critical review of the literature on pressure ulcer aetiology. J Wound Care. 2005; 14(2):87–90

Troy J, Karlnoski R, Downes K, et al. The use of EZ Derm® in partial-thickness burns: An institutional review of 157 patients. Eplasty. 2013; 13:e14

Werdin F, Tennenhaus M, Schaller HE, Rennekampff HO. Evidence-based management strategies for treatment of chronic wounds. Eplasty. 2009; 9:e19

Wounds UK. Effective debridement in a changing NHS: a UK consensus. London: Wounds UK. www.wounds-uk.com. Accessed December 29, 2017

Yager DR, Nwomeh BC. The proteolytic environment of chronic wounds. Wound Repair Regen. 1999; 7(6):433–441

Ye J, Mani R. A systematic review and meta-analysis of nutritional supplementation in chronic lower extremity wounds. Int J Low Extrem Wounds. 2016; 15(4):296–302

4 Negative Pressure Wound Therapy

Javier Buendia, Diego Marré, Marcus Castro Ferreira

Abstract

During the last decades, countless techniques, procedures, and dressings have been described in the field of reconstructive surgery; however, only a few have had as significant an impact as negative pressure wound therapy (NPWT). Complex wounds represent a major health issue in terms of patient morbidity and economic burden, and NPWT emerged as a reliable and effective treatment, thus becoming a fundamental tool for managing a wide array of wounds of varying etiologies and characteristics. Essentially, NPWT is composed of an interface material (usually a foam) that is applied directly onto the wound and covered and sealed with a plastic drape on top of which a suction device is connected. By removing exudate, enhancing blood flow, and decreasing bacterial load, NPWT stimulates the formation of granulation tissue and improves wound healing. The indications for NPWT are diverse, and its use is not restricted to plastic surgery; a number of other surgical specialties use NPWT as well. Nevertheless, it is surprising that the effects of this therapy remain to be fully elucidated, as are the optimal parameters that apply to different situations. This chapter discusses the origins of NPWT, its fundamental mechanisms, and the indications for it. Throughout, we provide some practical tips and tricks for using NPWT successfully in regions and wounds where it can be difficult to apply.

Keywords: angiogenesis, chronic wounds, granulation tissue, negative pressure wound therapy, reconstructive ladder

4.1 Introduction

Complex wounds are a challenging issue in health care, often translating into high treatment costs, long-term admissions, and uncertain evolution. Traditionally, wounds have been classified into acute or chronic according to their time of evolution. Notwithstanding the widespread use of this temporal classification, wounds may also be characterized as simple or complex, depending on parameters such as extension, kind of tissue affected, and the presence of comorbidities, among others.

Complex wounds may be defined as wounds that cannot be repaired by simple methods, such as direct closure, healing by secondary intention, or skin graft, thus requiring resurfacing by more sophisticated surgical procedures. The presence of exposed structures like tendon or bone, an unfavorable local environment, and comorbidities known to alter wound healing (e.g., diabetes, wound healing disorders, steroid treatment) may all influence wound complexity. Furthermore, complex wounds are frequently mistreated, leading to a torpid and long evolution; thus, in a number of cases, a complex wound becomes a chronic wound as well. In these complex and chronic scenarios, the wound's microenvironment usually exhibits a reduced mitotic index, increased proinflammatory chemokines, an absence of local growth factors, and an imbalance between extracellular matrix production and degradation. The role of the local microenvironment and its response to mechanical stimulus has gained increasing attention from both clinicians and researchers interested in wound healing.

The local alterations occurring in chronic wounds can have a significant impact on their healing capacity, making them more susceptible to complications. As reported by Mustoe et al., these wounds usually exhibit tissue hypoxia, bacterial contamination, ischemia–reperfusion damage, and altered cellular and systemic stress response in the elderly population. Taking into consideration these and other changes, Falanga proposed a new concept—wound bed preparation—in which favorable conditions are created for wound healing, including control of bioburden, reduction of exudate, debridement of necrotic tissue, and promotion of granulation tissue. In other words, the goal is to reset the wound-healing process back to the state of an acute wound. This concept is now considered the standard for wound care.

The use of negative pressure to alter the microenvironment and improve the bed of chronic and complex wounds was described more than 2 decades ago. Broadly referred to as negative pressure wound therapy (NPWT), this treatment modality has been shown to enhance healing of various types of wounds resulting from trauma, infection, congenital deformities, and tumors. The first report on the use of negative pressure as an aid to improve a wound's bed prior to skin grafting comes from Russia and was published in 1966 by Mirazimov.

Subsequently, in the 1980s and 1990s Davydov et al. published a series of case reports of infected wounds treated with negative pressure. Later on, Fleischmann et al. in Germany used this therapy for open fractures, osteomyelitis, and pressure ulcers. Even though these were all significant works, they did not have much international repercussion.

The studies published in 1997 by Morykwas, Argenta, and their colleagues were the first experimental and clinical papers published in English. Briefly, through experiments in pigs, these authors observed that, under negative pressure, wounds showed an increased blood flow and a decreased bacterial count, leading to the development of healthy granulation tissue. Additionally, in the clinical setting, NPWT was applied to 300 patients with complex wounds, with the authors reporting an impressive 99% of wound bed improvement by means of exudate control and granulation. Since then, a rapidly growing body of clinical and experimental evidence favoring the use of NPWT began to rise, leading clinicians and professionals alike to adopt NPWT as a standard of care for complex wounds in multiple centers worldwide.

The surging number of clinical trials and studies in this field have provided us with a more detailed understanding of the observed clinical effects as well as the mechanism of action at the tissue, cellular, and molecular levels. From a reconstructive point of view, the use of NPWT has somewhat revolutionized the classical approach to a number of wounds, to the point of being proposed by some as an established step on the reconstructive ladder. Moreover, this therapy has provided plastic surgeons with a tool that can turn a complex defect needing a technically demanding reconstruction to a wound amenable to repair with simpler techniques (▶Fig. 4.1).

> **Note**
>
> NPWT has altered the reconstructive ladder by offering simpler solutions to wounds and defects seemingly needing complex reconstructions.

4.2 Basic Science

As mentioned earlier, NPWT has had a tremendous impact on wound care and reconstructive surgery since its description and clinical application more than 2 decades ago. By allowing simpler methods of treatment for complicated wounds or serving as a reliable bridge between wounding and final reconstruction, NPWT has established itself as a fundamental tool in reconstructive surgery. Despite its proven clinical efficacy and established

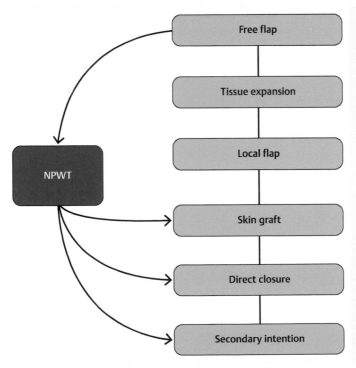

Fig. 4.1 In some cases, negative pressure wound therapy (NPWT) allows wounds needing complex reconstructions to be closed by simpler techniques.

mechanisms of action, some of the effects produced by negative pressure over the wound and surrounding tissues still remain controversial, especially at the molecular level. Experiments in animals and in vitro settings using bioreactors have yielded important insights; nevertheless the controlled situation of laboratory assays and species-specific molecular responses make it hard to fully extrapolate these findings into the clinical situation in which NPWT is applied to patients with comorbidities and complex wounds.

Regardless of the brand or manufacturer, there are four major components of any NPWT device: (1) a filler porous material or sponge placed into the wound, (2) a semipermeable dressing to isolate the wound environment and allow the vacuum system to transmit subatmospheric pressures to the wound surface, (3) a connecting tube, and (4) a vacuum system with a fluid collection canister. Under this basic configuration, the main effects of negative pressure on wounds are as follows:

- Wound deformation
  ° Macrodeformation
  ° Microdeformation
- Fluid clearance
- Improved blood flow and stimulation of angiogenesis
- Reduction of bacterial load

The formation of healthy granulation tissue and improved wound healing seen in wounds treated with topical negative pressure can be considered as the end result of the combination of the foregoing effects (▶ Fig. 4.2).

4.2.1 Wound Deformation

Macrodeformation

When disrupted, skin has a tendency to spread apart due to baseline tension forces. Immediately after application, NPWT induces centripetal wound contraction, which counteracts tissue's distraction forces, resulting in a macroscopic reduction of the wound's dimensions and the adequate contact between the wound bed and foam dressing. In this sense, it has been observed that polyurethane foams undergo an 80% volume reduction under -125 mm Hg of suction. Furthermore, a study in pigs showed that maximal wound contraction is already achieved at -75 mm Hg, whereas fluid removal is optimal at -125 mm Hg. These data illustrate the importance NPWT has in reducing the size of the wound. However, because this is mainly a mechanical effect, it is important to note that different degrees of macrodeformation will be obtained in different wounds, depending on the characteristics of tissues and their compliance.

Microdeformation

This type of mechanical stretch occurs at the tissue–foam interface, where tissue is drawn into the pores (commonly 400–600 μm), eliciting a proliferative response at the cellular level. Mechanotransduction describes the process by which cells transduce mechanical forces into biological signals and is believed to play a fundamental, yet understudied, role in the physiology of NPWT. When subjected to strain forces, cells proliferate as a consequence of cytoskeletal tension. In this sense, it is interesting that the 5–20% of strain elicited by NPWT is similar to the one required to induce cell division in vitro. Furthermore, as noted by Huang et al., the hostile environment of a chronic wound probably lacks the structural elements in the extracellular matrix that allow cells to effectively attach and elongate. If the ability to stretch is lost, the proliferative potential is dramatically reduced. NPWT is likely to deliver such strain to cells, inducing proliferation through different, yet effective,

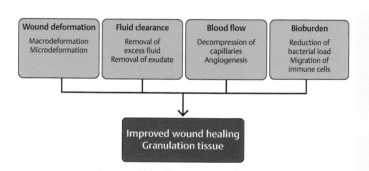

Fig. 4.2 The effects of negative pressure wound therapy.

mechanical and molecular signals. Genes involved in cellular proliferation, such as *myc*, *c-jun*, and *Bcl-2*, along with others encoding for extracellular matrix production and remodeling, are upregulated in response to stretch. McNulty et al. have elegantly simulated the mechanical microenvironment of NPWT by seeding fibroblasts into fibrin scaffolds and applying NPWT using Granu-Foam (KCI) dressing at −125 mm Hg. They observed a significant increase in the energetic status of cells, along with a rise in levels of transforming growth factor-β (TGF-β) and platelet-derived growth factor −α, −β (PDGF−α, PDGF−β), all of which may in part explain the remarkable formation of granulation tissue and improved wound healing associated with NPWT. Finally, it is noteworthy that cellular stretch induces not only proliferation but also cellular migration and differentiation, both of which are pillars in the process of wound healing.

4.2.2 Fluid Clearance

Edema is associated with a number of wounds of varying nature. Chronic wounds, traumatic injuries, and some abdominal wounds often exhibit significant fluid accumulation, which prevents closure on the one hand and impairs healing on the other. Tissue edema affects the natural biology of wound repair by different mechanisms. At a macroscopic level, edematous tissues often exhibit a reduced elasticity and capacity to be mobilized, precluding approximation of wound edges. Within tissues, undue buildup of extracellular fluid reduces the ability of cells to stretch and generate the tension necessary for proliferation. It likely compresses the already limited terminal vasculature at the wound edges, which further reduces blood flow, and it may also impair lymphatic drainage by oversaturating it. Furthermore, it must be noted that in some cases the accumulated fluid has an inflammatory profile and contains varying amounts of bacteria, which also affects wound healing.

As mentioned earlier, it has been observed that optimal fluid extraction with NPWT occurs at −125 mm Hg, which is one of the reasons why this pressure is often used. However, once most of the fluid has been removed, the high pressure may be reduced to a lower pressure that is more conducive to tissue growth. Looking at the different detrimental effects of fluid accumulation in wounds, it is possible to infer how NPWT, through its fluid-removal capacity, will positively affect the wound environment. First it reduces the edema that precludes approximation of borders in some wounds, such as fasciotomies and laparotomies with significant bowel swelling, making them more amenable to direct closure, or at least reducing their size (a feature shared with the macro-deformation effect explained earlier). Second, the removal of excess fluid from the interstitial space restores the cells' capacity to stretch and proliferate. Third, it improves blood flow by decompressing capillaries. Fourth, by removing excess fluid it is possible that the draining function of the lymphatic system is resumed. Fifth, the removal of exudate containing inflammatory cytokines and matrix metalloproteinases creates a more physiologic environment for wound healing to occur. As can be inferred, depending on the wound's characteristics, certain effects will predominate over others.

Finally, the ability to remove fluid from the wound and surrounding tissues has made NPWT an interesting therapeutic tool in cases of extravasation and venomous bites.

4.2.3 Improved Blood Flow and Stimulation of Angiogenesis

Pioneering experiments by Morykwas, Argenta, and their colleagues in a pig model showed a four-fold increase in blood flow in wounds treated with -125 mm Hg of NPWT. Studies thereafter have also reported on a paradoxical reduction of blood flow with pressures > 400 mm Hg. Although the increase in blood flow is probably secondary to the removal of fluid that decompresses and dilates blood vessels, the reduction observed at higher pressures is likely due to an increased extracellular pressure that eventually collapses capillaries. This possibility should be considered when one is selecting the amount of negative pressure to apply.

Vascularization is a fundamental and necessary element for wound healing and tissue formation. Studies showing a significant increase in granulation tissue in wounds treated with -125 mm Hg have attributed the accelerated formation of tissue to the improved blood flow elicited by negative pressure. Furthermore, negative pressure of up to -300 mm Hg has also been proven to increase blood flow in intact skin of healthy volunteers, whereas higher values fail to produce such an effect; blood flow returns to baseline values, though, interestingly, never below them. Considering these findings, and that negative pressure does not harm intact skin, it is likely that, when applied over a fresh flap (with a skin paddle), NPWT may enhance cutaneous blood flow of areas with presumably limited perfusion.

As already stated, the improved blood flow elicited by negative pressure is mainly due to a mechanical decompression of vessels within the wound. Nevertheless, apart from this mechanical effect, NPWT also generates an angiogenic response in the wound that leads to an overall increase in blood vessel density and vascularization. The temporary hypoxic environment that follows the application of negative pressure, which upregulates the expression of angiogenic growth factors (e.g., vascular endothelial growth factor A and hypoxia-inducible factor 1α), is what probably stimulates this phenomenon of neovascularization.

Noteworthy, the improved blood flow–neovascularization effect of NPWT has been exploited not only to enhance wound healing but also to enhance and accelerate the take of skin grafts and dermal substitutes.

4.2.4 Reduction of Bacterial Load

Even though there is conclusive data showing that wounds treated with NPWT exhibit reduced bacterial colonization when compared to control groups, or even that negative pressure is effective for infected wounds, the real effect of this therapy on bacterial burden remains debatable. Morykwas et al. in their initial studies observed that pig wounds inoculated with 10^8 *Staphylococcus aureus* or *S. epidermidis* had bacterial counts of less than 10^5 after 4 days of NPWT, which was significantly lower than wounds not treated with negative pressure. Other authors have reported on the successful treatment of infected wounds, some of them involving vascular artificial grafts, with the use of NPWT. In contrast, other studies have shown no effect on bacterial count or even an increase in *S. aureus* colonization in wounds treated with NPWT. Despite these results, it seems very plausible that by removing fluid and exudate, NPWT does help in reducing bioburden. Additionally, the improved blood flow elicited by this therapy may also assist in bacterial clearance by allowing more immune cells to reach the wound surface as well as by improving the delivery of systemic antibiotics to the wound site. Furthermore, as reported by Liu et al, the upregulation of cytokines such as interleukin (IL)-8 and IL-1β in response to the application of NPWT may trigger the migration of neutrophils to the wound and accelerate bacterial clearance.

To enhance the infection-control capacity of NPWT, some important modifications have been introduced to the system, such as silver-coated foams, combinations of the classic polyurethane foam and a silver dressing, and instillation.

4.3 Dressings and Parameters

As mentioned earlier, the four major components of any NPWT set comprise a filler porous material, a semipermeable dressing, a connecting tube, and a vacuum system. Sets from different manufacturers may vary, however, as to the porosity and composition of the filler material and the modalities of treatment that the vacuum system is able to provide in terms of intensity and waveform as well as the possibility of instillation. Most appliances are portable, and there are also disposable devices available for small wounds, which are very useful in an outpatient context.

4.3.1 Dressings

Gauze

Gauze provides minimum macrodeformation but good drainage. It can be used in multiple situations, though it is best indicated for superficial wounds. Gauze adheres to the wound surface more than other dressings, which can make its removal cumbersome and painful; applying a dressing along with petroleum jelly in combination with gauze will reduce its adherence, but it may reduce the therapy's effectiveness as well. Important advantages of gauze include its low cost and the possibility of creating custom-made systems.

Polyurethane Foam

Foams of multiple shapes and sizes (▶Fig. 4.3) are available to fit wounds of varying dimensions and configurations. Due to its flexible design, polyurethane foam easily adapts to the contours of deep and irregularly shaped wounds. Moreover, its open pore structure (133/400–600 µm) allows uniform distribution of negative pressure throughout the whole wound site and improves fluid drainage. The size and distribution of pores may vary across dressings from different manufacturers and also within each brand's products; selection of the proper dressing should thus be tailored to the wound's characteristics and the products available from the supplying company. Additionally, polyurethane ether foam dressings are hydrophobic, which enhances fluid removal. As described earlier, foam provides excellent macro- and microdeformation, which translates into macroscopic reduction of the wound surface and the promotion of cellular activity with the consequent formation of granulation tissue. An interesting modification introduced by KCI (San Antonio, TX) is the silver-coated polyurethane foam. As the name implies, this dressing has microbonded metallic silver uniformly distributed throughout its surface, providing an effective barrier to bacterial penetration. Silver ions are effective against aerobic, gram-negative, and gram-positive bacteria and may thus help in reducing wound infection.

Polyvinyl Alcohol Foam

WhiteFoam (KCI) (▶Fig. 4.3) has pores in the range of 60–270 μm and comes premoistened with sterile water, making it less adherent than other materials. Additionally, its higher tensile strength facilitates its placement in and removal from tunnels and undermined tissues, while its higher density restricts the in-growth of granulation tissue. Altogether, the reduced adherence and restricted tissue growth of polyvinyl alcohol foams make dressing changes less painful and more comfortable for patients, improving their tolerance and adherence to therapy. Furthermore, the characteristics just described also make WhiteFoam a useful dressing for exposed structures, such as blood vessels, or for situations in which negative pressure without formation of granulation tissue is desired, such as over skin grafts. Finally, it must be noted that, due to the dressing's higher density, higher values of negative pressure may be needed to ensure its proper functioning.

Abdominal Sponge Sets

An open abdomen is a potentially life-threatening condition for patients and a reconstructive challenge for surgeons. Early control of the exposed viscera and edematous tissues to achieve primary fascial closure is the main goal of treatment. Temporary closure techniques to isolate the abdominal contents from the external environment include the Bogotá bag and a three-layer construction described by Brock et al. consisting of a fenestrated polyethylene sheet between the abdominal viscera and the anterior parietal peritoneum; a moist, surgical towel over the sheet with two suction drains; and an adhesive drape over the entire wound, including a wide margin of surrounding skin. Similarly, The ABTHera system (KCI) includes a nonadhesive polyethylene sheet placed over the abdominal viscera, a fenestrated foam, a drape, and a suction system. Apart from effectively isolating the abdominal contents from the external environment and allowing rapid access for reentry without requiring sutures for placement, this system actively removes fluid, which reduces edema and intra-abdominal pressure. Additionally, the sponge elicits a centripetal force over the wound edges, which minimizes fascial retraction and loss of domain. In all, NPWT has radically changed the state of the art for open-abdomen treatment.

4.4 Parameters

The efficacy of NPWT in promoting wound healing has been largely accepted by clinicians and wound care personnel, yet high-level evidence demonstrating its effectiveness is scarce, and there is still much to learn about its mechanisms of action. In the future, we will hopefully have the data to assist clinicians in selecting the optimal parameters for specific wounds, including interface material as well as the amount and waveform of negative pressure. Advances in mechanobiology, the science of wound healing, the understanding of biofilms, and cell therapy will likely shed more light on the effects of NPWT and assist clinicians in the selection of the optimal parameters for different types of wounds, ultimately leading to improved care for our patients.

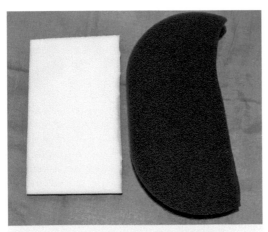

Fig. 4.3 Sponges. Polyvinyl alcohol (white) and polyurethane (black).

4.4.1 Pressure

The issue of how much negative pressure should be applied to a wound to optimize its healing capacity has been a matter of research and debate since the beginning. Despite advances, there is still a lack of defined practice parameters regarding pressure intensity, duration of treatment, and interval between dressing changes to provide the most efficient therapy. Thus, given the paucity of solid, evidence-based recommendations, most people are guided by their own experience and clinical judgment. In addition, the variable evolution of some wounds and the large number of factors affecting wound healing also make practice guidelines difficult to establish.

As discussed earlier in this chapter, the amount of negative pressure on a wound influences its contraction, blood flow, and fluid removal. Based on the landmark studies of Argenta and Morykwas, a protocol consisting of continuous suction at -125 mm Hg for the first 48 hours followed by an intermittent mode (e.g., 5 minutes on and 2 minutes off) for the remainder of the treatment may be considered as a standard. Nevertheless, the specific characteristics of each wound together with patient compliance need to be carefully evaluated in order to choose the best treatment option. An important, and probably underconsidered, aspect of negative pressure is that, although it stimulates granulation tissue formation across most of the wound's surface, at the edge it may actually induce hypoperfusion and result in ischemic tissue damage, which increases as the value of subatmospheric pressure rises. Additionally, the type of tissue has been shown to influence this effect, with the increase in blood flow occurring closer to the wound edge in muscle as compared to subcutaneous tissue (1.5 cm and 3 cm at -75 mm Hg, respectively). In conclusion and as a general consideration, the pressure value has to be high enough to allow for proper drainage, wound deformation, and occlusion of superficial bleeding, and at the same time, low enough to avoid generation of a large ischemic zone. The absolute value may vary between -75 and -125 mm Hg, depending on tissue and wound characteristics.

4.4.2 Modality

Some devices can be set to deliver negative pressure in different modalities, namely continuous, intermittent, and variable. In *continuous* pressure, the most widely used modality, the same pressure is permanently applied to the wound throughout the entire treatment. In *intermittent* therapy, the selected pressure is kept constant for a period of time (minutes) and periodically reduced (not to zero) for a short time, after which it returns to the preselected value (▶Fig. 4.4a). In the *variable* pattern, different values of pressure are applied continuously for longer periods of time, usually days (▶Fig. 4.4b). Some evidence suggests a higher efficacy of the intermittent and variable modes versus the continuous mode, although there are no solid, conclusive data supporting such a finding. It should also be noted that intermittent therapy is sometimes bothersome to patients in terms of the pain that each new suction produces as well as the noise of the device at the beginning of each cycle.

4.4.3 Instillation

Recently, instillation has been introduced as an adjunct to NPWT. With this method, the system delivers saline or any other active agent through the suction tube, thus providing a more favorable environment for wound healing and at the same time offering the advantages of a periodic washing effect. Even though NPWT is a closed dressing, some wounds may suffer dessication with suction; such wounds are the ones that would benefit the most from instillation. Despite its promising results, there is still little evidence supporting the use of instillation, and further research is warranted to determine its real potential as well as its indications.

> **Note**
>
> The wide variety of options for NPWT configuration must be carefully evaluated in order to customize the treatment for each wound.

4.5 Indications and Contraindications

The list of indications of NPWT is constantly growing as surgeons and wound specialists progressively apply it to an increasing array of different wounds, with a successful outcome in most cases. In this sense, it is fair to say that NPWT can be employed in virtually any open wound, provided that certain precautions are taken. Interestingly though, despite the broad list of indications, the one for which evidence is most robust are diabetic foot ulcers. ▶Table 4.1 summarizes the main indications for NPWT.

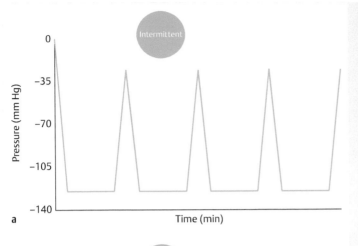

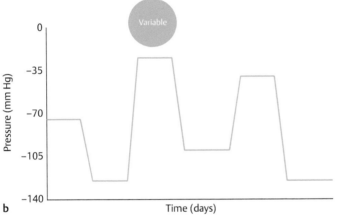

Fig. 4.4 Modalities of negative pressure wound therapy. **(a)** Intermittent. **(b)** Variable.

Table 4.1 Indications for negative pressure wound therapy

• Infected sternotomy	• Partial-thickness burns
• Degloving wounds	• Crohn's disease wounds
• Skin grafts	• Dehiscence wounds
• Traumatic wounds	• Free flap donor sites
• Surgical wounds	• Amputation stumps
• Pressure ulcers	• Hidradenitis suppurativa
• Open fractures	• Diabetic ulcers
• Venous stasis ulcers	• Chronic open wounds
• Fasciectomy wounds	• Dermal templates

Remember   **M!**

Despite the broad and continuously growing list of indications of NPWT, the most robust evidence supporting its use so far is in the treatment of diabetic foot ulcers.

Contraindications for NPWT are limited and mainly related to excess bleeding and infection. Caution must be exercised when using NPWT in bleeding wounds and/or anticoagulated patients, because the system may rapidly aspirate a large amount of blood, leading to potentially life-threatening hemodynamic complications. Also, this therapy should be used judiciously in grossly infected wounds because the closed system may serve as a favorable niche for bacterial replication. In these cases, thorough mechanical cleansing should be performed before the application of NPWT, and dressings should be changed every 24–48 hours, depending on the degree of contamination. Recently, with the introduction of instillation, complications related to infection seem to be decreasing. NPWT does not work on dead tissue, so all necrotic areas should be adequately debrided before treatment. Polyurethane foams should not be placed directly over exposed blood vessels (particularly vascular anastomoses), nerves, or the heart—negative pressure may stave the vessel walls and lead to severe bleeding. Moreover, some reports have suggested that when placed over an open sternum the negative pressure may pull the heart toward the bone's sharp edges, causing rupture of the right ventricle. Due to the effect that NPWT has on cellular proliferation, this therapy is also not recommended for tumoral wound beds. Likewise, negative pressure should not be used to treat fistulas in which the deep opening is unknown.

4.6 Tips and Tricks

4.6.1 Placing the Sponge

Adapting the foam dimensions to mirror the wound is an effective way to enhance granulation tissue formation using NPWT. Sponges have to be tailored to fit the wound contour as much as possible, trying not to overpack with sponge material.

At each dressing change, it is recommended to write on the drape the date of change plus any other important information, such as the number of pieces of sponge that have been placed inside. This facilitates communication with professionals performing future changes and improves patients' safety.

When using large pieces of the polyvinyl alcohol foam it is important to take into account that, due to the foam's high density and tensile strength, pressure may not be equally distributed, being lower farther from where the suction tube is placed. To solve this, a thin layer of polyurethane foam can be placed on top of the polyvinyl so that the pressure is delivered uniformly to the whole wound.

4.6.2 Pain Management

NPWT may cause pain during treatment and especially during dressing changes. Depending on the context, whether it is an inpatient or an outpatient, pain associated with this therapy can usually be managed successfully with oral or intravenous analgesics. For cases of persisting pain, progressive -25 mm Hg reductions in pressure until pain subsides is a common recommendation. It must be noted that the most painful part of therapy is usually the first suction. Thus patients under intermittent therapy may suffer with each new cycle; in such cases, changing to a continuous mode is highly recommended. When pain is associated with dressing changes, solutions that may make the procedure more comfortable for the patient include

switching to the less adherent polyvinyl alcohol foam, performing changes more frequently to avoid overgrowth of tissue into the sponge, placing a nonadherent dressing between the wound bed and the sponge to ease its removal, and infiltrating local anesthetic within the foam a few minutes prior to change. If the patient cannot tolerate the procedure despite all these measures, it may be wise to either program for changes under sedation or to interrupt NPWT and institute a new regime of wound care.

4.6.3 Wound Maceration

Maceration under the adherent drape may lead to fungal colonization/infection and complications thereof. The best option to avoid maceration is a proper technique. The wound edges and peripheral skin must be thoroughly cleaned and dried before applying the drape. The sponge should not exceed the wound edges, and the adherent drape should have no wrinkles or folds and should overlap onto intact skin for an adequate distance. There are several products available to protect skin or ensure proper adhesion of the drape during treatment. However, these should be used judiciously; oil-based products, for example, may reduce the drape's adherence.

4.6.4 Bridging

In most cases, the suction piece is placed right on top of the foam covering the wound. In some cases, however, the suction is applied from a remote site and needs to be "bridged" to reach the wound. The bridging technique has two main applications. First, it is a useful method to deliver suction from a more comfortable site to a less convenient one. For example, placing the suction piece right on top of a heel ulcer can be problematic for both the patient and the surgeon; instead, the suction can be placed at the midleg and bridged to the heel via a piece of foam. Secondly, the bridging technique can be applied when two or more different, but relatively close, wounds are treated at the same time. Here, each wound is set in the usual fashion, and a first large drape covering all wounds is applied. A hole is then made over each of the sponges, and a single piece of foam that bridges all of them is placed. The whole system is then covered with a second adherent drape, and the suction tube is installed at the desired site (▶ Fig. 4.5). It is important to note that the bridging foam must not be in direct contact with intact skin, which is what the first drape is used for.

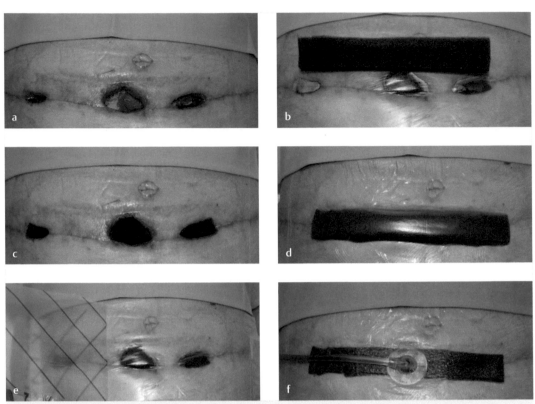

Fig. 4.5 Bridging technique. **(a)** Three different defects at the suture line following abdominal closure of a deep inferior epigastric perforator (DIEP) flap. **(c)** Each wound is filled with a sponge. **(e)** All wounds are covered with a plastic adherent drape. A small hole must then be made in the drape over each sponge. **(b)** The piece of sponge serving as the bridge is presented; it must be long enough to cover all wounds. **(d)** After putting the bridge over the wounds, the second drape is placed. **(f)** The suction tube is then placed over the bridge so that negative pressure is transmitted to all the underlying wounds.

4.6.5 Leakage

For NPWT to work properly, the sponge(s) must be completely sealed by the adherent drape, other wise negative pressure cannot be delivered to the wound. Leaks must then be promptly and effectively managed. When the leak is readily identified, placing a new piece of drape on top of it usually solves the problem. Unfortunately, in some cases, they are not easy to detect. Bar-Meir et al described the Maya technique based on instillation and subsequent rinsing of saline-diluted methylene blue dye onto the drape. The dye will color the dressing at the site of the leak.

There are different locations where placement of the dressing may be tricky and prone to leakage, such as the perianal and genital areas. An effective way of maintaining a closed suction system while at

the same time allowing permeability of the natural orifices is to replace the area that cannot be draped with a piece of plastic material, such as saline bags. The plastic is cut to fit the shape of the wound margin and sutured to it leaving a minimum of 5 cm of plastic beyond the wound edge. After the NPWT system is installed, the drape covering the sponge sticks to the plastic instead of the skin and nearby orifice. Once suction is initiated, the plastic piece can be folded toward the wound, keeping the orifice unobstructed (▶Fig. 4.6).

4.7 Clinical Applications

4.7.1 Case 1

A 64-year-old patient presented with a laparotomy incision infection with suspected abdominal

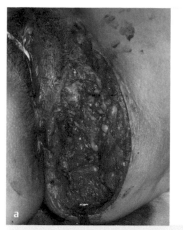
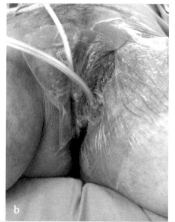
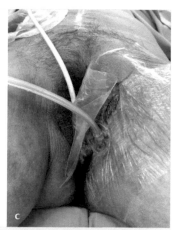

Fig. 4.6 Avoiding leaks in complicated areas. (a) Full-thickness defect near the perineal area. A "standard" negative pressure wound therapy dressing would have the adherent drape placed over the natural orifices and perineum. To circumvent it, a piece of plastic material (e.g., saline bag) is sutured to the wound edge facing the perineum. (b) Once the wound is filled with sponge, the adherent drape is placed over the plastic and not the skin so that proper a seal is obtained. (c) The plastic piece can be folded and unfolded to allow adequate permeability of orifices.

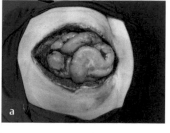
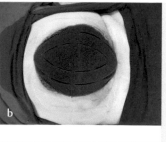
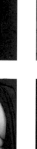
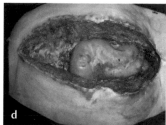

Fig. 4.7 (a–d) Case 1. See text for details.

compartment syndrome following bowel surgery (▶Fig. 4.7). The wound was aggressively debrided, resulting in a large, full-thickness defect of the abdominal wall with exposed, dilated bowel. The abdominal negative pressure wound therapy set was used as a bridge to final reconstruction to reduce the wound size, enhance fluid clearance, and reduce bioburden. Once the wound was reduced in size, edema had subsided, and healthy granulation tissue was obtained. Final closure was performed by means of a dual-mesh and component separation technique.

4.7.2 Case 2

A 74-year-old patient with multiple comorbidities was admitted to hospital from a nursing home after developing a grade IV pressure ulcer (▶Fig. 4.8). Initial debridement was carried out, and NPWT was started in order to prepare the wound bed before final reconstruction. With the patient's general condition optimized and the wound bed improved, a local rotation flap was used to cover the defect.

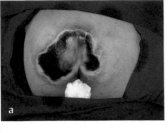
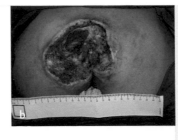

Fig. 4.8 (a–d) Case 2. See text for details.

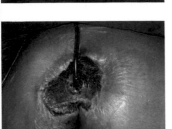
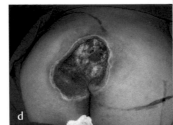

4.7.3 Case 3

A 44-year-old patient presented with a traumatic full-thickness wound on the dorsum of the left foot (▶ Fig. 4.9). Following surgical debridement, NPWT was applied for 72 hours to prepare the wound bed, after which a split-thickness skin graft was placed. To ensure its complete take, NPWT was applied to the skin graft for 5 days

4.8 Conclusions

Negative pressure wound therapy has established itself at the forefront of wound care. Either as definitive treatment or as a bridge before reconstruction, this system has provided surgeons of different subspecialties and professionals involved in wound care with an effective and reliable alternative for the management of a wide range of wounds. The ease of application and the existence of portable and disposable devices have expanded the use of NPWT to the outpatient setting, further increasing the patient population to which this therapy can be applied. Despite the proven clinical efficacy of NPWT, the underlying mechanisms leading to such effects remain to be fully elucidated, as are the ideal parameters for different kinds of wounds. Complications, though uncommon, can sometimes bring fatal consequences; it is therefore paramount to keep in mind the contraindications and precautions related to the use of NPWT.

4.9 Key Points

- NPWT is now a widely accepted method of wound care, especially for complex wounds.
- Even though it is used as a definitive treatment in some cases, NPWT is mostly regarded as an excellent alternative for wound bed preparation and/or temporary dressing prior to final reconstruction.
- In some situations, the use of NPWT may downscale the complexity of the final reconstruction.
- The mechanisms of action of NPWT have not been fully elucidated; however, evidence strongly points toward wound deformation, fluid clearance, improvement of blood flow, and possibly reduction of bioburden.
- Selection of parameters and materials should be carefully evaluated and selected depending on wound characteristics as well as the patient's comfort and compliance.
- Precautions and contraindications for using NPWT, although limited, must be thoroughly considered because misuse of this therapy may bring serious consequences.

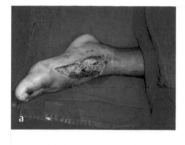
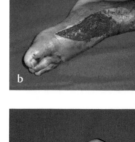
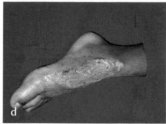
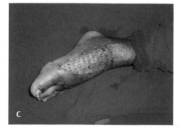

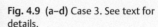

Fig. 4.9 (a–d) Case 3. See text for details.

Recommended Readings

Anagnostakos K, Mosser P. Negative pressure wound therapy in the management of postoperative infections after musculoskeletal tumour surgery. J Wound Care. 2014; 23(4): 191–194, 196–197

Argenta LC, Morykwas MJ. Vacuum-assisted closure: a new method for wound control and treatment: clinical experience. Ann Plast Surg. 1997; 38(6):563–576, discussion 577

Armstrong DG, Lavery LA; Diabetic Foot Study Consortium. Negative pressure wound therapy after partial diabetic foot amputation: a multicentre, randomised controlled trial. Lancet. 2005; 366(9498):1704–1710

Bar-Meir E, Tamir J, Winkler E. "Maya technique" for vacuum-assisted closure sealing. Plast Reconstr Surg. 2005; 116(3):931

Boone D, Braitman E, Gentics C, et al. Bacterial burden and wound outcomes as influenced by negative pressure wound therapy. Wounds. 2010; 22(2):32–37

Borgquist O, Ingemansson R, Malmsjö M. The influence of low and high pressure levels during negative-pressure wound therapy on wound contraction and fluid evacuation. Plast Reconstr Surg. 2011; 127(2):551–559

Brock WB, Barker DE, Burns RP. Temporary closure of open abdominal wounds: the vacuum pack. Am Surg. 1995; 61(1): 30–35

Davydov IuA, Abramov AIu, Larichev AB, Men'kov KG. Concept of clinico-biological control of the wound process in the treatment of suppurative wounds using vacuum therapy [in Russian]. Vestn Khir Im I I Grek. 1991; 146(2):132–136

Davydov IuA, Abramov AIu, Larichev AB. Substantiation of using forced early secondary suture in the treatment of suppurative wounds by the method of vacuum therapy [in Russian]. Vestn Khir Im I I Grek. 1990; 144(3):126–128

Davydov IuA, Abramov AIu, Larichev AB. Vacuum therapy in the prevention of postoperative wound infection[in Russian]. Vestn Khir Im I I Grek. 1991; 147(7–8):91–95

Davydov IuA, Larichev AB, Men'kov KG. Bacteriologic and cytologic evaluation of vacuum therapy of suppurative wounds [in Russian]. Vestn Khir Im I I Grek. 1988; 141(10):48–52

Davydov IuA, Larichev AB, Smirnov AP, Flegontov VB. Vacuum therapy of acute suppurative diseases of soft tissues and suppurative wounds [in Russian]. Vestn Khir Im I I Grek. 1988; 141(9):43–46

Davydov IuA, Larichev AB, Abramov AIu. Wound healing after vacuum drainage [in Russian]. Khirurgiia (Mosk). 1992(7–8): 21–26

Dumville JC, Hinchliffe RJ, Cullum N, et al. Negative pressure wound therapy for treating foot wounds in people with diabetes mellitus. Cochrane Database Syst Rev. 2013; 10(10):CD010318

Dumville JC, Webster J, Evans D, Land L. Negative pressure wound therapy for treating pressure ulcers. Cochrane Database Syst Rev. 2015(5):CD011334

Erba P, Ogawa R, Ackermann M, et al. Angiogenesis in wounds treated by microdeformational wound therapy. Ann Surg. 2011; 253(2):402–409

Falanga V. Classifications for wound bed preparation and stimulation of chronic wounds. Wound Repair Regen 2000; 8(5):347–352

Fernandez L, Norwood S, Roettger R, Wilkins HE III. Temporary intravenous bag silo closure in severe abdominal trauma. J Trauma. 1996; 40(2):258–260

Ferreira MC, Tuma P, Jr, Carvalho VF, Kamamoto F. Complex wounds. Clinics (Sao Paulo). 2006; 61(6):571–578

Fleischmann W, Lang E, Kinzl L. Vacuum assisted wound closure after dermatofasciotomy of the lower extremity [in German]. Unfallchirurg 1996; 99(4):283–287

Fleischmann W, Lang E, Russ M. Treatment of infection by vacuum sealing [in German]. Unfallchirurg. 1997; 100(4): 301–304

Fleischmann W, Strecker W, Bombelli M, Kinzl L. Vacuum sealing as treatment of soft tissue damage in open fractures [in German] Unfallchirurg .1993; 96:488–492

Garner GB, Ware DN, Cocanour CS, et al. Vacuum-assisted wound closure provides early fascial reapproximation in trauma patients with open abdomens. Am J Surg. 2001; 182(6):630–638

Glass GE, Murphy GF, Esmaeili A, Lai LM, Nanchahal J. Systematic review of molecular mechanism of action of negative-pressure wound therapy. Br J Surg. 2014; 101(13):1627–1636

Huang C, Leavitt T, Bayer LR, Orgill DP. Effect of negative pressure wound therapy on wound healing. Curr Probl Surg. 2014; 51(7):301–331

Janis JE, Kwon RK, Attinger CE. The new reconstructive ladder: modifications to the traditional model. Plast Reconstr Surg. 2011; 127 Suppl 1:205S–212S

Kim PJ, Attinger CE, Steinberg JS, Evans KK. Negative pressure wound therapy with instillation: past, present, and future. Surg Technol Int. 2015; 26:51–56

Lavery LA, La Fontaine J, Thakral G, Kim PJ, Bhavan K, Davis KE. Randomized clinical trial to compare negative-pressure wound therapy approaches with low and high pressure, silicone- coated dressing, and polyurethane foam dressing. Plast Reconstr Surg. 2014; 133(3):722–726

Lee KN, Ben-Nakhi M, Park EJ, Hong JP. Cyclic negative pressure wound therapy: an alternative mode to intermittent system. Int Wound J. 2015; 12(6):686–692

Lessing MC, James RB, Ingram SC. Comparison of the Effects of Different Negative Pressure Wound Therapy Modes-Continuous, Noncontinuous, and With Instillation-on Porcine Excisional Wounds. Eplasty. 2013; 13:e51

Li Z, Yu A. Complications of negative pressure wound therapy: a mini review. Wound Repair Regen 2014; 22(4):457–461

Liu D, Zhang L, Li T, et al. Negative-pressure wound therapy enhances local inflammatory responses in acute infected soft-tissue wound. Cell Biochem Biophys. 2014; 70(1):539–547

Llanos S, Danilla S, Barraza C, et al. Effectiveness of negative pressure closure in the integration of split thickness skin grafts: a randomized, double-masked, controlled trial. Ann Surg. 2006; 244(5):700–705

Malmsjö M, Gustafsson L, Lindstedt S, Gesslein B, Ingemansson R. The effects of variable, intermittent, and continuous negative pressure wound therapy, using foam or gauze, on wound contraction, granulation tissue formation, and ingrowth into the wound filler. Eplasty. 2012; 12:e5

Malsiner CC, Schmitz M, Horch RE, Keller AK, Leffler M. Vessel transformation in chronic wounds under topical negative pressure therapy: an immunohistochemical analysis. Int Wound J. 2015; 12(5):501–509

McNulty AK, Schmidt M, Feeley T, Villanueva P, Kieswetter K. Effects of negative pressure wound therapy on cellular energetics in fibroblasts grown in a provisional wound (fibrin) matrix. Wound Repair Regen. 2009; 17(2):192–199

Miller PR, Thompson JT, Faler BJ, Meredith JW, Chang MC. Late fascial closure in lieu of ventral hernia: the next step in open abdomen management. J Trauma. 2002; 53(5):843–849

Mirazimov BM. Free skin graft of the foot with vacuum preparation of the wound surface [in Russian]. Ortop Travmatol Protez. 1966; 27(10):19–22

Molnar JA, DeFranzo AJ, Hadaegh A, Morykwas MJ, Shen P, Argenta LC. Acceleration of Integra incorporation in complex tissue defects with subatmospheric pressure. Plast Reconstr Surg. 2004; 113(5):1339–1346

Morykwas MJ, Argenta LC. Nonsurgical modalities to enhance healing and care of soft tissue wounds. J South Orthop Assoc. 1997; 6(4):279–288

Morykwas MJ, Argenta LC, Shelton-Brown EI, McGuirt W. Vacuum-assisted closure: a new method for wound control and treatment: animal studies and basic foundation. Ann Plast Surg. 1997; 38(6):553–562

Morykwas MJ, Faler BJ, Pearce DJ, Argenta LC. Effects of varying levels of subatmospheric pressure on the rate of granulation tissue formation in experimental wounds in swine. Ann Plast Surg. 2001; 47(5):547–551

Morykwas MJ, Simpson J, Punger K, Argenta A, Kremers L, Argenta J. Vacuum-assisted closure: state of basic research and physiologic foundation. Plast Reconstr Surg. 2006; 117(7) Suppl:121S–126S

Murphy P, Lee K, Dubois L, DeRose G, Forbes T, Power A. Negative pressure wound therapy for high-risk wounds in lower extremity revascularization: study protocol for a randomized controlled trial. Trials. 2015; 16:504

Mustoe TA, O'Shaughnessy K, Kloeters O. Chronic wound pathogenesis and current treatment strategies: a unifying hypothesis. Plast Reconstr Surg. 2006; 117(7) Suppl: 35S–41S

Petkar KS, Dhanraj P, Kingsly PM, et al. A prospective randomized controlled trial comparing negative pressure dressing and conventional dressing methods on split-thickness skin grafts in burned patients. Burns. 2011; 37(6):925–929

Quyn AJ, Johnston C, Hall D, et al. The open abdomen and temporary abdominal closure systems–historical evolution and systematic review. Colorectal Dis. 2012; 14(8):e429–e438

Sartipy U, Lockowandt U, Gäbel J, Jidéus L, Dellgren G. Cardiac rupture during vacuum-assisted closure therapy. Ann Thorac Surg. 2006; 82(3):1110–1111

Saxena V, Hwang C-W, Huang S, Eichbaum Q, Ingber D, Orgill DP. Vacuum-assisted closure: microdeformations of wounds and cell proliferation. Plast Reconstr Surg. 2004; 114(5):1086–1096, discussion 1097–1098

Scherer SS, Pietramaggiori G, Mathews JC, Prsa MJ, Huang S, Orgill DP. The mechanism of action of the vacuum-assisted closure device. Plast Reconstr Surg. 2008; 122(3):786–797

Tarnuzzer RW, Schultz GS. Biochemical analysis of acute and chronic wound environments. Wound Repair Regen. 1996; 4(3):321–325

Timmers MS, Le Cessie S, Banwell P, Jukema GN. The effects of varying degrees of pressure delivered by negative-pressure wound therapy on skin perfusion. Ann Plast Surg 2005; 55(6):665–671

Verma H, Ktenidis K, George RK, Tripathi R. Vacuum-assisted closure therapy for vascular graft infection (Szilagyi grade III) in the groin-a 10-year multi-center experience. Int Wound J. 2015; 12(3):317–321

Wackenfors A, Sjögren J, Gustafsson R, Algotsson L, Ingemansson R, Malmsjö M. Effects of vacuum-assisted closure therapy on inguinal wound edge microvascular blood flow. Wound Repair Regen. 2004; 12(6):600–606

5 Local Anesthetics and Common Nerve Blocks

Pablo Monedero, Ismael González, Jesús Olivas

Abstract

A considerable number of plastic surgery procedures are done under local anesthesia with or without sedation; hence knowledge of their mechanism of action, dosages, and potential complications is of utmost relevance. Local anesthetics (LAs) block nerve conduction by binding to a modulated receptor located on the interior of the sodium channel, which prevents the increase in membrane permeability to sodium ions that would normally lead to a nerve impulse. The more potent and longer-acting LAs are more lipid soluble and show increased protein binding and less systemic absorption, but at the expense of having a higher potential for systemic toxicity. Even though systemic toxicity from LAs is an uncommon occurrence, when it occurs it should be managed promptly and effectively with supportive measures and intravenous (IV) administration of 20% lipid emulsion. LAs are used for field or regional blocks. Regional blocks supply anesthesia to a large territory with a comparatively small quantity of LA, avoiding the complications of general anesthesia and the systemic toxicity of large volumes of LA. Regional blocks in the face and limbs can be performed easily and effectively for a number of different procedures, such as wound closure, skin cancer excision and flap reconstruction, and nerve entrapment syndromes. This chapter describes the main aspects of the physiology of LAs and their use in the clinical setting, along with a technical description of the main blocks used in plastic surgery.

Keywords: local anesthetics, maximum dose, regional block, sedation, toxicity

5.1 Introduction

The first local anesthetic (LA), cocaine, was isolated from leaves of the coca plant in 1860. The medicinal use of coca was first investigated and described by Freud in 1884. Koller, an Austrian ophthalmologist, introduced the use of cocaine as a topical anesthetic for ophthalmologic procedures, and subsequently the clinical application of cocaine became widespread. The development of organic chemistry enabled the synthesis of procaine, another ester LA, analogue of cocaine, in 1905. In the 1940s lidocaine, the first amide LA, was introduced with fewer undesirable effects and deeper anesthesia than procaine. Bupivacaine was synthesized in 1957 with a longer duration of action. Levobupivacaine and ropivacaine were later introduced to reduce cardiac toxicity.

5.2 Basic Science

LAs block the generation and propagation of electrical impulses in nerves and other electrically excitable tissue. The nerve's action potential must be reduced by at least 50% before measurable loss of function is observed. Generation of action potentials primarily results from the activation of voltage-gated sodium channels (v-gSCs), the key target of LA activity. These channels are protein structures spanning the bilayer lipid membrane composed of structural elements, an aqueous pore, and voltage-sensing elements that control passage of ions through the pore. LAs act on the v-gSCs by modification of the lipid membrane surrounding them and by direct interaction with their protein structure. Binding sites to LAs are located on the intracellular side of the v-gSCs and possess stereoselectivity with preference for the R isomers, although S isomers have nearly equal efficacy with less potential for systemic toxicity. Depending on pK_a and environmental pH, LAs exist both as a lipid-soluble neutral form and as a hydrophilic charged form, with the ionized cationic form being clearly more potent. LAs must penetrate the lipid-rich nerve sheaths and cell membrane in order to reach the v-gSC. The binding site of LAs is located inside the channel pore and is not readily reachable from the extracellular side; therefore, in order to reach their binding site, LAs must first reach the intracellular space by crossing the nerve's membrane and diffusing through the lipid bilayer. Consequently, the potency of each LA is closely related to its lipid solubility and is dependent on pH. Most LAs have pK_a values slightly higher than physiologic pH. Alkalinization by addition of sodium bicarbonate to LA solutions increases their pH and shifts the equilibrium in favor of the neutral base forms, which facilitates translocation of the LA into the cytoplasm.

Nerve fibers show differences in susceptibility to LA blockade based on size, myelination, and length of fiber exposed to LA. In addition, a differential pattern of sensory block after application of LA to a peripheral nerve is observed. Temperature sensation is lost first, followed by sharp pain, and finally light touch. The quality of nerve blockade is determined not only by the potency of the individual LA but also by its concentration and volume. The latter is important because a sufficient length of axon must be blocked in order to prevent regeneration of the impulse in the adjacent node of Ranvier.

The onset of action of LAs depends on the route of administration and dosage (e.g., concentration). In peripheral nerve blocks (PNBs) where LA is injected in the vicinity of the target nerve(s), the amount of drug that reaches such nerve(s) will depend on diffusion of the drug and the proximity of injection. For a given route of administration, increasing the concentration can accelerate onset.

The duration of action of LAs is determined primarily by their protein binding. LAs with a high affinity for protein remain bound to the nerve membrane for longer periods of time. In other words, the higher the affinity for Na$^+$ channels binding, the longer the duration of the LA. Furthermore, duration of action is also influenced by the rate of vascular uptake of LA from the injection site.

5.3 Classification of Local Anesthetics

All currently available LAs consist of a lipophilic phenyl ring and a hydrophobic tertiary amine. In general, with increasing length of the carbon backbone of the tertiary amine, LAs exhibit greater lipid solubility, protein binding, potency, and duration of action. Based on the type of chemical bond, amide or ester, linking the phenyl ring with the tertiary amine, LAs are classified as amino-amides (articaine, bupivacaine, lidocaine, prilocaine, ropivacaine) or amino-esters (cocaine, chloroprocaine, procaine, tetracaine). Amide and ester LAs differ in their chemical stability, metabolism, and allergic potential. Amides are extremely stable, whereas esters are relatively unstable, particularly in neutral or alkaline solution. Amide compounds undergo enzymatic degradation in the liver, whereas ester compounds are hydrolyzed by plasmatic esterase enzymes. The metabolites of esters include p-aminobenzoic acid (PABA), which can occasionally induce allergic reactions. Allergies to amides are very rare.

Based on their chiral form, LAs are classified as single enantiomers or racemic mixtures. Enantiomers consist of two stereoisomers (left/sinister/S or right/dexter/R) that are mirror images of each other with respect to a specific chiral center. A racemic mixture contains equal amounts of the two enantiomers. The two forms possess different pharmacological properties that are of clinical importance. All currently available LAs are racemic mixtures, with the exception of lidocaine (achiral), levobupivacaine (S), and ropivacaine (S). Levobupivacaine's potency and efficacy are comparable to those of bupivacaine, but it has significantly less cardiac and central nervous system (CNS) toxicity, likely due to reduced affinity for subtypes of Na$^+$ channels expressed in brain and cardiac tissues.

5.4 Pharmacology

▶Table 5.1 and ▶Table 5.2 give an overview of the physicochemical properties, clinical use, and dosing of each agent. Recommended maximum doses given here relate to normal conditions (e.g., healthy individual weighing 70 kg). However, the dose must be tailored individually, depending on body weight and the patient's condition; reduced clearance of LAs associated with renal, hepatic, and cardiac diseases is the most important reason for lowering the dose of anesthetic in repeated or continuous administrations. Recommended maximum doses are orientative and do not constitute an absolute maximum dose because they are not evidence based. Furthermore, recommended maximum doses may vary according to injection technique, injection site (e.g., regions of high absorption), or single versus protracted injection. The common occurrence of CNS toxicity symptoms following infiltration of large volumes of lidocaine led to the recommendation of just 200 mg as the maximum dose. Epinephrine in concentrations of 2.5 to 5 µg/mL should be added to the LA solution when large doses are required, provided that there are no contraindications for the use of epinephrine.

The time to resolution of PNBs is extremely variable for different blocks, and between patients, even when all block-related factors are equal. When

Table 5.1 Physicochemical properties of selected local anesthetics

Local anesthetic	pK_a	Protein bound (%)	Relative potency for peripheral nerve block	Half-life (hours)
Lidocaine	7.9	64	1	1.6
Mepivacaine	7.6	77	2.6	1.9
Bupivacaine	8.1	95	3.6	3.5
Articaine	7.8	94	2.8	1
Ropivacaine	8.1	94	3.6	1.9
Chloroprocaine	8.7	6	0.5	0.1
Tetracaine	8.5	94	4	N/A

Table 5.2 Clinical use and recommended dosages of selected local anesthetics for local infiltration

Local anesthetic	Concentration (%)	Onset	Duration (hours)	Maximum single dose (mg)	Maximum dose with epinephrine (mg)
Articaine	4	Fast	1–2	400	500
Bupivacaine	0.25	Slow	2–8	175	225
Levobupivacaine	0.25–0.5	Slow	4–12	150	N/A
Lidocaine	0.5–2	Fast	1–3	300	500
Mepivacaine	0.5–2	Fast	2–4	400	500
Ropivacaine	0.5–1.5	Slow	5–8	250	N/A
Chloroprocaine	1–2	Fast	0.5–1	800	1,000
Tetracaine	0.5–2	Fast	1–3	20	N/A

patients are discharged from the operating area or from the hospital prior to complete resolution of the block, precautions should be taken to avoid injury to an insensitive limb and falls. Equipment such as slings, protective padding, and crutches may be needed. The duration of PNBs of short-acting agents, such as procaine and chloroprocaine, ranges from 30 to 60 minutes, whereas long-acting agents, such as bupivacaine and tetracaine, may remain active for nearly 10 hours. The rate of vascular uptake significantly affects LA duration of action because LAs can exert their anesthetic effect only as long as they remain at the site of deposition. Vasoconstriction slows the rate of vascular absorption and thus prolongs the duration of action. For this purpose, vasoconstrictive agents, such as epinephrine, are frequently added to LAs to increase duration. The prolongation of nerve block with vasoconstrictors is more prominent with LAs of intermediate duration, such as lidocaine and prilocaine, than with longer-acting agents, such as bupivacaine, possibly because the effect of long-acting LAs outlasts that of vasoconstrictors.

Caution
Getting the dose right
Local anesthetic concentration is expressed in percentage, so that
1% solution = 1 g of anesthetic in 100 mL of solution = 10 mg/mL
Hence, if the maximum recommended dose of, for example, lidocaine is 300 mg, then 30 mL of 1% solution would be the maximum to administer.

5.5 Toxicity and Complications of Local Anesthetics

Toxicity of LAs is the limiting factor in their clinical use. LAs are relatively safe if administered appropriately; however, significant systemic or localized toxicity can result from unintended intravascular or intraneural injection or if excessive doses are administered resulting in major systemic absorption. When epinephrine is added to LAs, intravascular injection will result in tachycardia and hypertension, which are useful signs that inadvertent intravascular injection has occurred. Rapid uptake of LA injected into a vascular area may also lead to systemic toxicity, which generally occurs immediately, but may become apparent > 10 minutes after injection.

Systemic toxicity manifests primarily in the cardiovascular and central nervous systems. The signs and symptoms of LA toxicity range from mild symptoms (ringing in the ears, metallic taste, tingling of the lips, and agitation) to severe neurologic (seizures) and cardiovascular signs (hypertension, hypotension, tachycardia, bradycardia, ventricular arrhythmias, and cardiac arrest).

The effect of LAs on the cardiovascular system is dual: by directly affecting cardiac myocytes and peripheral vascular smooth muscle cells, and indirectly by their action on the autonomic nervous system. The more potent, lipophilic LAs, such as bupivacaine, tetracaine, and etidocaine, are more cardiotoxic than the less lipophilic agents, such as procaine, prilocaine, and lidocaine

LAs readily cross the blood–brain barrier and generalized CNS toxicity may occur from systemic absorption or direct vascular injection. LAs' potential for generalized CNS toxicity approximately parallels their action potential blocking potency. Signs of generalized CNS toxicity are dose dependent, with low doses producing CNS depression, and higher doses resulting in CNS excitation and seizures. Increasing doses of LAs produce light-headedness, tinnitus, and tongue numbness, before the appearance of seizures, unconsciousness, and ultimately respiratory arrest and cardiovascular depression with heart arrest.

Treatment of LA systemic toxicity consists of IV administration of 20% lipid emulsion (1.5 mL/kg bolus, followed by 0.25 mL/kg/min infusion), together with supportive airway and hemodynamic management. Calcium channel blockers and β-blockers should be avoided; vasopressin is not recommended and initial doses of epinephrine should be small (10–100 µg IV). If there is no clinical improvement after 30 minutes, the bolus dose of lipid emulsion 1.5 mL/kg should be repeated and the continuous infusion increased to 0.5 mL/kg/min.

5.6 Allergic Reactions

Most adverse reactions to LAs are nonallergic and include psychomotor responses related to anxiety, sympathetic stimulation from pain or epinephrine, or toxic effects attributable to heightened sensitivity to known properties of the drug. However, two different types of allergic reactions have been described: allergic contact dermatitis and urticaria–anaphylaxis. Allergic contact dermatitis (type IV hypersensitivity) produces delayed swelling at the site of injection within 72 hours. Urticaria, anaphylaxis, and immediate allergic reactions (type I hypersensitivity), which typically begin within 1 hour of drug administration, are described in only a handful of case reports. Patients with suspected allergic reactions to LAs should be evaluated because most can tolerate other LA agents. An approach to safely precluding these reactions includes skin testing and controlled drug challenge.

5.6.1 Nerve Injury

Peripheral nerve injury is rare with PNBs. Related symptoms are transient, lasting days to months. Major complications resulting in permanent (> 6 months) nerve damage range between 0.015 and 0.09%. Most nerve injuries are believed to occur secondary to intraneural injection, which can be minimized if injection is halted and the needle withdrawn if undue resistance to injection is encountered or if the patient feels sharp pain or paresthesias. Additional risk factors for nerve injury include preexisting nerve pathology (including diabetes) and the use of standard longer-beveled needles. Symptoms of nerve injury are primarily sensory (pain, tingling, or paresthesia), though they may include a combination of motor and sensory deficits depending on the nerve involved and the severity of injury. Most symptoms resolve within 6 months; if symptoms are either severe or persistent, the patient should be referred to a neurologist.

5.6.2 Hematoma

Inadvertent puncture of nearby vascular structures can lead to perineural hematoma. It is prudent to avoid performing PNBs in patients with an abnormal coagulation status in anatomical locations in which application of pressure to the puncture site is not possible. The vast majority of hematomas can be controlled by directly pressing on the puncture site; rarely, surgical decompression may be required.

5.7 Adjuvants

Although many drugs have been added to LAs with the aim of decreasing onset time, increasing duration, increasing block density, or decreasing toxicity, they are not universally used because their side effects are felt to outweigh their benefits. The limited available evidence regarding potential adjuvants includes epinephrine, sodium bicarbonate, fentanyl, dexamethasone, and α2-agonists. Epinephrine is the most common vasoconstrictor added to PNBs, typically at a concentration of 1:200,000 to 1:400,000. It is used both to indicate rapid vascular uptake (e.g., during inadvertent intravascular injection an increase in heart rate of ≥ 20 bpm and/or an increase in systolic blood pressure ≥ 15 mm Hg after a dose of 15 µg of epinephrine should raise a suspicion of intravascular injection) and to decrease the LA's absorption, which may in turn reduce potential toxicity (in vascular areas) and prolong duration of the block. Side effects of epinephrine include tachycardia and a potential for ischemia to nerves and other tissues due to vasoconstriction. Consequently, in patients at risk of cardiac ischemia or those with possibly decreased perineural blood flow (e.g., postchemotherapy, diabetes, or vascular disease), it is reasonable to use lower concentrations (1:400,000). Sodium bicarbonate is used to reduce onset time of the LA effect. The quicker onset is most evident in LAs with commercially added epinephrine—which are formulated at a lower pH—but is often not of clinical significance. The addition of fentanyl or morphine to PNBs does not provide a clear clinical benefit. The addition of dexamethasone to LAs in PNBs was associated with longer duration of action in several trials. The addition of clonidine to LA for PNB prolongs the duration of sensory and motor blockade, albeit at the expense of a higher risk of hypotension, bradycardia, and sedation.

5.7.1 Benzodiazepines

Benzodiazepines (BDZs) enhance the effect of the neurotransmitter γ-aminobutyric acid (GABA) at the $GABA_A$ receptor, resulting in sedative, hypnotic, anxiolytic, anticonvulsant, and muscle relaxant properties. Used as systemic adjuvants to PNB, BDZs reduce anxiety and improve patient cooperation. According to their half-life, BDZs are categorized as short (midazolam, tetrazepam, or triazolam), intermediate (alprazolam, chlordiazepoxide, lorazepam, or lormetazepam), or long-acting (bromazepam, clonazepam, clorazepate, diazepam, or flunitrazepam).

BDZs are safe and effective for short-term use, although cognitive impairment and paradoxical effects, such as agitation, panic, aggression, or behavioral disinhibition occasionally occur. Low doses of short or intermediate BDZs are best titrated to optimize sedative effects.

BDZ overdose produces CNS depression with impaired balance, ataxia, and slurred speech. Severe symptoms include coma and respiratory depression. Supportive care is the mainstay of treatment of BDZ overdose. There is an antidote, flumazenil, which can be used to reverse excessive sedation of BDZs.

5.8 Essential Regional Blocks for Plastic Surgery

Regional nerve blocks provide anesthesia to a relatively large territory with small volumes of LA, thus avoiding potential complications of general anesthesia and the systemic toxicity associated with the administration of large volumes of LA. In addition, nerve blocks minimize patient discomfort, allowing a number of different procedures, such as local flaps in the face and limbs, debridement and suture of complex wounds, injection of botulinum toxin and limb surgery, with fast recovery. Herein we will describe the anatomy of cutaneous innervation of the face, scalp, ear, hand and wrist, and ankle and foot, followed by the technique of blocking the main nerves supplying these areas.

5.8.1 Face

The trigeminal nerve carries sensory information from the face through its three major branches: the ophthalmic nerve (V1), the maxillary nerve (V2), and the mandibular nerve (V3) (▶ Fig. 5.1). Whereas V1 and V2 are purely sensitive, V3 also carries motor axons that control muscles involved in biting and swallowing. The terminal branches of these nerves, namely supraorbital, supratrochlear (V1), infraorbital (V2), and mental nerve (V3), innervate the face and part of the scalp.

To successfully anesthetize their different territories, the nerves supplying the face should be located at the points where they exit the skull, which corresponds roughly with a mid-pupillary line going from the forehead to the mandible (▶Fig. 5.1). In general, only 2–3 mL of LA are enough to anesthetize a given territory, always remembering to inject in the vicinity of the nerve and aspirate first to prevent intravascular injection.

Supraorbital and Supratrochlear Nerves (V1)

The frontal nerve, a branch of the ophthalmic nerve, divides into the supraorbital and supratrochlear nerves. The former emerges from the supraorbital notch, whereas the latter exits the skull at a point just lateral to the bridge of the nose. Together these nerves supply the forehead and parietal scalp. To block these nerves, the supraorbital notch is first identified by palpation, and the needle is inserted pointing medially, injecting 2–3 mL of anesthetic. The needle is then advanced parallel to the brow toward the glabella, where another 2 mL are injected. Finally, the whole area is gently massaged to evenly distribute the anesthetic and favor its penetration

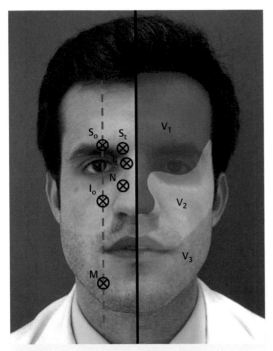

Fig. 5.1 Sensory innervation of the face. *Right half* showing cutaneous territories of trigeminal nerve divisions V1, V2, and V3. *Left half* depicting midpupillary line in red and location of supraorbital (S_o), supratrochlear (S_T), infratrochlear (I_T), external nasal (N), infraorbital (I_o), and mental (M) nerves.

into the nerve. If the glabellar area or the bridge or dorsum of the nose is not adequately numbed, then the infratrochlear nerve can be blocked by injecting 0.5 mL of LA at the junction of the nose with the medial canthus of the eye.

Infraorbital Nerve (V2)

The infraorbital nerve branches off the maxillary division of the trigeminal nerve and emerges onto the face at the infraorbital foramen, after which it divides into the palpebral, nasal, and labial branches. It can be blocked percutaneously or intraorally, with the latter approach being preferred due to reduced patient discomfort because it avoids puncturing the cheek, which is far more sensitive than the oral mucosa. A successful infraorbital block should provide adequate anesthesia to the lower eyelid, cheek, lateral nose, upper lip, and buccal gingivae of the maxillary anterior teeth and premolars. To begin, topical anesthetic can be applied to the mucosa at the level of the first superior premolar. With the patient looking straight ahead, the infraorbital foramen is located approximately 1 cm inferior to the ridge in the midpupillary line, leaving the third finger of the nondominant hand in place. Next, the upper lip is raised and the needle inserted between the first and second premolars (▶Fig. 5.2) and advanced. approximately 15 mm toward the foramen, making sure not to puncture the nerve. Two to three mL of LA are injected outside the foramen, and the area is gently massaged to allow spreading of the anesthetic. For procedures involving the upper lip and nasal ala, supplementary anesthesia may be necessary in some patients and can be provided by blocking the external nasal nerve (located between the nasal bone and the upper lateral cartilage) and maxillary frenulum, with approximately 0.5 mL of LA for each one.

Mental Nerve (V3)

The mental nerve branches off the inferior alveolar nerve and exits the mandible through the mental foramen to supply the chin and lower lip as well as the buccal gingivae of the mandibular anterior teeth and premolars.

Like the infraorbital nerve, the mental nerve can be blocked percutaneously or intraorally, with the latter being preferred for the same reasons as already described. The needle is inserted in the mucobuccal fold between the apices of the first and second premolars and advanced toward the mental

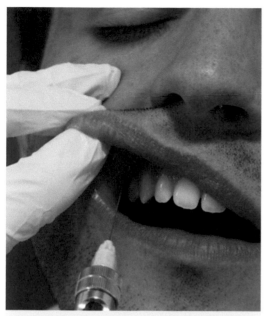

Fig. 5.2 Infraorbital nerve block, intraoral approach.

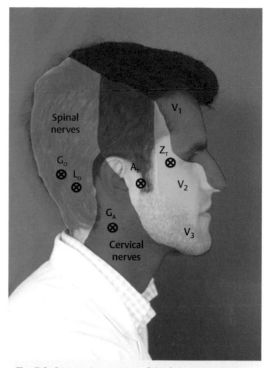

Fig. 5.3 Sensory innervation of the face and scalp, including trigeminal, cervical, and spinal nerve contributions. A_T, auriculotemporal nerve; G_A, greater auricular nerve; G_O, greater occipital nerve; L_O, lesser occipital nerve; Z_T, zygomaticotemporal nerve.

foramen, where 2–3 mL of LA are injected, followed by gentle massage to the area. If the lower lip or buccal gingivae are not completely numbed, applying LA into the mandibular frenulum is an option.

5.8.2 Scalp

SCALP is an acronym referring to its different layers, from superficial to deep, as follows:

S: Skin.

C: Connective tissue. This layer of adipose and connective tissue contains the main vessels and nerves supplying the scalp and is therefore where the LA should be delivered, always avoiding intravascular injection.

A: Aponeurosis (galea aponeurotica). The galea aponeurotica connects the frontalis muscle and the temporoparietal fascia anteriorly with the occipitalis muscle posteriorly.

L: Loose areolar connective tissue. This tissue provides a separation plane (e.g., subgaleal) for surgical flaps and traumatic avulsions.

P: Pericranium. This layer corresponds to the periosteum of the skull.

The cutaneous innervation of the scalp is supplied by the supratrochlear and supraorbital nerves (already described), the zygomaticotemporal (Zt) nerve, the auriculotemporal (At)

nerve, and the greater and lesser occipital nerves (G_O and L_O) (▶ Fig. 5.3):

Zygomaticotemporal Nerve

The Zt nerve is a terminal branch of the zygomatic nerve, which originates from the second division of the trigeminal nerve. The Zt nerve supplies a small area of the temporal scalp and the temple area. It is blocked by injecting 2–3 mL of LA in the concave surface of the posterior lateral orbital rim.

Auriculotemporal Nerve

The auriculotemporal nerve emerges from the posterior trunk of the mandibular nerve and supplies the temporal scalp. It is blocked by injecting 1–2 mL of LA approximately 1–2 cm anterior to the tragus.

Greater and Lesser Occipital Nerves

The G_O and L_O originate from the medial branch of the dorsal ramus of the second spinal nerve and supply all the occipital and part of the parietal scalp. They can be located and blocked in a line from the mastoid to the occipital protuberance, where the G_o is found at the junction of the lateral three quarters with the internal one quarter and L_o at the line's midpoint (▶Fig. 5.4).

5.8.3 Ear

The cutaneous innervation of the ear is complex. Several nerves contribute to it, including the auriculotemporal, greater auricular, and lesser occipital nerves. The conchal region is supplied by Arnold's nerve (branch of the vagus nerve) and sensory branches of the facial nerve, which make it a difficult area to anesthetize because these nerves cannot be blocked, and injections here are very painful and may lead to cartilage deformation (▶Fig. 5.5). The ear is usually anesthetized by a ring block, always making sure to avoid cartilaginous injections. For ear lobe procedures, the greater auricular nerve can be blocked by injecting 2 mL of LA subcutaneously into the posterior border of the sternocleidomastoid muscle, 2–3 cm inferior to the mastoid tip.

5.8.4 Hand and Wrist

The distal branches of the median, ulnar, and radial nerves provide cutaneous innervation to the hand and wrist (▶Fig. 5.6 and ▶Fig. 5.7). In the palm, the median and ulnar nerves divide into the common palmar digital nerves, which further subdivide into the proper palmar digital nerves running on each side of the fingers in association with the palmar digital arteries. The superficial branch of the radial nerve supplies the dorsum of the hand from the thumb to the radial half of the ring finger (▶Fig. 5.7).

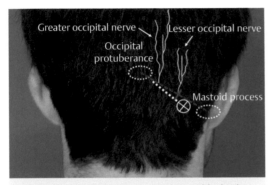

Fig. 5.4 Greater and lesser occipital nerve block. The red dotted line indicates the line from the mastoid process to the occipital protuberance, with its lateral and medial halves. The encircled *x* depicts the needle insertion point, and the white dotted line the site of anesthetic infiltration.

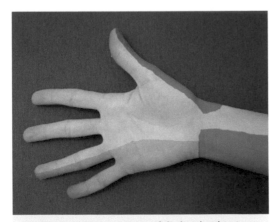

Fig. 5.6 Sensitive innervation of the hand, volar view. *Yellow*, median nerve; *green*, ulnar nerve; *red*, radial nerve; *pink*, medial antebrachial cutaneous nerve; *cyan*, lateral antebrachial cutaneous nerve.

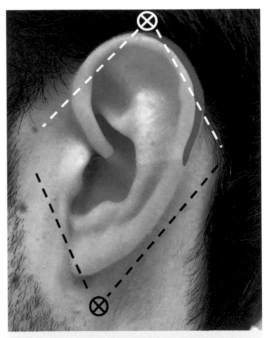

Fig. 5.5 Sensory innervation of the ear. *Green*, auriculotemporal nerve; *red*, lesser occipital nerve; *blue*, greater auricular nerve; *orange*, inferior branch of Arnold's nerve (from the vagus nerve) and the sensory branch of the facial nerve. The ring block technique for the ear. Encircled *x* indicates needle insertion points, and the dotted lines the site of anesthetic infiltration.

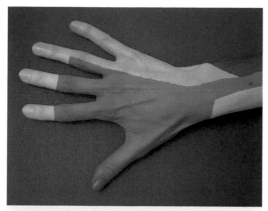

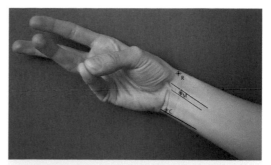

Fig. 5.8 Nerve blocks to the hand showing needle insertion points for the median (M), ulnar (C), and radial (R) nerves.

Fig. 5.7 Sensory innervation of the hand, dorsal view. *Yellow*, median nerve; *green*, ulnar nerve; *red*, radial nerve; *pink*, medial antebrachial cutaneous nerve; *cyan*, lateral antebrachial cutaneous nerve.

5.9 Median Nerve Block

In the wrist, the median nerve is located between the tendons of the flexor carpi radialis and palmaris longus and deep to the transverse carpal ligament. Approximately 3 cm proximal to the flexor retinaculum, the median nerve gives off a palmar cutaneous branch that supplies the thenar skin. To block the median nerve, the needle is inserted approximately 1.5 cm proximal to the wrist flexion crease, on the radial border of the palmaris longus (PL), at a 45-degree angle and pointing toward the index finger (▶ Fig. 5.8 and ▶ Fig. 5.9). The needle is then advanced distally until the transverse carpal ligament is penetrated, and 3–5 mL of LA are slowly injected. If paresthesias appear, the needle must be withdrawn a few millimeters prior to injection. Finally, 2 mL of LA are injected above the carpal ligament to block the palmar branch.

5.9.1 Ulnar Nerve Block

At the wrist, the ulnar nerve runs slightly dorsal and medial to the tendon of the flexor carpi ulnaris, being covered only by skin and fascia. It then enters Guyon's canal, where it divides into a superficial sensory branch and a deep motor branch. The palmar cutaneous branch arises from 4–5 cm proximal to the pisiform. The ulnar nerve can be anesthetized through a volar or medial (ulnar) approach. In the volar approach, the needle is inserted on the radial border of flexor carpi ulnaris tendon, whereas in the medial it is introduced in a medial to lateral direction beneath the flexor

carpi ulnaris just proximal to the styloid process of the ulna (▶ Fig. 5.8 and ▶ Fig. 5.9). For both, 2–4 mL of LA are injected, provided that no paresthesias are elicited and that the ulnar artery has not been entered. The dorsal cutaneous branch of the ulnar nerve arises approximately 5–6 cm proximal to the wrist crease and can be blocked by injecting 2 mL of LA at this point dorsal to the flexor carpi ulnaris.

5.9.2 Radial Nerve Block

In the distal forearm, the superficial (sensory) branch of the radial nerve exits between the brachioradialis and the extensor carpi radialis longus about 8–10 cm proximal to the radial styloid. Shortly after, the nerve divides into several branches with a relatively unpredictable distribution, which is why the radial nerve block is considered a field block requiring larger volumes of LA to obtain adequate anesthesia. The needle is inserted 1 cm proximal to the radial styloid in a radial-to-ulnar direction, and 4 mL of LA are injected in the subcutaneous plane. The needle is then reoriented as necessary to create a small lump of anesthetic over the dorsoradial aspect of the wrist.

5.9.3 Digital Nerve Block

Fingers can be blocked through a volar or dorsal approach, with the latter being less painful and therefore better tolerated by the patient. For a volar block, the needle is inserted on each side of the A1 pulley of the corresponding finger, injecting 2 mL of LA per side. Conversely, the dorsal approach is performed with the hand in pronation by inserting the needle on each side

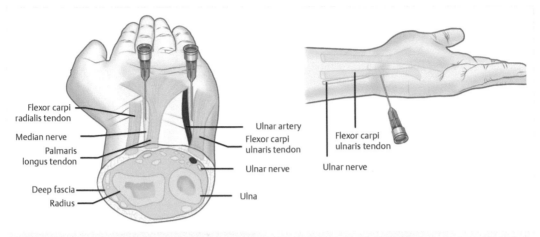

Fig. 5.9 Technique for median and ulnar nerve wrist block.

of the finger just distal to the metacarpophalangeal joint and injecting 2 mL of LA (with or without epinephrine). Another 2 mL of anesthetic are then injected dorsally to block the dorsal branches. This technique can be equally applied for toes.

Ankle and Foot

The distal branches of the tibial, peroneal, sural, and saphenous nerves provide cutaneous innervation to the foot and ankle. The plantar surface of the foot is innervated by the three distal branches of the tibial nerve (e.g., the medial plantar nerve, lateral plantar nerve, and medial calcaneal nerve), the sural nerve, and the saphenous nerve (▶ Fig. 5.10). The superficial branch of the peroneal nerve supplies the dorsal aspect of the foot and the anterolateral side of the leg, except for the first web space, which is innervated by the deep peroneal nerve. The posterolateral side of the leg and the lateral aspect of the fifth toe are supplied by the sural nerve, whereas the saphenous nerve innervates the medial aspect of the leg and foot (▶ Fig. 5.11).

Tibial Nerve

The tibial nerve and the posterior tibial artery run just anterior to the Achilles tendon before entering the tarsal tunnel, where the nerve runs posterior to the artery between the tendons of the flexor digitorum longus and flexor hallucis longus muscles.

With the patient in the supine position, the medial malleolus and the medial edge of the Achilles tendon are identified by palpation. The needle is inserted just medial to the tendon and advanced toward the tibial malleolus, injecting approximately 5 mL of LA in divided doses with frequent aspirations.

Saphenous Nerve

At the ankle, the saphenous nerve can be easily and effectively blocked by injecting 5 mL of LA in the subcutaneous tissue anterior to the medial malleolus and along the intermalleolar line.

Superficial Peroneal Nerve

This nerve runs in the subcutaneous tissue anterior to the lateral malleolus. Like the saphenous nerve, the superficial peroneal is blocked by a subcutaneous injection of 5 mL of LA in the tibial ridge along the intermalleolar line directed toward the fifth toe. Both the saphenous and the superficial peroneal nerve can be blocked from a single entry point.

Deep Peroneal Nerve

The deep peroneal nerve travels in association with the dorsalis pedis artery between the tendons of the extensor hallucis longus and the extensor digitorum longus to provide sensory innervation to the first web space. The patient is

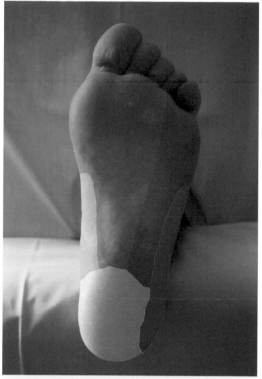

Fig. 5.10 Sensory innervation of the foot, plantar view. *Green*, saphenous nerve; *red*, sural nerve; *purple*, medial plantar nerve; *blue violet*, lateral plantar nerve; *yellow*, medial calcaneal nerve.

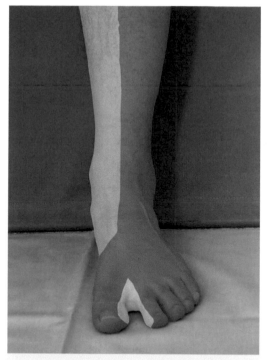

Fig. 5.11 Sensory innervation of the foot, dorsal view. *Green*, saphenous nerve; *red*, sural nerve; *purple*, superficial peroneal nerve; *yellow*, deep peroneal nerve.

asked to extend the toes in order to identify the tendons and the needle is then inserted deep between the extensor hallucis longus and the extensor digitorum longus, injecting 5 mL of LA.

Sural Nerve

The sural nerve runs in the subcutaneous plane between the lateral malleolus and the Achilles tendon, where injection of approximately 5 mL of LA results in effective anesthesia of the nerve's distal territory.

5.10 Conclusions

The use of LA is a well-established, effective, and safe method of delivering anesthesia. LA may be used alone for minor surgical procedures, or in combination with general anesthesia or intravenous sedation and analgesia for more complex, lengthy surgeries. LAs are chosen according to onset of action, duration of action, degree of motor blockade, and toxicity, all of which are influenced by the dosage and concentration of the LA as well as by the volume of the injection. The concentration of LA determines the rate of diffusion into the nerve, with higher concentrations providing more rapid onset of nerve block. LAs can be combined to decrease onset time while providing a longer duration of analgesia; however, such mixtures may lead to unpredictable blockade characteristics. Lidocaine and mepivacaine are typical examples of LAs with short duration of action (and generally quicker onset), whereas bupivacaine, levobupivacaine, and ropivacaine are examples of longer-acting agents. The recently approved formulation of slow-release liposomal bupivacaine has demonstrated the ability to provide prolonged analgesia, maintain a high safety profile in therapeutic doses, and decrease opioid requirements when compared with placebo in local infiltration applications for up to 24 hours.

Regional blocks are relatively easy and effective methods of providing anesthesia to a large territory with a comparatively small amount of anesthetic. These techniques are of great use for either emergency or elective procedures, precluding the need for sedation or other forms of deeper anesthesia in a number of cases. Knowledge of the regional anatomy and correct technique are paramount to avoid complications, such as intravascular injection, which can induce systemic toxicity of LA and intraneural injection, which may lead to permanent nerve damage.

5.11 Key Points

- Block duration is related to lipid solubility, the degree of vascularity of the tissue, and the presence of vasoconstrictors that prevent vascular uptake.
- Systemic toxicity has been reported despite negative aspiration for blood and the use of recommended dosages, so constant vigilance and preparation for treatment are essential.
- Bupivacaine has fallen out of favor due to its potential for serious toxicity and the availability of ropivacaine, which has a slightly decreased duration of action than bupivacaine but with an improved safety profile.
- Regional blocks of the face, scalp, and limbs provide anesthesia to a predictable anatomical territory, allowing a number of emergency and elective procedures, such as wound closure, scar revision, skin cancer excision, and local flap/graft reconstruction.
- Aspiration prior to injection, and needle withdrawal when paresthesias are elicited upon insertion, are key to preventing two of the most serious, yet infrequent, complications of regional blocks, namely intravascular and intraneural injection.

Recommended Readings

Ahlstrom KK, Frodel JL. Local anesthetics for facial plastic procedures. Otolaryngol Clin North Am. 2002; 35(1):29–53, v–vi

Becker DE, Reed KL. Local anesthetics: review of pharmacological considerations. Anesth Prog. 2012; 59(2):90–101, quiz 102–103

Chowdhry S, Seidenstricker L, Cooney DS, Hazani R, Wilhelmi BJ. Do not use epinephrine in digital blocks: myth or truth?

Part II. A retrospective review of 1111 cases. Plast Reconstr Surg. 2010; 126(6):2031–2034

Davies T, Karanovic S, Shergill B. Essential regional nerve blocks for the dermatologist: Part 1. Clin Exp Dermatol. 2014; 39(7):777–784

Davies T, Karanovic S, Shergill B. Essential regional nerve blocks for the dermatologist: Part 2. Clin Exp Dermatol. 2014; 39(8):861–867

Dickerson DM, Apfelbaum JL. Local anesthetic systemic toxicity. Aesthet Surg J. 2014; 34(7):1111–1119

Drake RL, Vogl AW, Mitchell AWM. Gray's Anatomy for Students. 3rd ed. Philadelphia, PA: Churchill Livingstone, Elsevier; 2014

Gadsden J. NYSORA local anaesthetics: clinical pharmacology and rational selection. 2013. http://tinyurl.com/hhlmw4k

Halldin CB, Paoli J, Sandberg C, Gonzalez H, Wennberg AM. Nerve blocks enable adequate pain relief during topical photodynamic therapy of field cancerization on the forehead and scalp. Br J Dermatol. 2009; 160(4):795–800

Harmon D, Barrett J, Loughnane F. Peripheral Nerve Blocks and Peri-Operative Pain Relief. 2nd ed. London: Saunders, Elsevier; 2011

Kaweski S; Plastic Surgery Educational Foundation Technology Assessment Committee. Topical anesthetic creams. Plast Reconstr Surg. 2008; 121(6):2161–2165

Lin Y, Liu S. Local Anesthetics. In: Barash PG, Cullen BF, Stoelting RK, Cahalan M, Stock C, eds. Clinical Anesthesia. 7th ed. Philadelphia, PA: Lippincott Williams & Wilkins; 2013:561–582

Lynch MT, Syverud SA, Schwab RA, Jenkins JM, Edlich R. Comparison of intraoral and percutaneous approaches for infraorbital nerve block. Acad Emerg Med. 1994; 1(6):514–519

Man D, Podichetty VK. Lipid rescue in resuscitation of local anesthetic-induced cardiac arrest in aesthetic surgery. Plast Reconstr Surg. 2010; 125(6):257e–259e

Neal JM, Mulroy MF, Weinberg GL; American Society of Regional Anesthesia and Pain Medicine. American Society of Regional Anesthesia and Pain Medicine checklist for managing local anesthetic systemic toxicity: 2012 version. Reg Anesth Pain Med. 2012; 37(1):16–18

Netter FH. Atlas of Human Anatomy. 5th ed. Amsterdam, Netherlands: Elsevier; 2010

Porter CJ, Frizelle FA. Use of local anaesthetic agents among New Zealand plastic surgeons—their practices and philosophies. Med Sci Monit. 2000; 6(1):194–197

Rosenberg PH, Veering BT, Urmey WF. Maximum recommended doses of local anesthetics: a multifactorial concept. Reg Anesth Pain Med 2004; 29(6):564–575, discussion 524

Schatz M. Allergic reactions to local anaesthetics. 2015. http://tinyurl.com/j7aarl7

Snoeck M. Articaine: a review of its use for local and regional anesthesia. Local Reg Anesth 2012; 5:23–33

Suzuki S, Koköfer A, Gerner P. Local anesthetics. In: Hemmings HC, Jr., Egan TD, eds. Pharmacology and Physiology for Anesthesia. Amsterdam, Netherlands; Elsevier; 2012:291–308

Uskova A, O'Connor JE. Liposomal bupivacaine for regional anesthesia. Curr Opin Anaesthesiol. 2015; 28(5):593–597

Weinberg GL. Lipid emulsion infusion: resuscitation for local anesthetic and other drug overdose. Anesthesiology. 2012; 117(1):180–187

6 Soft Tissue Infections and Antibiotics in Plastic Surgery

Cristina Aubá, José L. del Pozo

Abstract

Skin and soft tissue infections (SSTIs) include infections of skin, subcutaneous tissue, fascia, and muscle. Clinical presentation is variable, ranging from simple cellulitis to rapidly progressive necrotizing fasciitis. It is imperative to distinguish necrotizing from nonnecrotizing infections in order to avoid unnecessary delays of life- and limb-saving treatments. Eron's classification of SSTIs is based on the severity of local and systemic signs and provides information regarding the therapeutic approach for each category. Surgical site infections (SSIs) are the most common health care–associated infections, representing a considerable burden in terms of postoperative morbidity and mortality, delays in discharge, and hospital costs. Clinical management of SSIs is based on a combination of surgical, supportive, and antimicrobial therapies. On the other hand, infection is a leading cause of morbidity complicating breast implant surgery and is reported in 2–2.5% of interventions. Treatment goals are to eradicate infection and rescue the implant if possible. Several studies have revealed the presence of bacteria on the surface of breast implants and suggested an association between these findings and capsular contracture. The mechanisms of action, spectrum of activity, clinical uses, route of excretion, and toxic effects of the antimicrobial agents most commonly used in SSTIs are reviewed in this chapter.

Keywords: alloplastics infections, breast implant biofilm, broad-spectrum antimicrobials, capsular contracture, necrotizing fasciitis, skin and soft tissue infections, surgical site infections

6.1 Introduction

In this chapter skin and soft tissue infections (SSTIs) are addressed, with particular emphasis in general clinical and surgical management. In this sense, distinguishing severe from nonnecrotizing infections and knowing the main microorganisms involved, as well as the most commonly used antimicrobials, are crucial in the implementation of a prompt and effective therapy. In addition, the management of breast implant–associated infections is described, along with the role of biofilm and its relationship with capsular contracture.

6.2 Skin and Soft Tissue Infections

SSTIs include infections of skin, subcutaneous tissue, fascia, and muscle. Clinical presentation is variable, ranging from simple cellulitis to rapidly progressive necrotizing fasciitis. There are several factors that may predispose a patient to developing SSTIs, such as a breach in the epidermis, immunosuppression (malnutrition, hypoproteinemia, burns, diabetes mellitus, HIV infection), chronic venous or lymphatic insufficiency, and chronic neuropathy. On initial assessment it is imperative to distinguish necrotizing from nonnecrotizing infections to avoid delaying a treatment that may otherwise save a life or a limb.

> **Note**
>
> Infection, which is different from colonization, develops when microbial pathogenicity overcomes the host's immunological defenses.

6.2.1 Classification

SSTIs may be classified according to the layer of infection (►Table 6.1), severity of infection, and microbiological etiology. According to severity, the practice guidelines of the Infectious Diseases Society of America (IDSA) classifies SSTIs into five categories: superficial uncomplicated infections (e.g., impetigo, erysipelas, and cellulitis), necrotizing infections, infections associated with bites and animal contact, surgical site infections (SSIs), and infections in the immunocompromised host. Of note, Eron's classification, also based on the severity of local and systemic signs, incorporates information on management besides the clinical features of each group (►Table 6.2).

Table 6.1 Type of infection according to the layer of skin/soft tissue affected

Anatomical structure	Infection	Microbiological etiology
Epithelium	Varicella Measles	Varicella virus Measles virus
Keratin layer	Ringworm	Dermatophyte fungi
Epidermis	Impetigo	*Streptococcus pyogenes Staphylococcus aureus*
Dermis	Erysipelas	*Streptococcus pyogenes*
Hair follicles	Folliculitis, boils, carbuncles	*Staphylococcus aureus*
Sebum glands	Acne	*Propionibacterium acnes*
Subcutaneous fat	Cellulitis	β-Hemolytic streptococci
Fascia	Necrotizing fasciitis	*Streptococcus pyogenes* Mixed anaerobic infection
Muscle	Myositis Gangrene	Toxic strains of *Staphylococcus aureus* *Clostridium perfringens*

Table 6.2 Eron's classification of skin and soft tissue infections

Category	Clinical features	Management
Class 1	SSTI but no signs or symptoms of systemic toxicity or comorbidities	Drainage (if required) and oral antibiotics as outpatient
Class 2	Either systemically unwell or systemically well but with comorbidity that may complicate or delay resolution	Oral or outpatient intravenous antibiotic therapy; may require short period of observation in hospital
Class 3	Toxic and unwell (fever, tachycardia, tachypnea and/or hypotension)	Likely to require inpatient treatment with parenteral antibiotics
Class 4	Sepsis syndrome and life-threatening infection	Likely to require admission to intensive care unit, urgent surgical assessment, and treatment with parenteral antibiotics

6.2.2 General Management

The general management of SSTIs includes proper assessment of the indications for conservative or surgical treatment, the collection of samples for culture, and the instauration of an empirical or antibiogram-oriented therapy when needed. Uncomplicated SSTIs pose little risk to life and generally respond well to either source control (e.g., drainage or debridement) or a simple course of antibiotics, whereas complicated SSTIs, such as complicated abscesses, infected burn wounds, infected ulcers, infections in diabetics, and deep space wound infections, are often limb- or life-threatening conditions requiring surgical intervention.

Note

The timing of treatment initiation in skin and soft tissue infections is important for patient outcomes; failure to give antibiotics within 8 hours of presentation is associated with prolonged patient hospitalization.

Role of Swabs, Cultures, and Biopsies

Tissue biopsy or aspiration sampling of infected tissue is the *gold standard* for culture of SSTI and is especially important in cases of severe infection, systemic toxicity, or failure of initial therapy. A bacterial count of 10^5 organisms per gram of tissue has been regarded as the threshold for clinical infection. Swab cultures are probably the most commonly used method to determine the resistance pattern of skin pathogens in nursing home residents and are widely used in a number of other settings as well; however, they are controversial, especially when obtained from chronic wounds. If material superficial to the infected tissue is sampled, colonizers may be isolated. Furthermore, swab cultures should not be used to determine if a wound is acutely infected, but rather to identify potential pathogens when deep tissue biopsy is not elected.

Empirical Antibiotic Treatment

The microbiological diagnosis of any infection is ideally based on data from bacterial or fungal culture or serologic testing; however, it usually takes 24 to 72 hours for these results to become available, which is sometimes a prohibitively long period to wait without intervention. On the other hand, the most likely pathogens can usually be inferred from the clinical presentation. Thus, once pus samples are sent for culture and antimicrobial sensitivity testing, empirical oral or intravenous (IV) antimicrobial therapy should be started based on the severity of infection. A common approach is to use broad-spectrum antimicrobial agents as initial empirical therapy (sometimes involving a combination of antibiotics) so as to cover multiple possible pathogens commonly associated with the specific clinical entity.

Indications for IV antibiotics include a limb- or life-threatening severe soft tissue infection, signs and symptoms of systemic illness, immunosuppression, and elderly patients. The timing of initial therapy should be guided by the urgency of the situation. In critically ill patients, such as those in septic shock and febrile neutropenic patients, empirical therapy should be initiated immediately after or concurrently with collection of diagnostic specimens. In more stable clinical circumstances, antimicrobial therapy should be deliberately withheld until appropriate specimens have been collected and submitted to the microbiology laboratory. Premature initiation of antimicrobial therapy in these circumstances may suppress bacterial growth and preclude the opportunity of establishing an accurate microbiological diagnosis, which is critical in the management of these patients, who usually require several weeks to months of directed antimicrobial therapy.

> **Note**
>
> Microbiological diagnosis and susceptibility testing are of increasing importance in the current era of multidrug-resistant bacteria and have a major role in promoting appropriate prescription of antibiotics.

General Laboratory Workup

Patients with uncomplicated SSTIs do not usually require any investigations or hospital admission. However, patients with symptoms and signs of systemic compromise, including hemodynamic changes (e.g., tachycardia and hypotension) should undergo the following tests: blood culture and drug susceptibility, complete blood count with differential and creatinine, bicarbonate, creatine phosphokinase, and C-reactive protein levels. Additional investigations may be indicated depending on the severity of systemic illness. Once a pathogenic microorganism is identified in culture, most microbiology laboratories then run an antimicrobial susceptibility testing (AST), which measures the ability of a specific organism to grow in the presence of a particular drug in vitro and is performed using guidelines established by the Clinical and Laboratory Standards Institute. The goal of AST is to predict the clinical success or failure of the antibiotic being tested against a particular organism. Data are reported in the form of minimum inhibitory concentration, which is the lowest concentration of an antibiotic that inhibits visible growth of a microorganism, and interpreted by the laboratory as susceptible, resistant, or intermediate, according to Clinical and Laboratory Standards Institute criteria. A report of susceptible indicates that the isolated pathogen is likely to be inhibited by the usually achievable concentration of a particular antimicrobial agent when the recommended dosage for the particular site of infection is used.

Antibiogram-oriented Therapy

Once microbiological or antimicrobial susceptibility data are available, every attempt should be made to narrow the antibiotic spectrum. This is a critically important component of antibiotic therapy because it can reduce costs and toxicity and prevent the development of antimicrobial resistance in the community.

Bactericidal versus Bacteriostatic Therapy

A commonly used distinction among antibacterial agents is whether they are bactericidal or bacteriostatic. On the one hand, bactericidals, which cause death and disruption of the bacterial cell, include drugs that act primarily on the cell wall (e.g., β-lactams), cell membrane (e.g., daptomycin), or bacterial DNA (e.g., fluoroquinolones). Bacteriostatic agents, on the other hand, inhibit bacterial replication without killing the microorganism. Most bacteriostatic drugs, including sulfonamides, tetracyclines, and macrolides, act by inhibiting protein synthesis. The distinction is not absolute, and some agents that are bactericidal against certain organisms may be bacteriostatic against others and vice versa. Although in most cases this distinction is not significant in vivo, bactericidal agents are preferred in cases of serious infections, such as necrotizing fasciitis.

Use of Antimicrobial Combinations

Although single-agent antimicrobial therapy is generally preferred, a combination of two or more agents is sometimes recommended, such as to: (1) treat infections that are frequently caused by bacteria resistant to multiple antibiotics; (2) treat infections that are thought to be caused by more than one microorganism; and (3) prevent the development of resistant mutants in a bacterial population, which is generally the result of selective pressure from antimicrobial therapy.

Surgical Treatment

Some SSTIs require operative drainage or debridement, especially in cases where the bioburden is very high or in the presence of purulent collections (e.g., abscess), for which the penetration and activity of antimicrobial agents are often inadequate. Thus any abscess, regardless of size, must be drained for complete resolution. The drainage incision should be made parallel to a natural skin crease, at the most prominent part and going all the way into the abscess cavity. Care should be taken when incising abscesses near major vessels and nerves, where it is more prudent to access the cavity by blunt dissection. Any necrosed or unhealthy skin on the roof of the abscess should be excised completely. Necrotizing fasciitis is a surgical emergency, and early surgical treatment has been shown to optimize outcomes in these patients. Staged debridements until dermal bleeding is seen on the edges of the skin should be done in order to minimize damage to healthy tissue. Finally, there are no absolute contraindications for incision, drainage, and/or debridement of SSTIs. Patients whose physical condition is compromised should be stabilized and rendered fit for anesthesia before surgery.

6.2.3 Surgical Site Infections

SSIs are the most common health care–associated infection, representing a considerable burden in terms of postoperative morbidity and mortality, delays in discharge, and hospital costs (▶ Table 6.3). Since plastic surgery interventions have increased in number, frequency, and complexity, postoperative complications, particularly SSIs, have also increased. Data regarding incidence and risk factors for SSIs in plastic surgery are limited and sometimes refer to specific interventions. Moreover, according to current literature, SSI rates in plastic surgery interventions in relation to a specific preoperative contamination class are widely variable, ranging from 2 to nearly 20% in clean elective operations (e.g., excisional surgery and breast augmentation or reduction) and from 23 to 37% in clean-contaminated interventions (e.g., skin grafting of lower extremity vascular ulcers and burn wounds).

Table 6.3 Definition criteria for surgical site infection

Superficial incisional SSI	Occurs within 30 days postoperatively and involves skin or subcutaneous tissue of the incision and at least one of the following: 1. Purulent drainage from the superficial incision. 2. Organisms isolated from an aseptically obtained culture of fluid or tissue from the superficial incision. 3. At least one of the following signs or symptoms of infection: pain or tenderness, localized swelling, redness, or heat, and superficial incision is deliberately opened by surgeon and is culture positive or not cultured (a culture-negative finding does not meet this criterion). 4. Diagnosis of superficial incisional SSI by the surgeon or attending physician.
Deep incisional SSI	Occurs within 30 days after the operative procedure if no implant is left in place or within 1 year if implant is in place and the infection appears to be related to the operative procedure, involves deep soft tissues (e.g., fascial and muscle layers) of the incision, and the patient has at least one of the following: 1. Purulent drainage from the deep incision but not from the organ/space component of the surgical site. 2. A deep incision spontaneously dehisces or is deliberately opened by a surgeon and is culture positive or not cultured, and the patient has at least one of the following signs or symptoms: fever (> 38°C) or localized pain or tenderness (a culture-negative finding does not meet this criterion). 3. An abscess or other evidence of infection involving the deep incision is found on direct examination, during reoperation, or by histopathological or radiologic examination. 4. Diagnosis of a deep incisional SSI by a surgeon or attending physician.
Organ/space SSI	Involves any part of the body, excluding the skin incision, fascia, or muscle layers, that is opened or manipulated during the operative procedure. Specific sites are assigned to organ/space SSI to further identify the location of the infection (e.g., endocarditis, endometritis, mediastinitis, vaginal cuff, and osteomyelitis). Organ/space SSI must meet the following criteria: 1. Infection occurs within 30 days after the operative procedure if no implant is in place or within 1 year if implant is in place and the infection appears to be related to the operative procedure. 2. Infection involves any part of the body, excluding the skin incision, fascia, or muscle layers, that is opened or manipulated during the operative procedure. 3. The patient has at least one of the following: (a) purulent drainage from a drain that is placed through a stab wound into the organ/space, (b) organisms isolated from an aseptically obtained culture of fluid or tissue in the organ/space, (c) an abscess or other evidence of infection involving the organ/space that is found on direct examination, during reoperation, or by histopathologic or radiologic examination, and (d) diagnosis of an organ/space SSI by a surgeon or attending physician.

Source: Reproduced with permission from Stevens DL, et al. Practice guidelines for the diagnosis and management of skin and soft-tissue infections (Infectious Diseases Society of America Guideline). Clinical Infectious Diseases 2005;41:1371–1406.

Etiology

The normal skin flora comprises numerous species of microorganisms residing in the epidermis, which in the unwounded skin of a healthy individual are usually nonpathogenic. However, when skin is breached these microorganisms have the potential to penetrate into the dermis and subcutaneous tissue and cause infection. Infection, which is distinct from colonization, develops when microbial pathogenicity overcomes the host's immunological defenses. The majority of SSIs are monomicrobial and caused mainly by gram-positive or gram-negative bacteria, most often *Staphylococcus aureus*. The presence of methicillin-resistant *S. aureus* (MRSA) represents an important risk factor in the development of complications. SSIs can also be polymicrobial, in which case a synergistic effect may develop, increasing pathogenicity and complicating therapy.

Clinical Presentation

The severity of SSIs depends on a series of factors, and the clinical spectrum ranges from mild to life-threatening variants. SSIs are considered complicated SSTIs with potentially devastating consequences and therefore require early recognition and prompt management. Moreover, SSIs caused by highly pathogenic strains of common organisms (e.g., *S. aureus* expressing Panton–Valentine's leukocidin, or toxigenic strains of *Streptococcus pyogenes*) may present with systemic toxicity in immunocompetent individuals. These infections tend to spread rapidly and are considered medical emergencies necessitating urgent surgical debridement and high doses of antibiotics.

Diagnosis

Swabs of pus or tissue samples from open wounds usually provide the best diagnostic value. Samples from deeper tissues or exudate are the most appropriate for microbiological diagnosis and should be obtained after debridement and cleansing of superficial debris. Imaging techniques can provide structural information about deep tissue infections and differentiate necrotizing from nonnecrotizing infections by detecting the presence of edema along the fascial plane in the former. Radiography and computed tomography can be used to detect gas in tissues, which is indicative of necrotizing infection, whereas ultrasonography is useful for diagnosing and draining collections under direct vision. Magnetic resonance imaging has a particularly high sensitivity for the diagnosis of infections involving soft tissue and bone and can be used to determine the extent of deep tissue involvement.

Treatment

Management of SSIs involves a combination of supportive, antimicrobial, and surgical therapies (▶Fig. 6.1).

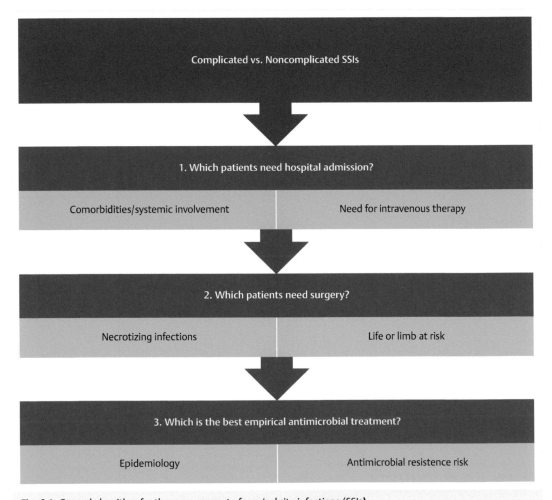

Fig. 6.1 General algorithm for the management of surgical site infections (SSIs).

In general, small abscesses are treated primarily by incision and drainage, with antibiotics indicated for patients who do not respond to these measures and those with either large collections or located in an area that is difficult to drain. Rapid progression of infection, signs of systemic illness, comorbidities, and immunosuppression are also indications for systemic antibiotic therapy. Negative pressure dressings, especially with silver- coated foams, can be used for infections with excessive exudate or for large wounds, always maintaining close vigilance on the wound and patient's evolution. Once infection is resolved, reconstructive procedures, including revascularization of critically perfused limbs, skin grafting, and flap closure may be needed. Regarding antibiotics, the timing of (effective) treatment initiation is critical—failure to give antibiotics within 8 hours of presentation is associated with prolonged patient hospitalization. Furthermore, the treating surgeon needs to be aware of microbial and patient factors that may render an empirical treatment inappropriate and guide therapeutic decisions accordingly. Inappropriate treatment, defined as the administration of an antimicrobial that has no activity against the isolated pathogen(s), is more likely in patients with a device-associated infection or an infection due to MRSA.

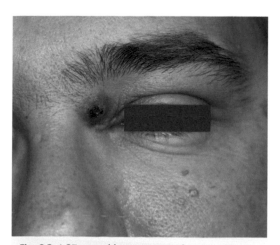

Fig. 6.2 A 27-year-old man came to the outpatient clinic with a 3-week history of a red, tender, pus-filled facial bump. Furuncles often rupture and drain spontaneously or following treatment with moist heat.

6.2.4 Nonnecrotizing Infections

Folliculitis, Furuncles, and Carbuncles

Furuncles are infections of the hair follicle, usually caused by *S. aureus*, in which suppuration extends through the dermis and into the subcutaneous tissue, leading to the formation of a small abscess (▶ Fig. 6.2). Folliculitis is characterized by a more superficial inflammation, with pus limited to the epidermis. Clinically, furuncles are inflammatory nodules with overlying pustules through which hair emerges. They often rupture and drain spontaneously or following treatment with moist heat. Infection involving several adjacent furuncles produces a carbuncle, which is seen as a coalescent inflammatory mass with pus draining from multiple follicular orifices. Carbuncles are typically larger and deeper than furuncles and develop most commonly on the back of the neck, particularly in diabetics. Most large furuncles and all carbuncles should be treated with incision and drainage. Systemic antimicrobials are usually unnecessary, unless fever or other evidence of systemic toxicity is observed.

Erysipela

Erysipela is an infection of the upper dermis that extends into the superficial lymphatics. Clinically, it presents as an erythematous indurated plaque with sharply demarcated borders. It is almost always caused by group A and B streptococci and less commonly by group G or C. In rare cases, other microorganisms, including *S. aureus*, *Streptococcus pneumoniae*, enterococci, and a variety of aerobic gram-negative bacilli, have been recovered from patients with erysipelas.

Cellulitis

Cellulitis is an acute, spreading, pyogenic inflammation of the dermis and subcutaneous tissue that lacks sharp demarcation from uninvolved skin. Prior to the introduction of *Haemophilus influenzae* type b conjugated vaccine in the immunization schedule, buccal cellulitis due to *H. influenzae* was responsible for up to 25% of cases of facial cellulitis in children between 3 and 24 months; today such disease is rare. Cellulitis is most commonly caused by β-hemolytic streptococci, especially groups A and B, and less often by groups C and G, as well as *S. aureus*.

Importantly, the incidence of community-acquired SSTIs due to MRSA is currently increasing.

Identifying the source of cellulitis (cutaneous, subjacent, or bacteremic) can provide clues as to the causative microorganism. Animal or human bites can cause cellulitis due to skin flora of the recipient or oral flora from the biter (e.g., *Pasteurella multocida*, *Erysipelothrix rhusiopathiae*). Specific pathogens should be suspected when infection follows exposure to seawater (*Vibrio vulnificus*), freshwater (*Aeromonas hydrophila*), aquacultured fish (*Streptococcus iniae*), or fish aquaria (*Mycobacterium marinum*). Subcutaneous injection of drugs (i.e., skin popping) can result in cellulitis due to unusual microorganisms, such as *Clostridium tetani*, *Clostridium botulinum*, *Clostridium sordellii*, *Clostridium novyi*, or *Bacillus cereus*. Cellulitis is not uncommon in lymphedematous arms following radical mastectomy and radiotherapy and in legs of patients who have had vein grafts harvested. Crepitant cellulitis is produced by either clostridia or non-spore-forming anaerobes (e.g., *Bacteroides* species, *Peptostreptococcus* species) either alone or mixed with facultative pathogens, particularly *Escherichia coli*, *Klebsiella* species, or *Aeromonas* species. Crepitant cellulitis of the left thigh may be associated with a colonic diverticular abscess. Though not frequently, cellulitis can occur secondary to bacteremia. Pneumococcal cellulitis of the face or limbs may occur in patients with diabetes mellitus, alcoholism, systemic lupus erythematosus, nephrotic syndrome, or hematological malignancy. Meningococcal cellulitis is rare and usually presents as periorbital cellulitis in children, whereas in adults it typically affects the extremities. Bacteremic cellulitis due to *Vibrio vulnificus* with prominent hemorrhagic bullae may follow the ingestion of raw oysters in patients with cirrhosis, hemochromatosis, or thalassemia. Bacteremia caused by gram-negative bacteria (e.g., *E. coli*, *Enterobacter* species, *Proteus* species) occasionally causes soft tissue infections, including cellulitis. *Pseudomonas aeruginosa* cellulitis may follow bacteremia in neutropenic patients, whereas less common opportunistic pathogens (e.g., *Helicobacter cinaedi*) may affect HIV patients.

Skin Abscesses

Cutaneous abscesses are collections of pus within the dermis and deeper layers. They usually present as tender, fluctuant, red nodules, often surmounted by a pustule and encircled by a rim of erythematous swelling. *S. aureus* is the sole pathogen in most cases, with a substantial number caused by MRSA strains. Skin abscesses can be polymicrobial, containing regional skin flora or organisms from adjacent mucous membranes. Incision and drainage of pus and debris, and probing of the cavity to break up loculations, provides effective treatment of these lesions.

Hidradenitis Suppurativa

Hidradenitis suppurativa (HS) is a chronic inflammatory, recurrent follicular disease affecting apocrine gland–bearing regions. It usually occurs in healthy adolescents and adults and is characterized by comedo-like follicular occlusion, mucopurulent discharge, and progressive scarring. Predisposing risk factors include genetic susceptibility, smoking, obesity, immunosuppression, hormonal changes (puberty, menstruation, menopause), and emotional and social stress. It has been suggested that HS is primarily a disease of the follicular epithelium that becomes secondarily infected, most commonly with *S. epidermidis* and *S. aureus*. Arthropathy is usually associated with HS. HS is classified in three stages, depending on the presence and extent of sinus tracts and scarring (Table 6.4). Diagnosis of HS is mainly clinical and is based on three main pillars: the presence of typical lesions, their characteristic distribution, and recurrence. Typical (primary) lesions include painful erythematous papules, nodules, or abscesses; draining sinuses; dermal contractures; or double-ended comedones. Regarding distribution, as already mentioned, HS affects areas containing apocrine glands, which include the axillae and groin, and perineal, perianal, and inter- and inframammary areas (▶Fig. 6.3).

> **Note**
>
> Diagnosis of hidradenitis suppurativa is based on the presence of typical lesions, characteristic distribution, and recurrence.

Treatment of HS starts with general recommendations, such as local hygiene and self-care, application of warm compresses with sodium chloride solution or Burow's solution, weight loss in obese patients, smoking cessation, and stress relief. A number of treatments have been described for HS, including topical clindamycin or resorcinol; oral tetracycline or a combination of clindamycin and rifampicin; intralesional (triamcinolone) and systemic steroids; anti-tumor necrosis factor-α (adalimumab);

Table 6.4 Hurley's classification of hidradenitis suppurativa and therapeutic alternatives for each stage

Stage	Clinical feature	Treatment
I	Abscess formation without sinus tract and cicatrization	Topical or oral antibiotics (tetracyclines, doxicyclines) Hormonal therapy Retinoids Botulinum toxin Radiofrequency treatment Corticosteroids
II	One or more widely separated recurrent abscesses with tract formation and scars	CO_2 laser ablation Immunosuppression therapies Surgery (limited excisions) Radiotherapy Radiofrequency
III	Multiple interconnected tracts and abscesses throughout an entire area	Radiotherapy Surgery (wide excisions)

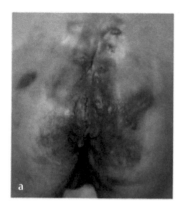

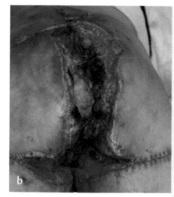

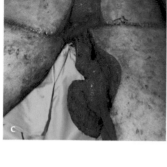

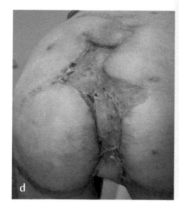

Fig. 6.3 A 58-year-old man presented with a history of recurrent episodes of perianal hidradenitis suppurativa requiring multiple interventions. (a) Preoperative view. (b) After wide surgical debridement of the affected tissue. Colostomy was required. Local rotation flaps were used, but wound dehiscence ensued, which was treated with negative pressure wound therapy (NPWT). (c) Post-NPWT. The defect was repaired with a pedicled gracilis myocutaneous flap and split-thickness skin grafts. (d) Postoperative view.

acitretin; surgical excision with or without reconstruction (depending on the extent of resection); and radiotherapy. Hurley's staging system provides a useful stratification of therapy according to severity (▶Table 6.4). Surgical treatment of HS may include drainage, simple excision with direct closure, or wide excision followed by secondary-intention healing, and local, regional, or free flaps. Skin grafting is generally not recommended, especially in the inguinoperineal region. Incision and drainage of purulent lesions is often required in the acute phase and provides short-term relief, but recurrent inflammation is almost the rule. An overall recurrence rate of 2.5% has been estimated, and it may be as high as 50% in the inguinoperineal region. For chronic and extensive disease, the most definitive surgical therapy is wide excision to deep fascia and flap reconstruction. Of note, intraoperative injection of methyl violet solution might aid in determining the extent of the sinus tracts prior to excision.

6.2.5 Necrotizing Soft Tissue Infections

Necrotizing soft tissue infections are the most aggressive SSTIs. There are two forms of necrotizing soft tissue infections: necrotizing fasciitis (NF) and Fournier's gangrene (FG), both of which are potentially limb- and life-threatening conditions requiring early recognition and emergent medical and surgical treatment.

Necrotizing Fasciitis

NF is a rapidly spreading infection that extends along the fascial planes (superficial and deep fascia), resulting in tissue necrosis. It may be polymicrobial (NF type 1) or caused by group A β-hemolytic streptococci (*Streptococcus pyogenes*), alone or in combination with other microorganisms, especially staphylococcus (NF type 2). Even though NF can occur anywhere in the body, it most commonly affects the lower extremities. Risk factors for this disease include diabetes, alcoholism, parenteral drug abuse, and history of trauma, surgery, or ulcers, through which microorganisms gain entry to the deep planes.

Clinical Findings

Clinically, NF presents as a sudden erythematous, swollen, and poorly demarcated area, with increased local temperature and severe pain that is typically disproportionate to local findings. These features, coupled with the presence of systemic toxicity, are highly suggestive of NF. As the disease progresses, the affected skin changes from a tense, painful erythematous patch to a dusky purple appearance, finally leading to skin breakdown, bullae, and gangrene, at which stage the lesions are no longer tender. High fever and systemic toxicity are common. Subcutaneous gas is often present in polymicrobial NF, especially in diabetics.

Laboratory Findings

Leukocytosis, along with elevation of acute phase reactants, is commonly seen in NF. Gram's stain of exudate or tissue can help in early identification of possible pathogens and should be obtained whenever possible. Blood cultures are frequently positive. The Laboratory Risk Indicator for Necrotizing Fasciitis score comprises a series of markers, including hemoglobin, glucose, creatinine, C-reactive protein, sodium, and white blood cell count, that help establish a diagnosis of NF with a 92% positive predictive value and a 96% negative predictive value (Table 6.5). Imaging findings indicative of NF include the presence of gas in an X-ray or signs of fasciitis, myositis, and edema

Table 6.5 The Laboratory Risk Indicator for Necrotizing Fasciitis score (LRINEC score) for distinguishing necrotizing fasciitis from other soft tissue infections

LRINEC score	
Variable	Score*
C-reactive protein (mg/L)	
< 150	0
≥150	4
Leukocytes (per mm³)	
< 15	0
15–25	1
> 25	2
Hemoglobin (g/dL)	
> 13.5	0
11–13.5	1
< 11	2
Sodium (mmol/L)	
≥ 135	0
< 135	2
Creatinine (mg/dL)	
< 1.6	0
≥ 1.6	2
Glucose (mg/dL)	
≤ 180	0
> 180	1

*A score > 6 is highly suggestive of necrotizing fasciitis.

along the fascial layers in a computed tomographic scan. Although laboratory and imaging tests are of great help, they should not delay treatment in cases with a clear clinical diagnosis of NF.

Management

Due to its rapid clinical course, early diagnosis of NF is crucial to reduce morbidity, and especially mortality, which approximates 24–34%. Early resuscitation, broad-spectrum antibiotics, and surgery are the main pillars of management. Immediate surgical debridement is essential and should be done promptly and aggressively; failure to remove all affected tissue results in further spreading of the infection. Empirical IV broad-spectrum antibiotics covering gram-positive and gram-negative aerobes and anaerobes should be used initially while awaiting for microbiology results. For group A streptococcal necrotizing fasciitis, penicillin alone or in combination with clindamycin can be used.

Fournier's Gangrene

Fournier's gangrene is a necrotizing fasciitis of the genitalia and perineum, which may extend to the lower abdominal wall and perianal area. Infection is usually polymicrobial, involving aerobic (*E. coli*, *Klebsiella* spp., enterococci) and anaerobic bacteria (*Bacteroides* spp., *Fusobacterium* spp., *Clostridium* spp., streptococci) that spread from local cutaneous, urogenital, or colorectal regions. Predisposing factors include diabetes mellitus, local trauma, paraphimosis, periurethral extravasation of urine, perianal or perineal infections (e.g., HS), and surgery (e.g., circumcision or herniorrhaphy). The clinical features of Fournier's gangrene are similar those of NF. Treatment is also based on fluid/electrolyte resuscitation, IV antibiotics, and surgery; however, mortality may be as high as 80% due to delayed diagnosis and treatment. The ultimate goal is to achieve complete wound healing while providing a reliable coverage and protection of the testicles with an acceptable cosmetic result. Nevertheless, marked sequelae related to the extent of fasciitis and debridements are not uncommon. Techniques described in the literature include healing by secondary intention, delayed primary closure, implantation of the testicle in a medial thigh pocket, residual scrotal skin mobilization, skin grafts, and pedicled and free flaps. Skin grafting or flap reconstruction is recommended for defects larger than 50% of the scrotum or extending beyond it. Currently, there is no evidence to support the use of flaps over the use of skin grafts for coverage of exposed testes.

Gas Gangrene

Gas gangrene is an acute and life-threatening infection characterized by fever, sudden onset of prominent pain, massive local edema, severe extensive *myonecrosis*, and accumulation of gas at the site of infection. It is usually caused by clostridia, particularly *Clostridium perfringens* in cases associated with muscle trauma. Nontraumatic clostridial myonecrosis is secondary to *Clostridium septicum* or even fungi in immunosuppressed hosts. Foul-smelling serosanguineous discharge from the wound and crepitus are typical findings of gas gangrene. Gram's stain usually shows gram-positive bacilli without spores—the presence of spores suggests *C. septicum*. Treatment includes early debridement to revert to the anoxic environment and prevent the infection from spreading, together with a combination of crystalline penicillin and clindamycin.

6.2.6 Pyomyositis

Pyomyositis is a primary pyogenic infection of skeletal muscle resulting from hematogenous spread and often progressing to abscess formation. It is generally located within the pelvis, affecting the gluteal, piriformis, and adductor muscles, where its non-specific clinical features, namely tumefaction, erythema, and pain, make its diagnosis difficult. While primary pyomyositis is caused mainly by *S. aureus* and sometimes *Streptococcus* spp., in secondary pyomyositis, gram-negative and anaerobic pathogens should be considered. Even though computed tomographic scan is the imaging technique of choice, magnetic resonance has higher sensitivity for muscle inflammation and fluid collection, making it a better alternative in the early stages, especially in immunocompromised patients, who are at higher risk of complications. Management depends on the stage of the disease. Incipient infections with diffuse inflammatory changes can be treated with antibiotics alone. However, 90% of patients present with an abscess at the moment of diagnosis, and in these cases early drainage in combination with IV antibiotics is indicated. Empirical antibiotic treatment is based on cloxacillin, penicillin G, vancomycin, and clindamycin.

6.2.7 Cutaneous Fungal Infections

Yeasts, mainly *Candida*, or dermatophytes cause common fungal skin infections. Although only *Candida* is part of the normal skin flora, both may cause infection under certain conditions, such as humid weather, tight or synthetic underclothing, poor hygiene, infrequent diaper or undergarment changes, altered immunity (e.g., diabetes or corticosteroids), pregnancy, obesity, or use of antibiotics. Unlike dermatophytes, *Candida* may invade deeper tissues, internal organs, and the bloodstream, causing life-threatening systemic candidiasis.

Candidiasis may be caused by any of *Candida's* species, most frequently *C. albicans.* It presents as a bright red, intensely itching or burning rash that generates a thick, white, and pasty residue on mucosa or skin. Small pustules may appear, especially at the edges of the rash. Dermatophyte infections are caused by different fungi (e.g., *Epidermophyton* spp., *Microsporum* spp.) resulting in ringworm or tinea. Dermatophytes feed on keratin present in skin, hair, and nails, and they can affect almost any part of the body. Some common sites include feet (tinea pedis or athlete's foot), the groin (tinea cruris or jock itch), scalp (tinea capitis), and beard area (tinea barbae). They usually present as an erythematous, scaly eruption, which may or may not be itchy. Asymmetry and an annular morphology are typical features of these lesions. Diagnosis of fungal infections is clinical and can be confirmed by scraping off a small amount of skin or residue with a scalpel or tongue depressor and having it examined under the microscope or grown in a culture medium. Treatment depends on location and extent of disease. Topical treatment includes creams or solutions containing miconazole, clotrimazole, oxiconazole, ketoconazole, econazole, ciclopirox, and nystatin. Oral fluconazole, ketoconazole, or itraconazole is indicated for patients with extensive disease.

6.3 Alloplastic Infections

Alloplastic materials are used routinely in plastic surgery, for both reconstructive and aesthetic purposes. Of the many complications that these products may have, infection is one of the most important in terms of the devastating consequences it may carry. Breast implants are the most frequently used alloplastic material, and infection is their leading cause of morbidity, reported in 2–2.5% of interventions. Unfortunately, alloplastic infection may be difficult to diagnose microbiologically, and specific diagnostic tools for breast implant infections are not yet available.

> **Note**
>
> From a clinical standpoint, it is important to differentiate infectious from noninfectious causes of breast implant failure. If infection is present, efforts should be done to isolate the pathogen in order to guide antimicrobial therapy.

6.3.1 Breast Implant Infection Microbiology and Pathogenesis

Infections related to breast implants are typically caused by skin flora, such as *S. aureus* and coagulase-negative staphylococci. Unusual microorganisms reported on a small number of cases include *Trichosporon beigelii*, *Pasteurella multocida*, *Clostridium perfringens*, and *Listeria monocytogenes* or *Granulicatella adiacens*.

Contamination of breast implants with the patient's skin microflora during surgery is the origin of most implant infections. Other less common pathogenic mechanisms include a contaminated implant, a contaminated surgical environment, skin-penetrating accidents, local soft tissue infections, breast trauma or massage, and seeding from a remote infection. Of note, adjuvant chemotherapy has been associated with a high rate of infection after reconstruction.

Implant-associated infection pathogenesis involves the interaction between microorganisms, the implant, and the host. Bacteria colonizing the surface of the implant have the capacity to form a *biofilm*, which is a layer composed of clusters of microorganisms embedded within a self-producing matrix of extracellular polymeric substance that anchors them to the implant's surface and protects them from host defenses and antimicrobial agents. The matrix contains channels that allow the flow of nutrients and waste. In addition, replicating bacteria are able to display cell-to-cell signaling (i.e., quorum sensing). Bacterial biofilms exhibit dramatically reduced susceptibility to antimicrobial agents as compared to free-floating (planktonic) cells of the same microorganism. A variety of potential antimicrobial resistance mechanisms have been proposed, including existence of altered growth rate inside the biofilm (e.g., persister cells), quorum sensing signaling systems, antimicrobial-destroying enzymes, stress response to hostile environmental conditions, overexpression of genes, and restricted antimicrobial penetration through the biofilm matrix. Consequently, the presence of biofilm often leads to failure of antibiotic treatment, in which case implant removal becomes the only way of effectively eradicating infection.

6.3.2 Clinical Presentation

Acute infections usually occur during the first month (average of 10–12 days after surgery), and present with erythema, swelling, warmth, pain, deformation, and, occasionally, wound dehiscence (▶Fig. 6.4). Discomfort and tension are associated with the presence of serosanguineous periprosthetic fluid. Fever and purulent drainage may be present. Additionally, patients may develop toxic shock syndrome, a life-threatening complication that occurs within 12–24 hours

after implant placement and is caused by toxin-producing strains of *S. aureus* and *S. pyogenes*. It courses with nausea, vomiting, watery diarrhea, myalgia, lethargy, and skin rash. Early recognition of this potentially fatal complication is paramount, and treatment is based on implant removal and IV antibiotics.

Late infections usually appear a few months to several years after implant placement and result from bacteremia and secondary colonization of the prosthesis (▶Fig. 6.5); therefore, any bacterial infection, including remote ones, represents a risk factor for implant infection and should be treated promptly. Likewise, invasive diagnostic procedures and surgery in patients with breast implants should be undertaken with proper antibiotic prophylaxis. The symptoms of late infections are less pronounced than those of acute ones and include moderate pain, mild erythema, slightly warm and stretched skin, and implant displacement. Drainage, which is nonpurulent, is not always present. In some cases infection may manifest with discomfort and fatigue only. Chronic inflammation, often linked to and stimulated by biofilm formation, increases the risk of developing capsular contracture.

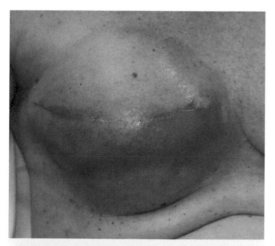

Fig. 6.4 Breast reconstruction in two stages with tissue expander and implant. Implant infection was observed 2 weeks after placement. Staphylococcus aureus was isolated. Conservative management with antibiotic treatment (e.g., levofloxacin 500 mg twice a day plus Rifampicin 600 mg twice a day) allowed implant salvage without surgical intervention.

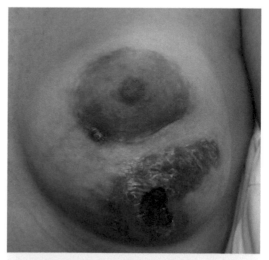

Fig. 6.5 A 25-year-old woman with tuberous breast deformity corrected by the Puckett technique and subglandular implants. Two months after surgery, the left implant became infected but was hidden by the patient. At the time of evaluation the implant was exposed, leaving no alternative but to remove it.

Role of Infection in Capsular Contracture

Capsular contracture refers to the thickening, contraction, and hardening of the physiological and normally thin layer of tissue (e.g., capsule) that the body forms around any foreign body, including breast implants. It is the most common and frustrating complication following breast implant surgery. The cause of capsular contracture remains to be fully elucidated, as are its prevention and treatment. A number of factors have been suggested, such as foreign body reaction, hematoma, and periprosthetic infection, including infection by nanobacterial-like particles. There is accumulating evidence supporting the hypothesis that subclinical infection is a cause of symptomatic capsular contracture; nevertheless, the relationship has not been firmly established. Several human studies have found bacteria on the surface of cultured implants, and an association between these findings and clinically significant capsular contracture has been suggested. Bacteria, predominantly *S. epidermidis*, were cultured from 56% (15/27) of implants surrounded by contracted capsules versus 18% (5/28) without capsular contracture. Similarly, bacteria were detected on 76% and 28% of implants with contractured and noncontractured capsules, respectively. Netscher et al cultured capsular tissue of 389 implants removed for reasons other than clinical infection; 24% of cases tested positive. Most of the organisms were coagulase-negative staphylococci and anaerobic diphtheroids, although fungi and other organisms were also detected. A comparative, prospective, blinded study of implants and capsules removed from patients with or without capsular contracture was conducted to investigate the association between biofilm and capsular contracture. Capsule and implant samples obtained during explantation were tested by routine culture, broth culture (after maceration and sonication for 20 minutes), and scanning electron microscopy.

During a period of 22 months, a total of 48 implant and/or capsular samples were studied from 27 breasts, of which 19 exhibited significant contracture (Baker's grade III/IV). Seventeen of these 19 capsules were positive, compared with only one of eight samples obtained from patients with minimal or no contracture. Other studies have also observed a significant association between capsular contracture and the presence of bacteria on the implant. Finally, studies assessing the efficacy of local antibacterial agents (e.g., povidone-iodine, cephalothin, bacitracin, cephalexin, and gentamicin) at the time of implantation have found significantly reduced rates of capsular contracture in treated implants/pockets, indirectly suggesting a role for bacteria in the pathogenesis of capsular contracture.

6.3.3 Diagnosis and Management

Once a diagnosis of implant infection is established, all efforts should be aimed at eradicating the causative pathogen and saving the implant if possible. The gold standard for diagnosis is a bacterial culture with an antibiogram. Periprosthetic fluid can be obtained by ultrasound-guided aspiration. Blood culture should be obtained in patients with suspected bacteremia. Empirical therapy with vancomycin is recommended, due to the high number of infections by β-lactam- resistant pathogens (MRSA and coagulase-negative staphylococci). Extended-spectrum cephalosporins or penicillins covering gram-negative pathogens should also be included. If fluid is negative in routine culture, an atypical mycobacterial infection must be suspected and therapy extended for 2 weeks in order to eliminate any unidentified pathogens. Although salvage of the implant may be possible with systemic antibiotics alone, removal is often required, especially if the patient's condition worsens or does not improve within 2 days of therapy. The removed implant must be analyzed for aerobic and anaerobic bacteria, mycobacteria, and fungi. Capsulectomy, though not mandatory, is recommended and usually performed. After implant removal, systemic antibiotics should be continued for 2 weeks, IV in severe infections. Despite the fact that immediate placement of a new implant after pocket irrigation with saline and povidone-iodine has been successful in selected cases, delayed reimplantation is generally advocated. The isolated pathogen and the time taken for eradication will dictate the optimal timing of reimplantation, which is usually performed 3 to 6 months after removal. Finally, the new implant should be placed in a different plane (i.e., submuscular) whenever possible.

Antimicrobial Prophylaxis

The risk of SSI is reduced from 14.4 to 5.8% in surgery without and with preoperative antibiotic prophylaxis, respectively. The guidelines for prevention of SSI provided by the Centers for Disease Control and Prevention (CDC) recommend antibiotic prophylaxis with a single dose of IV first- or second-generation cephalosporin prior to anesthesia and an intraoperative dose if surgery prolongs for 3 or more hours. In patients with allergies to β-lactam antibiotics, clindamycin or cotrimoxazole are recommended. Apart from preoperative antibiotic prophylaxis, an extended and advisable surgical practice includes irrigation of the implant and surgical pocket with an antiseptic or antibiotic solution. Continuation of prophylaxis beyond 24 hours in reconstructive cases has not been proven useful.

6.4 Antimicrobials for Skin and Soft Tissue Infections

This section discusses the spectrum of activity, mechanisms of action, and mechanisms of resistance of the antimicrobials most commonly used for SSTIs. Also discussed are their clinical uses, routes of excretion, and toxic effects.

6.4.1 Spectrum

Depending on the range of bacterial species susceptible to antimicrobials, antibacterials are classified as broad spectrum, intermediate spectrum, or narrow spectrum. Broad-spectrum antibacterials are active against both gram-positive and gram-negative organisms. Examples include tetracyclines, phenicols, fluoroquinolones, and third- and fourth-generation cephalosporins. Narrow- spectrum antibacterials have limited activity and are primarily useful against only particular species of microorganisms. For example, glycopeptides and bacitracin are effective against only gram-positive bacteria, whereas polymyxins are usually effective against only gram-negative bacteria. Aminoglycosides and sulfonamides are effective against only aerobic organisms, whereas nitroimidazoles are generally effective against anaerobes only.

6.4.2 Mechanisms of Action

The treatment of bacterial infections is increasingly complicated by the ability of bacteria to develop resistance to antimicrobial agents. Antimicrobial agents are often categorized according to their main mechanism of action, namely interference with cell wall synthesis (e.g., β-lactams and glycopeptides), inhibition of protein synthesis (macrolides and tetracyclines), interference with nucleic acid synthesis (fluoroquinolones and rifampin), inhibition of a metabolic pathway (trimethoprim-sulfamethoxazole), and disruption of bacterial membrane structure (polymyxins and daptomycin). Bacteria may be intrinsically resistant to one or more classes of antimicrobial agents, or they may acquire resistance by de novo mutation or via the acquisition of resistance genes from other organisms.

6.4.3 Mechanisms of Resistance

Antimicrobial resistance develops through a limited number of mechanisms: (1) permeability changes in the bacterial cell wall/membrane, which restricts antimicrobial access to target sites; (2) active efflux of the antimicrobial from the cell; (3) mutation in the target site; (4) enzymatic modification or degradation of the antimicrobial; and (5) acquisition of alternative metabolic pathways to those inhibited by the drug. Numerous antimicrobial resistance phenotypes result from the acquisition of external genes that may provide resistance to an entire class of antimicrobials. The versatility with which bacterial populations adapt to toxic environments, along with their facility in exchanging DNA, implies that antibiotic resistance is an inevitable biological phenomenon that will likely continue to be a chronic medical problem. Inappropriate use of antibacterial agents may create selective pressure for the emergence of resistant strains. Proper prescription of current antimicrobials and the continued development of new ones are vital to protect our patients against bacterial pathogens.

6.4.4 Antimicrobials Commonly Used in Soft Tissue Infections

The most common pathogens in SSTIs are β-hemolytic streptococci and *S. aureus*. Community-acquired MRSA infections are an emerging problem in the United States and Europe. These infections are typically resistant to β-lactams and erythromycin but are susceptible to trimethoprim-sulfamethoxazole, rifampicin, and sometimes clindamycin (▶Table 6.6). Community-acquired MRSA infections have a different genetic mechanism of resistance from hospital-acquired MRSA infections, and many of them contain Panton– Valentine's leukocidin gene, which is associated with significant local toxicity. The optimal management of community-acquired MRSA infections is not yet clear, but agents such as cloxacillin or cephalosporins are associated with clinical failure and should not be used. Currently, combinations of trimethoprim-sulfamethoxazole or clindamycin with rifampin are recommended for outpatient therapy. Inpatients may be treated with these parenterally or with therapies including vancomycin, daptomycin, or linezolid. Patients with lymphedema, or who have had saphenous vein harvesting for coronary artery bypass surgery, or those with tinea pedis, are predisposed to cellulitis, often due to

Table 6.6 Main antimicrobial drug dosages for skin and soft tissue infections

Antimicrobial	Dosage	Comment
Antibacterials		
Amoxicillin-clavulanate	875/125 mg twice a day	Some gram-negative rods are resistant; misses MRSA
Cefazolin	1 g every 8 h IV 50 mg/kg/d divided in 3 doses	For penicillin-allergic patients except those with immediate hypersensitivity reactions More convenient than nafcillin with less bone marrow suppression
Cephalexin	250 mg oral four times a day 25–50 mg/kg/d in 3–4 divided doses	
Cefuroxime	500 mg every 8–12 h	Good activity against *Pasteurella multocida*; misses anaerobes
Ceftriaxone	1 g every 12 h	
Ciprofloxacin	500 mg every 12 h	Good for anaerobes also human bite. Bacteriostatic; potential of cross-resistance and emergence of resistance in erythromycin-resistant strains; inducible resistance in MRSA
Clindamycin	300 mg three times a day 600 mg every 6–8 h	Good activity against staphylococci, streptococci, and anaerobes; misses *Pasteurella multocida*
Cloxacillin	1–2 g every 4 h IV 100–150 mg/kg/d in 4 divided doses	Inactive against MRSA
Colistin	5 mg/kg load, then 2.5 mg/kg every 12 h	Nephrotoxic; does not cover gram positives or anaerobes, *Proteus, Serratia, Burkholderia*
Daptomycin	4–6 mg/kg/d	Covers VRE, strains nonsusceptible to vancomycin may be cross-resistant to daptomycin
Doxycycline	100 mg twice a day 100 mg every 12 h	Excellent activity against *Pasteurella multocida*; some streptococci are resistant
Erythromycin	250 mg four times a day 40 mg/kg/d in 3–4 divided oral doses	Some strains of *Staphylococcus aureus* and *Streptococcus pyogenes* may be resistant
Ertapenem	1 g every 24 h IV	
Imipenem-cilastatin	500 mg every 6 h IV	
Levofloxacin	750 mg daily	
Linezolid	600 mg every 12 h	100% oral bioavailability Covers VRE and MRSA

Table 6.6 *(Continued)* Main antimicrobial drug dosages for skin and soft tissue infections

Antimicrobial	Dosage	Comment
Meropenem	1 g every 8 h IV	
Metronidazole	250–500 mg three times a day 500 mg every 8 h	Good activity against anaerobes; no activity against aerobes
Moxifloxacin	400 mg daily	
Mupirocin ointment	Apply to lesions twice a day	
Piperacillin-tazobactam	3.37 g every 6–8 h	Misses MRSA
SMX-TMP	160–800 mg twice a day 5–10 mg/kg/d of TMP component	Good activity against aerobes; poor activity against anaerobes
Vancomycin	30–60 mg/kg/d divided in 2–4 doses	Target serum concentrations of 15–20 µg/mL in severe infections
Antifungals		
Fluconazole	100–400 mg every 24 h 800 mg loading dose, then 400 mg daily	*Candida krusei* and *Candida glabrata* are resistant
Lipid complex amphotericin B	5 mg/kg/d	Not active against fusaria
Liposomal amphotericin B	3–5 mg/kg/d	Not active against fusaria
Posaconazole	400 mg twice a day with meals	Covers Mucorales
Voriconazole	400 mg twice a day × 2 doses, then 200 mg every 12 h 6 mg/kg IV every 12 h for 2 doses, followed by 4 mg/kg IV every 12 h	Accumulation of cyclodextrin vehicle with IV formulation with renal insufficiency

Abbreviations: IV, intravenous; MRSA, methicillin-resistant *Staphylococcus aureus*; SMX-TMP, sulfamethoxazole and trimethoprim; VRE, vancomycin-resistant enterococci.

streptococci, which is typically managed with an antistaphylococcal penicillin or first-generation cephalosporin. Unusual causes of soft tissue infection include *Eikenella corrodens* and oral anaerobes after human bites; *Pasteurella multocida* and *Capnocytophaga canimorsus* after animal bites; *A. hydrophila* after freshwater exposure or exposure to leeches; *V. vulnificus* after saltwater exposure; *Erysipelothrix rhusiopathiae* and *S. iniae* after fish exposure; and *Pseudomonas aeruginosa* after hot tub exposure.

Natural Penicillins

Agents include penicillin G (IV), penicillin V (oral), procaine penicillin (intramuscular [IM]), and benzathine penicillin (IM). Clinical uses of the natural penicillins include treatment of skin or soft tissue infections (when staphylococci are not suspected) caused by group A streptococci. These agents have short half-lives, necessitating frequent administration or continuous infusions (except long-acting IM formulations, such as penicillin G. benzathine and penicillin G procaine). They are renally excreted and

require dosage adjustment with renal dysfunction. Patients allergic to one penicillin should be considered allergic to all penicillins. Additionally, there is a cross allergenicity rate of 3–7% with cephalosporin compounds and some cross-allergenicity with carbapenems.

Aminopenicillins

The agents are ampicillin (IV and oral) and amoxicillin (oral). The advantages of amoxicillin over oral ampicillin are increased gastrointestinal absorption, decreased incidence of diarrhea, and dosage three times a day instead of four times a day. Their spectrum of activity extends the antibacterial spectrum of the natural penicillins to include certain strains of *E. coli*, and *Proteus mirabilis*. These agents have short half-lives and are excreted renally.

Penicillinase-Resistant Penicillins

Agents include methicillin (IV), nafcillin (IV), and cloxacillin (oral, IV). These are primarily used for treatment of group A streptococci and MRSA infections, which makes them useful agents for SSTIs caused by these organisms. The pharmacokinetic properties of these penicillins differ from the others in that they are the only penicillins that are not cleared renally. Similar to the natural penicillins, they have short half-lives and require frequent administration or continuous infusions. Prolonged use of these penicillins can induce transient neutropenia.

β-Lactamase Inhibitors

Agents in this group are amoxicillin-clavulanate, ampicillin-sulbactam, ticarcillin-clavulanate, and piperacillin-tazobactam. The spectrum of activity of the parent drug is increased by the addition of β-lactamase inhibitors (e.g., clavulanate and sulbactam). They have good activity against methicillin-susceptible staphylococci and group A streptococci, anaerobes, and some gram-negative organisms. Similar to other β-lactam agents, they are not active against MRSA. Clinical uses include coverage for mixed gram-negative, gram-positive, and anaerobic infections (including complicated skin or soft tissue infections) and empirical broad-spectrum therapy for polymicrobial infections.

Cephalosporins

Cephalosporins are not active against methicillin-resistant staphylococci or enterococci. First-generation cephalosporins are active against methicillin-susceptible staphylococci and most streptococci. Cefuroxime and the oral second-generation cephalosporins may be used for community-acquired SSTIs if MRSA is not involved. Third-generation cephalosporins can be used for nosocomial gram-negative infections or in combination with an anti-anaerobic agent (e.g., metronidazole) for polymicrobial infections. Ceftazidime is more active than any other third-generation cephalosporin against *Pseudomonas* spp. and is often used for nosocomial infections. Cefotaxime, cefuroxime, ceftizoxime, and the oral third-generation agents provide good coverage of community-acquired pathogens. Inducible resistance to ceftazidime and other cephalosporins can develop in *Enterobacter* organisms, and extended-spectrum β-lactamase–producing *E. coli* and *Klebsiella* spp. are an increasing problem.

Cefepime, a fourth-generation cephalosporin, has gram-positive activity similar to cefotaxime and gram-negative activity similar to or better than ceftazidime. Its spectrum includes *Pseudomonas* and *Enterobacter* species.

Carbapenems

Carbapenems (imipenem, meropenem, and ertapenem) have the broadest spectrum of activity of all antibiotics, covering gram-positive, gram-negative, and anaerobic organisms. They are commonly used as broad-spectrum empirical therapy, which can often be narrowed following reports of cultures and sensitivities. Ertapenem is considerably less expensive than the other carbapenems, while still providing a broad spectrum of activity. However, it does not provide good coverage of *Enterococcus* spp., *P. aeruginosa*, or *Acinetobacter* spp.

Vancomycin

IV vancomycin, a bactericidal glycopeptide antibiotic, has a spectrum of activity against most aerobic and anaerobic gram-positive organisms. It is the drug of choice for infections caused by MRSA, methicillin-resistant coagulase-negative staphylococci, ampicillin-resistant enterococci, highly penicillin-resistant *S. pneumoniae*, and *Bacillus* spp. Oral vancomycin is not absorbed and should not be used to treat systemic infections. Its most important toxic effect is ototoxicity. Nephrotoxicity can occur when it is coadministered with other nephrotoxic agents. "Red man" syndrome following vancomycin infusion is due to nonimmunologic release of histamine and does not constitute a true allergy.

Cotrimoxazole (Trimethoprim–Sulfamethoxazole)

Cotrimoxazole consists of two separate antimicrobials, trimethoprim and sulfamethoxazole, combined in a fixed (1:5) ratio. Both trimethoprim and sulfamethoxazole inhibit microbial folic acid synthesis and act synergistically when used in combination. Clinical uses of cotrimoxazole include the treatment of selected SSTIs. Hypersensitivity reactions to cotrimoxazole are common in patients with acquired immunodeficiency syndrome.

Fluoroquinolones

Agents include norfloxacin, ciprofloxacin, oflox-acin, levofloxacin, gatifloxacin, moxifloxacin, and gemifloxacin. Clinical uses of fluoroquinolones are quite broad and include treatment of gram-nega-tive aerobic infections, such as complicated SSTIs, and many resistant gram-negative organisms (e.g., nosocomial infections). The newer agents, moxi-floxacin, gatifloxacin, gemifloxacin, and levo-floxacin, are particularly well suited to treat community- acquired infections.

Linezolid

Linezolid is an oxalodinone that possesses ac-tivity against gram-positive bacteria, including MRSA, methicillin-resistant *Staphylococcus epi-dermidis*, vancomycin-resistant enterococci, and penicillin-resistant *S. pneumoniae*. Linezolid is not active against gram-negative bacteria, and it can be administered orally or IV. Linezolid is rapidly and extensively absorbed after oral dos-ing, with its bioavailability approaching 100%. Clinical uses of linezolid include treatment of re-sistant gram-positive bacterial infections. Many clinicians advise cautious use of this agent to pre-serve its activity against resistant gram-positive pathogens when there are few other available options. It is an alternative agent for the treat-ment of susceptible gram-positive infections in patients intolerant to first-line agents. Headache, diarrhea, and peripheral or optic neuropathy can also occur. Linezolid is also a weak monoamine oxidase inhibitor and may interact with some medications, such as selective serotonin reuptake inhibitors or monoamine oxidase inhibitor antidepressants.

Daptomycin

The spectrum of activity includes *S. aureus* (in-cluding methicillin-resistant strains), *Strepto-coccus pyogenes*, *Streptococcus agalactiae*, and *Enterococcus* spp. (including vancomycin-resistant strains). Toxicities of daptomycin include gastroin-testinal effects, hypersensitivity reactions, head-ache, insomnia, myalgias, and increase in creatine phosphokinase value. This agent is approved for complicated skin infections caused by gram-posi-tive pathogens. It may be of use in the treatment of vancomycin-resistant enterococci, but clinical data are currently scant.

Tetracyclines

Agents are short acting (tetracycline, chlortet-racycline, oxytetracycline), intermediate acting (demeclocycline, methacycline), and long acting (doxycycline, minocycline). Tetracyclines impair fetal bone growth and stain children's teeth and therefore should not be administered to pregnant women and infants. Enteric absorption is substan-tially decreased by coadministration with milk, antacids, iron, calcium, or compounds containing calcium, magnesium, or aluminum.

Tigecycline

Tigecycline is a novel glycylcycline antimicrobi-al that is structurally related to minocycline but with expanded activity. It is available for IV ad-ministration only. It is currently approved for com-plicated skin infections and will likely be of use against multiresistant pathogens, such as methi-cillin-resistant staphylococci, staphylococci with reduced susceptibility to vancomycin, vancomy-cin-resistant enterococci, and multidrug-resistant gram-negative organisms such as *Acinetobacter* or *Stenotrophomonas*.

Clindamycin

Clindamycin is active against aerobic and an-aerobic gram-positive microorganisms. Its clin-ical uses encompass the treatment of anaerobic infections (e.g., anaerobic and mixed head and neck, and pelvic infections), along with being a useful alternative for soft tissue infections. The combination of clindamycin and penicillin for necrotizing group A streptococcal or clostridial infections may be superior to either drug alone. For polymicrobial infections, it is commonly combined with a gram-negative active agent. Through the inhibition of protein synthesis, clin-damycin may reduce pyogenic toxin production. Antibiotic-associated diarrhea can occur in up to 20% of patients, including *Clostridium difficile* colitis in 1–10%.

Metronidazole

Metronidazole is quite active against most anaero-bic microorganisms, including *Bacteroides* species. It is often used in combination with other agents active against aerobes for mixed infections, includ-ing intra-abdominal infections.

6.5 Conclusions

SSTIs are part of any plastic surgeon's everyday practice; therefore knowledge of their general approach and management is paramount. Early recognition and prompt therapy, when indicated, are key in preventing the infection from spreading. In addition, by incorporating some of the basic principles of antimicrobials related to their mechanism of action, spectrum, and main indications, plastic surgeons should feel more confident in treating a number of infections seen in their practice. For more complicated scenarios, participation of an infectious disease specialist is mandatory because close communication with them provides an invaluable combination of medical and surgical knowledge that translates into the delivery of an effective targeted therapy, ultimately leading to improved patient outcomes.

6.6 Key Points

1. It is imperative to distinguish necrotizing from nonnecrotizing infections in order to avoid delays of treatment to save life and limb. Necrotizing fasciitis is a surgical emergency, and early surgical debridement optimizes outcomes in these patients.
2. Broad-spectrum antimicrobial agents are used as initial empirical therapy with the intent to cover multiple possible pathogens commonly associated with the specific clinical entity. Once the etiologic pathogen is identified, every attempt should be made to narrow the antibiotic spectrum to avoid resistance.
3. SSIs are considered complicated SSTIs requiring early recognition and prompt management. In some cases, SSIs may present with systemic toxicity in immunocompetent individuals.

4. Patients with breast implants presenting with a bacterial infection, even in distant places, should start antibiotic therapy. Likewise, invasive diagnostic procedures and surgery in patients with breast implants should be associated with antibiotic prophylaxis.
5. Although the implant can sometimes be salvaged by systemic antibiotics, breast implant infection often requires implant removal. Capsulectomy, though not mandatory, is advocated and usually performed. Immediate reimplantation is not advised.
6. Capsular contracture is the most common complication of breast implant surgery. Its cause, treatment, and prevention remain to be fully elucidated; nevertheless, infection has been suggested to have a role in its pathogenesis.
7. Depending on the range of susceptible microorganisms, antibacterials are classified as broad spectrum, intermediate spectrum, or narrow spectrum. Broad-spectrum antibacterials (e.g., tetracyclines, phenicols, fluoroquinolones, third- and fourth-generation cephalosporins) are active against both gram-positive and gram-negative organisms. Conversely, narrow-spectrum antibacterials have limited activity and are useful against only certain species of microorganisms.

Recommended Readings

Aabideen KK, Munshi V, Kumar VB, Dean F. Orbital cellulitis in children: a review of 17 cases in the UK. Eur J Pediatr. 2007;166(11):1193–1194

Abrahamian FM, Talan DA, Moran GJ. Management of skin and soft-tissue infections in the emergency department. Infect Dis Clin North Am 2008; 22(1):89–116, vi

Adams WP Jr, Rios JL, Smith SJ. Enhancing patient outcomes in aesthetic and reconstructive breast surgery using triple antibiotic breast irrigation: six-year prospective clinical study. Plast Reconstr Surg. 2006; 117(1):30–36

Alikhan A, Lynch PJ, Eisen DB. Hidradenitis suppurativa: a comprehensive review. J Am Acad Dermatol. 2009; 60(4):539–561, quiz 562–563

Baddour LM. Cellulitis syndromes: an update. Int J Antimicrob Agents. 2000; 14(2):113–116

Bickels J, Ben-Sira L, Kessler A, Wientroub S. Primary pyomyositis. J Bone Joint Surg Am. 2002; 84-A(12):2277–2286

Brown SL. Epidemiology of silicone-gel breast implants. Epidemiology. 2002; 13(Suppl 3):S34–S39

Burkhardt BR, Dempsey PD, Schnur PL, Tofield JJ. Capsular contracture: a prospective study of the effect of local antibacterial agents. Plast Reconstr Surg. 1986; 77(6):919–932

Darouiche RO. Treatment of infections associated with surgical implants. N Engl J Med 2004; 350(14):1422–1429

Del Pozo JL, Tran NV, Petty PM, et al. Pilot study of association of bacteria on breast implants with capsular contracture. J Clin Microbiol. 2009; 47(5):1333–1337

del Pozo JL, Auba C. Role of biofilms in breast implant associated infections and capsular contracture. Adv Exp Med Biol 2015; 831:53–67

del Pozo JL, Garcia-Quetglas E, Hernaez S, et al. Granulicatella adiacens breast implant-associated infection. Diagn Microbiol Infect Dis. 2008; 61(1):58–60

del Pozo JL, Patel R. The challenge of treating biofilm-associated bacterial infections. Clin Pharmacol Ther. 2007; 82(2):204–209

Dobke MK, Svahn JK, Vastine VL, Landon BN, Stein PC, Parsons CL. Characterization of microbial presence at the surface of silicone mammary implants. Ann Plast Surg. 1995; 34(6):563–569, 570–571

Drinka P, Bonham P, Crnich CJ. Swab culture of purulent skin infection to detect infection or colonization with antibiotic-resistant bacteria. J Am Med Dir Assoc. 2012; 13(1):75–79

Dryden MS. Complicated skin and soft tissue infection. J Antimicrob Chemother. 2010; 65(Suppl 3):iii35–iii44

Engemann JJ, Carmeli Y, Cosgrove SE, et al. Adverse clinical and economic outcomes attributable to methicillin resistance among patients with Staphylococcus aureus surgical site infection. Clin Infect Dis. 2003; 36(5):592–598

Eron LJ, Lipsky BA, Low DE, Nathwani D, Tice AD, Volturo GA; Expert panel on managing skin and soft tissue infections. Managing skin and soft tissue infections: expert panel recommendations on key decision points. J Antimicrob Chemother. 2003; 52(Suppl 1):i3–i17

Esposito S, Bassetti M, Borre' S, et al; Italian Society of Infectious Tropical Diseases. International Society of Chemotherapy. Diagnosis and management of skin and soft-tissue infections (SSTI): a literature review and consensus statement on behalf of the Italian Society of Infectious Diseases and International Society of Chemotherapy. J Chemother. 2011; 23(5):251–262

Figtree M, Konecny P, Jennings Z, Goh C, Krilis SA, Miyakis S. Risk stratification and outcome of cellulitis admitted to hospital. J Infect. 2010; 60(6):431–439

Guégan S, Lanternier F, Rouzaud C, Dupin N, Lortholary O. Fungal skin and soft tissue infections. Curr Opin Infect Dis. 2016; 29(2):124–130

Karian LS, Chung SY, Lee ES. Reconstruction of defects after fournier gangrene: A systematic review. Eplasty. 2015; 15:e18

Kjøller K, Hölmich LR, Jacobsen PH, et al. Capsular contracture after cosmetic breast implant surgery in Denmark. Ann Plast Surg. 2001; 47(4):359–366

Kohannim O, Rubin Z, Taylor M. Saline breast implant fluid collection and reactive arthritis in a patient with streptococcal toxic shock syndrome. J Clin Rheumatol. 2011; 17(2):89–91

Kujath P, Kujath C. Complicated skin, skin structure and soft tissue infections - are we threatened by multi-resistant pathogens? Eur J Med Res. 2010; 15(12):544–553

Liu C, Bayer A, Cosgrove SE, et al. Clinical practice guidelines by the infectious diseases society of america for the treatment of methicillin-resistant Staphylococcus aureus infections in adults and children: executive summary. Clin Infect Dis. 2011; 52(3):285–292

Lopez FA, Lartchenko S. Skin and soft tissue infections. Infect Dis Clin North Am. 2006; 20(4):759–772, v–vi

Marinella MA. Group C streptococcal sepsis complicating Fournier gangrene. South Med J 2005; 98(9):921–923

May AK. Skin and soft tissue infections. Surg Clin North Am. 2009; 89(2):403–420, viii

Moran GJ, Krishnadasan A, Gorwitz RJ, et al; EMERGEncy ID Net Study Group. Methicillin-resistant S. aureus infections among patients in the emergency department. N Engl J Med. 2006; 355(7):666–674

Morgan M. Treatment of MRSA soft tissue infections: an overview. Injury. 2011; 42(Suppl 5):S11–S17

Napolitano LM. Severe soft tissue infections. Infect Dis Clin North Am. 2009; 23(3):571–591

Netscher DT, Weizer G, Wigoda P, Walker LE, Thornby J, Bowen D. Clinical relevance of positive breast periprosthetic cultures without overt infection. Plast Reconstr Surg. 1995; 96(5):1125–1129

Pajkos A, Deva AK, Vickery K, Cope C, Chang L, Cossart YE. Detection of subclinical infection in significant breast implant capsules. Plast Reconstr Surg. 2003; 111(5):1605–1611

Pan A, Cauda R, Concia E, et al; Gruppo Italiano di Studio sulle Infezioni Gravi (GISIG) Working Group on Complicated Skin and Skin-Structure Infections. Consensus document on controversial issues in the treatment of complicated skin and skin-structure infections. Int J Infect Dis. 2010; 14(Suppl 4):S39–S53

Parada JP, Maslow JN. Clinical syndromes associated with adult pneumococcal cellulitis. Scand J Infect Dis. 2000; 32(2):133–136

Phillips BT, Bishawi M, Dagum AB, Khan SU, Bui DT. A systematic review of antibiotic use and infection in breast reconstruction: what is the evidence? Plast Reconstr Surg. 2013; 131(1):1–13

Pittet B, Montandon D, Pittet D. Infection in breast implants. Lancet Infect Dis. 2005; 5(2):94–106

Rieger UM, Mesina J, Kalbermatten DF, et al. Bacterial biofilms and capsular contracture in patients with breast implants. Br J Surg. 2013; 100(6):768–774

Sarkis P, Farran F, Khoury R, et al. Fournier's gangrene: a review of the recent literature [in French]. Prog Urol. 2009; 19(2):75–84

Slade DE, Powell BW, Mortimer PS. Hidradenitis suppurativa: pathogenesis and management. Br J Plast Surg. 2003; 56(5):451–461

Spear SL, Howard MA, Boehmler JH, Ducic I, Low M, Abbruzzesse MR. The infected or exposed breast implant: management and treatment strategies. Plast Reconstr Surg. 2004; 113(6):1634–1644

Stevens DL, Bisno AL, Chambers HF, et al; Infectious Diseases Society of America. Practice guidelines for the diagnosis and management of skin and soft-tissue infections [published correction appears in Clin Infect Dis 2006;15;42(8):1219]. (Note: Dosage error in article text). Clin Infect Dis. 2005; 41(10):1373–1406

Swartz MN. Clinical practice. Cellulitis. N Engl J Med. 2004; 350(9):904–912

Tognetti L, Martinelli C, Berti S, et al. Bacterial skin and soft tissue infections: review of the epidemiology, microbiology, aetiopathogenesis and treatment: a collaboration between dermatologists and infectivologists. J Eur Acad Dermatol Venereol. 2012; 26(8):931–941

Vandeweyer E, Deraemaecker R, Nogaret JM, Hertens D. Immediate breast reconstruction with implants and adjuvant chemotherapy: a good option? Acta Chir Belg. 2003; 103(1):98–101

Venturi ML, Attinger CE, Mesbahi AN, Hess CL, Graw KS. Mechanisms and clinical applications of the vacuum-assisted closure (VAC) Device: a review. Am J Clin Dermatol. 2005; 6(3):185–194

Virden CP, Dobke MK, Stein P, Parsons CL, Frank DH. Subclinical infection of the silicone breast implant surface as a possible cause of capsular contracture. Aesthetic Plast Surg. 1992; 16(2):173–179

Washer LL, Gutowski K. Breast implant infections. Infect Dis Clin North Am. 2012; 26(1):111–125

Wong CH, Khin LW, Heng KS, Tan KC, Low CO. The LRINEC (Laboratory Risk Indicator for Necrotizing Fasciitis) score: a tool for distinguishing necrotizing fasciitis from other soft tissue infections. Crit Care Med. 2004; 32(7):1535–1541

Zervos MJ, Freeman K, Vo L, et al. Epidemiology and outcomes of complicated skin and soft tissue infections in hospitalized patients. J Clin Microbiol. 2012; 50(2):238–245

7 Implants and Biomaterials

Marco Romeo, Chiara Distefano

Abstract

Biomaterials are materials intended to be physically, chemically, and functionally compatible with the biological system where they are implanted. For centuries, medicine and science have tried to replace and improve body parts through the implantation of foreign materials, from gold, glass, or wood to modern ceramics or even biological implants, with varying degrees of success. Although the perfect biomaterial is yet to be developed, any product implanted in the human body should fulfill a list of criteria ranging from biocompatibility to being noncarcinogenic, and it should have a mechanical resistance that suits the part that is being replaced. We are witnessing remarkable developments and advances in the production of synthetic materials as well as biological matrices, and with this a growing body of alternatives for a range of reconstructive and aesthetic needs. Although completely artificial products are still the mainstay of biomaterials, the current trend is progressively shifting toward the development of tissue-engineered substitutes, whereby biological scaffolds are seeded with cells to promote tissue and organ (re)generation to achieve complex functional structures. Injectable substances form an important part of the biomaterial field. Resorbable and permanent materials have been and continue to be used frequently for reconstructive and aesthetic purposes; therefore a thorough understanding of their composition, indications, and potential complications is paramount to any plastic surgeon to ensure their correct and safe use. This chapter describes the different classes of biomaterials and implants and outlines the main factors affecting the outcome of implantation.

Keywords: alloplastic, biomaterials, foreign body, implants, injectables, silicone

7.1 Introduction

Biomaterials and implants in modern times have a story, albeit a short one.

Yet, in human history there have been many attempts to use synthetic materials to replace parts and functions of the human body. In fact, it is possible to go back to the Mayan civilization (500 BC) to find some examples of dental implants with seashells achieving some degree of bone integration. Moreover, basic suturing has been a well-assumed concept since the time of the early Egyptians.

Sutures and dental replacements have been the two most investigated fields through the centuries. Despite the lack of knowledge about biology and materials, sutures were commonly used with a great deal of success for thousands of years.

Regarding materials, gold, glass, and even wood were commonly used 2,000 years ago by the Roman, Chinese, and Aztec civilizations.

In the last 2 centuries, invention of new materials (e.g., plastics) has given rise to many experiments, but given the lack of concepts of biocompatibility, the results were frustrating.

Modern history spans the two world wars, when polymethyl methacrylate (PMMA), Dacron, nylon, polyethylene, and high-molecular-weight steel were used for the first time in vascular and orthopaedic surgery.

The word *biomaterial* was introduced in the late 1960s and led to the formation of the Society for Biomaterials in 1975.

Since then, not only pioneering physicians but also researchers in all scientific fields have been conducting experiments and investigations to explore new materials and their compatibility with the human body.

This chapter describes the different classes of biomaterials and implants and their clinical application for successful implantation.

7.1.1 Basic Science

By definition, a biomaterial is any material engineered to be physically, chemically, or functionally similar to a biological material made to interact with a biological system. The purely artificial materials can also be considered biomimetic materials.

Biomaterials are usually classified as follows:
- Autograft: living tissue derived from a host
- Allograft: nonliving tissue derived from the same species (e.g., cadaveric tissues)
- Xenograft: nonliving tissue from different species (e.g., porcine or bovine tissue)
- Alloplast: synthetic material

This chapter does not discuss autografts.

The ideal biomaterial must fulfill a list of requirements to be successfully implanted with a low rate of complications. The first and most important feature is biocompatibility. According to Donaruma, biocompatibility exists when a biomaterial and a physiologic environment do not adversely significantly affect each other. In addition, biomaterials must produce no foreign-body inflammatory response, and they must be chemically inert, noncarcinogenic, nontoxic, nonallergenic, sterilizable, and resistant to mechanical strains. Biomaterials should not favor the growth of microorganisms, and it should be possible to fabricate them in the desired form. Also, temporary (degradable) implants must resorb in a predictable and nontoxic manner.

Some of these characteristics, such as chemical and inflammatory responses, are relative features that may be modulated according to a specific need.

7.1.2 Body Reaction to Biomaterials

Even the most biocompatible materials elicit a reaction from the host, which may eventually lead to implant failure or the development of a harmful, potentially lethal, outcome. Any biomaterial may thus trigger one or more of several responses, including inflammation and foreign body reaction, immunologic response, toxicity, thrombosis, cell migration, infection, and carcinogenesis.

Inflammation, defined as the reaction of a vascularized living tissue to injury, is the basic response toward any implant. Depending on the time span of activity it can be acute or chronic and eventually lead to a variable degree of fibrosis and the formation of a fibrous capsule as a result of foreign body reaction and isolation. The biocompatibility of a certain material is usually defined by the lowest possible inflammatory response that is limited in time and does not become chronic.

The immune response serves to protect the body from any agent (biological or synthetic) that is sensed as "nonself" and can be broadly divided into cellular and humoral. A humoral response with complement activation is largely involved in biomaterial reactions, with the complement mediating a local inflammatory response to the foreign body. When the cascade is abnormally activated, clinically relevant side effects ensue. Any material with low activation of the complement cascade is thus ideal for implantation. As a consequence of excessive inflammation due to artificial surface exposition, an imbalance between pro- and anticoagulation factors can occur at the site of implantation, leading to thrombus formation.

Lastly, implanted foreign materials might produce malignant neoplasia through either a direct cellular stimulation or secondary to chronic inflammation. Most cancers induced by implants are late sarcomas with rapid and local growth adjacent to the implant itself, with large surface materials likely posing a greater likelihood to develop this kind of tumor. Conversely, resorbable materials represent a minor risk. In any case, the incidence and rarity of these lesions together with the improvement of materials knowledge render prosthetic materials worthy of use, with more benefits than real risks.

7.2 Materials

7.2.1 Metals

Metals are among the materials most tolerated by the human body; thus they have been used for a long time, since the age of ancient Greece, long before modern research scientifically proved their safety.

Alloys are composed of different metals or a metal and another element. Given their stiffness, biocompatibility, radiotransparency, and resistance to stress various alloys (chromium-cobalt, steel, titanium) are used for bone fixation, joint prostheses, or sutures and staples. Outside the field of plastic and reconstructive surgery, alloys are used in the fabrication of complex devices, such as pacemakers and stents. Stainless steel (an alloy of iron, molybdenum, nickel, silicone, manganese, and chromium) was developed at the beginning of 20th century and proved to be reliable and flexible but rigid enough for plate fixation. Steel was later substituted by Vitallium (an alloy of cobalt, chromium, and molybdenum), developed in 1932 by Albert W. Merrick for the Austenal Laboratories, for its resistance to corrosion compared to steel. The resistance to corrosion was a sign of great progress because metal's erosion causes the release of toxic ions and possible mechanical failure, and it promotes inflammation. This alloy has also the rare feature of being compatible with magnetic resonance, though not to the same level as titanium.

Titanium is currently replacing all other metals due to its natural resistance to corrosion and its diamagnetic characteristics, which make it compatible with magnetic resonance. It can also be used as an alloy with vanadium and aluminum. Titanium is an abundant metal on earth; however, it is difficult and expensive to manufacture.

Gold and platinum are resistant to corrosion but have limited mechanical features. On the other hand, their high atomic number make them heavy enough to produce small heavy implants, such as those used for eyelid closure in facial palsy patients.

In addition, their ability to osseointegrate makes metals a very good material for dental implants and prosthetic limbs.

7.2.2 Polymers

The structure of polymers, as the name itself indicates, is constituted of a theoretically endless chain of a certain repeated molecule, which can have variable molecular weights, from low to high, and different properties according to specific features (▶Table 7.1). In addition, depending on their porosity, polymers interact differently with the surrounding tissues, in fact, macroporous polymers allow incorporation and encapsulation while nonporous polymers do not allow such phenomena.

Silicone

The most popular of polymers, silicone, is a synthetic material made of repeating units of siloxane, which is formed by a chain of alternating silicon and oxygen atoms combined with carbon and/or hydrogen. First described by Kipping in 1904, the amazing chemical properties of silicone allows it to be used in various forms: fluid, emulsion, compound, resin, and elastomer.

Silicone has a number of applications in medicine. In the 1940s, its hydrophobicity was employed to

Table 7.1 Polymer characteristics

Factors that influence polymer properties
Chemical composition
• Ester and amide links permit enzymatic degradation
• Cross linking increases viscosity
Length of chain
• Short chain: liquid
• Mid chain: gel
• Long chain: elastomer/solid

coat needles, syringes, and tubes to prevent coagulation of blood samples. The first published report of a silicone implant was in 1946, when Dr. Frank H. Lahey used a silicone elastomer for bile duct repair.

Examples of the use of silicone in hand surgery include the Swanson implants for metacarpophalangeal and interphalangeal joint arthroplasty and Silastic rods (Dow Corning) for tendon repair.

Liquid silicone has been used in the past for soft tissue augmentation, particularly in the field of cosmetic surgery; however, in 1992 the U.S. Food and Drug Administration banned this form of silicone for medical purposes, and its use should be condemned due to its severe adverse reactions, including inflammation, induration, discoloration, ulceration, migration, and granuloma formation.

In plastic surgery, silicone is widely used for manufacturing breast implants and other types of implants (e.g., gluteal, calf, pectoral). In 1962 Cornin and Gerow were the first to use silicone implants for breast reconstruction, and its use quickly expanded and popularized, in part due to the advantages of these implants compared to the foam-based implants available at that time. Initially, silicone implants were vacuum-molded, round-shaped implants with the anterior and posterior surfaces sealed together and a loop of Dacron mesh on the posterior aspect for fixation to the chest wall at the implantation site. Since their introduction, however, breast implants have undergone a number of changes. The first implants were made of liquid silicone encased within a silicone shell that frequently led to rupture and dispersion of silicone into the surrounding tissues. Implants are now made of cohesive silicone gel that has a consistency more similar to that of native breast tissue, with the important advantage that, if ruptured, the gel stays in place and no dissemination occurs. Cohesive silicone gel is used as filler for breast and gluteal implants, whereas the solid form is used for chin, malar, nasal, chest, and calf augmentation devices.

One of the most common complications associated with the use of implants for breast augmentation or reconstruction is capsular contracture, which refers to the thickening and contraction of the physiological fibrous layer of tissue that the body forms around the implant as part of the normal foreign-body reaction elicited by the device. The etiology of capsular contracture is multifactorial and not fully elucidated; nevertheless, in its most severe forms it can lead to

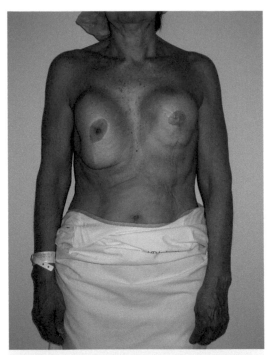

Fig. 7.1 Bilateral capsular contracture (Baker IV) in a patient with a previous breast augmentation.

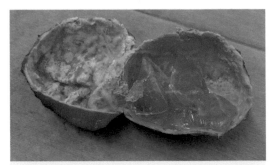

Fig. 7.2 Calcified capsules after removal. The wall was stone hard and required total excision.

prepared in forms of increasing strength and stiffness according to its density. Its porous and woven forms allow fibrovascular ingrowth and certain integration with the tissues. At the same time, this feature renders removal of the implant more difficult. Common applications of polyethylene in plastic surgery include the use of Medpor (Porex Surgical) for facial implants and orbital floor support (with or without an associated titanium mesh) and Marlex (Bard Davol Inc) for chest wall reconstruction.

Polypropylene

This polymer is made of a carbon backbone and side chains of hydrogen and methyl groups. Widely known by its commercial name, Prolene (Ethicon), polypropylene is mainly used for the fabrication of mesh for hernia repair and non-resorbable sutures.

Polyesters

Polyesters are polymers that contain the ester functional group in their chain. Mersilene (Ethicon) is a polyester mesh used for abdominal herniorrhaphy as well as chest wall reconstruction; Dacron, another polyester is used for vascular grafts and suture material. Polyester prostheses reinforced with polyurethane (Xomed, Medtronic) are also used for craniofacial reconstruction. Aliphatic polyesters are used for the fabrication of several sutures, including polyglycolic acid (Dexon, Covidien), polyglactin 910 (Vicryl, Ethicon), poliglecaprone 25 (Monocryl, Ethicon), and polyglyconate (Maxon, Medtronic), among others.

breast deformation and pain (▶Fig. 7.1), requiring implant removal/replacement and excision of the capsule (e.g., capsulectomy) (▶Fig. 7.2). It is worth noting that some studies have shown a lower incidence of capsular contracture when using polyurethane-coated implants. Another important concern regarding the use of breast implants is the possible association with the development of anaplastic large cell lymphoma. Common clinical findings include delayed onset (e.g., > 12 months following implantation) of fluid collection, the presence of a mass, and pathological lymph nodes. Patients with suspected breast implant–associated anaplastic large cell lymphoma should be should be managed within multidisciplinary teams to allow early diagnosis and treatment, which is frequently based on removal of the implant and complete excision of the tumor, capsule, and affected lymph nodes.

Polyethylene

Polyethylene is a nonresorbable, synthetic, relatively inert low-molecular-weight molecule

Polytetrafluoroethylene

Polytetrafluoroethylene (PTFE) is also known as Teflon, whereas expanded polytetrafluoroethylene (ePTFE) is more commonly known by its commercial name Gore-Tex and is a nonresorbable, inert, nonadhesive, and nonporous polymer. ePTFE is used for a number of clinical applications, including abdominal wall mesh, facial augmentation implants, slings for facial paralysis, suture coating, and vascular grafts, among others. Gore-Tex temporomandibular joint implants were withdrawn from the U.S. market due to their high complication rates, including extrusion and infection.

Polymethyl Methacrylate

PMMA is a hard, noncolored, nonresorbable, inert resin commonly used to replace missing bone. It is made intraoperatively by mixing a liquid methylmethacrylate monomer with a powdered methylmethacrylate polymer to form the resin, which is easily malleable to the desired shape; however, it produces an exothermic reaction reaching up to 80°C that lasts for approximately 10 minutes; therefore surrounding bone and soft tissues need to be irrigated to avoid damage. PMMA is most frequently used for craniofacial reconstruction, and its porosity allows bony ingrowth and slow antibiotic release. Its use as a permanent soft tissue filler has been fraught with complications as explained later in this chapter.

Polyacrylamide

This polymer is formed by repeating units of acrylamide and is most commonly known by the commercial names Aquamid and Bio-Alcamid. They are permanent soft tissue fillers used for facial or body augmentation that have the ability to attract and retain a great amount of water, mimicking human soft tissue consistency. Nevertheless, their use has been seriously questioned due to foreign body reactions and extrusion problems, which may appear years after injection.

Polyurethane

Polyurethane is made by the combination of urethane/polyether segments with different consistencies. It has become popular as a coating for breast implants, with some studies suggesting a lower incidence of capsular contracture.

Conversely, its use has raised concern about potential toxicity and carcinogenesis, although cancer associated with their use has yet to be demonstrated.

> **Note**
>
> Depending on porosity, polymers interact differently with the surrounding tissues, ranging from cellular and vascular ingrowth to no incorporation and encapsulation.

7.2.3 Ceramics and Glasses

Ceramics

Calcium ceramics are used for bone reconstruction because their osteoconductive features allow bone ingrowth and regeneration. The two main products include dicalcium phosphate ($CaHPO4$) and calcium hydroxyapatite $Ca10(PO4)6(OH)2$ [HA]. Their porosity can be modulated to enhance body fluid circulation (microporosity) or osteoconduction (macroporosity). On the downside, although they are very resistant to compression and torque forces, flaws and cracks may occur in load-bearing areas because of their porosity. Clinical applications of ceramics range from dental surgery to vertebral reconstruction, diaphysis bony repair, and cortical bone reconfiguration.

Bioglass

Bioactive glasses are classified as osteoconductive scaffolds with high osteoblastic activity because they stimulate in vivo formation of apatite on the outer surface, which promotes the formation and adhesion of bone. They can be combined with bone auto- and allograft, making bioglasses extremely interesting in bone repair and dental fixation.

The most common commercial product is Nova Bone (Porex Surgical) made with 45% sodium oxide, 45% silica dioxide, 5% calcium, and 5% phosphate.

In recent decades, mesoporous materials (pores with diameters between 2 and 50 nm) have become more appealing due to the fact that pore size and volume are adjustable, and surface properties are well defined. They have many potential applications, such as catalysis, adsorption/separation, and biomedicine. Mesoporous bioactive glass is superior to its nonmesoporous counterpart in terms of osseointegration.

7.2.4 Biological Implants

Biomaterials, usually derived from human or animal tissues, can be either degraded or incorporated into the host's tissue, which makes them different from any synthetic material. Higher biocompatibility results in minimal foreign body reaction with increased integration and vascularization, controlled production of anti-inflammatory cytokines, a lower risk of infection, and improved healing compared with synthetic materials. Two widely used classes of biological implants include acellular dermal matrix (ADM) and hyaluronic acid–based gels (HAGs). Depending on the use and the target tissue being repaired, these biological implants have been developed with variable features, such as mechanical resistance, tensile strength, and porosity.

Acellular Matrices

Acellular (also called decellularized) matrices processed from allogeneic or xenogeneic tissues are the most nature-simulating scaffolds. They have been used in tissue engineering of many tissues, including heart valves, vessels, nerves, tendons, and ligaments. This scaffolding approach removes the allogeneic or xenogeneic cellular antigens from the tissues, because they are the sources for immunogenicity upon implantation, but it preserves the extracellular matrix components, which are common among species and therefore immunologically well tolerated.

A decellularized tissue may be used as a scaffold for the fabrication of the tissue it originally came from (e.g., decellularized blood vessels for vascular grafts) or for the repair of a tissue other than its origin (e.g., acellular dermal matrices used for abdominal wall repair) can be used for homologous functions when it is used to replace an analogous structural tissue. The excellent biocompatibility of the decellularized matrices, coupled with the preservation of growth factors and extracellular matrix components further facilitates cellular invasion and remodeling.

In plastic surgery, the use of decellularized matrices, in particular those of dermal origin (e.g., ADM), have become increasingly popular in the management of a wide range of reconstructive problems, including their use as skin substitutes, for breast reconstruction, and for abdominal and chest wall repair. ▶ Table 7.2 summarizes the most common acellular dermal matrices and their use.

Breast Reconstruction

Breast reconstruction is currently one of the main uses of ADMs in plastic surgery because an implant can be placed at the time of mastectomy, with good coverage and without the need for tissue expansion. This enables an immediate reconstruction in cases that would otherwise be performed in a delayed fashion. Advantages of ADM in breast reconstruction include better breast-shape definition, prevention of implant decubitus on mastectomized skin, better implant isolation, and reduced likelihood of capsular contraction. Integration of the matrix into the surrounding tissues and increased vascularization are other relevant advantages of these products. Nevertheless, there are some relative limitations to the use of ADM in breast reconstruction, such as high rates of seroma requiring prolonged use of drains with antibiotic coverage, and the consequent risk of infection sometimes leading to removal of the implant. According to Lanier et al. and our own experience, stratification of patients by breast size is paramount, so that the smaller the breast, the lower the risk of seroma and infection and the better the aesthetic outcome.

Abdominal and Chest Wall Repair

Abdominal wall reconstruction is a complex challenge for both general and plastic surgeons. Eventration and large hernias can be treated by a component separation technique or using synthetic mesh made of polypropylene, polyethylene, PTFE, or absorbable materials like polyglactin 910 (Vicryl). All these materials, however, are vulnerable to infection and may require explanation if contaminated, and they do not become integrated as does ADM. Moreover, biological meshes prevent the risk of visceral adhesion.

Use of ADM in chest wall reconstruction is gaining popularity due to its low rate of infection, and it has been used for other applications, such as mediastinum sealing and diaphragm patching, among others.

> **Note**
>
> ADM should be included in each surgeon's armamentarium, but it must be used with caution. When reconstructing large breasts it might be better to switch to a different method of reconstruction.

Table 7.2 Acellular dermal matrices and hyaluronic acid gels in plastic surgery

Product type	Derivation	Applications
Alloderm (LifeCell)	Human	Burn wounds, abdominal, chest wall, and breast reconstructions, craniofacial repairs, hand reconstruction
Strattice (LifeCell)	Porcine	Abdominal and breast reconstructions
DermaMatrix (Synthes)	Human	Abdominal wall and breast reconstruction, facial reconstruction
FlexHD (Ethicon)	Human	Abdominal wall and breast reconstruction
Permacol (Covidien)	Porcine	Abdominal wall reconstructions, burn wounds, hand reconstruction, eyelid reconstruction, breast reconstruction
AlloMax (Bard)	Human	Breast reconstruction, hernia repair
Surgimend PRS (TEI Biosciences, Inc.)	Fetal bovine	Hernia repair, muscle flap reinforcement
Surgisis (Cook Medical)	Porcine	Abdominal and chest wall reconstructions, lip augmentation
Biobrane (Smith & Nephew)	Cadaveric acellular dermal matrix	Partial-thickness burns and donor sites
EZ Derm (Genzyme Corp.)	Porcine collagen, cross-linked porcine collagen	Partial-thickness burns; diabetic, pressure, and neuropathic ulcers
Integra (Integra LifeSciences Corp.)	Acellular silicone epidermal substitute over dermal scaffold of collagen and chondroitin-6-sulfate	Deep partial-thickness and full-thickness burns, postsurgical wounds, diabetic ulcers
OASIS Wound Matrix (Cook Medical, Inc.)	Porcine small intestine submucosa	Partial- and full-thickness burns; diabetic, venous, and pressure ulcers

Source: Data partially from Banyard DA, Bourgeois JM, Widgerow AD, Evans GR. Regenerative biomaterials: a review. Plast Reconstr Surg 2015;135(6):1740–1748.

7.2.5 Injectables

Collagen

Collagen is a protein normally present in skin, which gives support and integrity to skin. Its molecular components stay together thanks to cross-linked bonds sensitive to ultraviolet (UV) damage. Collagen turnover is regulated by exposure to UV rays, so that the net amount of collagen decreases with age and sun exposure. In 1978 the first collagen injection in eight patients using a mixture of human and bovine collagen gel led the way for collagen products all over the world. Currently, a number of alternatives are available in the market (▶Table 7.3). Early bovine-derived products required allergy testing before injection, with 3% of patients showing a positive result, which hampered the widespread use of these fillers and created the need to develop products that required no testing. Human-derived collagen was approved by the U.S. Food and Drug Administration (FDA) in 2003 under the names of Cosmoderm and Cosmoplast (▶Table 7.3).

Collagen injectable products may be used to correct superficial or deep wrinkles depending on viscosity of the product. When injected too superficially, there is a risk of granuloma formation, infection, and skin necrosis. On the other hand, injectables should not be used in people with autoimmune diseases, those who are pregnant or breastfeeding, or those who are allergic to or intolerant of any of the components of the product. Particular attention should be paid to people that are prone to hypertrophic or keloid scars. The injection technique must be accurate and in the right plane, and intravascular injection must always be avoided because it may lead to occlusion and ischemia.

Table 7.3 Collagen fillers from the first product on market to the most recent ones.

Year	Name	Composition	Manufacturer
1981	Zyderm I	35 mg/mL bovine collagen + 0.3% lidocaine	McGhan Medical
1983	Zyderm II	65 mg/mL bovine collagen + 0.3% lidocaine	McGhan Medical
1985	Zyplast	35 mg/mL cross-linked with gluterlaldehyde + 0.3% of lidocaine	McGhan Medical
2003	Cosmoderm I	35 mg/mL human-derived collagen	INAMED Corp.
2003	Cosmoderm II	65 mg/mL human-derived collagen	INAMED Corp.
2003	Cosmoplast	35 mg/mL cross-linked with glutaraldehyde human-derived collagen	INAMED Corp.
2008	Evolence	35 mg/mL cross-linked gel porcine-derived collagen	ColBar LifeScience Ltd.

> **Note**
>
> Human-derived and porcine-derived collagens are nowadays the most used injectable collagens, and they require no skin testing before treatment. Bovine derived collagens, such as Zyderm and Zyplast, require allergy testing prior to use.

Hyaluronic Acid

HA is a glycosaminoglycan normally present in the extracellular matrix that contributes significantly to fibroblast proliferation and migration into the skin, and it is involved in wound repair. HA, in particular, activates fibroblasts and draws liquids from the surrounding tissues, giving hydration to the skin. It is sensitive to UVA and UVB rays, so its degradation increases with sun exposure. In aesthetic medicine HA is the most popular injectable drug used for wrinkle correction and volume augmentation. HA has a relatively short life; therefore many laboratory techniques have been developed to enlarge its chain and make it more stable, creating a cross-linked HA. The higher the cross-linking, the more dense and stable the molecule is, allowing it to remain for longer periods.

In 2003 Restylane (Q-med) became the first FDA-approved HA product in the United States, and many others have followed or are pending approval (Teoxane, Teosyal, Filorga) but are commonly used in Europe. These fillers are made of nonanimal stabilized hyaluronic acids and HA chains stabilized by chemical agents. They have different concentrations of HA in their formulations. Although not cross-linked, HA formulations (e.g., Jalupro, Professional Derma SA) are used as biorevitalizers to correct superficial wrinkles. All other types of cross-linked HA fillers have increased viscosity and can be placed at dermal, subdermal, or supraperiosteal levels to correct superficial or deep wrinkles or give volume to different areas of the face, such as the cheeks, lips, and chin. As a dermal filler, HA is commonly prepared in a 1 or 2 mL ready-to-use syringe with a 27- to 32-gauge needle. After injection, the effect is readily seen from the first treatment and may last up to 12 months. The main side effect of aesthetic HA injections is granuloma formation, which can be treated with *Hyaluronidase*, an enzyme able to dissolve HA. It is not recommended for use in patients with autoimmune disease or during pregnancy.

High-molecular-weight HA has been used for volume enhancement of breasts and buttocks since the introduction of Macrolane in 2007 (Q-Med). However, its use in breast augmentation has been suspended in many countries due to the formation of encapsulated lumps, infection, and parenchymal fibrosis, which could impair breast cancer detection.

Hyaloglide (Fidia Advanced Biopolymers S.r.l.) is an auto cross-linked polymer derived from HA able to prevent adhesion formation in tendon and peripheral nerve surgery and is therefore used in hand surgery. It is formulated as a sticky and thick gel, working as a mechanical barrier between the repaired tendons and nerves and the skin above to prevent contact and adhesion during the early phases of healing.

Calcium Hydroxyapatite

Calcium hydroxyapatite (CaHA) is a synthetic injectable filler known as Radiesse (BioForm Medical, Inc.). The composition is 30% CaHA microspheres (the same composition as bone and teeth) suspended in a 70% carboxymethylcellulose aqueous carrier gel.

CaHA has been used in the past in many disciplines, such as maxillofacial surgery, ear, nose, and throat surgery, neurosurgery, orthopedics, and dentistry. The components are considered as normal components of the human body with biocompatibility tests demonstrating that injectable CaHA is biocompatible, nontoxic, nonirritating, and nonantigenic. Radiesse received FDA approval in 2006 for correction of facial fat loss (lipoatrophy) in patients with human immunodeficiency virus (HIV). CaHA is used mainly for correction of the middle and lower face, including oral commissure, marionette lines, mental crease, lateral chin, prejowl sulcus, and malar, submalar, and infraorbital augmentations. Following injection the gel is absorbed, whereas the microspheres of CaHA remain and are encapsulated by collagen, resulting in a highly biocompatible, long-lasting implant with a composition and consistency similar to adjacent tissues. So far there are no reports of calcification, osteogenesis, or foreign body reaction described with CaHA. When used as aesthetic filler, CaHA lasts up to 14–18 months. Finally, a proper injection technique is paramount for CaHA–if injected too superficially it may lead to visible and palpable dimples.

Poly-L-Lactic Acid

Poly-L-lactic acid (PLLA) is a biodegradable, synthetic polymer, which was granted approval for aesthetic facial volume correction and lipoatrophy in Europe in 2004. It can last up to 25 months and is thus considered a semipermanent option for volume correction. Sculptra (Sinclair IS Pharma) is an example of PLLA-based injectable dermal filler. This product should not be used for lip and periorbital augmentation, though it may be used for nonfacial correction, such as nipple reconstruction. Sculptra comes in vials that need to be reconstituted 24 hours before injection by adding 5 mL of sterile water. The mixture should be left overnight to slowly absorb water at room temperature. Before injection, it is optional to add 1 mL of lidocaine to the suspension to reduce pain during the injection, which should be carried out very slowly to avoid precipitation of the hydrogel suspension.

Polyacrylamide and Polyalkylimide

Polyacrylamide (Aquamid, Contura International) and polyalkylimide (Bio-Alcamid, Polymekon) are the most popular permanent fillers used in cosmetic surgery. Aquamid is composed of 97.5% sterile water and 2.5% of cross-linked acrylamide, whereas Bio-Alcamid is a frozen 4% acrylic alkylimide gel dissolved in 96% sterile water. Bio-Alcamid currently has European Community (EC) clearance in Europe but has yet to receive FDA clearance in the United States. Both work as an injectable liquid prosthesis able to elicit a reaction from the surrounding soft tissues, leading to the formation of a thin layer enclosing the material.

Bio-Alcamid and Aquamid have been used to treat lipoatrophy in patients with HIV thanks to their long-lasting results, the possibility of using large amounts of product in a single session, and their low rate of degradation. Both have shown satisfactory results in correction of HIV-related facial atrophy, in particular in the malar area (the main feature alteration in these patients).

Unfortunately, many side effects from the use of permanent fillers have been described, with foreign body reaction leading to granuloma formation being the main one. Other delayed complications include migration, infection, nodules, swelling, dysesthesia, chronic sinus, and migration into the lymphatic system. Many studies have demonstrated that the onset of these complications usually occurs 5 or 6 years following injection. A retrospective study showed complications in 4.8% of patients treated with polyalkylimide.

Migration usually occurs if the material is injected within a muscle or in a highly active anatomical area, whereas infection is due to impurities of the filler agent, implantation of large quantities, and biofilm formation. Minor traumas or low-grade infections may act as triggers for pathological immune reactions. Complications may be treated with the use of antibiotics, incision and drainage, and intralesional steroid injections. However, prevention is the only effective measure, and this includes using a proper aseptic technique, using small-gauge needles, avoiding the use of makeup, and using prophylactic antibiotics to prevent permanent contamination of the synthetic filler. It has been demonstrated that HIV patients treated with permanent fillers for facial lipoatrophy have a higher risk of complications after injection of permanent fillers, probably due to an altered cellular immune response that may result in a different reaction to permanent fillers themselves.

7.2.6 Glues and Adhesives

This group includes two types of adhesive—external (acrylate) and internal (fibrin) adhesives.

Acrylates are glues typically used for wound closure and repair of superficial lacerations, especially in children, because they avoid the need (and pain) of local anesthetic injection and are cheaper than a number of sutures. Several studies have showed that the aesthetic result is comparable to that obtained with traditional suturing. Acrylates have a risk of allergic reactions if used in large amounts, and there have been reports of exothermic reactions when the product comes in contact with some materials, such as cotton. Dermabond (2-octylcyanoacrylate) (Ethicon) is the most commonly used glue for wound repair. It works as both a skin adhesive and a microbial barrier with bacteriostatic properties. It is also used for skin graft edge fixation and nail adhesion to nail beds.

Fibrin adhesives (also called fibrin glue or fibrin sealants) are used mainly for hemostatic purposes in general surgery, gynecology, neurosurgery, and plastic surgery. Fibrin glue is made up of two components, fibrinogen and thrombin. When mixed just prior to application, these components form a fibrin clot that can be used as a hemostatic plug or to seal two raw surfaces together to reduce dead space. Because they are derived from human plasma, these products need to be processed to inactivate viruses and eliminate the risk of disease transmission. Their safety has been proved with no seroconversion noted for HIV, hepatitis A virus, hepatitis B virus, hepatitis C virus, Epstein–Barr virus, and cytomegalovirus. In addition, the fibrinogen component of Tisseel/Tissucol (Baxter Healthcare) contains bovine aprotinin, which may be immunogenic and therefore has the potential to elicit allergic or even anaphylactic reactions. Fibrin sealants have various uses in plastic surgery: seroma prevention, facelift surgery, and skin graft fixation. Even though there is little evidence to support its use fibrin glue may help to reduce seroma formation in patients after abdominoplasty or other body-contouring procedures. Moreover, a decrease in the total amounts of postoperative drainage has been reported. In facelift surgery it is commonly used to stop bleeding and facilitate adhesion of tissues, though no differences have been seen between glue and drains versus drains alone. Fibrin glue may also be used for skin graft fixation, where it yields higher rates of graft take, especially in difficult areas, such as folds and highly mobile zones. In microsurgery, fibrin glue is used to obtain a better sealing action and apposition after nerve coaptation and also to properly position and stabilize the vascular pedicle to prevent kinking after microsurgical anastomosis.

7.3 Implantation Tips and Pitfalls

Successful implantation of a biomaterial implies that a number of aspects have been considered, including factors relating to the patient, the site, the material, and the surgery itself.

A proper aseptic technique and sterility are of utmost importance. Prepping the implantation site requires thorough washing of the implantation pocket with antiseptic or antibiotic solutions, reducing the time of exposure of the implant to air, changing gloves before manipulating the implant, and limiting the use of drains. These measures are taken to reduce the risk of contamination and infection.

An implantable material should never be placed in a contaminated or infected site. Three to 6 months should be allowed before attempting implantation. Vascularization must be carefully assessed because not all tissues provide the same degree of coverage. When possible, it is always preferable to place implants under muscle or fascia. A previous history of radiation affects tissue vascularity and its ability to heal primarily and is a major risk factor of implant exposure, contamination, and infection. In addition, a meticulous surgical technique with attention to minimizing tissue trauma and properly developing the plane of implant insertion are also important.

The patient's comorbidities should also be assessed preoperatively, with particular attention to those affecting vascularization and wound healing, including a history of smoking, diabetes, and chronic use of steroids, among others.

In most cases, device failure becomes clinically evident by a constellation of clinical signs, including tenderness, swelling, erythema, deformation, pain, infection, fistula formation, and functional impairment. Imaging may also help to identify a potential complication. Ultrasound is noninvasive, quick, and inexpensive, but it yields limited information and is operator dependent. A computed tomographic scan provides fine morphological details but delivers a high dose of ionizing radiation, and it cannot be as accurate as magnetic resonance imaging, especially when detecting things like the presence of free silicone. Magnetic resonance imaging is the most expensive method, but it has the best multiplanar definition and is the method of choice for studying changes in soft tissues.

7.4 Clinical Applications

7.4.1 Case 1

A 46-year-old patient with right breast cancer had a mastectomy and immediate reconstruction with a tissue expander 2 years prior. Postoperatively, the expansion process had to be interrupted due to skin atrophy and risk of extrusion (▸ Fig. 7.3). To allow better coverage of the implant and be able to complete the expansion process it was decided to provide an extra soft tissue layer with a pedicled latissimus dorsi flap. At the time of surgery it was noted that the capsule was lying directly under the skin, and the expander itself was very close to the surface and at high risk

of extrusion (▸ Fig. 7.4). After providing proper muscle coverage with the latissimus dorsi flap the patient healed uneventfully and the expansion process was resumed (▸ Fig. 7.5).

7.4.2 Case 2

A 43-year-old patient with a bone sarcoma was treated by radiotherapy followed by wide local excision including the knee replacement using a titanium joint prosthesis (▸ Fig. 7.6). Given the history of radiotherapy, the implant was at high risk of exposure, and a decision was made to cover it with a medial gastrocnemius flap, which provided a thick layer of fresh (non irradiated), well vascularized muscle (▸ Fig. 7.7). Thanks to the gastrocnemius muscle coverage, the knee prosthesis did not become exposed despite some minor superficial skin breakdown.

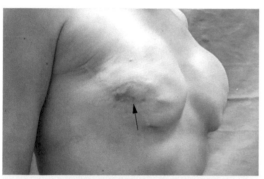

Fig. 7.3 Soft tissue atrophy due to lack of muscle coverage of the tissue expander. The arrow points where the expander can be palpated and seen by transparency.

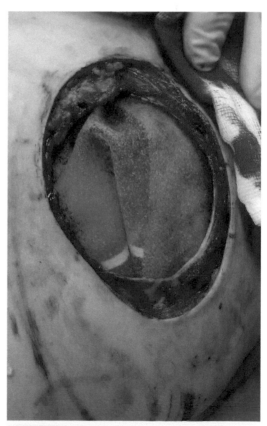

Fig. 7.4 Following excision of damaged skin it is possible to see how superficial the expander was and the minimal thickness of the skin and capsule.

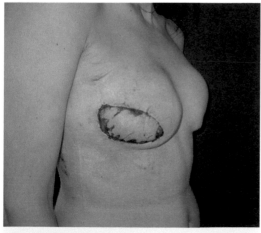

Fig. 7.5 The defect repaired with a pedicled latissumus dorsi flap with a skin paddle.

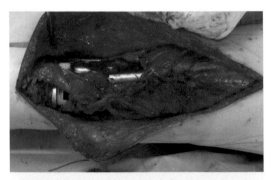

Fig. 7.6 A knee prosthesis placed after osteosarcoma excision barely covered by the pes anserinus.

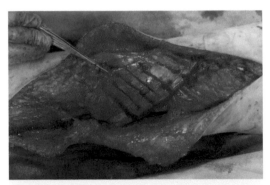

Fig. 7.7 A medial gastrocnemius flap was raised and turned to achieve complete coverage of the prosthesis. The fascial layer was incised to expand the muscle surface.

7.5 Conclusions

The use of biomaterials forms part of the daily practice of virtually every surgeon and in particular plastic surgeons. The collaboration of surgeons and scientists is fundamental to improve the quality, longevity, and overall safety of implanted materials. Alloplastic materials can and do serve a great purpose in both reconstructive and aesthetic surgery; however, their use can also lead to serious complications and unpleasant medicolegal issues. As surgeons we have the obligation to inform our patients of the potential risks of foreign material implantation so they can make an informed decision on the matter. Furthermore, careful preoperative assessment is important to identify possible factors that may place the implant at risk of exposure, infection, or failure.

7.6 Key Points

- The ideal biomaterial must produce no foreign-body inflammatory response. It must be chemically inert, noncarcinogenic, nontoxic, nonallergenic, and sterilizable, and it should not favor the growth of microorganisms.
- Inflammation is the most important phenomenon that will lead to either implant incorporation or rejection. An inflammatory reaction may be desired if it is mild and short in time.
- Polymers are an extremely versatile class of compounds, but each one should be used according to its composition and chemical and physical properties. They must be chosen carefully, depending on their use.
- Bioglass are the best compounds for bone integration; however, they can be fragile and prone to breakdown when submitted to heavy loads.

- Selection of a biomaterial must consider its use and mechanical features and the life-expectancy of the material. The benefits of implantation must always outweigh the inherent risks.
- Placement of implants under well-vascularized tissue is fundamental to prevent extrusion, contamination, and infection. Radiotherapy severely impacts tissues' quality and their ability to heal and is therefore a major risk factor for failure.

Recommended Readings

Alessio R, Rzany B, Eve L, et al. European expert recommendations on the use of injectable poly-L-lactic acid for facial rejuvenation. J Drugs Dermatol. 2014; 13(9):1057–1066

Banyard DA, Bourgeois JM, Widgerow AD, Evans GR. Regenerative biomaterials: a review. Plast Reconstr Surg. 2015; 135(6):1740–1748

Bleichrodt RP, de Vries Reilingh TS, Malyar A, van Goor H, Hansson B, van der Kolk B. Component separation technique to repair large midline hernias. Oper Tech Gen Surg. 2004; 6(3):179–188

Bobbio A. The first endosseous alloplastic implant in the history of man. Bull Hist Dent. 1972; 20(1):1–6

Borschel GH, Huang Y-C, Calve S, et al. Tissue engineering of recellularized small-diameter vascular grafts. Tissue Eng. 2005; 11(5–6):778–786

Castel N, Soon-Sutton T, Deptula P, Flaherty A, Parsa FD. Polyurethane-coated breast implants revisited: a 30-year follow-up. Arch Plast Surg. 2015; 42(2):186–193

Cavallaro A, Lo Menzo E, Di Vita M, et al. Use of biological meshes for abdominal wall reconstruction in highly contaminated fields. World J Gastroenterol. 2010; 16(15): 1928–1933

Chun YS, Verma K, Rosen H, et al. Implant-based breast reconstruction using acellular dermal matrix and the risk of postoperative complications. Plast Reconstr Surg. 2010; 125(2): 429–436

Costerton JW, Montanaro L, Arciola CR. Biofilm in implant infections: its production and regulation. Int J Artif Organs. 2005; 28(11):1062–1068

Daghighi S, Sjollema J, van der Mei HC, Busscher HJ, Rochford ETJ. Infection resistance of degradable versus non-degradable biomaterials: an assessment of the potential mechanisms. Biomaterials. 2013; 34(33):8013 8017

Dessy LA, Troccola A, Ranno RLM, Maruccia M, Alfano C, Onesti MG. The use of poly-lactic acid to improve projection of reconstructed nipple. Breast. 2011; 20(3):220–224

Donaruma LG. Definitions in biomaterials, D. F. Williams, Ed., Elsevier, Amsterdam, 1987, 72 pp., J Polym Sci C Polym Lett 1988;26(9):414–422

Dorozhkin S. Calcium orthophosphate-based bioceramics. Materials (Basel). 2013; 6(9):3840–3942

Drake DB, Ferguson RE Jr. Fibrin sealants in microvascular surgery: current status. J Long Term Eff Med Implants. 2001;11(1–2):65–72

FDA Press Release. Physicians to stop injecting silicone for cosmetic treatment of wrinkles. 1992

FDA Update on the Safety of Silicone Gel-Filled Breast Implants, Center for Devices and Radiological Health US Food and Drug Administration. 2011

Fowble B, Park C, Wang F, et al. Rates of reconstruction failure in patients undergoing immediate reconstruction with tissue expanders and/or implants and postmastectomy radiation therapy. Int J Radiat Oncol Biol Phys. 2015; 92(3):634–641

Frame J, Kamel D, Olivan M, Cintra H. The in vivo pericapsular tissue response to modern polyurethane breast implants. Aesthetic Plast Surg. 2015; 39(5):713–723

Garcia O Jr, Scott JR. Analysis of acellular dermal matrix integration and revascularization following tissue expander breast reconstruction in a clinically relevant large-animal model. Plast Reconstr Surg. 2013; 131(5):741e–751e

Ge PS, Imai TA, Aboulian A, Van Natta TL. The use of human acellular dermal matrix for chest wall reconstruction. Ann Thorac Surg. 2010; 90(6):1799–1804

Glasberg SB, Light D. AlloDerm and Strattice in breast reconstruction: a comparison and techniques for optimizing outcomes. Plast Reconstr Surg. 2012; 129(6):1223–1233

Gorczyca DP, Gorczyca SM, Gorczyca KL. The diagnosis of silicone breast implant rupture. Plast Reconstr Surg. 2007; 120(7, Suppl 1):49S–61S

Greenhalgh DG. The use of dermal substitutes in burn surgery: acute phase. Wound Repair Regen. 2014; 22(1):1–2

Hall S. Axonal regeneration through acellular muscle grafts. J Anat. 1997; 190(Pt 1):57–71

Headon H, Kasem A, Mokbel K. Capsular contracture after breast augmentation: an update for clinical practice. Arch Plast Surg. 2015; 42(5):532–543

Kadouch JA, Kadouch DJ, Fortuin S, et al. Delayed-onset complications of facial soft tissue augmentation with permanent fillers in 85 patients. Dermatol Surg. 2013; 39(10):1474–1485

Kunjur J, Witherow H. Long-term complications associated with permanent dermal fillers. Br J Oral Maxillofac Surg. 2013; 51(8):858–862

Lanier ST, Wang ED, Chen JJ, et al. The effect of acellular dermal matrix use on complication rates in tissue expander/implant breast reconstruction. Ann Plast Surg. 2010; 64(5):674–678

López-Noriega A, Arcos D, Izquierdo-Barba I, Sakamoto Y, Terasaki O, Vallet-Regí M. Ordered mesoporous bioactive glasses for bone tissue regeneration. Chem Mater. 2006; 18(13):3137–3144

Mahabir RC, Butler CE. Stabilization of the chest wall: autologous and alloplastic reconstructions. Semin Plast Surg. 2011; 25(1):34–42

Middleton MS, McNamara MP Jr. Breast implant classification with MR imaging correlation: (CME available on RSNA link) Radiographics. 2000; 20(3):E1

Ocampo-Candiani J, Sobrevilla-Ondarza S, Velázquez-Arenas L, Vázquez-Martínez OT. Complication of a polyalkylimide implant in a patient with facial trauma. Dermatol Surg. 2008; 34(9):1280–1282

Oswald A-M, Joly L-M, Gury C, Disdet M, Leduc V, Kanny G. Fatal intraoperative anaphylaxis related to aprotinin after local application of fibrin glue. Anesthesiology. 2003; 99(3):762–763

Prestwich GD. Hyaluronic acid-based clinical biomaterials derived for cell and molecule delivery in regenerative medicine. J Control Release. 2011; 155(2):193–199

Ratner BD, Hoffman AS, Schoen FJ, Lemons J. Biomaterials Science: A Multidisciplinary Endeavor. Biomater Sci. 2004:1–20

Russell NS, Scharpfenecker M, Hoving S, Woerdeman LAE. Consequences of Radiotherapy for Breast Reconstruction. Selected Topics in Plastic Reconstructive Surgery, InTechopen, 2011

Santanelli di Pompeo F, Laporta R, Sorotos M, et al. Breast implant-associated anaplastic large cell lymphoma: proposal for a monitoring protocol. Plast Reconstr Surg. 2015;136(2):144e–151e

Sbitany H, Serletti JM. Acellular dermis-assisted prosthetic breast reconstruction: a systematic and critical review of efficacy and associated morbidity. Plast Reconstr Surg. 2011; 128(6):1162–1169

Schelke LW, van den Elzen HJ, Canninga M, Neumann MH. Complications after treatment with polyalkylimide. Dermatol Surg. 2009; 35(Suppl 2):1625–1628

Silvers SL, Eviatar JA, Echavez MI, Pappas AL. Prospective, open-label, 18-month trial of calcium hydroxylapatite (Radiesse) for facial soft-tissue augmentation in patients with human immunodeficiency virus-associated lipoatrophy: one-year durability. Plast Reconstr Surg. 2006; 118(3, Suppl):34S–45S

Slater NJ, van der Kolk M, Hendriks T, van Goor H, Bleichrodt RP. Biologic grafts for ventral hernia repair: a systematic review. Am J Surg. 2013; 205(2):220–230

Smith S, Busso M, McClaren M, Bass LS. A randomized, bilateral, prospective comparison of calcium hydroxylapatite microspheres versus human-based collagen for the correction of nasolabial folds. Dermatol Surg. 2007; 33(Suppl 2):S112–S121, discussion S121

Spear SL, Sher SR, Al-Attar A, Pittman T. Applications of acellular dermal matrix in revision breast reconstruction surgery. Plast Reconstr Surg. 2014; 133(1):1–10

Toman N, Buschmann A, Muehlberger T. Fibrin glue and seroma formation following abdominoplasty [in German]. Chirurg. 2007; 78(6):531–535

Widgerow AD. Bioengineered matrices—part 2: focal adhesion, integrins, and the fibroblast effect. Ann Plast Surg. 2012; 68(6):574

Zhao D, Feng J, Huo Q, et al. Triblock copolymer syntheses of mesoporous silica with periodic 50 to 300 angstrom pores. Science. 1998; 279(5350):548–552

111

8 Principles of Osteosynthesis

Pedro Bolado, Jorge Bonastre, Luis Landin

Abstract

Bone tissue is derived from various embryological lineages which follow a process of either intramembranous or endochondral ossification. Bone is formed of organic and inorganic fractions composed of cells, proteins, and minerals that provide its physiological and structural characteristics. The organization of intrinsic collagen fibers determines whether bone tissue matures to become woven or lamellar. Bone consolidation can be direct or indirect. The latter occurs through five overlapping phases of callus formation. Fracture treatment should include reduction, absolute or relative stabilization, fixation of the fragments, and rehabilitation. However, fracture treatment is not exempt from complications, such as infection, delayed union, nonunion, and malunion. Distraction osteogenesis is a procedure that uses the process of generating new bone tissue between osteotomized bone fragments and can be used when other forms of bone fracture treatment or congenital malformations fail to provide enough bone length. This chapter presents the current knowledge of bone microanatomy and fracture pathophysiology, which constitute the foundations for bone healing and synthesis, and gives a comprehensive review of the most commonly used surgical techniques for fracture fixation and its complications.

Keywords: bone microanatomy, distraction osteogenesis, fracture stabilization, ossification, osteomyelitis, osteosynthesis devices, pseudarthrosis

8.1 Basic Science

8.1.1 Mechanisms of Ossification

Osteogenesis is the process of bone formation. The skeletal components are derived from three embryological lineages. Neural crest cells give rise to the pharyngeal arches and the axial skeleton; paraxial mesoderm forms the craniofacial skeleton and most of the axial skeleton through the division of the somites; and finally, the limbs' skeleton develops from the lateral plate mesoderm.

Differentiation of mesenchymal tissue into bone can follow an intramembranous or an endochondral mechanism. Intramembranous ossification is characterized by direct bone formation in a connective tissue membrane in the absence of cartilage. It occurs in flat bones, in the fracture callus, and in distraction osteogenesis. Endochondral ossification occurs through a cartilage intermediate, called the primary ossification core in the embryonic period, and a secondary ossification core after birth. This type of ossification occurs in long bones and in the fracture callus as well.

8.1.2 Bone Composition

Bone tissue consists of two essential components, namely extracellular matrix (ECM) and cells. The ECM contains an organic phase and a mineral fraction. The cells constitute a small percentage included in the organic fraction of bone tissue.

The organic fraction of the ECM constitutes 30% of dry bone mass and is mainly formed by three protein groups: collagenous, noncollagenous, and glycoproteins. Collagenous proteins form the osteoid, which is the chief element of bone matrix, and provide elasticity and flexibility. Collagen type I is organized in a fibrillar form and has a mineralization potential, providing bone elasticity and tensile strength. Hydroxyproline is a major component of collagenous proteins, and its increased urinary levels reflect bone resorption. Noncollagenous proteins include osteocalcin, a linear peptide hormone produced by osteoblasts during bone formation and incorporated into the bone matrix, and bone morphogenetic proteins (BMPs), which are involved in the formation of new bone, cartilage, and connective tissue. Finally, proteoglycans and glycoproteins form the fundamental amorphous substance that surrounds cells and collagen. They are composed mainly of hyaluronic acid chains bounded to subunits of chondroitin sulfate and keratin sulfate.

The inorganic or mineral phase accounts for 50–70% of bone composition and is responsible for providing mechanical rigidity and strength to the ECM. It is formed by hydroxyapatite crystals consisting of 80% tricalcium phosphate and 10% calcium carbonate.

Different growth factors, such as the Wnt family and BMPs, stimulate mesenchymal stem cell differentiation into osteoblastic progenitors, such as pro-osteoblasts, which then become osteoblasts and ultimately osteocytes. These cells are all located in the endosteal and periosteal layers. Osteoblasts are found on the surface of bone, and their main function is osteoid production. They also synthesize alkaline phosphatase and osteocalcin and have receptors for parathyroid hormone (PTH), $1,25(OH)_2$-vitamin-D, glucocorticoids, prostaglandins, and estrogens. Osteocytes are found within the bone matrix and constitute 90–95% of the cellular component. They develop from the osteoblasts located in the lacunae and are characterized by large cytoplasmic processes that extend radially through the osteons and to the canaliculi, allowing communication with other osteocytes and osteoblasts. Osteocytes are key in regulating homeostasis of extracellular calcium and phosphorus.

Osteoclasts are located in the trabecular bone surface in spaces called Howship's lacunae and at the head of the cortical perforating cones. They are activated by osteoblasts to exert their main function, which is to lyse bone. The contact zone of their cell membrane has a hairy pattern that increases the area of resorption. Once in contact with the bone surface, the osteoclast's cell membrane delimits an area fixed and sealed by integrins, where pH is reduced through a proton pump, and acid proteases are released, dissolving the mineral matrix and degrading the collagen component.

8.1.3 Bone Microanatomy

Depending on the organization of collagen fibers, two types of bone can be identified: woven and lamellar. Woven bone owes its name to its characteristically irregular organization of cells and collagen fibers, which, together with its increased water content, make it highly deformable and flexible. Woven bone is the primary or immature bone found in the skeletons of embryos and newborns, and it is gradually replaced by mature (e.g., lamellar) bone during skeletal growth. In adults woven bone may persist as part of the ear bones, tendon and ligament insertions, and cranial bone sutures. In addition, woven bone is the first to appear in the callus of healing fractures.

Lamellar bone, also called secondary or mature bone, completely replaces woven bone by 4 years of age and is organized in a specific and regular pattern according to the supported loads. Cortical bone is a type of lamellar bone forming 80% of an adult's skeleton. It is formed by a set of elementary functional units called osteons, composed of a series of concentrically arranged bone plates. At the center of each osteon, blood and lymphatic vessels and nerves run through the haversian canals, which interconnect with each other and with the periosteum through Volkmann's canals. The spaces between the osteons are occupied by interstitial lamellar systems (▶ Fig. 8.1).

The periosteum is a well-vascularized layer that covers the outermost part of cortical bone and is divided into an outer sheet, composed of poorly active fibrous tissue; and an active inner layer or cambium layer, lying in direct contact with the cortical bone surface and rich in osteoblast cells, which orchestrate callus formation and repair of bone following fracture.

Cancellous bone forms 20% of the skeleton and consists of a set of bony trabeculae arranged in a randomly oriented three-dimensional network that provides load support. The spaces between the trabeculae are occupied by bone marrow and fatty tissue. Cancellous bone has lower rigidity than cortical bone, but a metabolic activity that is eight times higher (▶ Fig. 8.1).

> **Note**
>
> The cambium layer is rich in osteoblasts. It activates after a fracture and forms the fracture callus.

8.1.4 Bone Healing

A fractured bone can heal or consolidate directly or indirectly depending on fracture treatment and stability. Direct, primary, or cortical consolidation takes place in anatomically reduced fractures with absolute stability. It is produced by the passage of vessels through the bone contact areas and osteoblastic apposition of new bone in areas of no contact. Direct consolidation occurs without callus formation.

Indirect or secondary consolidation occurs in fractures treated with flexible fracture stabilization, which allows interfragmentary mobility. Indirect consolidation occurs through callus formation along a set of five overlapping phases, namely hematoma, inflammation and angiogenesis, reparative, ossification, and remodeling. In the first phase of hematoma, the blood clot releases interleukins-1 and -6 (IL-1 and IL-6) and tumor necrosis factor-α (TNF-α) that

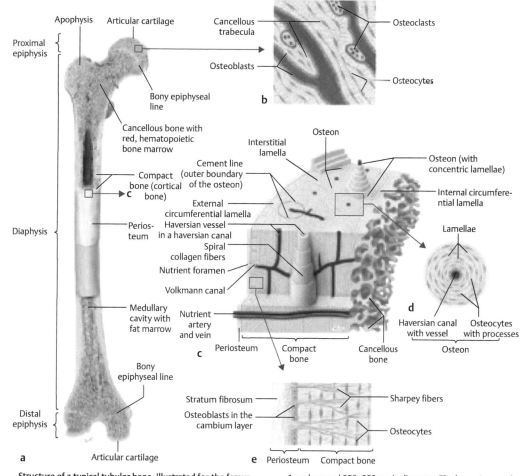

Fig. 8.1 Bone microanatomy. (Reproduced from Schuenke, Schulte, and Schumacher, Atlas of Anatomy, 2nd edition, ©2014, Thieme Publishers, New York. Illustration by Karl Wesker/Markus Voll.)

Structure of a typical tubular bone, illustrated for the femur
a Coronal saw cuts have been made through the proximal and distal parts of an adults femur (without sectioning the midshaft region).
b Detail from a: The sectioned areas display the lamellar architecture ("lamellar bone") of the cancellous trabeculae. The lamellae are arranged in contiguous plates, similar to plywood. Since the cancellous trabeculae do not have an actual vascular supply and are nourished by diffusion from the adjacent medullary cavity, the trabeculae attain a thickness of only about 200–300 μm.
c Detail from a: Three-dimensional representation of compact bone, whose structural units consist of vascularized osteons approximately

1 cm long and 250–350 μm in diameter. The haversian canals, which tend to run longitudinally in the bone, are connected to one another by short transverse and oblique Volkmann canals and also to the vessels of the periosteum and medullary cavity.
d Detail from c: Demonstrating the microstructure of an osteon. The haversian canal at the center is surrounded by approximately 5–20 concentric lamellar systems composed of osteocytes and extracellular matrix. The osteocytes are interconnected by numerous fine cytoplasmic processes.
e Detail from c: Showing the structure of the periosteum.

trigger the inflammation cascade. The inflammatory and angiogenesis phase then ensues with neutrophils, macrophages, and lymphocytes being recruited to the site of injury to remove debris and initiate repair. During this phase the initial hematoma is gradually replaced by a fibrin clot, and osteoclasts begin resorption of the bony ends. Vasodilation and hyperemia of the surrounding soft tissues promote

the formation of new capillaries that grow through the site of injury, and precursor cells begin to proliferate and differentiate into osteoblasts. Later in this phase, fibrin, collagen, and reticular fibers are replaced by granulation tissue. The reparative phase starts at the offset of inflammation and is characterized by the formation of a soft callus composed mainly of cartilage and varying amounts of connective tissue and

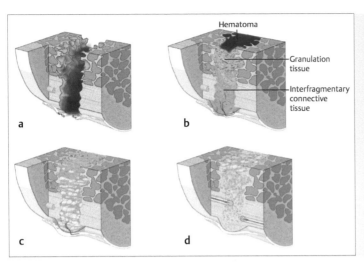

Fig. 8.2 Stages of bone callus formation during secondary fracture healing. **(a)** Hematoma filling the fracture gap. **(b)** Granulation tissue and connective tissue replacing the hematoma in the fracture gap with ingrowth of blood vessels. **(c)** Fibrocartilage replacing the connective tissue in the fracture gap. **(d)** Woven bone replaced by lamellar bone through haversian remodeling. (Reproduced from Ehrenfeld, Manson, Prein, Principles of Internal Fixation of the Craniomaxillofacial Skeleton Trauma and Orthognathic Surgery, ©2012, Thieme Publishers, New York.)

blood vessels, in response to mechanical and biological factors. The ossification phase starts at the third week to form the hard callus and lasts between 12 and 16 weeks, until the bony ends are firmly joined together. During this phase, the soft callus undergoes endochondral and intramembranous ossification. Finally, in the remodeling phase the immature woven bone with its irregular microstrucure is gradually replaced by mature, laminar, anisotropic bone in response to the mechanical load (▶ Fig. 8.2). According to Wolff's law, bones adapt to the load they are submitted to, so that with increasing loads, bones become thicker and stronger, whereas in situations of deceased loads, they become weaker and less dense.

> **Note**
>
> Bone callus is formed through five established phases: hematoma, inflammatory and angiogenesis, reparative, ossification, and remodeling.

8.2 Fracture Repair

The objective of fracture treatment is to promote consolidation and restore the bone's mechanical properties for maximum functional recovery. Different factors affect the process of bone regeneration, such as age, genetics, and mechanical factors.

8.2.1 Reduction

Anatomical relationships between bone fragments can be restored by open or closed manipulation.

The aim of anatomical reduction is to correct shortening, angulation, and rotation.

8.2.2 Stabilization

Fracture stabilization can be achieved by conservative (e.g., plasters) or surgical treatment. The objective is to reduce the mobility of the bony ends to allow bone healing. External fixators are not aimed at providing definitive stabilization, but rather a reasonable reduction until other issues are solved (e.g., vascular injury or soft tissue reconstruction).

Types of Stability

The biological response and the type of consolidation occurring at the fracture site are highly dependent on the degree of relative or absolute stabilization yielded by the selected treatment. For example, fractures stabilized with a plaster or elastic fixation (e.g., Kirschner wires), undergo secondary consolidation. Relative stability allows microscopic movements between the fragments following load application. Techniques of relative stability include intramedullary nailing, which controls fracture angulation and displacement, but not rotation. The addition of locking screws (e.g., locked intramedullary nailing) can help to correct shortening and rotation. Bridging plates fixed with locked screws provide relative stability by bridging the area of greater comminution while maintaining length and alignment. Finally, external fixators

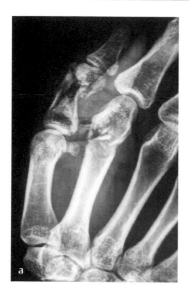
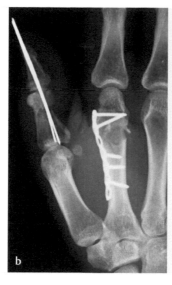

Fig. 8.3 (a) Comminuted fracture of the proximal phalanx of the thumb and second metacarpal. (b) Thumb fixation with Kirschner wires and second metacarpal fixation with 2-mm bridging plate.

can correct bone alignment, but the stiffness of the frame is limited because the rods are fixed to pins several millimeters or even centimeters above the fracture (▶Fig. 8.3).

Absolute stability is achieved with rigid fixation by interfragmentary compression at the fracture site resulting in primary or direct consolidation. Techniques of absolute stability include compression screws or plates that transform rotational forces into linear fracture compression, and tension bands that convert distraction tensile forces into compression forces at the fracture site.

> **Note**
>
> Absolute stability results in primary consolidation, whereas relative stability leads to fracture healing through callus formation (e.g., secondary consolidation).

8.2.3 Fixation

Osteosynthesis Devices

Kirschner wires are available in different diameters, from 0.8 to 3 mm. They are versatile and can be used in any small bone fracture, but comminuted fractures are their primary indication. Wires can be inserted through a closed or open approach, causing minimal trauma to the surrounding tissues, and they may be used as temporary or

definitive fixation providing relative stability to the fracture. One of their limitations is that they do not allow interfragmentary compression.

Screws are helical devices that convert rotational forces into linear motion (▶Fig. 8.4). *Cortical screws* are designed to penetrate through the rigid and hard structure of cortical bone. They have a narrow thread pitch with closely spaced threads. *Cancellous screws* are designed to fix epiphyseal and metaphyseal cancellous bone and osteoporotic bone. The threads are more separated so that with each 360-degree turn the screw advances a longer distance. In addition, the thread (external) diameter is comparatively larger than the inner (core) diameter.

Screws can also be self-tapping or self-drilling. Self-tapping screws have a taplike flute in their leading threads, which allows them to tap their own hole as they are driven into, but need bone drilling prior to insertion. Self-tapping screws are not recommended for use as lag screws. Self-drilling screws have a preliminary drill-like fluted tip that allows insertion without predrilling of bone (▶Fig. 8.4). Some self-tapping screws are also self-drilling.

Lag or compression screws provide reduction between two fragments and achieve absolute stability. The principle of lag screws is based on making the screw glide without purchase through the proximal fragment and thread through the distal fragment so that, with each turn, the distal fragment is brought against the proximal

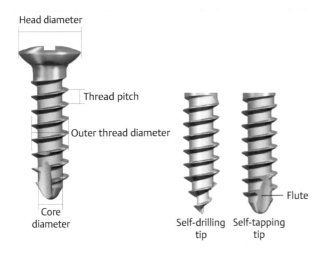

Head diameter

Thread pitch

Outer thread diameter

Core
diameter

Self-drilling
tip

Self-tapping
tip

Flute

Fig. 8.4 General configuration of screws and differences between self-tapping and self-drilling screws. (Reproduced from Ehrenfeld, Manson, Prein, Principles of Internal Fixation of the Craniomaxillofacial Skeleton Trauma and Orthognathic Surgery, ©2012, Thieme Publishers, New York.)

fragment. This can be obtained either with partially threaded screws or by overdrilling the near cortex (▶Fig. 8.5). It is very important to place the screw perpendicular to the fracture line; otherwise a shear plane can preclude proper reduction. Generally a screw should be tightened to only two-thirds of its strength to allow resistance to any additional functional loading. Compression screws are available in diameters from 1 to 2.7 mm. They are best used in long spiral fractures, and their use in short oblique fractures is ill advised. Cannulated compression screws are a variable-pitch type of headless implant that are placed within the bone by using a thin guidewire. These screws are tapered with a differential thread pitch to increase compression as the screw is advanced (▶Fig. 8.6). Their main use includes scaphoid fracture fixation, but they can also be used in joint arthrodesis and small tubular bone nonunions.

Intramedullary nails act as internal splints, making contact with bone at three points: the entry, the narrowest segment of the medullary canal, and the epiphyseal cancellous bone at the nail's distal end. Locked intramedullary nailing is based on placing perpendicular screws to the nail, which prevent its displacement inside the medullary canal and stabilize the fragments together.

Plates are usually indicated in simple diaphyseal fractures to provide interfragmentary compression. They are also used in anatomically reduced articular fractures, for buttressing epiphyseal and metaphyseal fractures, and for bridging comminuted fractures. Plate fixation brings the bony ends into direct contact, allowing direct consolidation. Desperiostization prior to plate application should be as limited as possible to avoid bone devascularization. Otherwise delayed fracture consolidation and remodeling may result in cortical porosis under the plate. To prevent this drawback, low contact plates have been developed (see later discussion).

Any plate can be used to provide any of the five key functions of plates, namely, neutralization, compression, support (buttressing), bridging, and tension band. Neutralization removes the loading forces from a fracture site by spanning it and transmitting these forces through the plate rather than through the fracture. An interfragmentary compression screw can be added to provide greater stability. Plates produce compression at the fracture site providing absolute stability, such as in transverse fractures. Compression plates' holes have an oval and inclined surface configuration. Once the fracture has been reduced, the plate is secured to the bone by placing screws in a neutral position (e.g., in the center of the plate hole) on one side of the fracture. A screw is then placed eccentrically on the other side of the fracture to produce bone displacement and fracture compression (▶Fig. 8.7). In addition, the holes' oval design allows placing an angulated screw as an interfragmentary compression screw. Supporting plates are used as a buttress in metaphyseal or epiphyseal shear fractures of long bones by placing the screws in the central location of the oval hole. A tension band transforms tensile forces into compressive ones. When an axial compression is

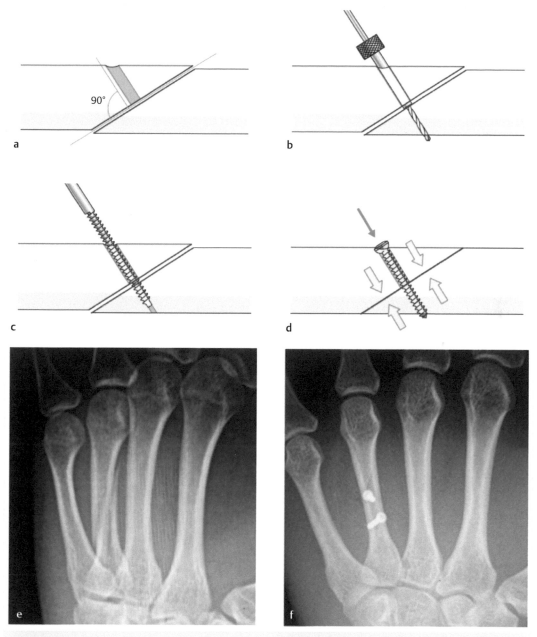

Fig. 8.5 Compression (lag) screw technique. **(a)** Anatomical fracture reduction. **(b)** Drilling of a glide 2.4 mm hole perpendicular to the fracture line in the near cortex. **(c)** Drilling of a concentric 1.8-mm hole in the opposite cortex. **(d)** Application of a 2.4 mm screw. **(e)** Spiral fracture of the fourth metacarpal. **(f)** Rigid fixation using 2-mm compression screws. (a–d: Reproduced from Rüedi, Buckley, Moran, AO Principles of Fracture Management. 2nd edition, ©2007, Thieme Publishers, New York.)

applied to a curved tubular long bone it provides tension on the convex cortex and compression on the opposite concave cortex. For a plate to act as a tension band, it must meet the following conditions: it must be applied on an eccentrically loaded bone; the plate must be placed on the

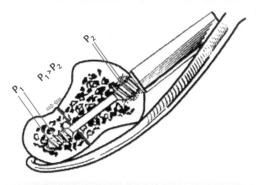

Fig. 8.6 Diagram showing scaphoid fracture fixation with cannulated compression screw. Differential pitch of the leading thread (P_1) and trailing thread (P_2) draws the bone fragments together to produce compression at the fracture line. (Reproduced from Plancher, Master Cases Hand and Wrist Surgery, ©2004, Thieme Publishers, New York.)

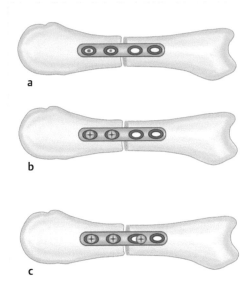

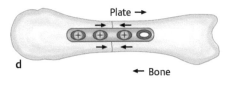

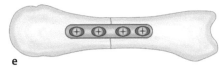

Fig. 8.7 Compression plate surgical technique. (a, b) Two centered screws secure the plate to the bone. An eccentrically drilled hole is made at the other side the fracture line. (c) A screw is inserted in the eccentrically drilled hole. (d) Screw tightening produces translation of the plate and bone in opposite directions, resulting in compression at the fracture line. (e) Fixation completed.

tension (convex) surface; the plate must be able to tolerate tensile forces; and the cortex opposite the plate must be intact and able to support compression forces (▶Fig. 8.8).

There are different types of plates. Old dynamic compression plates provided compression, neutralization, or tension band functions. They evolved to low-contact dynamic compression plates, which reduced plate–bone contact by 50%, thus preserving periosteal circulation. Modern locking compression plates permit screwing to the plate at a fixed angle by a thread in the screw head, which provides greater rigidity to the system, reduces the chance of osteosynthesis removal or loss of reduction, and increases resistance to axial loads. Locking compression plates cannot be bent to match bone anatomy. Locked head screws do not allow compression and can only be placed in the predetermined direction by the thread of the plate. Therefore a standard screw should be used to attain compression, and then locked screws can provide further support.

The design of the holes has evolved to combine the benefits of dynamic compression plates and locked screw plates. Plates with polyaxial screws tolerate some variability in the angle at which the screw is fixed to the plate, which allows placing the screw in different directions and offers high versatility. Reconstruction plates have a groove on both sides between the holes, allowing three-dimensional bending to adapt the plate to complex bone surfaces.

8.2.4 Rehabilitation

After fracture fixation, controlled rehabilitation should be indicated as early as possible to achieve full restoration of previous function. While rigid internal fixation facilitates early rehabilitation, fractures treated conservatively or by elastic fixation are difficult to rehabilitate before plaster or implant removal. Fracture consolidation may be positively or negatively influenced by a number of factors, as summarized in ▶Table 8.1.

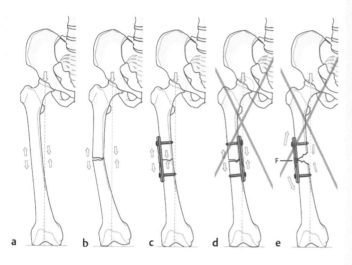

Fig. 8.8 The tension band principle illustrated on a femur fracture. (a) The femur is an eccentrically loaded bone with distraction (tensile) forces on the lateral cortex and compression on the medial side. (b) When fractured, the lateral gap opens while the medial side is compressed. (c) A correctly placed plate (e.g., on the side with tensile forces) will be under tension when loaded, producing compression at the fracture site, provided that the medial cortex is intact. (d) A plate placed on the wrong side (e.g., the compression surface) does not close the fracture gap and does not provide stability. (e) If the medial side is not intact, the tension band principle cannot work due to lack of buttressing. (Reproduced from Rüedi, Buckley, Moran, AO Principles of Fracture Management. 2nd edition, ©2007, Thieme Publishers, New York.)

Table 8.1 Modifying factors of bone consolidation

	Stimulators	Inhibitors
Mechanical	Axial compressive load, mechanical stability, electromagnetic stimulation	Distraction and shear forces, mechanical instability, soft tissue interposition
Metabolic	Blood supply, growth factors, hyperbaric oxygen, calcitonin, vitamin D, insulin, thyroid hormones	Corticosteroids, diabetes mellitus, chemotherapy, radiotherapy, protein malnutrition, smoking, nonsteroidal anti-inflammatory drugs, quinolones
Other		Tumors, infection

8.3 Complications

8.3.1 Infection/Osteomyelitis

Osteomyelitis is an inflammatory process caused by infection from a pyogenic source. It is usually caused by *Staphylococcus epidermidis* and *Staphylococcus aureus*, but *Streptococcus, Enterococcus, Escherichia coli, Proteus*, and *Pseudomonas* can also be responsible. Hematogenous osteomyelitis is usually acute and seen in young children, whereas direct inoculation osteomyelitis is commonly caused by a penetrating injury or open trauma and is commonly seen in adults. Bone infection is most frequent where necrotic bone remains (sequestrum). Its incidence is highly variable, depending on patient comorbidities and fracture presentation, being 2% in close tibia fractures and up to 20–40% in Gustilo type III open fractures. Initial symptoms include pain, fever, poor wound healing, tenderness, and warmth. Fistulae and nonhealing ulcers are usually present in chronic cases. Erythrocyte sedimentation rate and C-reactive protein have high negative predictive values. Plain radiographs usually present geodes, osteolysis, periosteal reaction, and implant loosening. Conventional radiography is the first imaging diagnostic test and is considered specific but not sensitive because changes in roentgenograms may take several weeks to appear. Computed tomography is often used in chronic cases to show sequestra, whereas magnetic resonance has high sensitivity and specificity to detect early cases (< 24 hours) of bone necrosis. A common algorithm for imaging diagnosis of osteomyelitis is to obtain plain radiographs looking for geodes and lytic lesions, and then confirm diagnosis by magnetic resonance. Definitive diagnosis of osteomyelitis is made by *positive cultures obtained from at least six bone samples*. Osteomyelitis is usually graded according to the Cierny–Mader classification (▶ Table 8.2).

Table 8.2 Cierny–Mader classification system for adult osteomyelitis

Type I	Medullary	Confined to the intramedullary surface of the bone
Type II	Superficial	True contiguous focus lesion
Type III	Localized	Full-thickness defect, cortical sequestration and/or cavitation
Type IV	Diffuse	Through-and-through process requiring intercalated resection of bone

Note

Magnetic resonance is the gold standard image test for detecting bone infection, but definitive diagnosis is made by positive bone cultures.

Treatment of osteomyelitis is based on two pillars: surgical debridement and systemic antibiotics. To achieve successful wound healing, bacterial count should be $< 10^5$ bacteria per gram of tissue. If infection is associated with the presence of osteosynthesis material, debridement and a 6-week antibiotic course are recommended in acute cases. Surgical debridement includes removing necrotic bone and sinus tracts until healthy pinprick bleeding bone is obtained. Multiple staged debridements and a 6-week antibiotic course are often needed to treat chronic osteomyelitis. Cement spacers allow local antibiotic delivery when a bone defect results from debridement. Later on, once infection resolves, removal of the spacer and bony reconstruction will be needed in these patients. In addition, removal of the osteosynthesis material is advisable in cases when further synthesis is no longer required and infection remains.

8.3.2 Delayed Union, Nonunion, Pseudarthrosis, and Malunion

Bone consolidation depends on various factors (▶Table 8.1), of which stability of the bony reconstruction and bone vascularization are key. Fracture vascularization depends on the extent of

injury and the vascular anatomy of the fractured bone. For example, bones like the scaphoid have a higher risk of avascular necrosis of the proximal pole following a fracture through the waist or proximal pole because most of the blood supply to the scaphoid enters distally. Likewise, damage caused by the traumatic injury, open fractures with significant soft tissue loss, and iatrogenic extensive desperiostization for osteosynthesis may all reduce bone vascularity and hamper consolidation.

Three major principles should be considered to achieve bone union: healthy vascularized soft tissue cover; absolute stability; and anatomical bone apposition following reduction or reconstruction. In the absence of a healthy soft tissue envelope, well vascularized tissue obtained from regional sources or by microsurgical free tissue transfer must be brought to the site of repair following debridement of all nonviable and poorly vascularized remnants. In addition, absolute mechanical stability and good, if not anatomical, alignment should be aimed. Finally, if after surgical debridement of unhealthy bony ends, bone apposition is not achieved primarily, then it needs to be provided surgically by bone shortening, grafting, transport, or vascularized transfers.

Note

Optimization of bone union is based on the presence of a healthy, well vascularized soft tissue envelope, absolute stability, and anatomical-reduction.

The exact amount of time it will take a fracture to consolidate is hard to determine. Delayed union occurs when a fracture requires more time than usual to achieve consolidation, which may range from 3 to 6 months, depending on the bone concerned and the type of fracture. Even though there is no pain and no pathological movement at the fracture site, complete bone union is not observed, and the fracture is still visible in plain radiographs, although progression over time is observed.

Nonunion occurs when no consolidation is observed. Weber and Cech classified nonunions as hypertrophic or atrophic, depending on the vascularity of the bony ends. Atrophic nonunion is caused by poor vascularization of the fracture fragments, which appear thin and sharp. Treatment requires bone grafts or even bone flaps in refractory cases. Hypertrophic nonunion occurs as a consequence of excessive mobility at the fracture site due to poor bone stabilization. Bony ends look widened in an "elephant foot" appearance, and treatment includes bone debridement and proper stabilization.

Pseudarthrosis is defined by a complete incapacity to achieve bone consolidation due to definitive failure of the osteogenetic process. After 6 to 8 months from the initial fracture, a fluid-filled cavity with a pseudosynovial membrane is formed, with painless and abnormal mobility at the fracture site. The incidence of pseudarthrosis is approximately 3–4%, being more frequent in longer bones, and up to 30% in Gustilo type III open tibial fractures. Treatment of pseudarthrosis involves bone debridement, apposition, and fixation as already mentioned (▶ Fig. 8.9).

Malunion occurs when the fractured bone is improperly aligned after consolidation, resulting in shortening, twisting, rotation, or bending. In the absence of functional impairment, treatment might not be necessary; however, if malunion has clinical relevance, appropriate alignment must be restored, which normally requires rotation, subtraction, or additional osteotomies, together with new fracture stabilization and/or bone grafts.

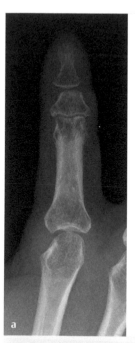 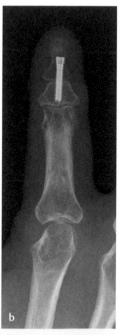

Fig. 8.9 (a) Distal phalanx pseudarthrosis of an Allen III replanted second finger. (b) Result after bone refreshment and stabilization with a cannulated screw.

8.4 Distraction Osteogenesis

Distraction osteogenesis consists of a low-energy osteotomy followed by gradual distraction of the bone fragments with a mechanical device. First described by Codivilla in 1904, early attempts had significant bone and soft tissue complications, until the 1950s, when Ilizarov developed the concept and principles of distraction osteogenesis. He found that tissues exposed to slow, steady traction became metabolically active and experienced growth and regeneration during distraction. Distraction osteogenesis may be a long process that requires commitment from both the patient and the surgeon. Candidates for bone transport are those with acute or chronic long bone defects > 2–3 cm, smaller bony defects that are excessively debilitated by prolonged absence of weight bearing on the affected limb, and individuals with recalcitrant infected nonunions. Bone transport involves preparation of the bony defect by resecting all infected and/or necrotic bone, and reshaping the bony ends following an acute injury. The cortical osteotomy must be made with low-energy methods, usually percutaneous drill holes connected by an osteotome, leaving the periosteum as well as the intramedullary contents and their blood supply intact. Care should be taken to avoid excessive disruption of the surrounding soft tissues. The most common frame design consists of a ring frame connected by threaded rods with proximal and distal reference wires. The docking site must be precisely aligned for union to occur. The transport ring is driven by four rods. Olive wires are used to align the proximal ring fixation block. Distraction of the transported bone should begin after a brief latent period of 1 to 3 weeks to allow for early callus formation and should follow a rate of approximately 1 mm per day. If a free flap has been used in the reconstruction, distraction should be deferred for 3 weeks. Close monitorization with frequent radiographic assessment is advisable in order to modify the distraction rate in case of premature consolidation or poor callus formation. After achieving the desired length, the device should remain in place for 1 month for every 1 cm of bone advancement. Despite careful technique and excellent patient cooperation, high complication rates are reported, including deep infection, nonunion, fracture after device removal, malunion, joint stiffness, tendon unbalance, and nerve palsy. Contraindications to bone transport include comorbidities, such as diabetes, inability to tolerate a prolonged treatment due to poor cooperation, head injury or mental illness, and soft tissue compromise. Advanced age can be considered as a relative contraindication, because bone transport has been successfully used in patients older than 60.

Distraction osteogenesis can be used to treat congenital anomalies, such as congenital short femur, congenital hip luxation, or congenital hemiatrophy. It has been described to treat developmental anomalies such as Albright's and Pierre–Robin's syndromes, epiphyseal dysplasia, or neurofibromatosis. It is also used in cases of osteomyelitis and posttraumatic bone losses of the phalanges, tibia, and femur more frequently.

8.5 Conclusions

Proper fracture care is a must for the plastic surgeon involved in trauma care and procedures involving bone reconstruction. Thorough knowledge of bone anatomy and physiology and bone consolidation pathophysiology constitutes an essential foundation. Fracture pattern and patient-related factors must be carefully considered in order to offer the best treatment option. Different solutions are available for operative management; therefore a careful preoperative plan should be designed to obtain excellent reduction, good stabilization, and proper fixation with the desired implant, which will together optimize surgical outcomes and increase the chances of consolidation.

Due to the wide knowledge currently available on fracture treatment, all those interested in expanding the concepts and principles described in this chapter are referred to dedicated textbooks and literature reviews on the topic.

8.6 Key Points

- Ossification can be divided into intramembranous and endochondral ossification.
- Two types of bone, woven and lamellar, are distinguished depending on bone tissue organization. Lamellar bone includes both cortical and cancellous bone.
- Depending on fracture treatment and stability, primary and secondary consolidation are distinguished.
- Secondary consolidation occurs through callus formation and is divided into five phases:

hematoma, inflammatory and angiogenesis, restorative, ossification, and remodeling phases.
- Fracture treatment should follow reduction, fixation, and rehabilitation.
- Different types of osteosynthesis devices, such as wires, screws, nails, and plates, are available for internal fixation.
- Osteomyelitis can be either hematogenous or the result of a wound, and is usually caused by *Staphylococcus epidermidis* or *Staphylococcus aureus.*
- Osteomyelitis treatment is based on debridement and systemic antibiotics.
- A healthy soft tissue envelope, mechanical stability, and bony apposition are the mainstays to achieving bone union.
- Complications related to bone union include delayed union, nonunion, and malunion.
- Depending on the vascularity of the bone ends, nonunions can be classified as hypertrophic or atrophic.
- Malunion is defined as inaccurately aligned bone consolidation.
- Distraction osteogenesis consists of a low-energy osteotomy followed by a gradual distraction of the bone fragments with a mechanical device that results in the generation of new bone between the fragments.

Recommended Readings

Ai-Aql ZS, Alagl AS, Graves DT, Gerstenfeld LC, Einhorn TA. Molecular mechanisms controlling bone formation during fracture healing and distraction osteogenesis. J Dent Res. 2008; 87(2):107–118

Belsky MR, Eaton RG, Lane LB. Closed reduction and internal fixation of proximal phalangeal fractures. J Hand Surg Am. 1984; 9(5):725–729

Boyle WJ, Simonet WS, Lacey DL. Osteoclast differentiation and activation. Nature. 2003; 423(6937):337–342

Brinker MR. Nonunions: evaluation and treatment. In: Browner BD, Levine AM, Jupiter JB, Trafton PG, Krettek C, eds. Skeletal Trauma: Basic Science, Management and Reconstruction. Vol 1. Philadelphia, PA: Saunders; 2003:507–604

Brinker MR, O'Connor DP. Outcomes of tibial nonunion in older adults following treatment using the Ilizarov method. J Orthop Trauma. 2007; 21(9):634–642

Cierny G III, Mader JT. Approach to adult osteomyelitis. Orthop Rev. 1987; 16(4):259–270

Codivilla A. On the means of lengthening, in the lower limbs, the muscles and tissues which are shortened through deformity. 1904. Clin Orthop Relat Res. 1994(301):4–9

Derek MK. Congenital anomalies of the lower extremity. In: Canale ST, Beaty JH, eds. Campbell's Operative Orthopaedics. Philadelphia, PA: Elsevier; 2013:1061–1074

Fakhry M, Hamade E, Badran B, Buchet R, Magne D. Molecular mechanisms of mesenchymal stem cell differentiation towards osteoblasts. World J Stem Cells. 2013; 5(4):136–148

Faran KJ, Ichioka N, Trzeciak MA, Han S, Medige J, Moy OJ. Effect of bone quality on the forces generated by compression screws. J Biomech. 1999; 32(8):861–864

Haidukewych GJ, Ricci W. Locked plating in orthopaedic trauma: a clinical update. J Am Acad Orthop Surg. 2008; 16(6):347–355

Hak DJ, Stewart RL. Tension band principle. In: Rüedi TP, Buckley RE, Moran CG, eds. AO Principles of Fractture Management. 2nd ed. Stuttgart; Thieme; 2007:249–256

Hanel DP, Lu TS, Weil WM. Bridge plating of distal radius fractures: the Harborview method. Clin Orthop Relat Res. 2006; 445(445):91–99

Hatzenbuehler J, Pulling TJ. Diagnosis and management of osteomyelitis. Am Fam Physician. 2011; 84(9):1027–1033

Huiskes R, Ruimerman R, van Lenthe GH, Janssen JD. Effects of mechanical forces on maintenance and adaptation of form in trabecular bone. Nature. 2000; 405(6787):704–706

Ilizarov GA. The principles of the Ilizarov method. Bull Hosp Jt Dis Orthop Inst. 1988; 48(1):1–11

Ilizarov GA. The tension-stress effect on the genesis and growth of tissues. Part I. The influence of stability of fixation and soft-tissue preservation. Clin Orthop Relat Res. 1989(238):249–281

Ilizarov GA. The tension-stress effect on the genesis and growth of tissues: Part II. The influence of the rate and frequency of distraction. Clin Orthop Relat Res. 1989(239):263–285

Klaue K, Fengels I, Perren SM. Long-term effects of plate osteosynthesis: comparison of four different plates. Injury. 2000; 31(Suppl 2):S-B51–62

Kwong FNK, Harris MB. Recent developments in the biology of fracture repair. J Am Acad Orthop Surg. 2008; 16(11):619–625

Perren SM. Evolution of the internal fixation of long bone fractures. The scientific basis of biological internal fixation: choosing a new balance between stability and biology. J Bone Joint Surg Br. 2002; 84(8):1093–1110

Provot S, Schipani E. Molecular mechanisms of endochondral bone development. Biochem Biophys Res Commun. 2005; 328(3):658–665

Safoury Y. Treatment of phalangeal fractures by tension band wiring. J Hand Surg [Br]. 2001; 26(1):50–52

Sakai K, Doi K, Kawai S. Free vascularized thin corticoperiosteal graft. Plast Reconstr Surg. 1991; 87(2):290–298

Salgado CJ, Becker DB, Armijo BS, Duncan AN, Chim H. Management of chronic osteomyelitis. In: Pu LQ, Levine JP, Wei FC, eds. Reconstructive Surgery of the Lower Extremity. Vol 2. St. Louis, MO: Quality Medical Publishing; 2013:893–908

Sánchez-Duffhues G, Hiepen C, Knaus P, Ten Dijke P. Bone morphogenetic protein signaling in bone homeostasis. Bone. 2015; 80:43–59

Snow M, Thompson G, Turner PG. A mechanical comparison of the locking compression plate (LCP) and the low contact-dynamic compression plate (DCP) in an osteoporotic bone model. J Orthop Trauma. 2008; 22(2):121–125

Wheeler DL, McLoughlin SW. Biomechanical assessment of compression screws. Clin Orthop Relat Res. 1998(350):237–245

9 Essentials of Dermatology for Plastic Surgeons

Isabel Irarrazaval, Pedro Redondo

Abstract

The skin is the body's largest organ. It is organized in layers that contain different kinds of cells and structures, which can give rise to a multitude of lesions of varying characteristics. Is it important for plastic surgeons to have a basic knowledge of the clinical features and management of the most common skin lesions, especially those with potential for malignant degeneration and amenable to surgical treatment. Additionally, a number of lesions, including premalignant and some malignant ones, can be treated with nonsurgical modalities, which generally result in less morbidity and which plastic surgeons should be familiar with to avoid overindication of surgical treatment in some cases. Nonmelanoma skin cancers, namely basal cell carcinoma and squamous cell carcinoma, are the most frequent cancers in humans. Their treatment is based mainly on surgical excision and reconstruction (when required), making them an important part of the collaboration between dermatologists and plastic surgeons in a number of institutions. Proper assessment of risk factors is paramount in the therapeutic approach and posttreatment follow-up of a patient with skin cancer.

Keywords: basal cell carcinoma, immunosuppression, Mohs micrographic surgery, skin cancer, squamous cell carcinoma, surgical excision

9.1 Structure and Function of the Skin

The skin is the body's largest organ, accounting for approximately 15% of the total body weight. It is a dynamic structure, with constant cellular replacement. It is composed of two main layers, the epidermis and the dermis, each of which contains different strata. Adnexal structures, including glands and hair follicles, are embedded within these layers. The skin performs numerous functions, the main ones being to serve as the interphase in our interaction with the external environment; to provide a protective barrier against various forces (mechanical, chemical, thermal), ultraviolet (UV) radiation, and microorganisms; to synthesize vitamin D; and to facilitate thermoregulation. According to coloration and tanning pattern, the skin is classified into six different phototypes (▶ Table 9.1).

9.1.1 Epidermis

The most superficial layer of the skin, the epidermis is organized into five strata (▶ Fig. 9.1). The epidermis contains two kinds of cells: keratinocytes and nonkeratinocytes. The stratum basale or germinativum contains a pool of proliferative cells that divide and become keratinocytes, which undergo progressive differentiation as they ascend through the stratum espinosum, granulosum, lucidum, and corneum until they are completely detached from the skin's surface. Nonkeratinocytic cells reside in the basal layer and have special functions, namely antigen presentation (Langerhans'cells); pigmentation and UV protection (melanocytes); and touch sensation (Merkel's cells).

9.1.2 Dermis

Deep to the epidermis lies a mesoderm-derived layer called the dermis, which makes up for approximately 90% of the skin's thickness and provides its tensile strength, elasticity, and healing abilities. The dermis is divided into papillary (superficial) and reticular (deep) layers. Importantly, the regenerative properties of

Table 9.1 Fitzpatrick's classification of skin phototypes

Phototype	Skin color	Sun exposure
I	White	Always burns, never tans
II	White	Usually burns, tans minimally
III	Beige	Burns moderately, tans gradually
IV	Brown	Burns minimally, tans easily and moderately
V	Dark brown	Rarely burns, tans very easily
VI	Black	Never burns, tans very easily

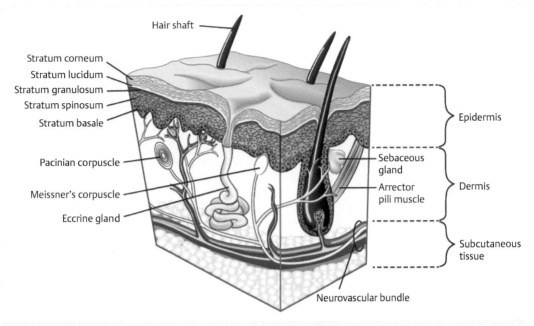

Fig. 9.1 Cross-sectional anatomy of the skin. (Reproduced from Papel, Facial Plastic and Reconstructive Surgery, 4th edition, ©2016, Thieme Publishers, New York.)

the skin depend on the integrity of the papillary dermis—when this layer is affected, wounds often exhibit poor healing and scarring. The cellular compartment of the dermis includes fibroblasts, which produce extracellular matrix components (e.g., collagen, elastin, and structural proteoglycans), immune mast cells, and histiocytes.

The dermal–epidermal junction (DEJ) is lined entirely by a basement membrane, which consists of a specialized aggregation of attachment molecules that act both as a barrier and as communicating channels between the two layers. Abnormalities in the DEJ result in rare conditions, such as bullous pemphigoid and epidermolysis bullosa. Also, with aging, the DEJ tends to become flatter, a phenomenon partly responsible for some of the distinctive features of aged skin.

9.1.3 Subcutaneous Layer

Also called the hypodermis, the subcutaneous layer lies beneath the dermis and is composed mainly of adipose tissue. Blood vessels and nerves running in this plane branch out to supply the overlying dermal plexuses (see Chapter 15).

9.1.4 Skin Appendages

Skin appendages include hair follicles, nail units, sweat glands, and sebaceous glands. Although these structures are all derived from embryonic epidermis, they reside in and are supported by the dermis. Sebaceous glands are present throughout the skin except on the palms of the hands and the soles of the feet. They produce sebum that drains into the hair follicles. While small in children, sebaceous glands enlarge and become active at puberty. Apocrine sweat glands reside in the areolae, axillae, inframammary folds, pubis, and anogenital region. Like sebaceous glands, apocrine sweat glands do not become active until puberty. Eccrine sweat glands (true sweat glands) are distributed throughout the whole body, with their highest density found on the palms and soles.

9.2 Basic Lesions of the Skin

The skin is an area in which a myriad of different lesions can appear. This chapter summarizes the most elemental and common ones (▶Table 9.2 and ▶Table 9.3).

Table 9.2 Primary lesions

Lesion	Elevation	Diameter	Description
Macule	Flat	< 1 cm	
Patch	Flat	> 1 cm	
Papule	Elevated	< 1 cm	
Plaque	Elevated	> 1 cm	Sometimes not visible but palpable
Nodule	Elevated	0.5–2 cm	Usually solid; dermis, may extend to subcutis
Tumor	Elevated	> 2 cm	
Vesicle	Elevated	< 1 cm	Filled with clear fluid (bulla > 1 cm)
Pustule	Elevated	< 1 cm	Filled with purulent fluid

Table 9.3 Secondary lesions

Lesion	Description
Crust	Dried remains of serum, blood, pus, or exudate
Scale	Accumulation of desquamating layers of stratum corneum
Ulceration	Full-thickness loss of the epithelium (erosion loss of superficial layers)
Atrophy	Thinning of the skin (epidermis atrophy thin and wrinkled, dermis atrophy depressed skin)

9.3 Skin Biopsies

Biopsy specimens are a fundamental part of the diagnostic approach of any skin lesion. Depending on the lesion's characteristics and suspected diagnosis, different techniques may be used. In order to optimize the result, the selected technique must ensure that sufficient tissue from the area of interest (where the abnormalities are expected) is obtained, while producing the least discomfort and cosmetic disturbance.

9.3.1 Shave Biopsy

Shaving is a simple method of obtaining samples of lesions suspected of affecting only the top layers of the skin (epidermis and superficial dermis). Using a scalpel parallel to the surface of the skin, the lesion is shaved off and the wound left to heal by secondary intention or treated by electrocauterization or topical hemostatic agents (e.g., 20% aluminum chloride, Monsel's solution [20% ferric subsulfate], 35% trichloroacetic acid, or silver nitrate).

Deep shaving is a variant in which more tissue is obtained by changing the angle of the blade to reach the mid to deep dermis.

9.3.2 Punch Biopsy

This is a convenient and quick method of obtaining a representative full-thickness sample. It is performed with a circumferentially shaped blade with diameters ranging from 2 to 10 mm. Depending on the diameter of the wound, it may be left to heal by secondary intention or closed with a single stitch. Importantly, punch biopsies of < 3 mm may not obtain sufficient tissue to establish an accurate pathological diagnosis.

9.3.3 Incisional Biopsy

Incisional biopsies imply taking a sample of the lesion by standard surgical technique using a scalpel and, in most cases, closure with sutures. This is a good alternative when removal of the entire lesion is likely to leave a significant aesthetic defect. When possible, normal skin should be included in the specimen to allow for comparison on histological examination.

9.3.4 Excisional Biopsy

This technique removes the entire lesion en bloc and represents the ideal method because it allows examination of the whole lesion—its full architecture and depth as well as its relationship with the layers of the skin. In some cases, however, the morbidity of performing a complete excision precludes the use of this technique.

9.4 Nonsurgical Treatment Modalities

Over the last decade, nonsurgical therapies for benign and malignant disorders of the skin have gained increasing popularity, mainly due to their reduced morbidity and superior cosmetic results compared to surgery. Although these techniques are mostly indicated and performed by dermatologists, plastic surgeons need to be familiar with their indications and limitations so as to be able to inform patients on the full range of options for a given lesion and avoid unnecessary surgical resections where possible. Finally, patients treated with these modalities should be closely followed because a number of lesions may respond partially or not respond at all, in which case escalation to a more aggressive therapy is warranted.

9.4.1 Cryodestruction

Also referred to as cryotherapy or cryosurgery, this technique involves destruction of skin lesions by direct application of a cryogenic agent, such as liquid nitrogen. Cryodestruction is effective against actinic keratoses, viral warts, and seborrheic keratosis.

9.4.2 Photodynamic Therapy

This procedural field therapy consists of the application of a topical photosensitizer (5-aminolevulinic acid or methyl aminolevulinate) followed by irradiation with a light source, which induces a phototoxic reaction that destroys abnormal cells. It is effective in the management of multiple actinic keratoses and squamous cell carcinoma (SCC) in situ, as well as some types of basal cell carcinoma (BCC). Secondary effects during and shortly after the application of light include erythema, edema, and a burning sensation, which can be quite painful in some cases. A new modality of photodynamic therapy, daylight–photodynamic therapy, uses exposure to natural daylight instead of an artificial light source.

9.4.3 Laser CO$_2$

This modality is described in Chapter 10.

9.4.4 Topical Treatments

Topical 5-Fluorouracil

This chemotherapeutic agent is a pyrimidine analogue, which acts by inhibiting thymidylate synthase, thus blocking DNA and RNA formation, especially in rapidly dividing cells.

5-Fluorouracil (5-FU) works best as a field treatment for actinic keratoses and SCC in situ, but it is relatively ineffective for BCC. Signs indicative of therapeutic success following application of 5-FU include inflammation, erythema, and erosions in dysplastic lesions. Conversely, undesired effects of this therapy include contact irritant or allergic dermatitis, phototoxicity, and scarring from ulceration. Patients may also experience pain, pruritus, and burning at the site of application.

Imiquimod

Imiquimod (Aldara, Medicis Pharmaceutical or Zyclara, Valeant Pharmaceuticals) is an immune response modifier with antitumoral and antiviral properties, which has shown to be effective in the treatment of genital warts, superficial BCC, and actinic keratosis, among others. Common side effects include skin irritation and erythema. In addition, although rare, flu-like symptoms and lymphadenopathies have also been reported following treatment with this product.

Topical Diclofenac

This nonsteroidal anti-inflammatory drug acts by inhibiting cyclooxygenase-2 (COX-2), which results in a reduction of prostaglandin synthesis and ultimately avoids suppression of the immune system. It is effective as a field treatment for actinic keratoses, but lesions slowly recur upon interruption of application. The most common reported adverse events (> 1%) are reactions at the site of application and irritant, allergic, or phototoxic contact dermatitis.

Ingenol Mebutate

Ingenol mebutate is a new topical therapy, the main advantage of which is the short treatment period (2–3 days) compared with the aforementioned methods. Its dual mechanism of action includes a chemoablative effect, which induces rapid cellular necrosis within a few hours of application and a long-lasting immunostimulatory effect that eliminates residual dysplastic cells through a neutrophil-mediated, antibody-dependent, cellular cytotoxic effect. This therapy is most effective against actinic keratoses and is currently under investigation for SCC in situ and BCC. The most common side effects include erythema, scaling, and crusting.

Deep Chemical Peels

The application of a chemical agent to the skin causes controlled destruction of the epidermis, with or without the dermis, leading to exfoliation and removal of superficial lesions, followed by regeneration of new epidermal and dermal tissues. Indications for chemical peeling include pigmentation disorders, superficial acne scars, ageing skin changes, and benign epidermal growths, such as seborrheic keratosis, actinic keratosis, sebaceous hyperplasia, warts, and milia. According to depth of penetration, chemical peels are classified as superficial, medium, and deep. Deep peels are performed with phenol-based solutions.

Peels may be complicated by hyper- or hypopigmentation, erythema, hypertrophic scarring and keloids, infections, and milia formation. In addition, deep peels may produce cutaneous atrophy, cardiac arrhythmias, and, very rarely, toxic shock syndrome. Contraindications are the presence of active cutaneous bacterial, viral, or fungal infection; a tendency to keloid formation; facial dermatitis; and patients taking photosensitizing medications or those with unrealistic expectations.

9.5 Benign Skin Tumors

Benign skin tumors include an extensive list of lesions of varying appearances, the full review of which is beyond the scope of this chapter. Instead, the focus here is on the most frequent tumors and on those of clinical interest to plastic surgeons.

There is currently no formal classification for benign lesions, which sometimes hampers communication and learning.

9.5.1 Epidermal Lesions

Seborrheic Keratosis

Formerly known as senile warts, seborrheic keratoses (SKs) are one of the most common lesions found in the adult and elderly populations. They are benign, sharply demarcated lesions, often with a waxy or verrucous, "stuck-on" appearance and may develop anywhere on the body. They are usually asymptomatic, but some patients may complain of itching. SKs vary in size and clinical appearance, ranging from a few millimeters to centimeters and can present as macular, papular, or verrucous lesions with a tan to black coloration.

Moreover, some SKs may simulate melanocytic neoplasms. SKs are mostly removed for cosmetic reasons by shave excision, curettage, and cryotherapy. The rarely occurring sign of Leser–Trélat is associated with an internal malignancy and involves the sudden appearance of multiple SKs.

Keratinocytic Epidermal Nevi (or Verrucous Nevus)

Epidermal nevi can be divided into organoid nevi (e.g., nevus sebaceous) and nonorganoid (keratinocytic) nevi. Keratinocytic epidermal nevi (frequently referred to simply as epidermal nevi) are benign, congenital tan to brown warty papules or plaques. They are either present at birth or become evident during early childhood and usually adopt a linear configuration on the extremities, although they may occur anywhere on the body. Histologically, epidermal nevi show hyperplasia of epidermal structures. They can be treated by surgical excision or laser therapy and other nonsurgical modalities. The epidermal nevus syndrome represents a sporadic association of epidermal nevi (usually extensive) with abnormalities in other organ systems.

Nevus Sebaceous (Nevus of Jadassohn)

This tumor consists of a hamartoma containing a combination of abnormalities of different skin components (epidermis, hair follicles, sebaceous and apocrine glands). It is usually located on the scalp and other areas of the head and neck. Although it may not be readily noticed, in most cases nevus sebaceous is present at birth or develops during early childhood, presenting as a small, flat, hairless, well-circumscribed yellowish linear or oval lesion. As the child grows, the lesion expands proportionately until puberty, when, as a result of androgen hormones, it becomes a waxy, verrucous, thick plaque (▶ Fig. 9.2). An episode of local trauma may also trigger this change. Lastly, usually during adulthood, different tumors begin to appear within the lesion. Although most of these are benign (e.g., trichoblastoma, syringocystadenoma papilliferum and trichilemmoma), malignant degeneration into BCC and less frequently SCC can also occur in a small number of patients (< 2.5%). Therefore, nevus sebaceous is a lesion that should be removed surgically. Although there is no

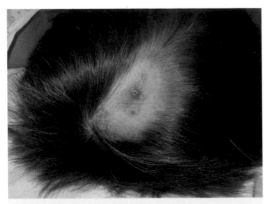

Fig. 9.2 Sebaceous nevus of Jadassohn.

real indication during childhood, excision before adolescence is strongly advocated because of its increased risk of malignant transformation and for cosmetic reasons, because these lesions are often located in aesthetic areas and, as already mentioned, they tend to grow during this period of age. Finally, the appearance of multiple nevi sebaceous may be associated with cerebral, ocular, and skeletal abnormalities as part of the epidermal nevus syndrome.

Acrochordon

These are benign, small, pedunculated, skin-colored or brownish papules, often located in folds. They have been associated with diabetes and an abnormal lipid profile. Indications for removal of these lesions are purely aesthetic. Shaving is the preferred method of excision.

9.5.2 Melanocytic Lesions (Usually Pigmented)

Ephelides or Freckles

Frequently seen in children and fair-skinned people, freckles are small, pigmented, uniform macules, appearing in sun-exposed areas that typically fade during winter months. Histologically, these lesions show a normal number of melanocytes with increased activity leading to the accumulation of melanin in basal keratinocytes.

Café au Lait Macules

Café au lait macules are sharply demarcated pale brown macules >n 5 mm in size. They are usually present at birth or appear shortly after. Isolated lesions have no clinical significance; however, multiple lesions (> 5) may be associated with underlying conditions, such as neurofibromatosis and other genetic disorders. Histologically these lesions show increased melanogenesis due to an excessive number of melanosomes, with a normal number of melanocytes.

Lentigines

Lentigines are acquired pigmented lesions, larger and better defined than freckles. The most common form, solar lentigines, arise in the middle-aged population and are induced by UV light; thus their preference for sun-exposed areas like the face and hands. Normal solar lentigines should be distinguished from lentigo maligna and lentigo maligna melanoma. Lesions that have appeared recently, showing different colors in their surface or with irregular borders, should be evaluated by a dermatologist to rule out malignancy.

Histologically there is a localized proliferation of melanocytes, specially at the tips of elongated rete ridges.

Nevi

The word *nevus* (pl. *nevi*) describes merely a cluster of cells. In order to classify nevi, attention should be paid to the type of cells contained within the lesion as well as their location within the layers of the skin.

Melanocytic Nevus

Melanocytic nevi are the most frequent melanocytic tumors. They are acquired lesions consisting of a concentration of nevus cells (slightly altered melanocytes). Clinically, they appear as round macules or flat papules, homogeneously colored, with regular borders and a diameter < 6 mm. According to where the nests of cells are located, melanocytic nevi are classified as junctional (at the epidermal–dermal junction), intradermal (dermis), and compound (elements of both junctional and intradermal). Junctional nevi usually present as flat brown macules, whereas intradermal nevi appear as fleshy, dome-shaped, skin-color to dark brown papules. The number of common melanocytic nevi depends on age (they usually develop at puberty), skin phototype (higher incidence in Caucasians), genetic background, immunosuppression, and UV light exposure.

Contrary to common belief, nevi are rarely premalignant, and, in fact, melanoma typically arises as a new lesion rather than developing from preexisting ones.

Dysplastic and Atypical Nevus

The terms *dysplastic nevus* and *atypical nevus* are frequently treated as synonymous; nevertheless, such equivalency is incorrect from a basic conceptual view as well as from a clinical standpoint. *Atypia* describes the clinical appearance of a nevus, whereas *dysplasia* refers to the presence of altered cells on histopathological analysis. Thus not all atypical nevi exhibit dysplasia on histological assessment, and, in turn, some common nevi can well be regarded as dysplastic following analysis. Atypia is based on the observation of one or more of the following clinical features, commonly summarized as ABCDE: *a*symmetry, *b*order irregularity, *c*olor variability, *d*iameter > 6 mm, *e*volution experiencing growth or changes. Conversely, dysplasia is classified as mild, moderate, or severe, depending on the degree of cellular alteration (cellular atypia).

Understanding the association between atypical nevus/dysplastic nevus and melanoma is fundamental for anyone involved in the diagnosis and management of these lesions. In the first place, as already stated, there is robust evidence showing that melanoma develops more frequently de novo rather than from a preexisting lesion, regardless of whether it was a common, dysplastic, or atypical nevus. Furthermore, studies of nevus-derived melanomas show similar proportions arising in dysplastic and common nevi. Secondly, despite widespread belief, most dysplastic nevi in the general population do not progress to melanoma but remain stable or regress. However, the presence of dysplastic nevi does constitute an important marker for an increased risk of melanoma, and in consequence any patient with such a lesion should be referred to a skin specialist for a complete physical examination and close follow-up. Regarding management, the recommendations are not to excise every atypical (irregular) nevus, but only those clinically suspicious for melanoma. Once removed, those showing mild or moderate dysplasia may be observed like common nevi regardless of margin status, whereas reexcision is indicated for those with severe dysplasia or when the pathologist cannot fully distinguish between dysplastic nevus and melanoma.

Blue Nevus

Blue nevi are well-circumscribed, homogeneous, blue-gray to blue-black round papules, often < 1 cm in size. Histologically, blue nevi are composed of a collection of melanocytes in the dermis. Conservative treatment is recommended for this tumor unless changes are observed (e.g., size, color, symptoms, etc.), in which case excision removing the superficial and deep dermis all the way to the subcutaneous tissue is indicated. Of note, primary nodular or metastatic melanoma may clinically and dermoscopically mimic blue nevus.

Halo Nevus

Common benign, asymptomatic lesions characterized by a central melanocytic nevus surrounded by a peripheral halo of hypopigmentation. With time, the central nevus usually disappears. These lesions do not require any treatment, although they should be reviewed in cases of morphological changes or symptoms.

Spitz's Nevus

This is a benign, usually acquired melanocytic lesion, frequently reported in children and young people and one of the main differential diagnoses of melanoma. Spitz nevus appears predominantly in the head and neck and presents as a solitary, dome-shaped, round to oval, reddish to dark brown papule, as large as 1 cm in diameter. Although Spitz's nevus has specific dermoscopic features, there are cases in which neither dermoscopy nor histopathology can reliably distinguish a Spitz's nevus from melanoma. Surgical excision is indicated for all spitzoid lesions appearing after puberty. Lesions without signs of atypia in patients younger than 12 years can be managed conservatively with digital dermoscopic monitoring.

Congenital Melanocytic Nevus

Congenital melanocytic nevi (CMN) appear at birth or shortly after. Based on size, CMN are classified as small (< 1.5 cm), intermediate (1.5–19.9 cm), large (> 20 cm), and giant (> 40 cm). They typically occur on the trunk, presenting initially as a flat, pigmented patch that changes over time, when darker macules and papules and sometimes hair begin to appear, giving the lesion an unsightly mottled and heterogeneous aspect (▸Fig. 9.3). The three main concerns about CMN are its potential for malignant transformation into melanoma, its association with neurocutaneous melanosis, and its unaesthetic appearance. Regarding malignant degeneration, the risk of melanoma in CMN depends mostly on size—for small and medium lesions the risk is < 1% risk, whereas for large lesions it is < 5%. Importantly, most CMN-derived melanomas appear before 15 years of age. Neurocutaneous melanosis is associated with giant lesions and other factors, such as satellite nevi or multiple CMN, male sex, and head and neck and dorsal midline location. Neurocutaneous melanosis can affect different regions of the central nervous system and become life threatening in some cases.

Treatment of CMN, especially large and giant, is based on surgical excision, mainly to reduce the risk of malignancy and improve cosmesis. Although highly recommended, whether surgery reduces the incidence of malignant melanoma remains unproven. The unaesthetic appearance of CMN constitutes in many cases the main reason for surgical excision due to the significant psychological impact that these

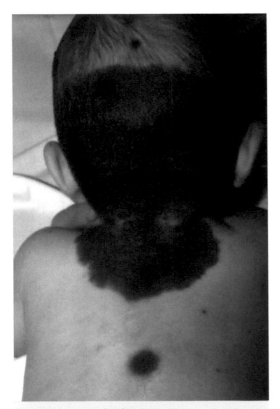

Fig. 9.3 Congenital melanocytic nevus.

lesions cause, especially large ones. Surgery usually involves serial excision, tissue expansion, and flap coverage. Alternatives to surgical excision have been described, such as dermabrasion, curettage, electrosurgery, andlasers, which could be a good option when morbidity from surgical excision is unacceptable and for cases in which the main concern are the thick hairs growing on the surface of the lesion.

Nevus of Becker

Nevus of Becker typically appears on the shoulder and back of males (5:1) during puberty, presenting as a unilateral, gradually enlarging, and usually hypertrichotic melanocytic lesion (also considered as a hamartoma).

Nevus of Ota

Nevus of Ota is a unilateral, blue-brown facial patch most usually distributed along the territory of the first and second branches of the trigeminal nerve. This type of nevus is more common in Asians and dark-skinned races. Histologically it is characterized by the presence of elongated melanocytes scattered among collagen bundles of the reticular dermis. Treatment usually involves the use of laser therapy, namely Q-switched neodumium:ytrium-aluminum-garnet.

Nevus of Ito

Exhibits the same clinical and histological features as nevus of Ota, differing from it in its area of involvement (posterior shoulder and areas innervated by posterior supraclavicular and lateral cutaneous brachial nerves).

Mongolic Blue Spot (Congenital Dermal Melanocytes)

These lesions are more common in Asian and dark-skinned individuals, presenting as bluish-gray patches with indistinct margins on the lumbosacral area. They typically disappear by childhood and therefore require no treatment.

9.6 Fibrous Tumors

9.6.1 Dermatofibroma

Indurated minimally elevated to dome-shaped papule or nodule with a yellowish to reddish-brown surface that appears in adulthood, more commonly on the lower extremities. Dermatofibromas usually exhibit a positive dimple sign (apparent downward movement of the tumor when pressed at the edges).

9.6.2 Neurofibroma

Neurofibromas are asymptomatic skin-colored, protuberant to pedunculated, soft or rubbery papule-nodules, usually < 2 cm in size. Neurofibromas appear more commonly as solitary lesions; in the presence of multiple lesions neurofibromatosis 1 or 2 must be ruled out. Regardless, they are usually treated by simple excision.

9.7 Miscellaneous

9.7.1 Epidermal Cyst

Usually but incorrectly called sebaceous cysts, epidermal cysts are a proliferation of epidermal cells within a circumscribed dermal space containing an accumulation of foul-smelling keratinous debris with a central pore. Epidermal cysts are located most often on the face, neck, and trunk, where they appear as a fluctuant, flesh colored nodule with a visible punctum (pore), which is usually a useful distinguishing feature from lipomas. They are mostly asymptomatic but may become inflamed or infected, resulting in pain and tenderness. Uninfected cysts can be excised with their surrounding capsule, whereas infected ones are treated by incision and drainage of any purulent material, followed by a course of antibiotics and excision of the remaining capsule/cyst once infection and inflammation have subsided (see Chapter 12 for further details).

Trichilemmal (pilar) cysts are epidermal cysts of the scalp and are managed as already described.

9.7.2 Mucocele

Mucoceles are the most common lesions of the oral cavity and result from mechanical trauma to minor salivary glands. They appear most frequently in the lower lip and cheek mucosa and may be seen at any age, with a concentrated incidence around the second decade of life. Clinically, mucoceles are characterized by a painless, semitranslucent, soft submucosal nodule with multiple cycles of swelling, rupturing, and refilling. Surgical excision is recommended in most cases.

9.7.3 Mucous Cyst

Mucous cysts (also called myxoid cysts) are soft, shiny, viscous-filled nodules appearing in the distal interphalangeal joint in relation to the presence of an osteophyte. In some cases the cyst may compress the nail matrix, resulting in nail plate depression and grooves. Treatment of mucous cysts involves surgical excision, including removal of the underlying osteophyte. Even though they usually appear on one side of the joint, the opposite should be explored during surgery to rule out the presence of occult cysts.

9.7.4 Angiomas

Eruptive angiomas, also known as ruby spots or senile or cherry hemangiomas, are benign tumors of capillary vessels. They appear as isolated or multiple, bright red, dome-shaped to polypoid, sharply demarcated papules up to several millimeters in diameter.

9.7.5 Milium Cysts

Benign, small, white, superficial cysts (< 3 mm in size) appearing most commonly on the face. They are extracted using a sharp instrument, such as a 14-gauge needle or a no. 11 scalpel blade.

9.7.6 Dermoid Cysts

These are congenital lesions developing from the entrapment of endodermal and mesodermal remnants along the lines of embryonic fusion. With time they tend to become progressively larger due to accumulation of debris within the cyst. They are most commonly seen along the supraorbital ridge, lateral brow, or nasal midline (▶Fig. 9.4). Lesions along the nasal midline should be investigated by magnetic resonance and/or computed tomographic scan prior to removal in order to rule out intracranial extension as well as glioma, meningocele, and encephalocele. Surgical excision is the recommended treatment.

9.7.7 Pilomatrixoma

These are small, benign tumors derived from the hair matrix, most commonly seen in the head and

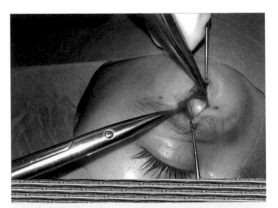

Fig. 9.4 Excision of a dermoid cyst located on the supraorbital rim. The supraorbital nerve is seen running on the surface of the cyst (case courtesy of Dr. Bernardo Hontanilla).

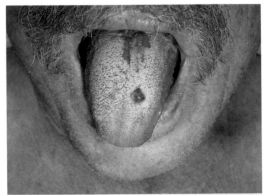

Fig. 9.5 Pyogenic granuloma on the tongue.

neck and upper limbs of younger patients. Clinically, they appear as a flesh-colored, white, or bluish papule or nodule, which is firm on palpation due to calcification. Pilomatrixomas are usually solitary lesions; multiple ones have been associated with myotonic dystrophy and Gardner's syndrome. Despite its benign nature, locally aggressive and even metastatic lesions have been reported, which is why surgical excision is the treatment of choice.

9.7.8 Pyogenic Granuloma

Pyogenic granuloma is a benign, abrupt, vascular proliferation that develops spontaneously or following local trauma, burn, or insect bite. They frequently appear on the head and neck or upper limb as a soft, reddish, pedunculated papule or nodule characterized by easy bleeding. The main differential diagnosis of a solitary pyogenic granuloma is Spitz's nevus in children, whereas in adults amelanotic melanoma should be ruled out, especially those appearing on the nail bed. Treatment options include surgical excision, curettage, and electrodessication and laser therapy (▶ Fig. 9.5).

9.8 Premalignant Lesions

9.8.1 Actinic Keratoses

Actinic keratoses (AKs) represent one of the most common premalignant lesions of the skin. Their usual form of presentation is that of a scaly,

erythematous papule with a hyperkeratotic texture. They exhibit slow growth and can range from a small (1–3 mm) papule to a large plaque but with little infiltration. AKs are sometimes better identified by touch rather than visual inspection. Risk factors for AK include advanced age, fair skin, cumulative sun exposure, and immunosuppression. The clinical importance of AK lies in its potential to progress into invasive SCC. Overall, the risk of malignant transformation of AK is low, though highly variable (0.1–20%). However, it is known that the risk of developing SCC increases with the number of AKs (more than five AKs) and that the great majority of SCCs originate from a preexisting AK. Unfortunately, to date there are no reliable methods for predicting which lesions will undergo malignant transformation, which is why the recommendation is to treat them all.

> **Note**
>
> Although a small proportion of AKs progress to invasive SCC, the vast majority of SCC develops from a preexisting AK.

9.8.2 Cutaneous Horn

Cutaneous horns are well-circumscribed, conical, dense, hyperkeratotic protrusions, appearing more commonly on sun-exposed skin. Although they arise most frequently from benign lesions, such as SK, we have deliberately included them in this section because, on occasion, cutaneous horns develop from premalignant (e.g., actinic keratosis) or malignant (e.g., SCC) areas. This fact explains why cutaneous horns should be treated by complete surgical excision, with exhaustive histopathological examination of the base.

9.8.3 Leukoplakia

Leukoplakia is defined as a white patch or plaque that cannot be characterized clinically or pathologically as any other disease, and represents the most common premalignant lesion of the oral cavity. Use of tobacco and alcohol is strongly associated with the development of leukoplakia. Clinically, it usually presents as a flat thin white patch in the oral cavity, which rarely exhibits histopathological abnormalities. Overall, malignant transformation of leukoplakia is rare, but attention should be paid to suspicious lesions in which the risk of development into SCC is higher. Management of leukoplakia ranges from tobacco and alcohol cessation and close observation to, more commonly, local destruction (e.g., laser) plus observation or surgical excision.

9.8.4 Erythroplasia

Erythroplasia is defined as a bright red, velvety patch that cannot be characterized clinically or pathologically as being caused by any other condition. In contrast to leukoplakia, the presence of dysplasia on histopathological analysis is very common in erythroplasia; therefore these lesions should be treated by wide surgical excision in all cases. Erythroplasia of Queyrat is a form of SCC in situ, appearing on the glans and prepuce of the uncircumcised male. Clinically it appears as a solitary or multiple erythematous, well-demarcated, velvety patches or plaques. Treatment options include surgical excision, 5-FU, and photodynamic therapy.

9.9 Nonmelanoma Skin Cancers

Nonmelanoma skin cancers (NMSCs) are the most common human neoplasms. Even though the term NMSC includes a variety of tumors (e.g., Merkel's cell carcinoma, adnexal tumors, cutaneous lymphomas, and other rare tumors), it mainly refers to BCC and SCC, because these are by far the most common skin cancers, with BCC being three to six times more frequent than SCC. Hereafter, the term NMSC will be used to name BCC/SCC exclusively, unless otherwise specified.

The epidemiology of NMSC is both alarming and economically significant; not only are these the most common cancers but their overall incidence is rapidly increasing as well. Whereas in Europe it is estimated that 700,000 new cases of NMSC are diagnosed each year, in the United States this figure rises to 2.8 million. As suggested by Lewin, the increasing incidence is probably multifactorial and includes the aging of the general population, changes in sun exposure habits, higher solar radiation due to environmental changes, migration phenomena, and the higher number of patients taking immunosuppressant drugs. SCC and BCC most commonly affect people over 60 years of age; nevertheless, during the last decade there has been a steady increase in the incidence of BCC in younger people, particularly women.

The clinical features and presentation of BCC and SCC are different; however, they do share similarities in their history, which is usually highly suggestive of NMSC. These patients often present with a new lesion with a changing pattern over the last couple of months, or an old one that has changed its appearance over the same period. Therefore, together with a detailed history, a thorough physical examination is needed, noting not only new lesions but also old ones that may have changed.

Nowadays there are a number of therapeutic alternatives for NMSCs, depending on their clinical and histological characteristics, but the mainstay of treatment continues to be surgical excision with safe margins, which offers excellent curative rates and low recurrence.

As explained later in this chapter, metastatic spread is extremely rare in BCC and infrequent in SCC, which translates into a favorable prognosis in the vast majority of cases. However, both BCC and SCC can be locally aggressive and may infiltrate soft tissues and underlying supportive structures, resulting in severe disfigurement and a significant impact on quality of life in some cases. Additionally, recent evidence suggests that the mortality rates of SCC might have been underestimated, a fact that strongly highlights the need for proper and complete excision of the primary lesion.

9.9.1 Risk Factors

The development of NMSC has been associated with genotypic, phenotypic, and environmental factors. Of all, sun exposure is by far the most important risk factor, especially in fair-skinned people. Not surprisingly, 80% of NMSCs develop in sun-exposed areas, particularly the head and neck. UVB radiation damages both DNA and RNA, which leads to the generation of mutagenic photoproducts. UVA, in turn, though far from benign, is less harmful than UVB. Of note, it has been suggested that, whereas cumulative sun exposure is strongly associated with SCC, the same does not fully apply to BCC, for which intermittent sun exposure and exposure during childhood might be more important. This feature explains, in part, why BCC may appear in both young and advanced-age individuals, whereas SCC develops almost exclusively in older people. Factors other than UV light exposure accounting for a small minority of NMSC include arsenic, ionizing radiation therapy, chronic wounds, and scars. In addition, the development of SCC may be enhanced by the combination of sun exposure plus cigarette smoking and human papilloma virus infection. Immunosuppressed patients are at particular risk of developing NMSCs. Caucasian recipients of solid-organ transplantation under lifetime immunosuppressive therapy need to be regularly checked because the incidence of BCC and SCC in them increases more than 10-fold and 65-fold, respectively, which dramatically inverts the 3–6:1 BCC:SCC ratio seen in the general population. Genetic syndromes that strongly predispose to NMSC include xeroderma pigmentosum, oculocutaneous albinism, dystrophic epidermolysis bullosa, and Gorlin's syndrome, among others. Patients with Gorlin's syndrome carry a mutation in the PCTH1 tumor-suppressor gene of the hedgehog pathway, which makes them highly susceptible of developing multiple and early-onset BCC, as well as other cutaneous and noncutaneous neoplasms. Other environmental and genetic risk factors for NMSC are summarized in ▶ Table 9.4.

9.9.2 Basal Cell Carcinoma

BCC is both the most common skin malignancy and the most frequent neoplasm in humans. It usually presents as a pink, skin-colored, or even pigmented, slowly growing lesion, most frequently in the head and neck of older people. The main histological features of BCC include the presence of basaloid tumor cells clusters with a characteristic peripheral nuclear palisading at the margins of tumor nests. Additionally, a variable inflammatory infiltrate and ulceration are observed in some cases. In 1978, Wade and Ackerman described 26 different histopathological types of BCC. Although the clinical appearance of these different subtypes helps to guide the initial approach, what really defines the lesion and its management is the pathologist's report. In this sense, any surgeon

Table 9.4 Risk factors for basal cell carcinoma and squamous cell carcinoma

	SCC	BCC
Ultraviolet light	✓	✓
Ionizing radiation	✓	✓
Chemical (arsenic)	✓	✓
Human papillomavirus	✓	
Cigarette smoking	✓	
Xeroderma pigmentosum	✓	✓
Nevoid basal cell carcinoma syndrome (Gorlin)		✓
Bazex syndrome		✓
Others (oculocutaneous albinism, epidermodysplasia verruciformis, dystrophic epidermolysis bullosa, Muir–Torre syndrome	✓	
Nevus sebaceous		✓
Rombo syndrome		✓
Chronic nonhealing wounds and ulcers	✓	✓
Discoid lupus, lichen planus, lichen sclerosus, porokeratosis	✓	
Immunosuppression (organ transplantation, inflammatory chronic diseases, chronic lymphocytic leukemia, AIDS)	✓	✓

Source: Reproduced with permission from Narayan D. Benign and malignant tumors of the skin. In: Guyuron B, Eriksson E, Persing JA, eds. Plastic Surgery Indications and Practice. Philadelphia: Saunders; 2009;119–146.

involved in the treatment of BCC must be familiarized with the main histological subtypes with regard to their aggressiveness and prognosis. Furthermore it is important to note that, in up to 40% of the cases, a lesion may present with a combination of two or more histological patterns, in which case the most aggressive component dictates its biological behavior and surgical management.

The following are the most frequent clinical subtypes of BCC:
- Nodular (50–65%): This subtype is the most common form of BCC. It is usually located in the head and neck region, presenting as a solitary, pearly, telangiectatic nodular papule with rolled borders (▶ Fig. 9.6). The rapid enlargement of some nodular BCCs causes ischemia of the most apical portion, leading to ulceration and bleeding. This feature gives them the classical appearance of a

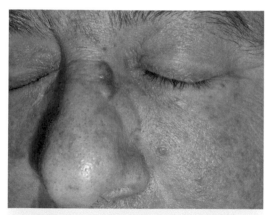

Fig. 9.6 Nodular basal cell carcinoma on the lateral aspect of the nose. Note also xantelasmas on both upper eyelids.

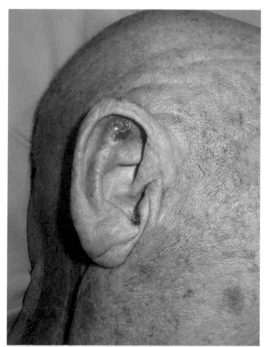

Fig. 9.7 Ulcerated (ulcus rodens) basal cell carcinoma on the posterior crus of the helix of the right ear.

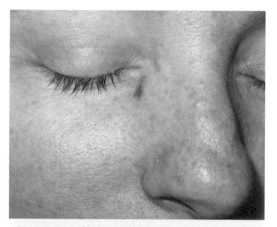

Fig. 9.8 Superficial spreading basal cell carcinoma on the inner canthus of the right eye.

"rodent ulcer" (ulcus rodens), which is generally associated with a more locally aggressive behavior (▶Fig. 9.7). An important differential diagnosis of nodular BCC is amelanotic melanoma, which is fortunately far less common.

- Superficial spreading (10–15%): Clinically, superficial BCC presents as a scaly, slightly shiny, erythematous patch most often in the upper trunk and shoulders (▶Fig. 9.8). In some cases a pearly rim is observed surrounding the lesion. While ulceration of a superficial BCC is rare, minor erosions and crusts are frequently seen on its surface. Due to its clinical appearance, superficial BCCs may be confused with similar-looking lesions, such as AKs, eczema, fungal infection, and psoriasis. An important feature of this type of BCC is its confinement to the epidermis without dermal extensions, which makes it a tumor of low aggressiveness, susceptible to treatment with nonsurgical therapies as explained later in this chapter.
- Pigmented (5%): Characterized for its melanin-derived pigmentation, this variant of BCC presents most commonly as pigmented nodular papules, in which case their main differential diagnosis is nodular melanoma.
- Sclerosing, morpheaform, or fibrosing (2%): This is regarded as the most aggressive variant of BCC. It usually presents as a slow-growing, ill-defined, scarlike plaque in the face, and is characterized by a strong tendency to invade the deep layers of the skin, which makes its complete removal challenging and its recurrence rates the highest of all subtypes (▶Fig. 9.9).
- Fibroepithelioma of Pinkus (< 1%): A very rare subtype, fibroepithelioma of Pinkus is considered an indolent BCC, usually presenting as a warty-looking lesion on the trunk.

Additional histopathological subtypes include basosquamous BCC, which is an aggressive combination of BCC and SCC, and micronodular BCC, a destructive

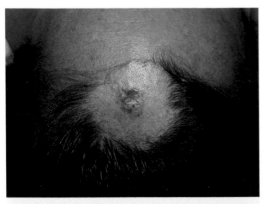

Fig. 9.9 Sclerosing basal cell carcinoma on the anterior scalp.

Table 9.5 Risk factors for recurrence of basal cell carcinoma

- Diameter > 2 cm
- Head and neck, particularly around nose, ears, and eyes ("mask area")
- Sites of prior radiation
- Recurrent tumor
- Breslow thickness > 2 mm
- Ill-defined borders
- Aggressive clinical/histological subtype: morpheaform, infiltrating, micronodular, basosquamous
- Perineural invasion
- Immunosuppression

variant composed of small islands of tumor cells diffusely scattered in the dermis, which explains their subclinical spread and high rates of recurrence.

Risk Stratification Assessment

The knowledge and understanding of the risk factors for recurrence and metastasis are essential because they not only influence the outcome but also guide the choice of treatment. BCC is classified as high-risk or low-risk depending on the following factors (▶Table 9.5):
- Diameter: BCCs > 2 cm have a higher chance of recurring.
- Location: BCCs located in the face are more likely to recur, regardless of treatment modality (▶Fig. 9.10). Although location and diameter are normally considered independent

factors, the National Comprehensive Cancer Network stratifies size in relation to location, so that the following are considered high-risk factors:

- Diameter ≥ 6 mm on "mask area" of the face (which is considered a high risk location)
- Diameter ≥ 10 mm on moderate risk locations, including forehead, cheeks, neck, and scalp
- Diameter ≥ 20 mm on trunk and extremities

BCCs arising in sites of prior radiotherapy are also considered high-risk tumors.
- Recurrent tumors: Incompletely excised primary BCCs located on the face recur in up to 40% of cases. Surgical clearance is more difficult to achieve in recurrent versus primary BCC.
- Depth of invasion: Tumors with a Breslow thickness > 2 mm are considered at high risk of recurrence. Likewise, invasion of underlying fat, fascia, muscle, cartilage, or bone makes it difficult to correctly assess the extent of spread, which may lead to incomplete removal.
- Ill-defined borders: Tumors with poorly defined borders have greater subclinical extension, which is difficult to assess macroscopically, leading to higher rates of incomplete excisions and recurrence.
- Clinicohistological subtypes: Morpheaform, infiltrating, micronodular, and basosquamous subtypes are aggressive histopathological variants characterized by their invasive behavior and higher rate of recurrence.
- Perineural invasion: Although rare in BCC (< 0.5%), perineural invasion is associated with a higher risk of recurrence.
- Immunosuppression: As stated earlier, immunosuppressed patients are at higher risk of developing NMSC. Now, not only is their incidence increased, but tumors are more likely to recur and metastasize as well.

Workup and Treatment

If a diagnosis of BCC is suspected, then a thorough complete physical examination should be undertaken to rule out concomitant tumors and melanoma. If a biopsy is required prior to complete excision, then one needs to make sure that the specimen includes deep (reticular) dermis, especially when a more deeply invasive process is suspected, because tumors with infiltrative histology

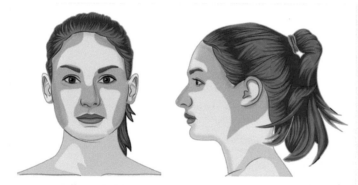

Fig. 9.10 Diagram depicting the "H" zone of the face, which includes the upper lip, nose, periorbital region, temple extending to the mandibular angle, preauricular area, ear, and postauricular region. These areas are sites of embryonic fusion planes that run perpendicular to the skin surface, allowing deeper invasion of the tumor. Skin cancers, particularly basal cell carcinoma, developing in the H zone, are believed to have a higher risk of recurrence.

are sometimes present in the deeper dermis only. Although BCC rarely metastasizes, it can be locally aggressive and destructive in the long term (locally advanced BCC). For cases in which extensive involvement of underlying structures is suspected, imaging should be considered to determine the extent of tumor spread and decide on the best excisional/reconstructive strategy.

Once the diagnosis of BCC is established, the tumor should be stratified as low risk or high risk in order to decide on the best therapeutic plan, keeping in mind that the goal of treatment will always be complete clearance with maximum preservation of function and the best possible cosmetic outcome. In this sense, the mainstay of treatment continues to be surgical excision; nevertheless, nonsurgical alternatives, including 5-FU, imiquimod, cryotherapy, and photodynamic therapy, offering less morbidity and better aesthetic results, are available for low-risk superficial tumors. It should be noted though, that the rates of complete removal with these techniques are not as high as with surgery, albeit recurrences of low-risk tumors are more easily managed.

> **Note**
>
> The clinical and surgical margins must be clearly delineated before injection of local anesthetic as infiltration distorts the tissues and hinders proper demarcation.

Low-Risk Basal Cell Carcinoma

For tumors < 2 cm in diameter, located on the trunk or extremities and without aggressive clinical or histological features, *excision with 4 mm margin* is recommended. If margins are positive on histopathological examination, then Mohs micrographic surgery (MMS) is recommended in all cases except for tumors located in the "L" zone, which may be treated by standard reexcision.

Curettage and electrodessication are also considered first-line treatment options for superficial variants. However, curettage and electrodessication, or any treatment other than surgical excision, should not be used for tumors located in hair-bearing areas like the scalp, pubis, axilla, and beard due to their potential for infiltrating hair bulbs and spreading therefrom. Finally, for elderly patients or those with severe comorbidities in whom surgery is not an option, external beam radiotherapy can be employed.

High-Risk Basal Cell Carcinoma

Due to their higher chance of subclinical extension, invasiveness, and recurrence, high-risk BCCs are best treated using MMS. In addition, MMS, or any technique that thoroughly analyzes deep and peripheral margins prior to closure, is particularly recommended for tumors appearing in the face, where maximal preservation of health tissue is desired. If for any reason the margins cannot be assessed before wound closure/reconstruction, then wide excision with a 10–15 mm margin with immediate closure and postoperative histopathological assessment may be considered.

If following MMS a positive margin is reported, then reexcision of that margin should be performed; alternatively, radiotherapy may be administered. Radiotherapy is also indicated for locally advanced cancer that escapes surgical management and for tumors showing perineural invasion (▶Table 9.6). It is important to note, though, that the real benefit of radiotherapy in these cases

Table 9.6 Indications for radiotherapy in NMSC

- High-risk BCC and SCC with positive margins after Mohs surgery
- BCC and SCC with extensive perineural or large nerve involvement
- SCC with lymph node metastasis
- NMSC and DFSP in patients unable to undergo surgery[a]
- Patients with DFSP and positive margins in whom further resection is not feasible
- Merkel's cell carcinoma

Abbreviations: BCC, basal cell carcinoma; DFSP, dermatofibrosarcoma protuberans; NMSC, nonmelanoma skin cancer; SCC, squamous cell carcinoma.
[a] This indication is subjective depending on the case and the extent of surgery needed.

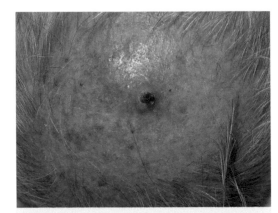

Fig. 9.11 Squamous cell carcinoma on the vertex of the scalp.

is controversial, and there is no conclusive evidence supporting its use at this time.

Alternative treatments for patients with locally advanced or metastatic BCC in whom surgery is inappropriate are vismodegib or sonidegib, two oral, smoothened antagonists, which block the hedgehog pathway.

9.9.3 Squamous Cell Carcinoma

Compared to BCC, SCC in the general population is less frequent but more aggressive. Additionally, unlike BCC, SCC almost always arises from a precursor lesion, namely AKs (solar keratoses) and SCC in situ. In fact, it has been suggested that actinic keratoses and SCC are part of the same keratinocyte dysplasia continuum. It is important to note that, although more than 90% of SCCs arise from a previous actinic keratosis, less than 10% of actinic keratoses actually progress to SCC. Also, a small proportion of SCCs arise in sites of chronic wounds or ulcers (e.g., Marjolin's ulcer), chronic radiation dermatitis, and infrared irradiation, these tumors are usually associated with a worse prognosis. Clinically, in most cases SCC presents as an erythematous hyperkeratotic papule or nodule with ill-defined borders and an adherent crust on sun-exposed areas of older people (▶Fig. 9.11). With time, the lesion usually becomes progressively more tender and bleeds easily. Other forms of presentation include exophytic verrucous-like lesions, which can be locally deeply invasive but less likely to metastasize, and an ulcerative form, characterized by its invasiveness and higher rate of lymph node spread. Histologically SCC is characterized by aggregations of pleomorphic eosinophilic keratinocytes arising from the epidermis and extending into the dermis. Of note, the degree of keratinization depends on cellular differentiation—a well-differentiated tumor will contain more keratinous pearls than a less or nondifferentiated specimen.

Risk Stratification Assessment

As with BCC, it has been demonstrated that proper management of the primary lesion reduces the rates of recurrence of SCC. However, while a number of large-scale studies and guidelines have attempted to stratify SCC, there is still no consensus on the list of risk factors for recurrence, the definition of high-risk SCC, or a clear estimation of prognosis. This lack of evidence and unanimity makes the decision-making process difficult in relation to staging, primary therapy, and indication of adjuvant treatment. Not surprisingly, the management of SCC is quite varied, even among experienced clinicians. Furthermore, the fact that SCC has a significantly higher metastatic rate than BCC makes this lack of consensus a remarkably important issue, which is being actively addressed by a number of groups. The most important stratification systems come from the National Comprehensive Cancer Network, the American Joint Committee on Cancer (7th edition), the Union for International Cancer Control, and the Brigham and Women's Hospital. Although these four systems differ from one another, for this chapter we have opted to list all the risk factors mentioned in them so as to provide the average clinician with "red-flags" for tumors necessitating a more thorough workup and management due to their higher risk of recurrence, metastasis, and disease-specific death (▶Table 9.7).

- Diameter: As with BCCs, SCCs with a diameter > 2 cm have a higher chance of recurring.
- Location: The ears, lip, and temple have been regarded as high-risk areas for SCC. As with BCC, location and diameter have also been combined as follows:
  ○ Diameter ≥ 6 mm on ears, lip, and temple, genitalia, hands, and feet
  ○ Diameter ≥ 10 mm on forehead, cheeks, neck, and scalp
  ○ Diameter ≥ 20 mm on trunk and extremities

SCCs arising in sites of previous radiotherapy also exhibit a higher risk of recurrence. Likewise, those appearing in chronically injured skin, such as chronic wounds, ulcers, scars, and burned sites are usually much more aggressive and likely to recur.

- Rapid growth: This feature should alert the clinician to the aggressiveness of the tumor and its chances of recurring.
- Depth of invasion: Thickness > 2 mm or invasion beyond the papillary dermis portends a greater likelihood of recurrence.
- Ill-defined borders: As in BCC, subclinical extension is difficult to assess macroscopically in poorly defined tumors, which leads to incomplete excisions and higher rates of recurrence.
- Histology: Tumors with poorly differentiated histology, an acantholytic or mucin-production pattern, or aggressive subtypes (e.g., adenoid, adenosquamous, desmoplastic, and infiltrative) are all considered to have a high risk of recurrence.

- Perineural and lymphovascular invasion: This is much more frequent in SCC and may be present on histological sections or clinically in the form of neuralgic pain, paresthesia, anesthesia, or muscular palsy. Because these tumors present most commonly in the face, the affected nerves are usually sensitive branches of the trigeminal nerve or motor fascicles of the facial nerve. Regardless of whether it is symptomatic or not, perineural invasion is associated with a worse prognosis; hence a more radical resection should be performed. Furthermore, the larger the affected nerve, the worse prognosis becomes.
- Immunosuppression: Previously we have mentioned how immunosuppressed patients are at higher risk of developing NMSC, particularly SCC. Increased susceptibility depends on the etiology of immunosuppression, with solid organ transplant recipients > chronic lymphocytic leukemia > small-cell lymphocytic lymphoma > other types.

Thompson et al have recently published a meta-analysis on the risk factors for recurrence, metastasis, and disease-specific death in cutaneous SCC and found statistical significance for diameter > 20 mm; Breslow thickness > 2 mm; invasion beyond subcutaneous fat; perineural invasion; location on the temple, ear, and lip; poor differentiation; and immunosuppression. Furthermore, the authors suggest tumor depth to be the factor associated with the highest risk ratio of local recurrence and metastasis, and tumor diameter greater than 20 mm the factor with the highest risk ratio of disease-specific death.

Workup and Treatment

Apart from complete skin examination, regional lymph node basins must be explored in patients with (suspected) SCC because > 80% of SCC metastases are lymphatic, and their involvement influences management. Imaging should be requested in patients with disease extending beyond subcutaneous fat and those with perineural invasion. For the latter, magnetic resonance imaging is recommended as the best imaging modality.

Low-Risk Squamous Cell Carcinoma

Excision with 6 mm margins and postoperative histological assessment are recommended for low-risk SCC. The increase in surgical margins

Table 9.7 Risk factors for recurrence of squamous cell carcinoma

- Diameter > 2 cm
- Head and neck, particularly *ears,lips*, and *temples*; sites of previous radiation; *mucosal surfaces*; *genitalia*; and *chronically injured skin*, including *scars, wounds, ulcers*, or *burned sites*
- *Rapid growth*
- Recurrent tumor
- Breslow thickness > 4 mm
- Ill-defined borders
- *Histologic features: loss of differentiation, adenoid,adenosquamous,desmoplastic* and *infiltrative subtypes*
- Perineural and *lymphovascular invasion*
- Immunosuppression

Note: In italics are features that are either absent or modified in the basal cell carcinoma list.

with respect to the 4 mm advocated for BCC is because the borders of SCC are less defined and harder to assess clinically; taking an extra 2 mm improves the rates of complete clearance. Positive margins of tumors located in the L zone are best managed by reexcision, whereas for the rest of the areas, MMS is recommended. The rate of recurrence of incompletely excised SCCs can be as high as 50% or more. As with BCC, nonsurgical therapies as well as curettage and electrodessication can be used in low-risk SCC with the same precautions as for hair-bearing areas. Finally, for elderly patients unable to sustain surgery, radiotherapy is advocated. In the author's opinion, however, these patients benefit more from a complete local destruction under local anesthesia (which very rarely cannot be done), leaving the wound to heal by secondary intention than from radiotherapy, because this group of patients of advanced age and sometimes limited mobility will likely be more troubled by having to attend multiple sessions of radiotherapy than by the postoperative recovery of a relatively minor procedure.

High-Risk Squamous Cell Carcinoma

The management of high-risk SCC is very similar to its BCC counterpart. Due to their high rate of recurrence if incompletely excised and the greater potential for lymphatic spread, complete removal of high-risk SCC is of utmost importance. Hence, MMS or any technique providing complete assessment of deep and peripheral margins is indicated. If MMS cannot be performed, then wide excision with postoperative margin assessment should be done. In the presence of perineural involvement, adjuvant radiotherapy is recommended following surgical excision.

Lymph Nodes

Patients with clinically palpable or suspicious nodes on radiological assessment should undergo fine needle or core biopsy. Cases with positive nodes should be referred to a multidisciplinary unit and undergo further staging investigations. These patients will most probably necessitate regional lymph node dissection and adjuvant radiotherapy. Furthermore, in most cases with cervical node involvement, the parotid gland is affected as well (60–80%). Parotid infiltration as a direct extension of SCC has a poor prognosis, and recommendations are to perform a superficial parotidectomy in cases where the cancer extends into the parotid fascia.

For tumors presenting several high-risk features, some authors have recommended sentinel lymph node biopsy or prophylactic node dissection; however, solid evidence supporting the use of either surgery is lacking.

> **Note**
>
> To date, there is no robust and conclusive evidence supporting the use of radiotherapy, sentinel lymph node dissection, and prophylactic node dissection in high-risk SCC.

9.9.4 Prognosis and Follow-Up

Prognosis of BCC and SCC is usually excellent after surgical excision, particularly in the former due to its unlikeliness to metastasize. SCC, however, presents with nodal involvement in 3.7–5.2% of cases, and approximately 2% of patients die of SCC. Although low in percentage, especially if compared to other cancers, this figure does become relevant when it is transformed to the absolute number of patients that it represents. In the United States, for example, the upper limit of SCC's mortality approaches the lower one for melanoma.

Follow-up of NMSC must be strict during the first 5 years because it is estimated that 30–50% of patients will develop another one of these cancers within the next 5 years, meaning they have 10 times the risk of the general population. Besides, these patient almost always present with varying degrees of sun damage, which increases their risk of developing melanoma as well. Furthermore, most of SCC's recurrences and metastases appear within 24 months of initial treatment, although some studies have described dissemination to occur at later time points, between 5 and 10 years. Frequency of follow-up then depends on the type of tumor and the presence of high-risk features. In this sense, patients with BCC should undergo complete physical examination once or twice during the first 24 months and have yearly visits thereafter. SCC, in turn, requires revision every 3–6 months during the first 2 years, and then every 6–12 months. Organ transplant recipients will need a closer follow-up regime due to their higher chance of developing more tumors, usually of increased aggressiveness, following the appearance of the first one.

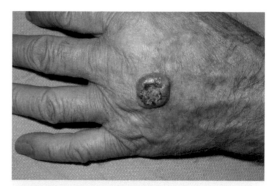

Fig. 9.12 Keratoacanthoma on the dorsum of the left hand.

9.9.5 Bowen's Disease

This condition describes the presence of SCC in situ. Histologically, these lesions exhibit full-thickness epidermal dysplasia without dermal invasion, hence their in situ denomination. It is estimated that approximately 3–5% of these lesions progress to invasive SCC. Bowen's disease more commonly affects older individuals and has a predilection for the lower limbs, face, and neck. It shares the same risk factors as AK, of which long-term sun exposure is also the most important. Clinically, Bowen's disease usually presents as a slowly enlarging, sharply defined erythematous plaque with a scaly or crusted surface. Treatment of Bowen's disease may include surgical excision, curettage, and surgery as well as nonsurgical, less invasive alternatives, such as cryotherapy, photodynamic therapy, topical imiquimod, 5-FU, and ablative laser.

9.9.6 Keratoacanthoma

Keratoacanthoma (KA) is a fast-growing atypical proliferation of differentiated squamous epithelia, which regresses spontaneously over the course of several weeks, usually leaving behind an atrophic scar. Clinically, KA appears as a dome-shaped, erythematous nodule with a crater-like central keratotic core, frequently seen on sun-exposed areas of elderly, fair-skinned people (▶ Fig. 9.12). KAs are usually 10–20 mm in size, although they can grow as big as 20 cm. Development of multiple KAs may

be seen in a number of conditions, such as individuals taking BRAF inhibitor. The main concern with KA is its borderline position between benignity and malignancy. An adequate biopsy specimen including the center (if not the whole) of the lesion and subcutaneous fat must be obtained to allow proper examination of both the cellular component and the lesion's full architecture. Conversely, inadequate samples may be mistakenly regarded as SCC. Although some controversy remains regarding the optimal management of KA, surgical excision is strongly recommended. Some destructive forms of craniofacial KAs exist and should be considered. Observation may be an alternative provided that clear signs of regression are already present. Otherwise, if a KA is left untreated, assuming that it will undergo spontaneous involution, two things may occur: malignant transformation (unlikely yet possible) or exaggerated growth (not possible to predict), which can potentially leave an unsightly scar after complete regression.

9.9.7 Marjolin's Ulcer

This disease involves the malignant degeneration of chronically inflamed, scarred, or traumatized skin. Although most commonly associated with burn scars, Marjolin's ulcer may arise from several other chronic wounds, such as pressure sores, venous stasis ulcers, hidradenitis suppurativa, vaccination scars, traumatic wounds, and others. Malignant transformation is usually in the form of SCC, though BCC and melanoma have been reported as well. Pathogenesis of Marjolin's ulcer is multifactorial and includes promotion of malignant degeneration by toxins released from damaged tissues; a greater susceptibility of injured skin to carcinogens; and lymphatic obstruction, which hampers adequate immune system vigilance and tumor suppression. According to time of onset since injury, Marjolin's ulcer is classified as acute (< 12 months), in which BCC is more commonly found, and chronic (> 12 months), where degeneration into SCC is more frequent. In either case, tumors developing from chronic wounds are usually aggressive, with higher rates of local recurrence and lymph metastases than primary cutaneous cancers. In this sense, malignant degeneration should be suspected in any long-standing wound not responding to proper care or that has undergone recent changes. For histological analysis, incisional biopsy of suspicious areas, including a segment of normal skin, is recommended. Finally, treatment usually involves wide local resection and graft or flap reconstruction.

9.9.8 Merkel's Cell Carcinoma

Merkel's cell carcinoma is a rare, highly aggressive cutaneous tumor with high recurrence rates and metastatic behavior. It is commonly seen in fair-skinned elderly patients (> 65 years) with a history of chronic sun exposure. Immunosuppression secondary to hematological malignancies, organ transplant, and HIV are major risk factors as well. Patients presenting with a diagnosis of Merkel's cell carcinoma should undergo a complete preoperative workup, including physical examination of the skin and lymph nodes and imaging to rule out regional and distant spread. Sentinel lymph node biopsy is also recommended for patients without palpable nodes. Treatment of Merkel's cell carcinoma is based on wide local excision, regional lymph node dissection (if palpable nodes or positive sentinel node), and adjuvant radiotherapy and chemotherapy in some cases. Prognosis is somewhat ominous, with a mortality rate higher than melanoma and an overall 5-year survival rate of 30–64%.

9.9.9 Dermatofibrosarcoma Protuberans

Dermatofibrosarcoma protuberans (DFSP) is a low-grade malignant sarcoma of fibroblast origin. Clinically, DFSP manifests as a slow-growing indurated plaque that can eventually transform into a firm, violaceous to red-brown, painless nodular plaque, most commonly on the trunk or upper limbs. Though the plaque usually appears de novo, DFSP may also develop over a preexisting scar or previously traumatized areas. Differential diagnosis includes keloid scars, large dermatofibromas, epidermal cysts, and morphea. DFSP invades local tissues through finger-like projections, which can lead to incomplete removal and subsequent recurrences. Although distant metastases are rare, the risk increases after several recurrences, a fact that underscores the importance of performing a complete primary excision. Lesions suspicious for DFSP should be biopsied (deep subcutaneous or incisional). If there is a diagnosis of DFSP, surgical excision with margin assessment (MMS or delayed MMS) prior to closure has shown remarkable oncologic clearance with very low rates of recurrence. If following surgical removal positive margins are still found, external radiotherapy is indicated. Finally, imatinib mesylate has been approved for recurrent and metastatic DFSP showing the t(17;22) translocation.

9.9.10 Leiomyoma and Leiomyosarcoma

Leiomyoma is an abnormal proliferation of smooth muscle clinically characterized by a firm, smooth-surfaced, skin-colored, or pinkish-brown, occasionally painful, intradermal nodule, 0.5–3 cm in diameter, appearing during adolescence or late adulthood. Multiple leiomyomas may be a manifestation of Reed's syndrome (multiple cutaneous and uterine leiomyomas associated with kidney cancer). Their malignant counterparts, leiomyosarcomas, are much less common but difficult to distinguish clinically. Growth, ulceration, an irregular shape, and the presence of pain are suggestive of malignancy, which should be ruled out with a biopsy. Treatment of leiomyosarcomas involves wide local excision or MMS.

9.9.11 Cutaneous Angiosarcoma

These are rare malignant, vascular tumors accounting for < 1% of all sarcomas. They show a special predilection for elderly males, appearing most commonly on the face and scalp or in areas of chronic lymphedema or previous radiotherapy. Stewart–Treves's syndrome describes the appearance of an angiosarcoma in long-standing chronic lymphedema secondary to any cause, including mastectomy and lymph node dissection, congenital causes, and others. Clinically, angiosarcoma presents as an enlarging bruise-like patch, a blue-violaceous nodule, or an unhealed ulceration. The mainstay of treatment is wide local excision followed by wide field radiotherapy.

9.10 Conclusions

The skin may be affected by a large number of lesions of benign, premalignant, and malignant nature. Although plastic surgeons should be familiar with the most common skin lesions, their knowledge should probably be focused on those needing surgical treatment, due to either their malignant potential or their size, because in many cases the excision of these lesions leaves behind a defect needing reconstruction with methods of varying complexity. BCC and SCC are the most common skin cancers, for which sun exposure is one of the most important risk factors. A number of other conditions predisposing to the development of these cancers have been described as well, with immunosuppressed patients being at particular risk. Even though prognosis is good in the vast majority of cases, some tumors or patients may exhibit certain factors of increased aggressiveness that require a more meticulous approach regarding preoperative assessment, margin of surgical excision, and postoperative follow-up. Optimization of outcomes of BCC/SCC treatment is based on a correct surgical excision and thorough histopathological analysis. Good and fluent communication between the ablative surgeon and pathologist is therefore of utmost importance to correctly identify any positive margins needing further excision. Finally, it is important to know the role that radiotherapy and other treatments, such as the hedgehog pathway inhibitor vismodegib, have in the overall management of BCC and SCC.

9.11 Key Points

- UV radiation constitutes the main risk factor for nonmelanoma skin cancer, especially in fair-skinned individuals. Although cumulative sun exposure causes most SCC, BCC is associated with a combination of cumulative and intense occasional exposure.
- Immunosuppressed patients are at particular risk of developing NMSC, with the incidence of SCC overcoming that of BCC.

- BCC and SCC are classified as low risk or high risk based on a number features inherent to the tumor itself and the patient, which ultimately determine treatment and prognosis. These should not be confused with risk factors associated with the development of skin cancer.
- The mainstay of treatment of BCC and SCC is surgical excision with margins. These will vary depending on the tumor's risk stratification (e.g., high risk or low risk).
- Nonsurgical modalities have a role in the treatment of superficial lesions; however, their rate of success is inferior compared with surgery.
- Recurrent tumors are more difficult to eradicate than primary ones and should ideally be treated with MMS or a modality that involves margin assessment prior to closure/reconstruction.
- Skin cancers in aesthetic areas should be treated with MMS to reduce morbidity while optimizing oncologic clearance.
- Postoperative follow-up should be tailored according to the nature of the tumor and its risk of recurrence (high risk vs. low risk). Immunosuppressed patients should be followed more closely due to their risk of developing more tumors and tumors of increased aggressiveness.

Recommended Readings

Alikhan A, Ibrahimi OA, Eisen DB. Congenital melanocytic nevi: where are we now? Part I. Clinical presentation, epidemiology, pathogenesis, histology, malignant transformation, and neurocutaneous melanosis. J Am Acad Dermatol. 2012; 67(4):495.e1–495.e17, quiz 512–514

Australian Cancer Network. Basal cell carcinoma, squamous cell carcinoma (and related lesions)—a guide to clinical management in Australia. Cancer Council Australia and Sydney; 2008. http://www.cancer.org.au/content/pdf/HealthProfessionals/ClinicalGuidelines/Basal_cell_carcinoma_Squamous_cell_carcinoma_Guide_Nov_2008-Final_with_Corrigendums.pdf

Axell T, Holmstrup P, Kramer IRH, et al. International seminar on oral leukoplakia and associated lesions to tobacco habits. Community Dent Oral Epidemiol. 1984;12:145–154

Baker SR, Swanson NA, Grekin RC. An interdisciplinary approach to the management of basal cell carcinoma of the head and neck. J Dermatol Surg Oncol. 1987; 13(10):1095–1106

Baxter JM, Patel AN, Varma S. Facial basal cell carcinoma. BMJ. 2012; 345:e5342

Bichakjian CK, Lowe L, Lao CD, et al. Merkel cell carcinoma: critical review with guidelines for multidisciplinary management. Cancer. 2007; 110(1):1–12

Bichakjian CK, Olencki T, Aasi SZ, et al. Basal Cell Skin Cancer, Version 1.2016, NCCN Clinical Practice Guidelines in Oncology. J Natl Compr Canc Netw. 2016; 14(5):574–597

Brodland DG, Zitelli JA. Surgical margins for excision of primary cutaneous squamous cell carcinoma. J Am Acad Dermatol. 1992; 27(2 Pt 1):241–248

Chen AC, Martin AJ, Choy B, et al. A phase 3 randomized trial of nicotinamide for skin-cancer chemoprevention. N Engl J Med. 2015; 373(17):1618–1626

Christenson LJ, Borrowman TA, Vachon CM, et al. Incidence of basal cell and squamous cell carcinomas in a population younger than 40 years. JAMA. 2005; 294(6):681–690

Chu MB, Slutsky JB, Dhandha MM, et al. Evaluation of the definitions of "high-risk" cutaneous squamous cell carcinoma using the American Joint Committee on Cancer staging criteria and National Comprehensive Cancer Network guidelines. J Skin Cancer. 2014; 2014:154340

Connolly SM, Baker DR, Coldiron BM, et al; Ad Hoc Task Force. Ratings Panel. AAD/ACMS/ASDSA/ASMS 2012 appropriate use criteria for Mohs micrographic surgery: a report of the American Academy of Dermatology, American College of Mohs Surgery, American Society for Dermatologic Surgery Association, and the American Society for Mohs Surgery. J Am Acad Dermatol. 2012; 67(4):531–550

Copcu E. Marjolin's ulcer: a preventable complication of burns? Plast Reconstr Surg. 2009; 124(1):156e–164e

Duffy K, Grossman D. The dysplastic nevus: from historical perspective to management in the modern era: part I. Historical, histologic, and clinical aspects. J Am Acad Dermatol. 2012; 67(1):1.e1–1.e16, quiz 17–18

Duffy K, Grossman D. The dysplastic nevus: from historical perspective to management in the modern era: part II. Molecular aspects and clinical management. J Am Acad Dermatol. 2012; 67(1):19.e1–19.e12, quiz 31–32

Dunn M, Morgan MB, Beer TW. Perineural invasion: identification, significance, and a standardized definition. Dermatol Surg. 2009; 35(2):214–221

Farhi D, Dupin N, Palangié A, Carlotti A, Avril MF. Incomplete excision of basal cell carcinoma: rate and associated factors among 362 consecutive cases. Dermatol Surg. 2007; 33(10):1207–1214

Ferrara G, Gianotti R, Cavicchini S, Salviato T, Zalaudek I, Argenziano G. Spitz nevus, Spitz tumor, and spitzoid melanoma: a comprehensive clinicopathologic overview. Dermatol Clin. 2013; 31(4):589–598, viii

Griffiths RW. Keratoacanthoma observed. Br J Plast Surg. 2004; 57(6):485–501

Gualdi G, Monari P, Apalla Z, Lallas A. Surgical treatment of basal cell carcinoma and squamous cell carcinoma. G Ital Dermatol Venereol. 2015; 150(4):435–447

Gurudutt VV, Genden EM. Cutaneous squamous cell carcinoma of the head and neck. J Skin Cancer. 2011; 2011(2011):502723

Herrero JI, España A, Quiroga J, et al. Nonmelanoma skin cancer after liver transplantation. Study of risk factors. Liver Transpl. 2005; 11(9):1100–1106

Hsu MC, Liau JY, Hong JL, et al. Secondary neoplasms arising from nevus sebaceus: A retrospective study of 450 cases in Taiwan. J Dermatol. 2016; 43(2):175–180

Ibrahimi OA, Alikhan A, Eisen DB. Congenital melanocytic nevi: where are we now? Part II. Treatment options and approach to treatment. J Am Acad Dermatol. 2012; 67(4):515.e1–515.e13, quiz 528–530

Idriss MH, Elston DM. Secondary neoplasms associated with nevus sebaceus of Jadassohn: a study of 707 cases. J Am Acad Dermatol. 2014; 70(2):332–337

Irarrazaval I, Redondo P. Three-dimensional histology for dermatofibrosarcoma protuberans: case series and surgical technique. J Am Acad Dermatol. 2012; 67(5):991–996

Jensen P, Hansen S, Møller B, et al. Skin cancer in kidney and heart transplant recipients and different long-term immunosuppressive therapy regimens. J Am Acad Dermatol. 1999; 40(2 Pt 1):177–186

Karia PS, Jambusaria-Pahlajani A, Harrington DP, Murphy GF, Qureshi AA, Schmults CD. Evaluation of American Joint Committee on Cancer, International Union Against Cancer, and Brigham and Women's Hospital tumor staging for cutaneous squamous cell carcinoma. J Clin Oncol. 2014; 32(4):327–334

Krengel S, Scope A, Dusza SW, Vonthein R, Marghoob AA. New recommendations for the categorization of cutaneous features of congenital melanocytic nevi. J Am Acad Dermatol. 2013; 68(3):441–451

Kricker A, Armstrong BK, English DR, Heenan PJ. Does intermittent sun exposure cause basal cell carcinoma? a case-control study in Western Australia. Int J Cancer. 1995; 60(4):489–494

Kwiek B, Schwartz RA. Keratoacanthoma (KA): An update and review. J Am Acad Dermatol. 2016; 74(6):1220–1233

LeBlanc DM, Ramanadham SR, Wells DD. Basal cell carcinoma, squamous cell carcinoma and melanoma. In: Janis JE, ed. Essentials of Plastic Surgery. Boca Raton, FL: CRC Press; 2014:176–194

LeBoeuf NR, Schmults CD. Update on the management of high-risk squamous cell carcinoma. Semin Cutan Med Surg. 2011; 30(1):26–34

Lewin JM, Carucci JA. Advances in the management of basal cell carcinoma. F1000Prime Rep. 2015; 7:53

Lindelöf B, Sigurgeirsson B, Gäbel H, Stern RS. Incidence of skin cancer in 5356 patients following organ transplantation. Br J Dermatol. 2000; 143(3):513–519

Madan V, Lear JT, Szeimies RM. Non-melanoma skin cancer. Lancet. 2010; 375(9715):673–685

Mehrany K, Weenig RH, Lee KK, Pittelkow MR, Otley CC. Increased metastasis and mortality from cutaneous squamous cell carcinoma in patients with chronic lymphocytic leukemia. J Am Acad Dermatol. 2005; 53(6):1067–1071

Mohan SV, Chang ALS. Advanced Basal Cell Carcinoma: Epidemiology and Therapeutic Innovations. Curr Dermatol Rep. 2014; 3:40–45

Moloney FJ, Comber H, Conlon PJ, Murphy GM. The role of immunosuppression in the pathogenesis of basal cell carcinoma. Br J Dermatol. 2006; 154(4):790–791

Muranushi C, Olsen CM, Green AC, Pandeya N. Can oral nonsteroidal antiinflammatory drugs play a role in the prevention of basal cell carcinoma? A systematic review and meta-analysis. J Am Acad Dermatol. 2016; 74(1):108–119.e1

Narayan D. Benign and malignant tumors of the skin. In: Guyuron B, Eriksson E, Persing JA, eds. Plastic Surgery Indications and Practice. Philadelphia, PA: Saunders; 2009; 119–146

NCCN Guidelines version 01.2016 Basal and Squamous Cell Skin Cancers. National Comprehensive Cancer Network, 2016.

Ong CS, Keogh AM, Kossard S, Macdonald PS, Spratt PM. Skin cancer in Australian heart transplant recipients. J Am Acad Dermatol. 1999; 40(1):27–34

Ross AS, Schmults CD. Sentinel lymph node biopsy in cutaneous squamous cell carcinoma: a systematic review of the English literature. Dermatol Surg. 2006; 32(11):1309–1321

Rosso S, Zanetti R, Martinez C, et al. The multicentre south European study 'Helios'. II: Different sun exposure patterns in the aetiology of basal cell and squamous cell carcinomas of the skin. Br J Cancer. 1996; 73(11):1447–1454

Rowe DE, Carroll RJ, Day CL Jr. Prognostic factors for local recurrence, metastasis, and survival rates in squamous cell carcinoma of the skin, ear, and lip. Implications for treatment modality selection. J Am Acad Dermatol. 1992; 26(6):976–990

Rünger TM. How different wavelengths of the ultraviolet spectrum contribute to skin carcinogenesis: the role of cellular damage responses. J Invest Dermatol. 2007; 127(9):2103–2105

Schöllkopf C, Rosendahl D, Rostgaard K, Pipper C, Hjalgrim H. Risk of second cancer after chronic lymphocytic leukemia. Int J Cancer. 2007; 121(1):151–156

Thompson AK, Kelley BF, Prokop LJ, Murad MH, Baum CL. Risk factors for cutaneous squamous cell carcinoma recurrence, metastasis, and disease-specific death: A systematic review and meta-analysis. JAMA Dermatol. 2016; 152(4):419–428

Wade TR, Ackerman AB. The many faces of basal-cell carcinoma. J Dermatol Surg Oncol. 1978; 4(1):23–28

Wolf DJ, Zitelli JA. Surgical margins for basal cell carcinoma. Arch Dermatol .1987; 123(3):340–344

10 Laser Therapy: Principles and Applications in Skin Diseases

Maider Pretel, Ester Moreno-Artero

Abstract

The term *laser* is an acronym for *light amplification by stimulated emission of radiation*. Lasers deliver monochromatic, coherent, collimated, and high-intensity beams of light. In contrast, intense pulsed light devices are filtered flashlamps that emit polychromatic, noncoherent light in a broad range of wavelengths, being less powerful than lasers. The theory of selective photothermolysis, which states that the laser energy can be absorbed by a defined target chromophore, leading to its controlled destruction without significant damage to the surrounding tissue, is one of the most important concepts to understand why laser light can be used for targeted therapeutic purposes. Wavelength, pulse duration, energy density, chromophores of the skin (oxyhemoglobin, melanin, and water), fluence, irradiance, and spot size are laser parameters that influence clinical outcomes in the use of lasers for the treatment of different skin diseases, including vascular lesions, pigmentation disorders, melanocytic lesions, and skin resurfacing. These parameters have to be accurately taken into account for preventing undesirable effects, such as scarring, hypo-/hyperpigmentation, or alopecia. There are different modes of how laser light can be delivered: in a continuous wave (CW), such as the CW CO_2 and older argon technology; quasi-CW, including the potassium-titanyl-phosphate, copper vapor, copper bromide, krypton, and argon-pumped tunable dye lasers; or a pulsed wave mode, such as long pulse-duration pulsed-dye laser and Q-switched ruby, alexandrite, or neodymium:yttrium-aluminum-garnet lasers (nanosecond pulse durations). The choice of laser should be made on the basis of the individual absorption characteristics of the target chromophore.

Keywords: laser, selective photothermolysis, skin disorders, vascular, pigment, hair, resurfacing

10.1 Introduction

The term *laser* is an acronym for *light amplification by stimulated emission of radiation*. Laser light represents a part of the electromagnetic spectrum of energy and has several properties that are different from other light sources. Lasers deliver monochromatic, coherent, collimated, and high-intensity beams of light. In contrast to sunlight, which encompasses a wide spectrum of wavelengths, laser light is monochromatic, which means that it emits light of only one clearly defined single wavelength of a very narrow band of wavelengths. Laser light waves are in phase with respect to space and time (coherence). A laser beam has a defined narrow beam diameter with no divergence, which virtually does not increase even with increasing distance (collimation). Finally, these light sources can emit light with very high intensity.

In contrast, intense pulsed light (IPL) devices are filtered flashlamps that emit polychromatic, noncoherent light in a broad range of wavelengths. Thus IPL devices are dimmer and less powerful than lasers.

Most lasers used in dermatology generate light within the visible (400–760 nm), near-infrared (760–1400 nm), mid-infrared (1,400–3,000 nm), and infrared (> 3000 nm) range but rarely in the ultraviolet range (200–400 nm) of the electromagnetic spectrum.

All laser systems are composed of the laser medium, the optical cavity, and a power source. The laser medium, which can be a solid (e.g., ruby, neodymium:yttrium-aluminum-garnet [Nd:YAG], or alexandrite), a liquid (e.g., dye), or a gas (e.g., argon, krypton, or carbon dioxide), determines the wavelength of the emitted light. The optical cavity, which contains the laser medium, serves as a resonator in which the laser process occurs.

10.2 Basic Science

10.2.1 Laser–skin Interactions

When laser light reaches the skin, it may interact with the tissue in four different ways: it can be absorbed, reflected, scattered, or transmitted. Only light that is absorbed will exert a detectable clinical effect. The amount of light that penetrates deeply into the skin is dependent upon light scattering and absorption by chromophores, which are the specific light-absorbing targets. The three main chromophores in the skin are melanin, (oxy)hemoglobin, and water. Tattoo ink is the main external chromophore of importance in laser dermatology.

The amount of light that is absorbed by the specific chromophore depends on the wavelength used and whether it corresponds to the specific absorption spectrum of the respective chromophore. When choosing a laser for a certain indication, not only the absorption maximum of the target chromophore needs to be taken into account, but also the depth of penetration of the chosen laser wavelength in order to actually be able to reach the target within the tissue.

10.2.2 Selective Photothermolysis

The theory of selective photothermolysis, proposed by Anderson and Parrish in 1983, is one of the most important concepts to explain laser–tissue interactions and why laser light can be used for targeted therapeutic purposes. It states that the laser energy can be absorbed by a defined target chromophore, leading to its controlled destruction without significant damage to the surrounding tissue. To achieve this, a number of principles concerning wavelength, pulse duration, energy density, and chromophores of the skin need to be applied.

Wavelength

The wavelength of the laser light needs to correspond to the absorption maximum or lie within the absorption spectrum of the respective target chromophore. Moreover, it should be of sufficient length to penetrate to the depth of the target.

Pulse Duration

The pulse duration (PD) of the laser heavily affects the likelihood of achieving the desired clinical effect. The PD of the laser beam must be equal to or shorter than the thermal relaxation time (TRT) of the target chromophore. TRT is defined as the time required for 90% of an object to cool to 50% of the temperature achieved immediately after the laser exposure without conducting heat to the surrounding tissue. The TRT is heavily influenced by the size of the target. Large objects lose heat much more slowly than small objects. Different blood vessels have different TRTs: capillaries have a TRT

Table 10.1 Thermal relaxation times of important laser targets

Structure	Size (μm)	TRT (approx.)
Tattoo ink particle	0.5–4	10 ns
Melanosome	0.5–1	250 ns
Blood vessels	50	1 ms
	100	5 ms
	200	20 ms
Hair follicle	200	10–100 ms

of tens of microseconds, port-wine stain (PWS) venules have a TRT of tens of milliseconds, and leg veins of hundreds of milliseconds (▶Table 10.1). Small pigmented targets (e.g., melanosomes within pigmented melanocytes in a nevus of Ota) are best treated with short (submicrosecond) pulses, whereas larger pigmented targets (e.g., hair follicles) have longer TRTs and are best treated with longer (millisecond) pulses.

If a structure is heated for a period equal to or shorter than its relaxation time, the resultant damage is confined to the target object alone, reducing the risk of scarring. Conversely, if an object is heated for longer than its thermal relaxation time, thermal diffusion leads to heating of surrounding structures.

Note

If a structure is heated for a period equal to or shorter than its relaxation time, the resultant damage is confined to the target object alone, reducing the risk of scarring.

Energy Density

The energy density delivered by the laser beam, also referred to as fluence, must be high enough to actually destroy the target chromophore within the defined pulse duration but should also be at a level that minimizes collateral tissue damage. Energy density is measured in joules per centimeter squared (J/cm^2).

Chromophores of the Skin

The three main endogenous chromophores in the skin are melanin, hemoglobin, and water. Each of these chromophores has its own absorption spectrum and absorption peak.

Melanin has a wide spectrum of absorption, which slowly decreases from the ultraviolet to the near infrared range (300–1,000 nm). The absorption spectrum of hemoglobin ranges from 400 to 600 nm, whereas oxyhemoglobin shows its maximum absorption peak at 418 nm, followed by smaller peaks at 548 and 577 nm. These absorption peaks can be targeted specifically, in order to minimize absorption by competing chromophores.

Water shows increasing absorption, starting at mid-infrared and increasing toward the infrared portion of the electromagnetic spectrum.

10.3 Therapeutic Parameters

Wavelength and pulse duration are the most important laser settings that govern the effects of laser light on skin. Fluence, irradiance, and spot size are additional laser parameters that influence clinical outcomes.

10.3.1 Fluence

Fluence is a measurement of the amount of light energy delivered per unit area. For most pulsed lasers used to treat vascular lesions, the fluences range from 3 to 15 J/cm². For IPL in vascular lesions, higher fluences are required, ranging from 15 to 30 J/cm². The destruction of very large structures, such as hair follicles, requires high fluences (20–50 J/cm²) due to the amount of tissue that has to be heated. The 1,064 nm Nd:YAG laser in vascular lesions also requires the use of high fluences (> 100 J/cm²). The target chromophore in telangiectasias (oxyhemoglobin) has low affinity for this wavelength, and delivery of high amounts of energy is necessary to heat the target tissue.

10.3.2 Spot Size

Spot size is the diameter of the beam of light emitted from the laser that hits the skin. In general, the depth of penetration of laser energy increases with wavelength until the mid-infrared region of the electromagnetic spectrum. Scattering of light occurs to a greater degree with small spot sizes. Thus the energy that enters the target tissue is attenuated far more rapidly with the use of small spot sizes than with the use of large spot sizes. Spot size is most important when targeting structures in the mid to deep dermis with long pulsed lasers. For targets in the epidermis or upper dermis, spot size is less important.

10.3.3 Other Considerations

Skin Cooling

Epidermal melanin is an undesired chromophore when treating dermal targets. Excessive heating of the epidermis can lead to epidermal damage, resulting in hypopigmentation or hyperpigmentation. Epidermal damage can be minimized through the use of skin cooling, and this is especially important with darkly pigmented skin. There are three basic types of skin cooling: precooling, parallel cooling, and postcooling, which correspond to extracting heat from the skin before, during, and after the laser exposure, respectively.

All cooling methods extract heat at the skin surface via a cooling agent (gas, liquid, or solid). For spray cooling, a cold liquid is used (e.g., liquid fluorocarbon is sprayed on the skin). Solid contact cooling often consists of a cold sapphire window held against the skin, through which laser or IPL energy is delivered.

Safety

Laser safety is a significant concern for the patient, physician, and clinical staff. Eye injuries and blindness may occur rapidly and painlessly. Blindness can occur even if only 1% of the beam is reflected into the eye from shiny metal, glass, or plastic surfaces. The highest risk occurs with near-infrared Q-switched lasers. Lasers and IPL sources used for hair removal can target the retina and uveal tract. Anterior eye injury from lasers or IPL sources usually occurs with treatment of the lower eyebrow or vascular lesions near the eye (without an eye shield properly in place). An opaque laser eye shield covering the patient's cornea will not prevent damage if the laser or IPL directly impacts exposed sclera. Long-pulse, near-infrared laser light can penetrate through the eyelid and damage the eye. Proper use of laser-protective eyewear (including eye shields) is mandatory in laser surgery. Wraparound glasses and goggles are rated by optical density (OD) at specific wavelengths. For dermatological lasers, proper protection is an OD ≥ 4 at the wavelength of the laser being used. Color of the goggles is not an indicator of level of protection.

Fire and explosions may occur when lasers are in use. Drapes, clothing, dry hair, and plastic materials, including endotracheal tubes, can be ignited, especially when oxygen is in use. The greatest risk is with the CO_2 and erbium:YAG lasers used for skin resurfacing and ablative fractional treatments. To prevent fire, it is highly recommended that any hair near the treatment field be moistened and makeup removed when one is working around eyelids. Alcohol, acetone, or other flammable skin-cleaning solutions must be allowed to completely dry before laser use. Intraoperative oxygen concentration should be reduced to < 40%. A fire extinguisher and water should be readily available.

Laser-generated "plume materials" may be inhaled, particularly with resurfacing or vaporization of hair during its removal. To avoid laser plume biohazards smoke evacuators and good ventilation are the most effective measures. Submicrometer surgical filter masks provide some protection when worn properly.

10.4 Types of Laser

Laser light can be delivered by either a continuous wave or a pulsed wave. The continuous-wave (CW) light is emitted over an uninterrupted period of time with a constant beam of light. CW lasers, such as the CW CO_2 and older argon technology, emit a constant beam of light with long exposure durations that can result in nonselective tissue injury.

Quasi-CW mode lasers, including the potassium-titanyl-phosphate (KTP), copper vapor, copper bromide, krypton, and argon-pumped tunable dye lasers, shutter the CW beam into short segments, producing interrupted emissions of constant laser energy. These lasers may be associated with higher incidences of hypertrophic scarring and textural changes.

Truly pulsed lasers can be either very short pulsed, with nanosecond pulse durations (as in Q-switched ruby, alexandrite, or Nd:YAG lasers), or long pulsed, with pulse durations within the millisecond range (e.g., the pulsed-dye laser [PDL]). The short pulse durations limit the thermal spread of the heat and therefore decrease the likelihood of scarring.

Because cutaneous lasers have different clinical applications related to their specific wavelengths and pulse durations, the choice of laser should be made on the basis of the individual absorption characteristics of the target chromophore (▶ Table 10.2).

10.5 Clinical Applications

The following section describes the use of lasers for the treatment of different skin diseases, including vascular lesions, pigmentation disorders, melanocytic lesions, and skin resurfacing.

10.5.1 Vascular Lesions

Oxyhemoglobin is the target chromophore in vascular lesions, and its absorption peaks are found at wavelengths 418, 512, and 577 nm, which corresponds to the yellow area of the electromagnetic spectrum. For this reason the lasers most frequently used in the treatment of vascular lesions, although not the only ones, are the KTP (532 nm), the PDL (577–600 nm), and the Nd:YAG (1,064 nm) lasers. Other lasers that can be used include the argon-pumped tunable dye laser (577, 585 nm), the copper bromide vapor laser (578 nm), and the krypton laser (568 nm). When one is treating vascular lesions, consideration should be given to the fact that, because melanin has a wider absorption spectrum that includes visible and infrared light, at these wavelengths absorption also occurs by epidermal melanocytes and, in general, by the whole epidermis, with the subsequent risk of hypopigmentation and scarring. The depth and thickness of the type of blood vessel targeted, as well as the patient's skin phototype, are therefore important factors to take into account in the treatment of vascular lesions.

Port-Wine Stains

PWSs are a type of vascular malformation affecting 3 of every 100 newborns and are present at birth. Normally they present as pale pink macules or spots, which may occur singly or multiply at any anatomical site, although they are more common on the head and neck. They may have psychological and social consequences, which in some cases makes early treatment in childhood advisable. Depending on their location they may be associated with certain syndromes with systemic involvement (e.g., Sturge–Weber's syndrome when their distribution follows the ophthalmic division of the trigeminal nerve or Klippel–Trénaunay–Weber's syndrome when they are located in the extremities and accompanied by soft tissue hypertrophy and venous malformations).

It is essential to differentiate PWSs from nevus simplex or salmon patches, also known as flammeus neonatorum, angel's kisses, or stork bites, which are pink macules or spots that characteristically fade during the first year of life in 50% of patients.

The size and location of the lesion determine the response to the laser treatment. Thus lesions located

Table 10.2 Lasers commonly used in dermatology

Laser	Wavelength (nm)	Mode	Pulse duration(s)	Target chromophore	Indications
Pulsed dye	585–600	Pulsed	$(0.45–40) \times 10^{-3}$	Hemoglobin	Telangiectasias, port-wine stains, scars, verrucae, pyogenic granuloma
Potassium-titanyl-phosphate (KTP)	532	Quasi-continuous wave	10^{-3}	Hemoglobin	Facial telangiectasias
Long-pulsed neodymium:yttrium-aluminum-garnet (Nd:YAG)	1,064	Pulsed	$(1–200) \times 10^{-3}$	Hemoglobin	Leg and facial telangiectasias and venulectasias, blue reticular veins, venous lakes, venous malformations
Q-switched alexandrite	755	Pulsed (ns)	10^{-7}	Melanin Black and green tattoos	Lentigines Black and green tattoos
Q-switched Nd:YAG	1,064	Pulsed (ns)	10^{-8}	Black tattoos	Nevi of Ota Black tattoos
Q-switched frequency-doubled Nd:YAG	532	Pulsed (ns)	10^{-8}	Melanin Red tattoos	Lentigines Red tattoos
Q-switched ruby	694	Pulsed (ns)	3×10^{-8}	Melanin Black and green tattoos	Lentigines Black and green tattoos
Diode	800	Pulsed	10^{-3}	Melanin	Hair removal
Alexandrite	755	Pulsed	10^{-3}	Melanin	Hair removal Pulsed-dye laser–resistant vascular lesions
Carbon dioxide	10,600	Continuous wave/pulsed	$10^{-5}–10^{-3}$	Water	Resurfacing, scars, ablation of epidermal lesions
Erbium:YAG	2,940	Pulsed	$(3–100) \times 10^{-4}$	Water	Resurfacing, scars, ablation of epidermal lesions

on the distal part of extremities and the centrofacial region (the area innervated by the second branch of the trigeminal nerve: the medial area of the cheeks, the lower eyelid, nose, and upper lip) usually respond worse to treatment than those located on the periphery of the face (in descending order: forehead, upper eyelid, lateral malar region, or jaw) and the neck. In addition, the earlier the treatment is performed, the better the response, even at ages of less than 6 months. As for the characteristics of the vessels, lesions with deep vessels with thicker walls show a poorer response to treatment. In contrast, the greater the extent of the lesion, the better the response to the laser will be. In any case, treatment of PWSs requires multiple sessions (after 8–10 sessions a lightening of 80% or more is achieved).

Most PWSs are superficial, with the vessels located at a mean depth of 0.46 mm. Two patterns of PWS located on the extremities can be defined: the better-defined geographic pattern (▶ Fig. 10.1) and the blotchy pattern with less well defined edges. The former are at greater risk of becoming hypertrophic, thick, darker, and deeper and are sometimes associated with soft tissue hypertrophy and lymphatic malformations. In such cases, in order to increase laser penetration, larger spot sizes should be used together with greater fluences and wavelengths. The PDL was created specifically for this disorder and initially emitted light at a wavelength of 577 nm. Currently, the pulsed-color laser, which uses the liquid medium rhodamine, emits short pulses of light flashes with a wavelength between 585 and 595 nm. Although this reduces absorption by the chromophore, penetrance is greater, which in turn makes it more effective in the treatment of PWSs. Many authors recommend using fluences of between 4 and 15 J/cm², with spot sizes of

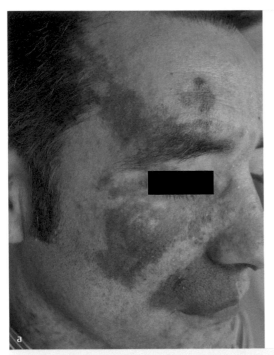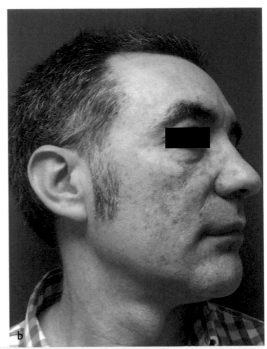

Fig. 10.1 **(a)** A 39-year-old man with a port-wine stain on the right hemiface. **(b)** Result after 12 sessions with a pulsed-dye laser.

between 7 and 12 mm. The ideal situation would be to begin with fluences of 5 or 5.5 J/cm² and a spot size of 7 mm and to gradually increase these by 0.5 J/cm² at each subsequent treatment session at intervals of 3 or 4 months.

The fact that the pulses of light are of short duration, between 1.5 and 10 ms, increases the selectivity of the laser as it acts only on the vessel and not on the surrounding tissue. This limits thermal damage as the time of thermal relaxation of the vessels ranges from 1 to 10 ms. The deeper the capillaries are and the thicker their wall, the longer the pulses will need to be (a maximum of 3 ms, except for bluish or purple nodular lesions, in which case pulses of up to 10 ms should be used). Thus, in large-caliber vessels short pulses are needed to apply a large amount of heat in a short space of time, which increases the risk of purpura.

Some studies have demonstrated IPL to be more effective in the lightening of these types of lesions. Other lasers used include the CO_2, the KTP 532 nm, and the long-pulsed Nd:YAG 1,064 nm laser.

The short-term complications arising from treatment with PDL, IPL, or any other type of vascular laser are normally limited to purpura (▶ Fig. 10.2) and hemorrhagic crusting lesions, with IPL showing lower incidence of purpura. In the long term, abnormalities in pigmentation are the most frequent adverse effect. Because the absorption spectrum of melanin includes visible and infrared light, at the wavelengths used by vascular lasers absorption also occurs by melanocytes in the epidermis and in general by the whole epidermis, with the subsequent risk of hypopigmentation and development of scarring. Furthermore, although permanent hyperpigmentation has not been reported, postinflammatory hyperpigmentation is not infrequent, especially in patients with a dark phototype (phototype III or higher). The use of hydroquinone, alpha-hydroxy acids, azelaic acid, and/or kojic acid is usually necessary in the treatment of hyperpigmentation following inflammation.

The development of hypertrophic and keloid scars is less frequent but may be favored by the concomitant or recent use of oral retinoids, and therefore it is advisable to delay laser treatment 1 or 2 years after treatment with oral isotretinoin has been completed.

Finally, in order to avoid the classic "chessboard" pattern resulting from alternating areas of treated

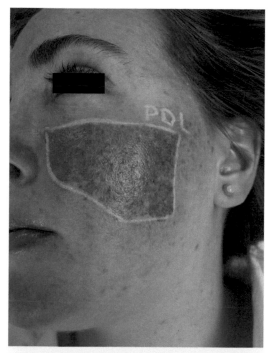

Fig. 10.2 Purpura immediately after treatment of a couperosis with a pulsed-dye laser with a fluence of 8.5 J/cm² and a pulse duration of 2 ms with a spot size of 7 mm.

and untreated skin, we recommend making several passes with the laser and in different directions, with 15% overlapping pulses.

Infantile Hemangiomas

Hemangiomas are the most frequent tumors in childhood, affect girls more frequently, usually appear shortly after birth, and grow rapidly in the first years of life, with full and subsequent spontaneous regression in most cases. Anetodermas, together with the formation of fibrous fatty tissue and telangiectasias, are often residual lesions. Hemangiomas may be superficial and bright red in color or deep and bluish or mixed in color. They can be segmental or focal, and their progression includes a proliferative phase, a static phase, and a final involutional phase.

A general consensus exists on the indication to treat those hemangiomas that may be life threatening or cause recurrent ulceration, bleeding, or infection and those that grow quickly or distort vision, airway, anatomy, or physiological functions. In addition, treatment is indicated for lesions that will likely resolve only partially, those with sequelae, or those associated with congestive heart failure. Currently, and although in most cases observation and watchful waiting are sufficient, because of the difficulty of predicting the degree of and time to involution in individual cases, it would seem reasonable to use propranolol at early ages for those hemangiomas that are large or are accompanied by functional abnormalities.

Treatment of hemangiomas with PDL remains controversial as does its efficacy in reducing the proliferative phase; however, it appears that for ulcerated hemangiomas PDL could reduce pain and favor healing—key factors to bear in mind given that 5% and 11% of hemangiomas become ulcerated during the proliferative phase. Nevertheless, it should be noted that laser treatment can potentially induce ulceration in hemangiomas.

PDL lasers have been shown to be effective in the treatment of superficial hemangiomas in the proliferative and involutional phases. The penetration limit of this laser (1.2 mm) does not render it very useful in the treatment of deep lesions. In such cases, useful options would be IPL and, in deep lesions, the Nd:YAG 1,064 nm laser. However, the latter leads to damage of the surrounding tissue and favors the formations of scars due to its lack of specific absorption by the oxyhemoglobin. Argon lasers are of limited use given their low penetrance (< 1 mm) and the high risk of hypertrophic scarring that accompanies their uses. The KTP 532 nm laser may be used in superficial hemangiomas. CO_2 lasers are used, particularly in the treatment of hemangiomas located in high-risk areas in which the aim is to avoid substantial bleeding, such as laryngeal or oral lesions. Finally, IPL (550, 570, or 590 nm wavelengths) can be used effectively in the treatment of hemangiomas with satisfactory results.

Telangiectasias

Telangiectasias are dilated capillaries, arterioles, or venules. Clinically, they are classified into simple or linear, arboriform, vascular, or papular spider veins.

Linear or arboriform facial telangiectasias are frequently found on the cheeks and dorsum of the nose. They vary in size between 0.1 and 1 mm in diameter and are common in healthy individuals as well as in association with skin disease, such as couperosis, chronic sun damage, connective tissue disorders, surgical scars, prolonged application of topical corticosteroids, and liver disease, among others. Linear facial telangiectasias respond favorably to PDL treatment, which is the treatment of choice.

According to the thickness of the vessel wall, telangiectasias can be classified into narrow caliber (0.1–0.4 mm) and large caliber (> 0.4 mm). Clinically, narrow-caliber lesions are usually reddish in color, whereas large-caliber lesions show a bluish coloration. This is an important issue because when the diameter of the vessel wall is greater than 0.4 mm, longer pulses of between 20 and 40 ms are required. Furthermore, vessels larger than 0.2 mm in diameter usually require multiple treatment sessions.

In general, 3 to 10 mm spot sizes can be used. When working with purpuric doses, fluences ranging from 5 to 8.5 J/cm^2 should be used, with multiple short pulses of 0.45 ms. Two strategies to avoid purpura secondary to treatment include using a single longer pulse (10 ms) with a fluency greater than those used with purpuric doses (9 J/cm^2), or using two or three short pulses, even of 0.45 ms with a lower fluency (4–5 J/cm^2).

KTP 532 nm lasers are an effective alternative to PDLs, resulting in fewer side effects, with less edema, erythema, and pain. IPL with a cutoff filter of 550 to 560 nm is also a valid option for facial telangiectasias. Nonpurpuric long-pulsed PDL has been proved to be more effective than treatment with microsecond 1,064-nm Nd:YAG laser. Argon lasers are an effective treatment for this type of lesions; however, they result in the development of depressed scars, hypopigmentation, hyperpigmentation, and recurrence, and hence their use has become obsolete. Similarly, CO_2 lasers are not used due to the resulting damage in the dermis. This type of laser is not selective, and surrounding tissue is also destroyed.

For vessels that are larger in caliber, deeper or bluish in color, an Nd:YAG 1,064 nm can be used. This wavelength has a low absorption by hemoglobin, which must be corrected with high fluences (70–100 J/cm^2), pulse durations of between 20 and 30 ms, and a beam diameter of between 3 and 5 mm. Among the side effects associated with the treatment with Nd:YAG 1,064 nm lasers, the formation of blisters and atrophic scars or hypopigmentation is not uncommon.

Nevus Aracneus

Nevus aracneus is a subtype characterized by the presence of dilated capillaries around a central arteriole. It is more frequent between the ages of 7 and 10 years. Between 50 and 75% of the childhood lesions undergo spontaneous regression. However, the incidence among adults is 15%. It responds to treatment with PDL (two or three short pulses with fluences ranging from 6.5 to 7.5 J/cm^2), and adverse effects are rare.

Telangiectasias and Venulectasias

Telangiectasias and venulectasias of the lower extremities are dilated capillaries and venules that affect a significant part of the general population. They are usually fine reddish or bluish vessels with a diameter of between 0.2 and 2 mm and result from the inadequate venous drainage of the lower limbs, caused by poor communication between the deep and superficial venous systems due to hormonal, genetic, trauma-related, or age-related factors. The treatment of choice is currently sclerotherapy. However, the difficulty involved in cannulating the narrowest vessels makes them a target for PDLs (with fluences between 6 and 7.5 J/cm^2) or KTP. Laser treatment would also be indicated in patients with a history of adverse reactions to sclerosing substances, lack of response to sclerotherapy, needle phobias, ankle veins, or telangiectatic matting. The main limitations in the use of these lasers are postinflammatory hyperpigmentation (occurring in 20–40% of cases with PDLs) and the impossibility of treating vessels of more than 1 mm in thickness located at a depth of more than 1 mm, due to the lower penetrance of the wavelengths used by such lasers. Some authors have suggested, as an alternative in these cases, the use of Nd:YAG lasers, although we believe that the pain and the greater risk of hypopigmentation and scar formation render its use less advisable.

Perhaps the best therapeutic option with the best results is the combination of laser treatment, sclerotherapy, and, when necessary, phlebectomy.

Venous Malformations of the Head and Neck

Venous malformations are congenital low-flow vascular lesions. They may be hereditary, although they are most often spontaneous. On the head and neck they are violet-blue, soft, compressible, non-pulsatile masses that usually expand when venous return is blocked. This type of vascular malformation never involutes. On the contrary, they grow larger throughout life, not due to vascular proliferation but in relation to increases in venous pressure. Depending on their location and size they may cause both aesthetic and/or functional problems, such as dysphagia, dysphonia, peripheral facial paralysis, and blindness. In these cases, surgery is usually limited due to the risk of impairing or worsening the function of the anatomical structures affected by the venous malformation or of causing facial disfiguration or important cosmetic defects. Sclerotherapy followed or not by surgery is a useful therapeutic option although it may cause side effects, such as dysphagia, dysphonia, facial paralysis, hemorrhage, ulceration (especially in deep malformations), scarring, blistering, infection, unilateral blindness, hemoglobulinuria, deep vein thrombosis, and, rarely, pulmonary thromboembolism.

For superficial venous malformations located on the skin or mucosae, treatment with Nd:YAG 1,064 nm laser may be sufficient (▶ Fig. 10.3). In case of recurrence, laser treatment or either surgery or sclerotherapy or both could be repeated.

In deeper venous malformations, however, laser treatment could have a role as a neoadjuvant treatment in combination with surgery and/or sclerotherapy. This is because the Nd:YAG laser acts not only on the vascular endothelium but also on the collagen of the dermis, thus generating an increase in fibrous tissue and, as a result, notably reducing the risk of ulceration associated with sclerotherapy.

For the treatment of cutaneous venous malformations, certain authors have proposed the use of fluences between 80 and 100 J/cm^2, pulses of 15–20 ms, and a spot size of 7 mm in diameter. In the case of lesions located on mucosae, fluences around 100 J/cm^2 are recommended, and for glomuvenous malformations around 80 J/cm^2 should be used.

It is worth highlighting that, unlike treatment with PDLs in which the purpura reveals the tissue response to treatment, with Nd:YAG lasers there is no clinical parameter to indicate this. Furthermore, whitening of the skin must be avoided because it is the clinical manifestation of underlying thermal damage. This is not applicable to the mucosae.

Rosacea

Rosacea is a skin and vascular condition characterized by the association of telangiectasias, facial papules and pustules, and rhinophyma, with or without added ocular abnormalities. Not all the elements that make up the disorder are always present. Its cause is unknown, but it seems that the parasite *Demodex folliculorum* could be involved in the pathogenesis of the inflammatory lesions of rosacea. Telangiectasias are dilations of dermal capillaries as a consequence of reduced structural integrity of the dermis and the angiogenesis linked to the characteristic inflammation. The definitive treatment for couperosis is PDL.

For treatment purpuric (fluences between 5.5 and 6.5 J/cm^2 with pulses of 0.45 ms) or subpurpuric doses (two or three passes with fluences of between 7 and 9 J/cm^2 and pulses of 6 to 9 ms) may be used

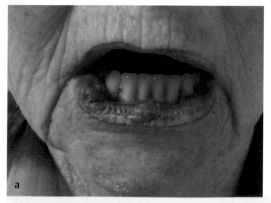
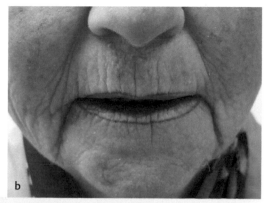

Fig. 10.3 (a) A 75-year-old woman with a venous malformation on the lower lip. (b) Result after two sessions with an Nd:Yag laser with a fluence of 80 J/cm^2 and a pulse duration of 40 ms with a spot size of 5 mm (b).

(►Fig. 10.4). Results are usually good, and the side effects are practically nonexistent except for purpura resulting from the extravasation of blood following the rupture of the blood vessel wall.

10.5.2 Poikilodermia of Civatte

Poikilodermia of Civatte arises as a consequence of sustained actin damage and is very often associated with photosensitization due to chemical agents, in particular fragrances. It is characterized by the presence of irregular hyperpigmented plaques with telangiectasias and skin atrophy located on the lateral aspects of the neck and the upper part of the thorax.

Treatment with PDL and KTP lasers and, more recently, fractionated ablative and nonablative lasers, is efficient, although sometimes the Gaussian distribution of the light beam in this type of lesion may give rise to a "honeycomb" appearance to the skin, characterized by a network of relatively untreated skin around central areas with an improved appearance due to treatment. This problem may be resolved by making several passes in different directions.

If PDLs are used, we recommend not to use fluences greater than 6J/cm² due to the risk of scarring. The ideal solution is to use fluences between 5 and 6 J/cm², with pulses of between 0.45 and 0.5 ms when hyperpigmentation is predominant and of 1.5 to 2 ms when erythema is an issue. Three to five sessions are normally required for lightening of the lesions.

IPL is perhaps the treatment of choice because it improves not only the telangiectasias but also the hyperpigmentation and has a low incidence of side effects. Most authors recommend performing a first session using a filter of 515 nm and fluences of 22 to 25 J/cm², in two pulses of 2.4 and 4 ms separated by 10 ms.

10.5.3 Pyogenic Granulomas

Pyogenic granuloma is a very frequent vascular proliferation, usually presenting as a single sessile or pedunculated, rapidly growing, wine-red lesion with a friable surface that tends to bleed or ulcerate. Among the different types of laser, PDL (fluences between 6.5 and 9 J/cm²) and long-pulsed Nd:YAG lasers are the treatment of choice. Normally, several treatment sessions are required, but, because each session produces further trauma, this is often impractical. Other useful options include IPL and argon and alexandrite lasers. Cauterization and vaporization with CO_2 represent the first lines of treatment in the excision of the papular component, after which, if necessary, a PDL may be used to eliminate the residual macular component.

10.5.4 Venous Lakes

These are papulonodular lesions 2–10 mm in diameter, elastic, bluish or violet in color, which are found especially on the lips and are due to dilated venules located in the superficial dermis. The treatment of choice is long-pulsed Nd:YAG laser with fluences between 100 and 140J/cm², and pulses of between 20 and 40 ms. One single session is usually sufficient. Scarring is one potential complication after laser treatment of these lesions, especially in those with a diameter of greater than 5 mm.

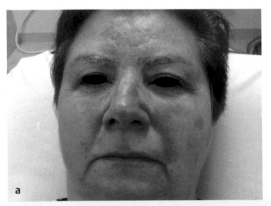 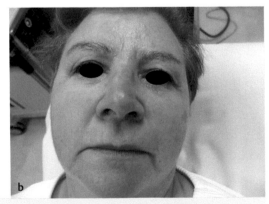

Fig. 10.4 (a) A 68-year-old woman with diffuse facial erythema secondary to rosacea. (b) Cosmetic result after a single session of a pulsed-dye laser following two passes at 7 J/cm² with a pulse duration of 6 ms and 10 ms with a spot size of 10 mm.

10.5.5 Common Verrucae

These are benign lesions associated with the human papilloma virus. Although it is not a first-line treatment, they respond favorably to PDL. Fluences of 7–7.5 J/cm² can be used. Flat warts can disappear with a single pulse of treatment, whereas hypertrophic warts usually require two to four sessions.

10.6 Pigmentation Disorders

Laser treatment of pigmented lesions began to develop following the creation of Q-switched lasers capable of very short pulses lasting between 4 and 100 ns and with a high energy. The absorption spectrum of melanin is very wide and includes visible and infrared light (600–1,200 nm). In the treatment of pigmented lesions it is therefore essential to classify them according to their location into epidermal, dermal, or mixed. Thus pigmented lesions found in the epidermis can be treated with lasers that reach the superficial dermis, such as the KTP 532 nm laser, whereas deeper pigmented lesions will require lasers that use greater wavelengths, such as the Q-switched ruby laser and alexandrite and Nd:YAG 1,064 nm lasers.

10.6.1 Ephelides and Lentigines

Ephelides and lentigines are lesions caused by an increase in melanosomes in epidermis. As already pointed out, the laser treatment of choice for epidermal pigmented lesions is the KTP 532 nm laser. Diode lasers that produce an 800 nm light have also been used in the treatment of this kind of lesion as well as Q-switched ruby and alexandrite lasers. The latter are more useful in the treatment of deeper pigmented lesions, such as nevi of Ota and Ito as well as congenital nevi in which the accumulation of pigment is found in the dermis. In the treatment of ephelides and lentigines, due to the location of the melanin, the Q-switched ruby laser offers greater absorption than alexandrite lasers and therefore is somewhat more effective, although this greater absorption by normal melanocytes in the dermis will also result in hypopigmentation. This is probably beneficial in patients with light-colored skin but may be a problem in those with higher phototypes.

10.6.2 Nevi of Ota and Ito

In these cases, unlike the lesions just described, the pigment is deeper; thus the Q-switched alexandrite laser not only reaches deeper layers than the Q-switched ruby laser, which per se makes it more effective, but also absorption by the normal melanocytes in the epidermis is lower, thus creating a lower risk of hypopigmentation. The Q-switched Nd:YAG laser is also used in treatment of this type of pigmentary lesions (▶Fig. 10.5). A recent study comparing the efficacy and toxicity rates of the Q-switched alexandrite and the Q-switched Nd:YAG lasers has demonstrated that the former has a higher rate of pigment clearance and a lower complication rate.

10.6.3 Acquired or Congenital Benign Melanocytic Nevi

The treatment of choice for melanocytic nevi with clinical and/or dermoscopic characteristics of atypia is excision to allow histological analyses and assessment of margins. Laser treatment is thus reserved to clinically benign lesions, especially unresectable or disfiguring ones (▶Fig. 10.6), in patients without a personal or family history of melanoma and after always following biopsy and anatomopathological analysis of the lesion. In general, the nevi found in the papillary dermis respond relatively well to treatment, whereas deeper ones, which show associated hair follicles, are more difficult to eradicate. Congenital nevi, in particular, respond worse to laser treatment, due to their greater depth, and recurrence is not infrequent. In any case, it appears that response is based on the dermal fibroplasia over the melanocytes, which could mask a potential malign transformation of the lesion. The lasers most widely used are Q-switched ruby, alexandrite, and Nd:YAG 532 nm.

10.6.4 Café-au-lait Spots and Nevus Spilus

Café-au-lait spots are caused by a greater amount of pigment in the melanocytes and keratinocytes of the basal layer of the epidermis. They are found very frequently as isolated lesions in the general population, although when they appear in numbers greater than six and associated with other clinical manifestations, neurofibromatosis should be ruled out. They may also appear in McCune–Albright's syndrome, Bloom's syndrome, Fanconi's anemia, ataxia-telangiectasia, Bannayan–Riley–Ruvalcaba's syndrome, among others. Q-switched

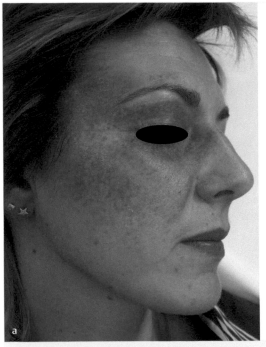
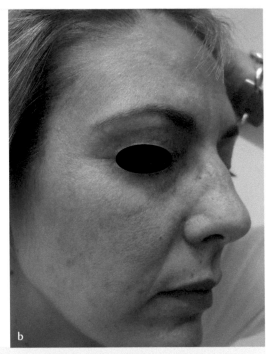

Fig. 10.5 (a) A 38-year-old woman with a history of nevus of Ota. (b) Result after eight sessions with a neodymium:yttrium- aluminum-garnet Q-switched laser at 8 J/cm² with a spot size of 3 mm.

ruby, alexandrite, and Nd:YAG 352 nm are the lasers most frequently used.

Nevi spilus are pigmentocellular nevi over an underlying café-au-lait spot. PDL, erbium YAG (Er:YAG), Q-switched Nd:YAG, Q-switched ruby laser, and Q-switched alexandrite laser have been used for these lesions.

10.6.5 Melasma

Melasma is a disorder of unknown etiology in which both genetic and hormonal (pregnancy, use of hormonal anticonceptives) and exogenous factors (ultraviolet light) appear to be involved. Cases of melasma are classified as epidermal, dermal, or mixed depending on whether the melanin is distributed in the basal and suprabasal layers of the epidermis, in the melanophages, or in both, respectively. The first are highlighted with a Wood lamp light. The treatment of choice is topical depigmenting agents (hydroquinone, retinoids, and chemical peels). Q-switched lasers result in an inflammatory state that exacerbates and even perpetuates the problem. Er:YAG lasers may improve the clinical appearance of the melasma initially, but postinflammatory hyperpigmentation is not infrequent. Among all the lasers, those of the fractionated, nonablative type are perhaps the best treatment option, especially for high phototypes (III–IV) in which response rates of between 75 and 100% have been reported. This response appears to be linked to a greater absorption of hydroquinone in the epidermis and dermis. However, in spite of this initial clinical improvement, melasma tends to recur after treatment.

10.6.6 Becker's Nevus

This is a hamartoma that usually appears in childhood or adolescence on the shoulder, arm, or upper part of the trunk. It is usually dark brown in color, sometimes with multiple hair follicles, and has smooth muscle tissue among its components. Given that melanin is located both in the epidermis and the dermis, this type of lesion may benefit from treatment with Q-switched lasers, such as the alexandrite and ruby lasers. However, both incomplete lightening and recurrences are possible.

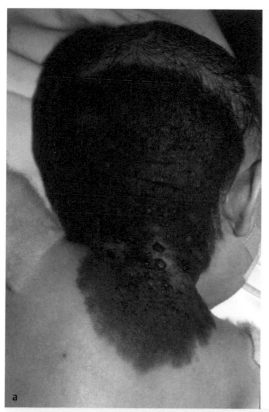

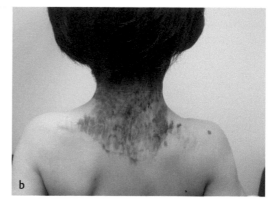

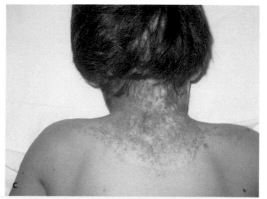

Fig. 10.6 (a) A 9-month-old boy with a giant congenital nevus in the occipital and posterior cervical region and the back. (b) Result after several serial resection operations. (c) Appearance after 15 palliative sessions with an alexandrite Q-switched laser at 10 J/cm² with a spot size of 3 mm.

10.6.7 Hyperpigmentation following Inflammation or due to Other Causes

Fractional photothermolysis with low density and low energy appears to be a current option that is useful in the treatment of postinflammatory hyperpigmentation. However, Q-switched ruby, alexandrite, and Nd:YAG lasers should be used with caution because they are capable of causing hyperpigmentation themselves.

In contrast, hyperpigmentation resulting from sclerotherapy is due to the extravasation of blood and the deposition of hemosiderin, as a result of which Q-switched ruby, alexandrite, and Nd:YAG have been used successfully in the treatment of this type of lesion.

Some drugs, such as amiodarone, minocycline, or imipramine, are capable of inducing a type of hyperpigmentation that may be due to the deposition of hemosiderin, melanin, or both. Q-switched ruby and Nd:YAG 1,064 nm lasers have been successfully used in its treatment.

10.7 Laser Hair Removal

Hypertrichosis, or an increase in body hair beyond the normal range, can be a source of emotional stress. If the excess hair is a cosmetic or psychosocial problem for the patient, a variety of treatment modalities, including laser surgery, are available. The long-pulsed ruby (694 nm), the long-pulsed alexandrite (755 nm), and the diode (810 nm) lasers have wavelengths (red to near-infrared) and pulse times targeted to melanin found in the melanosomes of the hair bulb and the hair itself. Therefore, the laser energy absorbed by the melanosomes is released as heat and subsequently damages the surrounding follicle. Pulse durations in the millisecond domain cause enough thermal damage for complete and confined follicular disruption. IPL has also been reported to be effective in the treatment of hypertrichosis. For dark-skinned patients or those with tanned skin, the millisecond Nd:YAG lasers (1,064 nm) are more appropriate because their longer wavelengths result in less absorption by epidermal melanin.

Laser hair removal has expected side effects, such as perifollicular erythema and edema, and has the potential for more serious complications, such as pigmentary alterations or even scarring if excessive treatment fluences are used.

10.8 Skin Resurfacing

Resurfacing lasers were first designed to remove or reduce wrinkles by injuring superficial skin and allowing a new layer of collagen to form at the dermal–epidermal interface. Among resurfacing lasers, there are ablative and nonablative lasers as well as fractionated and nonfractionated lasers. Nonfractionated lasers act on the entire projected surface area of the treated skin, whereas fractionated lasers target an equally distributed portion of the projected area. Ablative lasers vaporize tissue and therefore are more aggressive compared with the gentler nonablative lasers that leave the skin intact. Although ablative lasers result in far more down time and a more difficult recovery process, they remain the lasers that produce the most dramatic outcomes. Ablative lasers retain a higher risk of potentially severe damage in the form of scarring, discoloration, and infections of the skin by bacteria, viruses, or fungi.

Antiviral medications (e.g., valacyclovir, famciclovir) should be initiated prophylactically (even in the absence of prior herpetic infection) to prevent the possibility of a generalized herpetic infection in the denuded skin, especially if the treated region involves perioral skin or adjacent areas. Antibiotic coverage, particularly against staphylococci, may be prudent but is much debated. Antifungal prophylaxis with fluconazole (a single-dose 200 mg tablet) given during the early postoperative period has been demonstrated to prevent candidal infection and may promote reepithelialization.

10.8.1 Ablative Nonfractionated Lasers

Ablative skin resurfacing removes the epidermal layer, producing the most dramatic laser-treated results for skin resurfacing. The lasers quickly superheat water molecules in the skin tissue so that, when water turns into gas, the skin cells are vaporized in a precise skin-peeling effect. This effect promotes collagen formation and retraction of the dermis and epidermis to tighten the skin. The original devices had serious side effects, including scarring and difficult wound healing. However, the most recent generation of ablative lasers—particularly the fractionated ablative lasers—have been able to reduce the trauma from treatment and decrease downtime while still allowing for effective resurfacing.

These lasers were originally developed to treat photodamage and acne scarring and have remained the most effective treatment. Treatment of acne scarring is a common indication for ablative lasers. In general, CO_2 lasers achieve better results for acne scarring than the traditional Er:YAG laser. Elevated or distensible acne scars are most amenable to resurfacing, compared to ice-pick and nondistensible scars, which are often resistant.

Focal ablation has been effectively used for resurfacing elevated, irregular epidermal lesions, such as seborrheic keratoses, epidermal nevi, and verrucae. Additionally, benign hyperplasias or neoplasms with an elevated component can be "debulked" (e.g., hypertrophic scars, rhinophyma, microcystic lymphatic malformations, adnexal tumors [including syringomas and angiofibromas], and xanthomas). Other possible indications for both the CO_2 and Er:YAG lasers could be actinic keratosis, actinic cheilitis, epidermal nevus, or acantholytic diseases (Hailey–Hailey's disease and Darier's disease) (▶ Fig. 10.7).

10.8.2 Ablative Fractional Lasers

The most recent generation of ablative lasers are the fractional ablative lasers, which came into use around 2007. These lasers have been able to reduce trauma and decrease downtime while retaining resurfacing power. In addition, fractional ablative lasers are much safer than their nonfractionated counterparts, but they may still be associated with significant risk of potential damage in the form of scarring, discoloration, and skin infection.

The main use of these lasers is for mild skin tightening to battle laxity and rhytides. However, these lasers can also treat photodamage, atrophic acne scars, hypopigmented scars, and depigmentation.

Two lasers are normally used for ablative resurfacing, both in their fractionated and nonfractionated

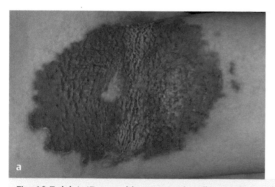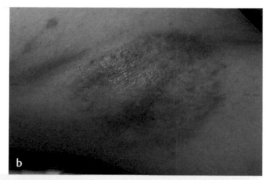

Fig. 10.7 **(a)** A 47-year-old patient with axillary Hailey–Hailey's disease. **(b)** Outcome 1 year after treatment with carbon dioxide laser skin resurfacing. Note the postinflammatory hyperpigmentation with no evidence of recurrence.

forms: the CO_2 laser and the Er:YAG laser. Both the CO_2 and the Er:YAG lasers have wavelengths in the infrared portion of the electromagnetic spectrum; thus the chromophore is predominantly water.

Carbon Dioxide Laser

The CO_2 laser emits light at a wavelength of 10,600 nm in the far infrared spectrum. The initial CW CO_2 laser, which targeted intracellular and extracellular water with subsequent nonspecific thermal tissue injury, produced unacceptable cosmetic consequences. By redesigning the laser to deliver much higher peak fluences (> 5–7 J/cm²) in a much shorter time, or pulse duration (1 ms), it became possible to vaporize superficial layers of skin without creating excessive nonselective thermal damage. This change enabled physicians to resurface facial skin, vaporize cutaneous lesions, and improve scars while limiting the risk of scarring that was associated with the traditional CW CO_2 lasers. Furthermore, the hemostasis caused by the laser produces a bloodless field and therefore good visualization.

Erbium: Yttrium-Aluminum-Garnet Laser

The Er:YAG laser emits light at a shorter wavelength (2,940 nm) than the CO_2 laser. This wavelength corresponds to a peak in water absorption and is 16 times more strongly absorbed by water within the skin cells; hence its use to selectively vaporize soft tissue. The Er:YAG laser also has a very short pulse duration, which further limits damage to surrounding areas. In addition to finer ablation and shortened healing time, pigmentary changes are also less common, making it beneficial

for highly pigmented individuals. However, hemostasis is not complete, causing pinpoint bleeding at the dermal–epidermal junction, and the amount of skin tightening appears to be less than that after treatment with the CO_2 laser.

10.9 Conclusions

The term *laser* is an acronym for light amplification by stimulated emission of radiation. The principal indications for laser in dermatology, mainly for cosmetic purposes, are vascular lesions, such as PWSs, venous lakes, and telangiectasias; epidermal and dermal pigmented lesions; and removing or reducing wrinkles, photodamage, atrophic acne scars, or hypopigmented scars. The lasers most frequently used in the treatment of vascular lesions are the KTP (532 nm), the PDL (577–600 nm), and the Nd:YAG (1,064 nm). For the epidermal and dermal pigmented lesions, the KTP 532 nm laser, and the Q-switched ruby laser or the alexandrite and Nd:YAG 1,064 nm lasers, respectively, are the most used. To injure superficial skin and allow a new layer of collagen to form at the dermal–epidermal interface, the fractional CO_2 laser and the Er:YAG laser are the most recent generation of ablative lasers. Wavelength, pulse duration, energy density, chromophores of the skin (oxyhemoglobin, melanin, and water), fluence, irradiance, and spot size are laser parameters that have to be accurately taken into account for preventing undesirable effects, such as scarring, hypo-/hyperpigmentation, or alopecia. Thus the choice of laser should be made on the basis of the individual absorption characteristics of the target chromophore.

10.10 Key Points

- *Laser* is the acronym for *light amplification by stimulated emission of radiation.*
- Lasers deliver monochromatic, coherent, collimated, and high-intensity beams of light, whereas intense pulsed light (IPL) devices emit polychromatic, noncoherent light in a broad range of wavelengths.
- The three main endogenous chromophores (specific light-absorbing targets) in the skin are melanin, hemoglobin, and water. Each of these chromophores has its own absorption spectrum and absorption peak.
- The theory of selective photothermolysis states that the laser energy can be absorbed by a defined target chromophore, leading to its controlled destruction without significant damage to the surrounding tissue.
- Wavelength, pulse duration, energy density, chromophores of the skin (oxyhemoglobin, melanin, and water), fluence, and spot size are laser parameters that influence clinical outcomes in the use of lasers for the treatment of different skin diseases.
- Oxyhemoglobin is the target chromophore in vascular lesions, and its absorption peaks are found at wavelengths 418, 512, and 577 nm.
- The lasers most frequently used in the treatment of vascular lesions are the KTP (532 nm), the PDL (577–600 nm), and the Nd:YAG (1064 nm).
- Melanin is the target chromophore in pigmented lesions; its absorption spectrum is very wide and includes visible and infrared light (600–1,200 nm).
- Epidermal pigmented lesions can be treated with lasers that reach the superficial dermis, such as the KTP 532 nm laser, whereas dermal pigmented lesions will require lasers that use greater wavelengths, such as the Q-switched ruby laser, alexandrite laser, and Nd:YAG 1,064 nm laser.
- Resurfacing lasers are designed to injure superficial skin and allow a new layer of collagen to form at the dermal–epidermal interface. The most recent generation of ablative lasers are the fractional ablative lasers: the CO_2 laser and the Er:YAG laser. The main use of these lasers is for mild skin tightening to battle laxity and rhytides. However, these lasers can also treat photodamage, atrophic acne scars, hypopigmented scars, and depigmentation.

Recommended Readings

Allevato M, Boixeda P. Educación cotinua láser en Dermatología (1ª parte). Act Terap Dermatol. 2006;29:6

Anderson RR, Parrish JA. Selective photothermolysis: precise microsurgery by selective absorption of pulsed radiation. Science. 1983; 220(4596):524–527

Bolognia JL, Jorizzo JL, Schaffer JV. Bolognia Textbook of Dermatology. 3rd ed. Barcelona, Spain: Mosby Elsevier; 2012

Cantatore JL, Kriegel DA. Laser surgery: an approach to the pediatric patient. J Am Acad Dermatol. 2004;50(2):165–184, quiz 185–188

Castiñeiras I, Del Pozo J, Mazaira M, Rodríguez-Lojo R, Fonseca E. Actinic cheilitis: evolution to squamous cell carcinoma after carbon dioxide laser vaporization. A study of 43 cases. J Dermatolog Treat. 2010;21(1):49–53

Dierickx CC, Casparian JM, Venugopalan V, Farinelli WA, Anderson RR. Thermal relaxation of port-wine stain vessels probed in vivo: the need for 1–10-millisecond laser pulse treatment. J Invest Dermatol. 1995;105(5):709–714

Dover JS, Margolis RJ, Polla LL, et al. Pigmented guinea pig skin irradiated with Q-switched ruby laser pulses. Morphologic and histologic findings. Arch Dermatol. 1989;125(1):43–49

Garzon MC, Huang JT, Enjolras O, Frieden IJ. Vascular malformations: Part I. J Am Acad Dermatol. 2007;56(3):353–370, quiz 371–374

Garzon MC, Huang JT, Enjolras O, Frieden IJ. Vascular malformations. Part II: associated syndromes. J Am Acad Dermatol. 2007;56(4):541–564

Goldman MP, Fitzpatrick RE. Cutaneous Laser Surgery: The Art & Science of Selective Photothermolysis. 2nd ed. Maryland Heights, MO: Mosby Elsevier; 1998

Kar H, Gupta L. Treatment of nevus spilus with Q switched Nd:YAG laser. Indian J Dermatol Venereol Leprol. 2013; 79(2):243–245

Lazzeri D, Larcher L, Huemer GM, et al. Surgical correction of rhinophyma: comparison of two methods in a 15-year-long experience. J Craniomaxillofac Surg. 2013;41(5):429–436

Morelli JG. Use of lasers in pediatric dermatology. Dermatol Clin. 1998;16(3):489–495

Minsue Chen T, Wanitphakdeedecha R, Nguyen TH. Carbon dioxide laser ablation and adjunctive destruction for Darier-White disease (keratosis follicularis). Dermatol Surg. 2008;34(10):1431–1434

Nanni CA, Alster TS. Complications of carbon dioxide laser resurfacing. An evaluation of 500 patients. Dermatol Surg. 1998;24(3):315–320

Pretel-Irazabal M, Lera-Imbuluzqueta JM, España-Alonso A. Carbon dioxide laser treatment in Hailey-Hailey disease: a series of 8 patients. Actas Dermosifiliogr. 2013;104(4):325–333

Papadavid E, Katsambas A. Lasers for facial rejuvenation: a review. Int J Dermatol. 2003;42(6):480–487

Scherer K, Waner M. Nd:YAG lasers (1,064 nm) in the treatment of venous malformations of the face and neck: challenges and benefits. Lasers Med Sci. 2007;22(2):119–126

Stier MF, Glick SA, Hirsch RJ. Laser treatment of pediatric vascular lesions: Port wine stains and hemangiomas. J Am Acad Dermatol. 2008;58(2):261–285

Savas JA, Ledon J, Franca K, Chacon A, Zaiac M, Nouri K. Carbon dioxide laser for the treatment of microcystic lymphatic malformations (lymphangioma circumscriptum): a systematic review. Dermatol Surg. 2013;39(8):1147–1157

Wheeland RG. Clinical uses of lasers in dermatology. Lasers Surg Med. 1995;16(1):2–23

Wang JI, Roenigk HH Jr. Treatment of multiple facial syringomas with the carbon dioxide (CO2) laser. Dermatol Surg. 1999;25(2):136–139

Yu P, Yu N, Diao W, Yang X, Feng Y, Qi Z. Comparison of clinical efficacy and complications between Q-switched alexandrite laser and Q-switched Nd:YAG laser on nevus of Ota: a systematic review and meta-analysis. Lasers Med Sci. 2016;31(3):581–591

Zenzie HH, Altshuler GB, Smirnov MZ, Anderson RR. Evaluation of cooling methods for laser dermatology. Lasers Surg Med. 2000;26(2):130–144

11 How to Set Up a Research Protocol in Plastic Surgery

Stefan Danilla, Ekaterina Troncoso Olchevskaia

Abstract

There has been a shift in the paradigm of medical practice, from a pragmatic approach to understanding and treating an illness to an evidence-based medicine approach. Evidence-based medicine uses the scientific method to answer clinical questions and generate knowledge. This process follows preestablished steps according to the scientific method, and starts with a question. The research question should be feasible, interesting, novel, ethical, and relevant. When one is designing a research protocol, it is important to establish what kind of question to ask: diagnostic, etiologic, prognostic, or therapeutic. There are many ways of answering each type of question; designing the best way to answer a given question generates more accurate, higher-level evidence. This chapter provides an overview of how to set up a research protocol in plastic surgery.

Keywords: diagnosis, etiology, prognosis, research protocol, research question, statistics, therapy

11.1 Introduction

We are surrounded by clinical questions in our daily practice. Is my patient sick? What is causing his/her sickness? Will it cause disability? Which treatment should I give him/her? Since 1992, there has been a shift in medical paradigms, and the traditional ways of responding to these questions have changed toward evidence-based medicine.

Evidence-based medicine uses the scientific method to answer clinical questions and places lower value on nonsystematic clinical experience. The scientific method is the process by which scientists attempt to construct a reliable and consistent representation of the world. It consists of four steps: (1) identification and description of a phenomenon, (2) formulation of a hypothesis to explain the phenomenon, (3) use of the hypothesis to predict future observations, and (4) experiments to test the predictions.

The search for the cause of diseases is one of the most important questions we face. Causation is an essential concept in the practice of epidemiology. For Rothman, "A cause is an act or event or a state of nature which initiates or permits, alone or in conjunction with other causes, a sequence of events resulting in an effect." Because the only way to know what causes a determined effect is the contrafactual model of causation, we can only talk about association or relation between a possible cause and an effect.

Statistical methods can be used to determine if two or more events are connected. In statistics, this is referred to as inference. There are many statistical tests for hypotheses that can determine the association, or lack thereof, between two or more events.

The scientific method in general and as applied in medicine follows a sequence of steps that begin with a research question and end with analysis and conclusions (▶ Fig. 11.1).

11.2 Clinical Question and Types of Study

Every protocol must start by asking a question. Questions arise from personal experience, problems encountered, knowledge, new ideas, new technologies, skepticism, imagination, observation, teaching, creativity, and so on. The work begins with formulating a good research question that is feasible, interesting, novel, ethical, and relevant (FINER).

A good clinical question has three parts: (1) patients or a population, (2) intervention and comparison, and (3) outcomes. This method of formulating a research question is called the PICO strategy (patient or problem, intervention or indicator, comparison, and outcome).

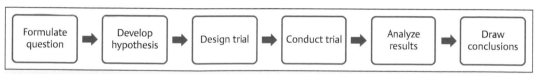

Fig. 11.1 Diagram of the scientific method.

Once a FINER question has been formulated, the next step is to perform a thorough bibliographic background to determine whether the question has been asked before, and, if so, to study any previous attempts to answer it. After gathering the relevant information, you should have an idea of how previous researchers have approached the problem, and with that knowledge decide which area of clinical epidemiology (diagnosis, prognosis, treatment, or etiology) applies to your question.

11.2.1 Diagnosis

When facing a patient with an illness, as doctors we have the difficult task of elaborating a correct diagnosis. Fortunately, we have diverse tests to help us rule out or confirm a diagnosis. These diagnostic tests have several features that allow us to decide how accurate the diagnosis will be after applying the test, and whether the test is even worth performing. These features are extracted from conclusions of diagnostic studies. So if you have developed a new diagnostic test and you want to prove its use and accuracy, you should conduct a diagnostic study.

11.2.2 Prognosis

On the other hand, if you already know the diagnosis of your patient, but you need to know the prognosis with or without treatment, you search for prognostic studies. These studies are designed to determine which course the disease will take.

11.2.3 Treatment

If you know your patient's diagnosis and prognosis, you will need to determine the most effective treatment to administer to maximize your patient's well-being. Treatment studies help answer these questions.

11.2.4 Etiology

It can be difficult to determine why a patient is diseased. Doing so requires a profound knowledge of the disease's pathophysiology. Etiology studies aim to find the cause of pathology.

A subgroup of studies that does not fit into any of the preceding categories includes clinical cases, case series, and presentations of surgical technique. These types of studies are the oldest and most popular types of medical literature worldwide. However, they are highly criticized because, with just one case or a small case series, authors may arrive at the wrong conclusions. In fact, these types of publications are rarely cited, so many journals reject them to avoid lowering their impact and credibility. Although the level of evidence of case reports and case series is at the lowest level of the evidence hierarchy (▶ Fig. 11.2), their "open format" makes them useful for providing atypical presentations of diseases, difficult and uncommon diagnoses, rare conditions, and novel surgical techniques. Also, because randomized clinical trials may exclude many patients, for example patients with polypharmacy or with more than two comorbidities, case reports and case series may help us to observe unknown effects of therapies on these patients. For surgeons, and especially plastic surgeons, clinical knowledge is more easily recalled when it arises from real-life reports.

11.2.5 Clinical Cases

Clinical case reports consist of a detailed description of the clinical record, treatment, complications, and follow-up of a single patient. You should highlight the special characteristics why you believe this particular case is worth reporting.

11.2.6 Case Series

Case series are similar to clinical case reports, but rather than reporting on a single patient they

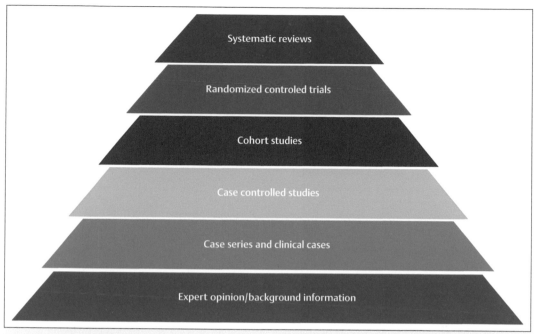

Fig. 11.2 Levels of evidence.

report on a group of patients with a similar characteristic. For a study to be considered a case series, it should include between 2 and 10 cases.

11.2.7 Surgical Techniques

Novel surgical techniques, such as face transplants and high-definition liposculpture, are commonly first reported in this type of report. These publications help to update the international surgical community about the latest surgical techniques.

All of these reports should come with a full research of the existing literature Novel surgical techniques, such as face transplants and high-definition liposculpture, are commonly first reported as surgical techniques.

11.3 Basic Components of a Research Protocol

Every research protocol includes at least the following sections (▶Table 11.1):

Research question: Research questions arise from many backgrounds, such as personal experiences, knowledge, and imagination. As mentioned earlier, a good research question must be feasible, interesting, novel, ethical, and relevant. Your research

Table 11.1 Common sections of a research protocol

Research question
Literature review
Objectives of the research
Population, patients, study center, inclusion and exclusion criteria
Intervention
Measurements
Statistics

question must be well formulated because the hypothesis, objectives, and methods will directly derive from it.

Literature review: Searching the literature for previous attempts to answer your research question, together with a complete knowledge of the disease's pathophysiology, is paramount to establishing the background of your research and to more properly designing your protocol.

Objectives: The objectives are declaratory statements that provide information about the type of study to be conducted, and they define the specific aims of the study. The primary objective should be coupled with the hypothesis of the study. Secondary objectives should state the aims to help.

Population, sample, study center, and inclusion and exclusion criteria: A population is a group of people that have a set of clinical, demographic, and temporal characteristics you want to study. Your patients should be a representative sample from the population you want to study. To help you select your patients you need to establish the inclusion and exclusion criteria. The *inclusion criteria* define the main characteristics of your target population. The *exclusion criteria* are used to remove patients that can alter the quality of the data or the interpretation of the results. Your *study center* is the health care center where patients are recruited. If you want your study to have a higher external validity (extrapolation to the broader population), or if you need to recruit patients faster, then you can design a *multicentric study.*

Intervention: The intervention you want to study must be well characterized. It may be a treatment or a disease, depending on the type of study you are conducting; also, depending on your design, the intervention can be assigned by the researcher (experimental study), or chosen by the patient or the patient's physician (observational study).

Measurements: The way you are going to measure your outcomes should be well defined and established. Your outcomes could be a clinical variable or an indirect variable. Clinical variables, such as death, complications, hospital admission, quality of life, are more significant, but you may not be able to measure them. In those cases you can use an indirect variable, such as biological markers. We strongly advise using patient-reported outcomes, such as the Body-QoL or the Breast-Q, for measuring outcomes in plastic surgery.

Statistics: Depending on the type of study you are conducting, statistical analysis can be used to describe your results or find association between interventions and outcomes.

11.4 Measuring the Accuracy of a Diagnostic Test

Establishing a correct diagnosis is an important part of our daily work. To reach the right diagnosis, we frequently need to perform some diagnostic tests. Nevertheless, to interpret the results of those tests you need to be familiarized with some basic principles about them.

First of all, establishing a diagnosis is an imperfect process, which gives as a result a probability of having the alleged illness. If you have a diagnostic test and the presence of illness, and you represent it on a 2 × 2 table (▶Fig. 11.3), then there will be patients correctly diagnosed (true-positive or true-negative), and patients erroneously diagnosed (false-positive or false-negative).

Because we do not know the truth, we use the best-known diagnostic method there is—the gold standard or the standard of comparison.

Sensitivity is defined as the proportion of individuals that are truly sick and have a positive result in the test, and *specificity* as the proportion of individuals that are truly healthy and have a negative result in the test.

Sensitivity and specificity are intrinsic properties of a test and are calculated with individuals we already know whether they are sick or not. But what we really need to know is, given the result of the test, if our patient is sick or not. The *positive predictive value* is defined as the probability of sickness of an individual with a positive result on the test. The *negative predictive value* is the probability of not being sick when the result of the test is negative. The main difference between sensitivity, specificity, and positive or negative predictive value is that sensitivity and specificity are intrinsic properties of the test, whereas predictive value depends on the population being tested.

If you want to do the math, you can look at the 2 × 2 table (▶Fig. 11.3) and see that sensitivity is a/(a + c), specificity is d/(b + d), positive predictive

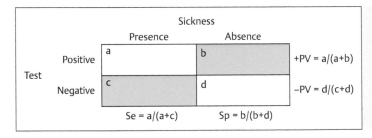

Fig. 11.3 Table 2 × 2, c and b are true results, and a and d are false results.

value is a/(a + b), and negative predictive value is d/(c + d). Another way to calculate the positive predictive value is

$$\frac{\text{sensitivty} \times \text{prevalence}}{(\text{sensitivty} \times \text{prevalence}) + (1 - \text{specificity}) \times (1 - \text{prevalence})}$$

When choosing a test, you want it to be both sensitive and specific (except if you want to reduce the false-negatives or the false-positives to a minimum), but as you elevate the sensitivity of the test you will have to sacrifice specificity, and vice versa. Therefore, if the result of your test is a continuous variable, you will need to find a cutoff point that can separate the normal from the abnormal, with a reasonable sensitivity and specificity. A good way to find this cutoff point is the receiver operator characteristic (ROC) curve (▶ Fig. 11.4). The closer the cutoff point is to the left superior corner, the better the test, as is also true with a larger area under the curve. Thus, when choosing a cutoff point, you want a value as close to the left superior corner as possible.

An alternative way to describe the accuracy of a test is the likelihood ratio. The likelihood ratio is the probability of having a test result in people with the disease, divided by the probability of having the same result in people without the disease. You have to express the likelihood ratio in terms of the odds, rather than as a probability.

11.5 Determining the Prognosis of a Disease

The prognosis is a prediction of the evolution of a disease after its onset. Patients and their family members want to know what is going to occur if the disease takes its natural or clinical course. The *natural course* of a disease describes the way patients with a given disease evolve if they are not treated, whereas the *clinical course* of a disease describes its evolution under medical attention.

When performing a prognostic study, you have to group a cohort of individuals with a given disease, follow them over time, and measure their clinical results. Some elements needed to execute a prognostic study are a sample, an inception cohort, follow-up, and outcome.

11.5.1 Sample

As with every study, you need your sample of patients to represent the population you are studying. It is important to accurately describe the characteristics of patients in your sample (age, severity of the disease, comorbidities, etc.), the environment they were identified in, and the way sampling was conducted.

11.5.2 Inception Cohort

You need to clearly define the point in the disease at which your patients are to be followed. It may be the moment when they first experience symptoms, the moment of diagnosis, or the beginning of treatment. What is most important is that you included all your patients at a uniformly early time in the disease. This is called an inception cohort.

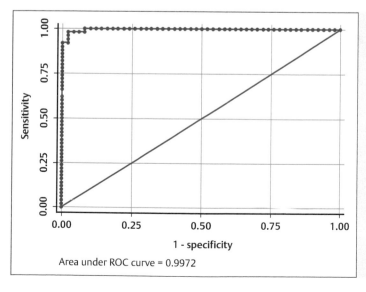

Fig. 11.4 Receiver operator characteristic (ROC) curve example.

Area under ROC curve = 0.9972

11.5.3 Follow-up

The follow-up should be as long as the necessary amount of time for your outcome to occur in most of your cohort. It depends on the pathophysiology of the disease and ranges from a few weeks (e.g., surgical site infections) to several years (e.g., recurrence of breast cancer).

11.5.4 Outcome

The chosen outcome has to be considered important in the course of the disease. The five most common outcomes evaluated in prognosis studies are called the five Ds: death, disease, discomfort, disability, and dissatisfaction.

Knowing this, you have to describe the course of the given disease. There are different ways to do this. The easiest way is to calculate the rate of proportion of patients that presented the outcome you are studying over a specific period of time (incidence). Commonly used rates for prognosis research are survival at 5 years, lethality, specific mortality, improvement, remission, and recurrence.

The problem with using rates is that it excessively summarizes the information, and you will miss the course of the disease. For example, if you look at the 5-year survival rate of a cohort of patients with a dissecting aortic aneurysm, and another one with lung cancer, both of them will have a 10% survival chance at 5 years. However, most patients with a dissecting aortic aneurysm will be deceased over the first few months, whereas patients with lung cancer will pass away steadily over time (▶Fig. 11.5).

To engage this problem survival curves were created. This is called survival analysis, and the best known method for doing the analysis is the Kaplan–Meier method. With the Kaplan–Meier method you can estimate the probability of surviving for a given length of time while considering time in many small intervals. If you look at ▶Fig. 11.6 you can see a typical Kaplan–Meier survival curve. The y-axis demonstrates the probability of survival, whereas the x-axis presents the time of follow-up after diagnosis. Intervals of time depend on the events. When a patient dies (or the outcome we are studying occurs), the probability of survival is calculated by dividing the number of patients who lived by the number of patients at risk of dying. When a patient is already dead or lost in a specific period of follow-up, that patient is no longer susceptible to dying, so you should not use that person to calculate the survival. Patients may be lost at any time during follow-up. This is called censure, and if it occurs, you need to stop counting these patients to calculate survival. Finally, it is important to keep in mind that, as time goes by, there will be fewer patients in the study (because they had the event or because they are censured), so survival estimation will be less precise over time, and this needs to be interpreted carefully.

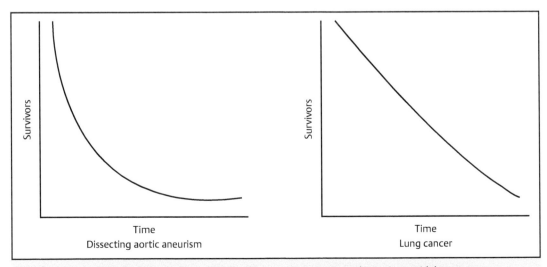

Fig. 11.5 Course of the disease in patients with dissecting aortic aneurysm and in patients with lung cancer.

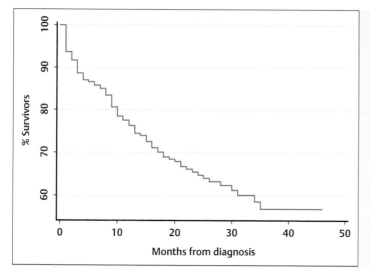

Fig. 11.6 Kaplan–Meier curve for stage IV breast cancer in a cohort of patients followed over 48 months.

11.6 Analyzing the Effectiveness of a Treatment

When diagnosing a patient with a certain disease, we need to establish a certain treatment. But, how does one choose the best treatment for a patient? Does the treatment really work? Does it have risks?

All of these questions start with an idea that we are going to call a hypothesis. A hypothesis is an affirmative sentence about the natural world for the purpose of performing empirical tests. A *treatment* can be defined as any intervention destined to improve the natural course of a disease. Treatments can have many forms, from a pill to psychological therapy. If you want to prove a hypothesis about a treatment, there are basically two methods to choose from: observational or experimental studies.

11.6.1 Observational Studies

Researchers observe what happens to patients exposed to an intervention, but they do not control the exposure. The major advantage of these studies is viability; the disadvantage is that the groups could have important biases that can generate the wrong conclusions.

11.6.2 Experimental Studies

Unlike with observational studies, the researcher assigns the intervention. When performed correctly, the researcher can isolate the true contribution of the treatment and can reduce biases to a minimum. When the treatment is assigned randomly, we say it is a randomized controlled trial, and it represents the best design for testing a treatment.

Randomized Controlled Trial

When performing a randomized controlled trial, first you have to select a sample of representative patients of your population with the condition you want to treat. Then you randomize all participants into two or more groups. The group that will receive the intervention, which is supposed to be better than the current therapy, is called the experimental group. The other group of patients, the control group, may receive placebos, current therapy, or the best treatment there is. Both groups are followed for a sufficient period of time for the outcome to occur. The results obtained in both groups are contrasted (compared) to determine if the new therapy works or if it is better than regular therapy. The following elements of a randomized controlled trial should be kept in mind.

Sampling

Patients need to fulfill specific selection criteria (inclusion and exclusion) to increase the homogeneity of the sample in the trial, increase internal validity, and clearly portray the effect of the intervention. *Inclusion criteria* define the main characteristics of the population you want to study, whereas *exclusion criteria* are used to exclude patients that can alter the quality of the data or the interpretation of the results. So exclusion criteria are *not* the opposite of inclusion criteria, and vice versa. However, you have to be careful not to be too strict, otherwise your trial will lose external validity, and you won't be able to extrapolate your results to the general population.

Intervention

When planning your intervention you should ask yourself three questions: (1) Is my intervention doable in a normal clinical practice? If the intervention is too expensive, or the patient has to take a pill every 2 hours, then your intervention is not feasible in the normal world. (2) Is the complexity of your intervention acceptable for normal clinical practice? Usually, a more complex and multidisciplinary approach has better results in the normal world, but it is harder to reproduce in an experimental study. (3) Does your intervention differ substantially from alternative therapies?Thus, it is reasonable to assume that the effect you are observing is due to the intervention.

Control Group

Your control group can have one of the following:

1. *No intervention:* This way you compare your therapy with the natural course of the disease.
2. *Observation only:* The main difference is that the patients are closely observed by the researchers. The Hawthorne effect, which refers to patients getting better just because they are in a clinical trial, is a commonly seen phenomenon.
3. *Placebo:* A placebo is every intervention that is duplicates the actual therapy but does not use the active compound. The placebo effect is a phenomenon in which patients' symptoms improve because they believe they are being treated.
4. *Standard therapy:* If an effective therapy already exists, and it is a standard treatment, you should compare your new therapy to that effective therapy. Otherwise it would be unethical not to treat a group of patients, knowing there is a proven therapy for the disease being studied.

Randomization and Group Assignment

Randomization is the best way to distribute baseline variables, such as age, gender, comorbidities, among the groups. For your study to be reliable it is important that you randomize your patients accordingly. Randomization ensures that each patient has the same probability of being assigned into any research group. There are many ways to randomize, such as flipping a coin or using computer software. Avoid pseudorandomization using birth dates, days of the week, and the like.

Blinding

Participants may change their behavior because they are in a clinical trial, which may induce biases. This can be avoided by using blinding or masking. There are basically four ways to blind your research:

1. Those responsible for allocating the patients into the groups should not know the group assignment.
2. Patients should not know which group they are in.
3. Physicians who see the patients should not know which group the patients are in.
4. When assessing outcomes, researchers should be unaware of the treatment groups.

It should be noted that the terms *simple, double,* and *triple blind* are confusing and should be avoided. The best thing is to describe your methods in detail.

Outcomes Assessments

The statistical tests that can be performed to analyze the results of a study are discussed later in this chapter. A simple way to describe the magnitude of the effect of a treatment is to use the following clinically useful measurements of the treatment consequences:

Absolute risk reduction = *Event rate in control group*
− Event rate in experimental group

Relative risk reduction
$$= \frac{Event\ rate\ in\ control\ group - Event\ rate\ in\ experimental\ gi}{Event\ rate\ in\ control\ group}$$

Number of patients needed to treat
$$= \frac{1}{Event\ rate\ in\ control\ group - Event\ rate\ in\ experimental\ group}$$

Analysis by Intention to Treat or Explanatory Trials

Some patients in your trial will not follow the treatment they were assigned to. As a result, you need to decide whether to analyze patients' results by the groups they were randomized to *(analysis by intention)*, or by the treatment they actually received *(explanatory trial)*. Your decision depends on what you want to prove. If you perform an intention analysis, your results will more closely resemble what happens in a normal practice. However, if you want to measure the real effect of your therapy, then you need to analyze your results by the actual treatment that your patients are receiving. The problem of doing this is that you will lose the randomization and will no longer be doing a randomized controlled trial. Therefore, our recommendation is to always perform an analysis by intention.

Phases of Therapy Studies

Therapy studies aimed at testing new drugs need to undergo the following phases:

1. *Phase I trials:* Try to identify the dose interval that is safe and well tolerated. This phase is performed in a very small group of patients.
2. *Phase II trials:* This phase provides preliminary information about the efficacy of the drug and the association between dose and efficacy. This phase also includes few patients.
3. *Phase III trials:* This phase provides final evidence on efficacy and common side effects. It is performed in a large group of patients.
4. *Phase IV (not a real phase):* This phase is referred to as postmarketing surveillance, and it helps in identifying uncommon side effects. It is applied to the general population.

11.7 In Search of the Cause of Your Patient's Disease

When you diagnose a patient with a given disease, you (and your patient) will probably want to know what caused it. As explained earlier, etiology studies assess the causality of a disease. It is not easy to prove the cause of an illness; if you perform a trial, you may find a relationship or association between a possible cause and an effect, but does it really mean that your alleged "cause" precedes the effect you are observing? And that this association did not happen the other way around? Over the years there has been an abundance of research addressing same questions.

Rothman defined *cause* as "an event, a condition, or characteristic that preceded the disease onset and that, had the event, condition, or characteristic been different in a specified way, the disease either would not have occurred at all."

11.7.1 Counterfactual Approach

The counterfactual approach hypothesizes what would have happened under conditions contrary to the actual ones. For example, if your patient with breast cancer undergoes surgery and dies, you have no way to know if your surgery caused her death because you can't reverse course and not operate to see if she lives. The problem with this approach is evident—it is not possible to go back in time; but it does serve as the basis for how we can perfect our studies to be as close as possible to a counterfactual approach (e.g., using randomization, performing cohort studies or randomized clinical trials).

11.7.2 Sufficient Cause and Component Causes

Early causal thinking tries to find single causes as explanations for the observed phenomena. For example, Koch, with the discovery of *Mycobacterium tuberculosis* in 1882, noticed that, without *Mycobacterium tuberculosis* it is not possible to develop tuberculosis; ergo, the cause of tuberculosis must be Koch's *bacillus*. However, diseases are caused by multiple factors. For example, if you have had a tuberculosis vaccine and you are young and healthy, it is less probable that you will develop tuberculosis, even if you are exposed to it.

A *sufficient cause* is "a complete causal mechanism, a minimal set of conditions and events that are sufficient for the outcome to occur." For example, components for having tuberculosis would be overcrowding, low immunity, being exposed to *Mycobacterium tuberculosis*, and other undiscovered component causes (▶Fig. 11.7). A *necessary cause* is one that "for the disease to occur must be present or must have occurred." In the same example, if you live in an overcrowded place and have low immunity, yet you have never been exposed to *Mycobacterium tuberculosis*, then it is impossible

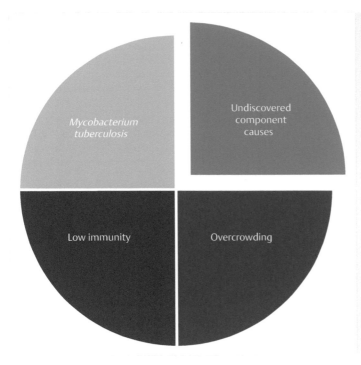

Fig. 11.7 Component causes for the sufficient cause for having tuberculosis. *Mycobacterium tuberculosis* would be a necessary cause.

Mycobacterium tuberculosis

Undiscovered component causes

Low immunity

Overcrowding

to get tuberculosis. By this model, treating a component of a sufficient cause could prevent the disease from occurring, so you should put your effort into finding these component causes.

11.7.3 Probabilistic Causation

In the probabilistic approach, a cause increases the probability that an effect will occur. For example, smoking increases the probability of developing lung cancer; therefore, smoking would be one of the causes of lung cancer. The problem with this approach is that it fails to explain why not every patient that smokes develops lung cancer.

11.7.4 Bradford Hill Considerations of Causation

In 1965 Sir Austin Bradford Hill suggested the following series of considerations to help us decide if an association between events is a causation association:

1. *Strength of association:* The stronger the association between an alleged cause and an effect, the more likely that it is because of a causative association. We can measure the strength of association by calculating the absolute risk or the relative risk.
2. *Consistency:* If a number of different investigations are performed in different periods of time, with a different population, in different environments, and they all come to the same conclusion, then it is probable that a causative association exists.
3. *Specificity:* When one variable causes an effect, and if the effect does not occur when the variable is eliminated, it is referred to as the specificity of the association. However, this characteristic should not be overemphasized because one cause can lead to many effects, and one effect may be the consequence of many causes.
4. *Temporality:* Causes must precede effects. This is indeed very obvious, but when performing a

transversal or a case-control study, it may not be that easy to find this temporal relationship of the association.

5. *Biological gradient:* If the association can reveal a biological gradient, or a dose–response curve, then it is more likely that a causative association exists.

6. *Plausibility:* Biological plausibility must exist. It is more probable that a causative association occurs if it concurs with our pathophysiological understanding of the disease.

7. *Coherence:* The interpretation of a causative association should not be conflicted with the generally known facts of the natural history and biology of the disease.

8. *Experiment:* The causative association is supported by experimental trials.

9. *Analogy:* In certain situations, it may be fair to judge the association between the cause and the effect by analogy.

11.8 What about the Analysis?

Because studies are conducted in a sample and not in the real population, statistical tests are used to translate the results over to the target population. In every study there are two types of errors: (1) a *systematic error*, which is due to bias and must be controlled in the study design; and (2) a *random error*, which occurs randomly (by chance).

Two approaches are used to deal with a random error. The first one is called hypothesis testing. The null hypothesis, or H_0, is the one the researcher is trying to reject in order to ascertain the alternative hypothesis, or H_1. Usually the null hypothesis is "no differences between the groups"; hence different statistical tests must be performed in order to reject it. In addition, when performing a statistical inference there are two possible types of error. Error type I, or α, occurs when the researcher rejects H_0 when it is actually true (e.g., the conclusion is that there are differences between the groups when the reality is that they are the same). Error type II, or β, occurs when the researcher accepts H_0 when it is actually false (e.g., the conclusion is that both

groups are the same when in reality they are different). Because it is worse to reject H_0 when it is true, every effort must to be made to control this type of error. The way to do this is to assign an "acceptable" value of error. In medical publications we assign this value to be < 10%; that is 5% in a two-tailed test, from where the typical p-value < 0.05 is derived. Other typical values are established at 20% or 2% (p-value < 0.1 or < 0.01). We recommend that you use the actual value. It is important to note that these results should be interpreted with care, because statistical significance does not always mean clinical significance. In very large samples you can have a statistically very significant result without it being clinically significant.

The other way to deal with random error is by estimation. Through this approach you can calculate the magnitude of the effect in your sample and estimate a range of results where the real value is in the target population. This range of values, or statistical precision, is expressed with a confidence interval, established by a common agreement in 95%. This means that your result has 95% probability of being between the confidence interval in the real population.

Some common statistical tests are summarize in ▶Fig. 11.8.

11.9 Key Points

- Every research project starts with a good research question: PICO strategy is the essential key.
- At the beginning one has to perform a thorough bibliographic background search. The question has probably been answered before.
- It doesn't matter which pathway of clinical epidemiology the question belongs in, as long as the design to answer it is as accurate and unbiased as possible.
- Statistical tests translate the results from the research to the target population; therefore, it is important to be meticulous in the analysis of results. Don't be afraid to consult with an expert in statistics to help you with the analysis.

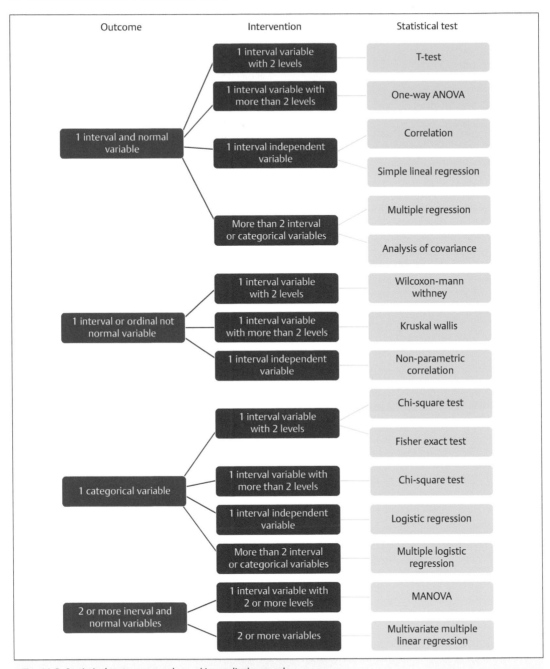

Fig. 11.8 Statistical tests commonly used in medical research.

Recommended Readings

Agha R, Rosin RD. Time for a new approach to case reports. Int J Surg Case Rep. 2010; 1(1):1–3

Altman DG. Analysis of survival times. Practical Statistics for Medical Research. CRC Press. 1990; 365

Choosing the correct statistical test. http://bama.ua.edu/~jleeper/627/choosestat.html

Choosing the correct statistical test in stata. http://www.ats.ucla.edu/stat/stata/whatstat/

Danilla S, Cuevas P, Aedo S, et al. Introducing the Body-QoL®: a new patient-reported outcome instrument for measuring body satisfaction-related quality of life in aesthetic and post-bariatric body contouring patients. Aesthetic Plast Surg. 2016; 40(1):19–29

Fletcher R, Fletcher SW. Clinical Epidemiology: The Essentials. Philadelphia, PA: Lippincott Williams & Wilkins; 2013:275

Guyatt GH, Rennie D. Users' guides to the medical literature. JAMA. 1993; 270(17):2096–2097

Höfler M. The Bradford Hill considerations on causality: a counterfactual perspective. Emerg Themes Epidemiol. 2005; 2(1):11

Kaplan EL, Meier P. Nonparametric estimation from incomplete observations. J Am Stat Assoc. 1958;53: 457–481

Maldonado G, Greenland S. Estimating causal effects. Int J Epidemiol. 2002; 31(2):422–429

Pusic AL, Klassen AF, Scott AM, et al. Development of a new patient-reported outcome measure for breast surgery: the BREAST-Q. Plast Reconstr Surg. 2009; 124(2):345–353

Renton A. Epidemiology and causation: a realist view. J Epidemiol Community Health. 1994; 48(1):79–85

Rothman KJ. Causes. Am J Epidemiol. 1976; 104(6):587–592

Section II
Techniques

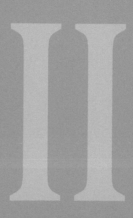

12 Basic Surgical Techniques, Sutures, and Wound Closure

Diego Marré, Tomas Gantz, Alex Eulufi

Abstract

Learning the principles and mastering the techniques of wound closure and suturing are essential to every surgical trainee, regardless of specialty. A good resultant scar begins with a properly designed incision, gentle and atraumatic handling of tissues, selection of the appropriate closure material, and correct reapproximation of the edges. The outcome of wound closure (i.e., the scar) is influenced by a number of factors, including location, shape, orientation, tension, contamination, patient-related factors, and surgical technique. Unfortunately, no matter how meticulous we are, poor scarring sometimes develops and must be addressed by various nonsurgical and surgical methods. In this regard, it is important to consider the amount of time since wounding and to set realistic goals with the patient. Scar revision is usually performed on fully or near-fully matured scars in order to optimize the benefits of the procedure. Scars needing intervention are usually managed conservatively for a period of 6–12 months, after which surgical treatments are available.

This chapter describes the basic aspects of wound suturing as they relate to suturing material and basic techniques. Different methods of scar revision are also discussed.

Keywords: needles, scar revision, scarring, suture, wound closure

12.1 Introduction

Plastic surgery is a broad and varied surgical specialty. Because plastic surgeons deal mainly with the repair and rearrangement of soft tissues, most of our procedures leave behind a mark, most commonly in the form of a scar, which is subject to scrutiny and judgment from patients and colleagues. Furthermore, an important part of our practice is correcting unpleasant "marks" left after another procedure (plastic or not). Additionally, not infrequently, patients with lacerations or who are to be operated by other surgical specialists, ask to be sutured by a plastic surgeon with the wish to obtain as fine a scar as possible. Excepting the

unreasonably demanding ones, these patients are right to some extent in that, unlike other surgical specialties, an ongoing aspect of a plastic surgeon's training is actually learning to achieve inconspicuous scars by identifying and managing all factors that may potentially affect wound healing and the final appearance of the resulting scar. Of all such factors, the one the surgeon has most (if not complete) control of is the surgical technique. This chapter describes the principles of wound closure, suturing techniques, and scar revision.

12.2 Sutures

Selection of the correct suture material is an important factor for the overall success of wound closure, regardless of its complexity. Unfortunately, however, proper education about and familiarization with the products available for tissue closure have fallen almost into oblivion in some areas and subspecialties. The main task for any suture in any tissue is to hold the edges together in correct apposition until healing is established. The choice of material will then be influenced not only by the type of tissue but also by the local and systemic conditions as well as the distraction forces that may occur during the healing process.

12.2.1 Classification of Sutures

Sutures can be classified according to different parameters as will be described here. There are different possible combinations, and, although the choice is usually based on training and personal preferences, it is important to consider certain factors that can guide selection of the best material (▶Table 12.1).

Resorbable/Nonresorbable

Sutures are classified as resorbable or nonresorbable depending on whether the organism will degrade it or not. Nonresorbable sutures do not undergo any processes of degradation; they remain in place indefinitely until they are removed. Resorbable sutures may be resorbed by

Table 12.1 Factors influencing the selection of suture material

Type of tissue
Anatomical area
Presence of or potential for contamination
Local inflammation
Tension of closure
Wound's healing capacity
Patient comorbidities, including wound-healing disorders

either proteolysis or hydrolysis. In *proteolysis*, the suture is digested by an enzymatic process of foreign body reaction, which generates a localized inflammation at the site of the stitch. In *hydrolysis*, the suture is gradually absorbed by the penetration of fluids and is thus less inflammatory than proteolysis. Resorbable sutures have established degradation rates; nevertheless, certain factors, such as contamination/infection, fever, and poor nutritional status may accelerate their resorption and as such should be considered when selecting the most appropriate material. Likewise, in areas with high enzymatic content, such as the stomach or cervix, faster degradation of resorbable sutures is observed.

> **Note**
>
> **Resorbable Sutures**
> The local environment, presence of contamination, inflammation, fever, and an altered nutritional status may accelerate the rate of degradation of resorbable sutures.

Monofilament/Braided

According to their configuration, sutures are classified as monofilament or braided (also called multifilament). Monofilament sutures are composed of s single thread. Due to the little resistance that tissues offer to the passing of monofilaments, these sutures are ideal for delicate structures, such as vessels and nerves, though they are used in various other tissues as well. Furthermore, because of their single-thread configuration, monofilaments usually elicit less reaction from the tissues and have a low risk of infection in comparison to their braided counterparts. One of the main shortcomings of monofilaments is their high packing memory—defined as the tendency of a suture to retain the shape it had in its original envelope—which makes it a little harder to manipulate and requires

more ties to secure the knot. Also, if improperly handled, monofilaments are more prone to developing cracks or weak spots, which could reduce their tensile strength.

Multifilament sutures consist of several strands braided together. Braided sutures have a higher friction coefficient and almost no memory, which facilitates their handling and increases knot security. Due to their multithread configuration, braided sutures have varying degrees of *capillarity*, defined as the ease with which fluids are wicked along the threads. Additionally, bacteria may home between the threads and spread into the wound site. This potential shortcoming needs to be considered when suturing wounds at risk of contamination or infection. In an attempt to lower such risk, some manufacturers have developed braided sutures coated with antibiotics; although their efficacy remains to be demonstrated. Another disadvantage of multifilaments is their "saw effect" as they pass through the tissues, which can be an issue when trying to close wounds with friable edges. Coating makes the suture less sharp and has been introduced by some manufacturers to reduce this effect.

Natural/Synthetic

Sutures may be of natural or synthetic origin. Natural threads include silk, linen, and collagen (more commonly known as catgut), the latter derived from either the serosal layer of beef (bovine) or the submucosal fibrous layer of sheep (ovine) intestines. Natural sutures were the first available in the market and continue to be used in a number of settings; however, they have some important disadvantages, including high capillarity, the generation of a sometimes strong inflammatory reaction, problems with tolerance, and loss of mechanical strength when wet. Synthetic materials on the other hand include the absorbable polyglycolic acid, polylactic acid, poliglecaprone 25, and polydioxanone as well as the nonabsorbables nylon, polyester, polyvinylidene fluoride (PVDF), and polypropylene. Synthetic sutures are more frequently used because they have overcome many of the shortcomings of natural sutures.

12.2.2 Tensile Strength

An important feature common to all sutures regardless of their composition or origin is tensile strength, which is defined as the strain, in kilos, that a given suture is able to sustain before breaking. During the first days following wound closure, the suture is primarily responsible for holding the wound edges together. As healing progresses, the tissues gradually regain their intrinsic tensile strength while the suture loses its own, with the rate of such loss varying across different materials. Thus selection of the most appropriate material must consider the balance between the healing capacity of the repaired tissue, the tension of closure, and the rate at which the suture loses its tensile strength. In this sense, tensile strength is usually expressed as the fraction of the original strength remaining at a given time (e.g., Vicryl [Ethicon] retains approximately 60% of its tensile strength at 14 days). Even though tensile strength is related to absorption, these are completely different terms that should not be used interchangeably. Of course, the faster a suture is resorbed, the faster it will lose its tensile strength; nevertheless, in some cases sutures that take longer to be absorbed lose their strength comparatively quickly, and sutures that remain in place (e.g., nonresorbable) still lose their strength over time. Finally, it is important to note that the knot is usually the weakest point of a stitch, meaning that the tensile strength at that point is reduced in relation to the rest of the suture. In addition, cracks and crushes from inappropriate handling may produce weak spots as well.

▶Table 12.2 summarizes the main sutures available today with regard to their permanence, configuration, origin, absorption, and tensile strength.

12.2.3 Gauges and Needle

The diameter or gauge of a suture can be expressed in two ways: according to the United States Pharmacopeia (USP) or the European Pharmacopeia (EP), with the former being the most widely used, ranging from 12–0 to 10. Simply and briefly, the higher the number *of zeros*, the thinner the suture is (e.g., 5–0 is thinner than 3–0). Conversely, for whole-numbered gradings (e.g., 0, 1, 2, 3, and 4), the higher the *number*, the thicker the suture (e.g., a 3 suture is thicker than a 1 suture) (▶Table 12.3).

Regarding needles, most sutures come already armed in their packaging, meaning they are already attached to a needle. Some sutures are double-armed; they are armed with two needles, one at each end of the thread. Needles are made of stainless steel alloy, which allows, to a certain extent, bending without breaking. Even though there are different types of needles, they all share the same basic structure, which includes a point, a body, and an eye or attachment zone. Additionally, there are four basic measurements that define the structure of a needle, namely the arc (also called the needle length), chord length, radius, and diameter (▶Fig. 12.1).

The needle's attachment zone may be eyed or swaged. Eyed needles must be threaded manually, offering the advantage of using any combination of needle and thread; however, manual threading can be difficult and time consuming for thinner sutures and carries the inherent risk of puncture during manipulation. In addition, the protrusion of the thread at each side of the eye may cause drag and may damage the tissue as it passes through. Swaged needless, on the other hand, are eyeless and have the suture already incorporated to them so that the attachment zone is thinner than the body of the needle, thus eliminating drag. Finally, there are sutures with a needle insertion system that allows easy removal by pulling on the thread without having to cut it (control release needle, Ethicon).

The body of the needle usually represents the fraction of a circumference with the curvature ranging from 5/8 to 1/4 of a circle, although other shapes, such as straight, hook-shaped, progressive/asymptotic, and ski-shaped needles are available as well. Regardless of their shape and curvature, needles can have three basic configurations: round, triangular, and spatula. With round-bodied needles the tissues are spread around the needle rather than being cut by it, making round-bodied needles ideal for closure of fascia, tendon, peritoneum, or friable tissues, among others. Triangular needles are also called cutting needles due to the presence of a sharp edge that cuts through the tissues. *Conventional cutting* needles have the apex of the triangle (e.g., the sharp edge) on the inside of the needle, whereas in *reverse cutting* needles the cutting edge is on the exterior of the curve, making them preferable for skin closure. Additionally, the reverse cutting configuration increases needle strength and makes it more resistant to bending. Spatulated needles have extremely sharp edges, which cause minimal trauma to the sutured tissues and are used mainly in ophthalmic surgery and microsurgery.

Table 12.2 Sutures

Material	Commercial name	Classification	Tensile strength (% retained)	Absorption	Tissue reaction
Polyglycolic acid	Dexon (Covidien)/Safil (Aesculap USA)/Assufil (Assut Europe)	Synthetic, absorbable, braided multifilament	35% in 14 days Lost in 30 days	Hydrolysis, 60–90 days	Minimal
Glycolid 90%/L-lactide 10%	Vicryl rapide (Ethicon)/Assufil fast	Synthetic, absorbable, braided	50% in 5 days	Hydrolisys, 40 days	Minimal
Glycolid 90%/L-lactide 10% (polyglactin 910)	Vicryl	Synthetic, absorbable, braided (size 8–0 through 3) and synthetic, absorbable, monofilament (size 10–0, 9–0)	60% remains after 2 weeks 30% remains after 3 weeks Lost within 30 days	Hydrolysis, minimal until day 40, complete in 60–90 days	Minimal
Glycolide/lactide (lactomer)	Polysorb (Medtronic)	Synthetic, absorbable, braided	80% in 14 days	Hydrolysis, 50–70 days	Minimal
Glycolide/dioxanone/ trimethylene carbonate (Glycomer 631)	Biosyn (Medtronic)	Synthetic, absorbable, monofilament	75% in 14 days	Hydrolysis, 90–120 days	Minimal
Glycolide/caprolactone/ trimethylene carbonate/ lactide (Polygytone 6211)	Caprosyn (Medtronic)	Synthetic, absorbable, monofilament	20–30% in 10 days	Hydrolysis, 60 days	Minimal
Polydioxanone	PDS II (Ethicon)	Synthetic, absorbable, monofilament	70% remains after 2 weeks 50% remains after 4 weeks 25% remains after 6 weeks Lost within 1 year	Hydrolysis, Minimal within 3 months, complete within 6–9 months	Minimal
Glyconate	Monosyn (Aesculap USA)	Synthetic, absorbable, monofilament	50% in 14 days	Hydrolysis, 60–90	Minimal
Poliglecaprone 25	Monocryl (Ethicon)	Synthetic, absorbable, monofilament	20–30% in 14 days	Hydrolysis, 90–120	Minimal
Poly-4-hydroxybutyrate	Monomax (B. Braun)	Synthetic, absorbable, monofilament	50% in 90 days	Hydrolysis, 1 year	

Table 12.2 *(Continued)* Sutures

Material	Commercial name	Classification	Tensile strength (% retained)	Absorption	Tissue reaction
Polyester	Ti-Cron (Covidien)/Dagrofil (Braun)/Synthofil (Aesculap)/PremiCron (Braun)	Synthetic, nonabsorbable, braided multifilament	No loss of tensile strength	–	Low
Nylon 6	Monosof (Medtronic)/Dermalon (Medtronic)/Dafilon (Braun)/Supramid (Braun)/Surgilon (Medtronic)	Synthetic, nonabsorbable, monofilament	Gradual loss of tensile strength over time	–	Minimal
Polypropylene	Prolene (Ethicon)/Surgilon (Covidien)/Surgipro (Medtronic)/Premilene (B. Braun)	Synthetic, nonabsorbable, monofilament	No loss of tensile strength	–	Minimal
Polybutester	Vascufil (Covidien)/Novafil (Medtronic)/Miralene (Braun)	Synthetic, nonabsorbable, monofilament	No loss of tensile strength	–	Minimal
Steel	Steelex (Aesculap USA)/steel	Synthetic, nonabsorbable, monofilament	No loss of tensile strength	–	Minimal
Collagen (plain)	Surgical gut (Ethicon)	Natural absorbable monofilament	Tensile strength lost at 7–10 days	Proteolysis, 70 days	Moderate
Collagen treated with chromium salt solution to resist degradation	Chromic gut (Ethicon)	Natural absorbable monofilament	Tensile strength lost at 3–4 weeks	Proteolysis, 90 days	Moderate (less than plain catgut)
Heat-treated collagen to accelerate degradation	Fast-absorbing surgical gut (Ethicon)	Natural absorbable monofilament	Tensile strength lost at 7 days	Proteolysis, 60 days	Moderate
Silk	Silkam (B. Braun)/Sofsilk (Covidien)/Mersilk (Ethicon)	Natural, nonabsorbable, braided multifilament	50% in 60 days	–	Moderate
Poly (ethylene terephthalate)	Ethibond Excel (Ethicon)	Synthetic, nonabsorbable, braided multifilament	No loss of tensile strength	–	Minimal
Linen	Linatrix (B. Braun)	Natural, nonabsorbable, braided multifilament	No loss of tensile strength	–	High

Table 12.3 Suture gauges

USP	Thread gauge (mm)
12–0	0.001–0.009
11–0	0.010–0.019
10–0	0.020–0.029
9–0	0.030–0.039
8–0	0.040–0.049
7–0	0.050–0.069
6–0	0.070–0.099
5–0	0.10–0.149
4–0	0.15–0.199
3–0	0.20–0.249
2–0	0.30–0.349
0	0.35–0.399
1	0.40–0.499
2	0.50–0.599
3+4	0.60–0.699
5	0.70–0.799
6	0.80–0.899
7	0.90–0.999
8	1.00–1.099
9	1.10–1.199
10	1.20–1.299

The point of the needle usually follows the shape of the body, except in tapered needles in which there is a sharp pointed tip but a blunt (round) body (▶Fig. 12.2).

12.2.4 Tissue Adhesives

As their name implies, these are biological adhesives derived from cyanoacrylate that have the ability to polymerize in the presence of moisture. This produces an adherent resistant band between the edges of adhesive contact, which facilitates wound edge apposition and healing. Because they provide very little or no tensile strength, the use of tissue adhesives is mainly restricted to the epidermal approximation of tension-free superficial cutaneous wounds. For deeper wounds, an adhesive may be used provided that the subcutaneous and/or dermal planes have been securely approximated with the use of sutures. Some commercially available tissue adhesives are LiquiBand (Cardinal Health), Histoacryl (B. Braun), Dermabond (Ethicon), Indermil (Covidien), and Leukosan (BSN medical).

12.3 Wound Closure

Wound closure is one of the first skills taught to any medical student or surgical trainee. There are several factors that influence the final outcome of wound closure, namely orientation, shape, location,

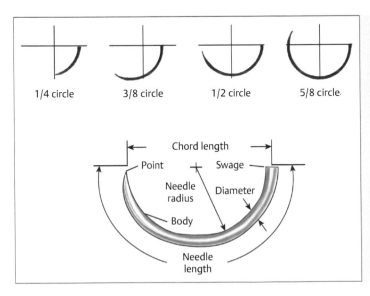

Fig. 12.1 Anatomy and curvature of a needle. (Reproduced from Janis, Essentials of Plastic Surgery, 2nd edition, ©2014, Thieme Publishers, New York.)

1/4 circle   3/8 circle   1/2 circle   5/8 circle

Chord length

Point   Swage

Needle radius   Diameter

Body

Needle length

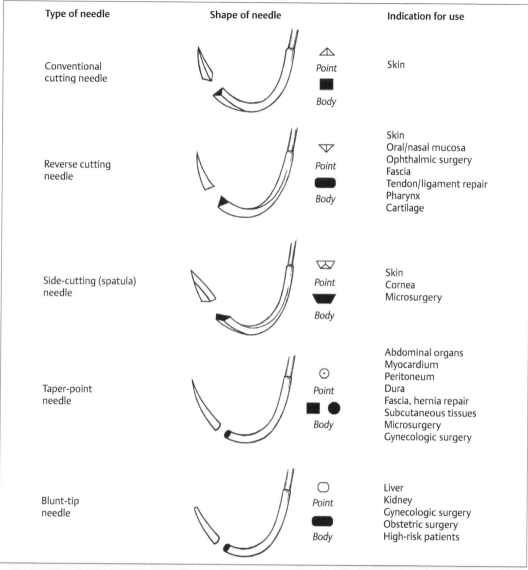

Type of needle	Shape of needle	Indication for use
Conventional cutting needle	Point / Body	Skin
Reverse cutting needle	Point / Body	Skin Oral/nasal mucosa Ophthalmic surgery Fascia Tendon/ligament repair Pharynx Cartilage
Side-cutting (spatula) needle	Point / Body	Skin Cornea Microsurgery
Taper-point needle	Point / Body	Abdominal organs Myocardium Peritoneum Dura Fascia, hernia repair Subcutaneous tissues Microsurgery Gynecologic surgery
Blunt-tip needle	Point / Body	Liver Kidney Gynecologic surgery Obstetric surgery High-risk patients

Fig. 12.2 Main configurations of suture needles. (Reproduced from Janis, Essentials of Plastic Surgery, 2nd edition, ©2014, Thieme Publishers, New York.)

tension, presence or risk of contamination/infection, patient-related factors, and surgical technique.

12.3.1 Orientation

All incisions leave a scar, without exceptions. Scars cannot be erased; instead they can be strategically hidden or, if on exposed areas, positioned to make them as inconspicuous as possible. With time they may even become less noticeable, but they do not disappear. Thus an important factor determining a scar's final aspect is orientation. During the 19th and 20th centuries several anatomists and surgeons studied the mechanical behavior of skin, some of them with a purely anatomical descriptive purpose and others with the aim of delivering a guide to placement of surgical incisions. That is how, not surprisingly, up to 36 different guidelines have been described. In 1962, Borges described the *relaxed skin tension lines* (RSTLs) as lines that follow the furrows formed when the skin is relaxed by pinching, muscle contraction, or joint mobility. These lines then became the main guideline for the placement of incisions, especially in the face. Perpendicular to RSTLs are the *lines of maximal extensibility* (LMEs), which, as the name suggests, indicate the direction at which skin has its greater mobility (▶ Fig. 12.3). It follows that, in order to obtain a scar as inconspicuous as possible, incisions should be made parallel to RSTLs and closed in the direction of LMEs. In addition, when planning facial incisions, the aesthetic units and subunits of this anatomical area should be considered (▶ Fig. 12.4). When we look at someone's face, we unconsciously expect a certain break at the margin between two different units. Hence, if the scar lies over such a line, it will be much less noticeable than if it lies within the unit. Moreover, in cases in which a block of tissue is excised, a better result is sometimes obtained by removing and replacing the whole subunit rather than a part of it, even if this involves removing healthy surrounding skin.

The orientation of surgical incisions (and resulting scars) is related not only to making them inconspicuous but also to avoiding any functional impairment. This concept is of utmost importance when planning incisions over joints or flexion creases. An incision must never cross perpendicularly over a joint or flexion crease because this might lead to contracture and restrict the joint's range of movement. Instead, zigzag, such as a Brunner type in the hand, or **S**-shaped incisions, such as those used for axillary and inguinal lymph node dissection, should be used (▶ Fig. 12.5).

> ## Note
>
> **Relaxed Skin Tension Lines**
> The relaxed skin tension lines described by Borges should not be confused with Langer's lines. Karl Langer was an anatomist who studied the direction of ellipses formed after stabbing a round-tipped awl into hundreds of cadavers. Langer's lines represent lines of tension (cleavage) and are different from RSTLs. In fact, in many areas, RSTLs and Langer's lines lie perpendicular to one another.

12.3.2 Shape

Semicircular scars can sometimes lead to swelling and bulging of tissue on the concave side, producing a step-off commonly referred to as a *trapdoor deformity*. The possible mechanisms leading to

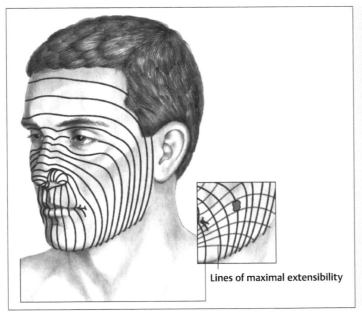

Lines of maximal extensibility

Fig. 12.3 Relaxed skin tension lines and lines of maximal extensibility. (Reproduced from Sherris, Larrabee, Principles of Facial Reconstruction, 2nd edition, ©2010, Thieme Publishers, New York.)

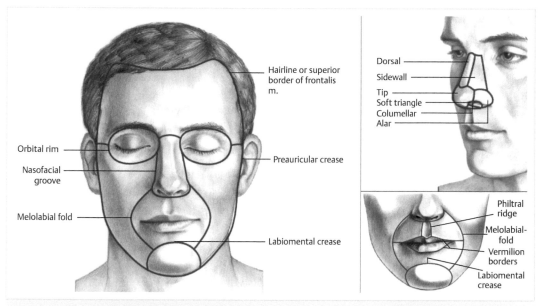

Fig. 12.4 The aesthetic units and subunits of the face. (Reproduced from Sherris, Larrabee, Principles of Facial Reconstruction, 2nd edition, ©2010, Thieme Publishers, New York.)

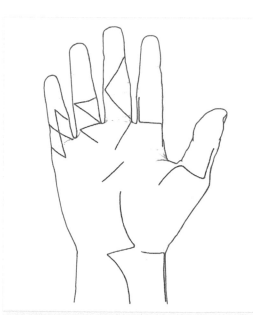

Fig. 12.5 Brunner-type (zigzag) and other hand incisions illustrating the principle of avoiding perpendicular scars across joint creases. (Reproduced from Pechlaner et al, Atlas of Hand Surgery, 2nd edition, ©2000, Thieme Publishers, Stuttgart.)

this include wound contraction along the curvilinear margin and disruption of venous and lymphatic drainage. *Pincushioning* is a similar phenomenon, often seen in round-shaped flaps in which the flap becomes bulgy inside an apparently constricted scar halo. Although this may sometimes lead to an unsightly result, in some cases it can be used favorably to re-create dome-shaped structures in areas such as the nose.

12.3.3 Location

The same incision, sutured using the same technique, might have a dramatically different outcome depending on the area of the body where it is done. The face is a very forgiving anatomical area because wounds generally heal very well, rarely become infected, and produce satisfactory scars. In contrast, other areas, such as the sternum and deltoid region, have a greater tendency to produce hypertrophic scarring and keloids. Extra care should then be exerted when suturing in these regions, avoiding any unnecessary damage to tissues and minimizing any additional inflammatory stimulus. Unfortunately, despite all measures, a keloid might still ensue; it is important to inform patients of this possibility during the preoperative consultation. Other potential zones of poor scarring are mobile areas, such as skin overlying joints. Even though a short period of immobilization following surgery helps to prevent dehiscence, stretch from subsequent joint motion might eventually produce a widened scar. In all these cases, because the origin of the problem is related to the wound's location, efforts to revise scars in these areas are usually futile; therefore the surgical indication needs to be discussed with the patient, with a warning that the surgical scar may be similar to or even worse than the original one.

12.3.4 Tension

As with any structure that is repaired by direct approximation of its borders, tension in wound closure should be avoided. Although a certain degree of tension can be accepted as long as it does not risk the viability of the wound edges, undue tension is unacceptable, even if direct closure is still possible. Just because the wound edges can be (forcibly) approximated does not necessarily mean that direct closure should be performed, especially in exposed areas, such as the face. Not infrequently, the rearrangement of local tissues will result in a much better functional and aesthetic outcome, even in the presence of added scars, which of course should be well planned in terms of length and orientation. Tension in a wound can significantly reduce blood supply to the wound edges, especially in active smokers, and poorly vascularized wound edges are at higher risk of dehiscence, marginal necrosis, and infection. On the other hand, for those wounds that do heal uneventfully, widening is likely to occur with time. Thus, for wounds in which closure without tension cannot be achieved even after generous tissue undermining, or may do so under excessive tension, a skin graft or flap should be considered.

Note

Wound Closure

In some cases, just because the edges of a wound can be approximated does not necessarily mean that direct closure should be performed; the rearrangement of local tissues can often produce a better functional and cosmetic result.

12.3.5 Contamination

Primary closure is possible in all clean wounds and most traumatic injuries, provided that adequate rinsing with saline is performed. For grossly contaminated wounds, such as farm, bite, and blast injuries, primary closure is contraindicated. Instead, these wounds should be thoroughly debrided of devitalized tissues and foreign bodies, cleansed with antiseptic soap and copious amounts of saline, and left open. A couple of approximating stitches can be placed to avoid significant retraction that might prevent direct closure afterward. Depending on the nature of the wound and the degree of contamination, the need for systemic antibiotics should be assessed. A second washout should be performed 48 hours later to assess evolution, particularly regarding signs of infection. At the time of closure, it is important to ensure that there are no clinical signs of infection and that bacterial count is less than 10^5 bacteria per gram of tissue. Wounds presenting 8–12 hours after the initial trauma might also have an important degree of contamination and devitalized borders. Thus either debridement (*Friedrich*) and primary closure or delayed closure as already explained should be performed. In areas of rich vascularization, such as the face and scalp, this window of time can extend to nearly 24 hours.

12.3.6 Patient Factors

Factors affecting wound healing are discussed in Chapter 2. Regarding scar appearance, apart from systemic and genetic predispositions that might per se influence the final result, another important aspect to consider is age. Children usually mount a more pronounced inflammatory response and therefore tend to heal faster, but their scars remain red and swollen for a longer period of time. Conversely, aged people usually take longer to heal and have decreased tensile strength, but in turn have less scarring and little contraction due to reduced elastin, decreased collagen synthesis, and less inflammation. These aspects need to be considered not only during wound closure but also at the time of suture removal and before resuming normal mobilization that might place the scar under tension.

12.3.7 Surgical Technique

Once the wound is ready for closure, the first thing that needs to be decided is which suture material to use. Selection of the suture material should be based on the specific tissue and wound requirements. As explained earlier, materials that are absorbed by hydrolysis elicit less of an inflammatory reaction and are therefore preferred in many situations. Consideration should also be given to the suture's structure; multifilament sutures should not be used in contaminated wounds because bacteria and other microorganisms may be captured between the threads, increasing the risk of infection. Tensile strength and absorption rate are also important. Depending on the anatomical area, the wound's tension, and the state of surrounding tissues, in some instances a fast-absorbing suture might be preferred, whereas in other scenarios the surgeon might be looking for an absorbable suture that remains in place and retains its strength for a longer period of time. However, regardless of the material used, it is important to know that wounded skin will never regain the tensile strength of normal skin. During the first few days after closure, the suture is the main thing responsible for keeping the wound edges together. At week 1, tensile strength is less than 5% of normal skin, steadily increasing to 10% at 2 weeks, 25% at 4 weeks, and 40% at 6 weeks, reaching its maximum of 80% at approximately 10 weeks. For any wound, once healed, most of the tensile strength is provided by the dermis, which is why proper approximation of this structure is essential during wound closure. Depending on the anatomical area and wound characteristics, the dermis may be sutured independent of the overlying epidermis using buried stitches (to be discussed) or

together with the epidermis using any of the stitch configurations described later in this chapter. Deep wounds involving subcutaneous tissue and fascia (superficial or deep) must be closed in a layered fashion.

All wounds should be closed by *everting* the edges because this ensures correct apposition of the dermis, which is essential to achieving proper wound healing. Wounds that look everted immediately after closure will always flatten, whereas inverted ones will remain that way, potentially leading to delayed healing and poor scarring. Eversion is achieved by passing the needle in a way that more tissue is captured at the depths than at the surface (▶ Fig. 12.6). Together with eversion, wound edges should also be properly aligned by recruiting a similar amount of tissue (in thickness and in depth) on each side of the wound. If unequal bites are taken, the edge with the thicker bite will overlap the one in front. Finally, because the knot is the most inflammatory component of the suture with the potential to capture microorganisms within it, placing it directly over the wound might increase the risk of infection. Instead it should lie on either side of the wound.

> **Note**
>
> **Tensile Strength**
> Wounded skin regains approximately 80% of its unwounded tensile strength.

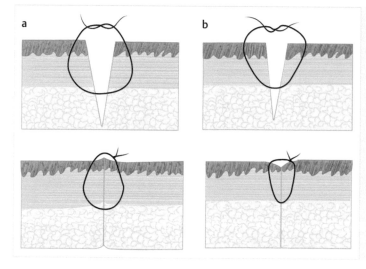

Fig. 12.6 Correct method of stitch placement to obtain eversion of wound edges. **(a)** The suture should capture more tissue in the depths than at the surface, which gives the stitch a slightly pear-shaped appearance. **(b)** Incorrectly placed stitches result in inversion of wound edges.

12.4 Suturing Techniques

The basic suturing techniques are explained in ▶ Table 12.4 and illustrated in ▶ Fig. 12.7. Although a brief written explanation and a diagram are useful to get an idea of each technique, nothing can replace practical hands-on learning both in inanimate models and in real surgery.

Table 12.4 Suturing techniques

Suture	Technical description	Advantages	Disadvantages
Simple interrupted	Needle is passed capturing more tissue in depth than in surface. Bites of equal width and thickness	Most commonly used; good for border eversion	Can be time consuming compared to running suture
Continuous running	Starts with simple stitch, cutting only the end without the needle. Running suture then proceeds along the wound. Knot at the end tied with last loop	Fast to perform; can provide hemostasis if done in a locked fashion	May be less precise than interrupted sutures; border approximation can be difficult to maintain in wounds under tension; if local infection or hematoma develops, cutting one stitch undoes the whole suture
Vertical mattress	Needle enters "far" from margin taking a deep bite in one edge and exits equally on opposite edge; on the way back, the needle is passed "close" to the margins and more superficial	Excellent border eversion and provides good hemostasis	Can produce ischemia of wound edges; leaves unsightly marks
Horizontal mattress	Needle is passed forward taking equal bites on both edges and brought backward in the same manner a couple of millimeters distal or proximal on the wound	Excellent border eversion; good for wounds that tend to invert; can be done in a running and locking fashion for tight closure	Can leave marks if tied too tightly; running-locking may produce ischemia of wound edges
Inverted dermal	Needle first penetrates dermis on the edge "close" to the surgeon with the needle pointing at surgeon and then passes through the opposite dermal border with needle facing away from surgeon; when knot is tied it lies on the deep side of the loop	Gold standard for dermal approximation; buried knot reduces epidermal erosion and suture exposure	Too many and too tight might compromise vascularization
Running subcuticular (intradermal)	Can start without a knot, with a buried knot or as a simple stitch; suture is passed through the dermis parallel to the skin in equal bites at both sides. The exit of each bite marks the entry point of the opposite; can finish with a buried knot, an external knot tying the suture end to itself, or no knot at all	Offers the best cosmetic result as it avoids marks on skin	The main purpose of this suture is to bring the epidermis together and facilitate epithelialization; therefore, it neither withstands tension nor everts wound edges; consequently, it must always be done in combination with a deeper layer of closure to provide tensile strength and eversion

Table 12.4 *(Continued)* Suturing techniques

Suture	Technical description	Advantages	Disadvantages
Skin adhesives	Main component, cyano-acrylate, is applied over approximated edges	Fast, atraumatic, very useful in children for superficial lacerations or epidermal layer of deeper wounds	Does not provide tensile strength nor produce eversion of wound edges
Skin tape	Must be placed over correctly aligned wound edges without tension	Fast, atraumatic	Does not provide tensile strength nor produce eversion of wound edges
Skin staples	Evert the edges using toothed forceps before placing the staple	Fast, produces little ischemia	Leaves unsightly marks if removed late

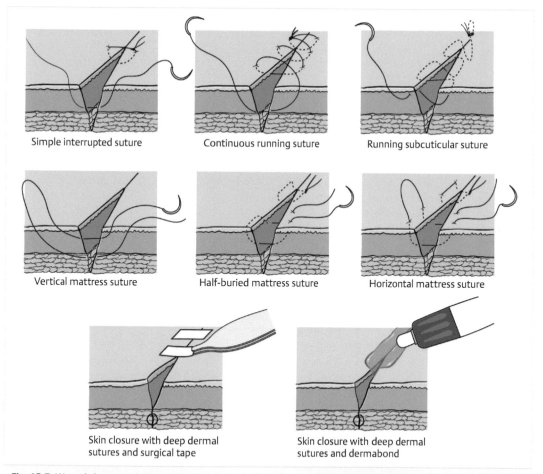

Simple interrupted suture

Continuous running suture

Running subcuticular suture

Vertical mattress suture

Half-buried mattress suture

Horizontal mattress suture

Skin closure with deep dermal sutures and surgical tape

Skin closure with deep dermal sutures and dermabond

Fig. 12.7 Wound closure techniques: simple interrupted; continuous running; running subcuticular (intradermal); vertical mattress; half-buried horizontal mattress; horizontal mattress; skin tapes. (Reproduced from Bullocks et al, Plastic Surgery Emergencies Principles and Techniques, 2nd edition, ©2017, Thieme Publishers, New York.)

12.4.1 Common Problems and Solutions in Wound Closure

Most wounds, incisional and traumatic, can be closed using the principles and techniques just described. However, not infrequently, in some wounds with a certain configuration or given characteristics, simple direct closure leads to skin redundancy, uneven alignment of edges, ischemic areas, and so forth. This section describes technical solutions to achieve proper border alignment in uneven wounds.

Problem: Borders of unequal length.

Solutions: This situation is produced when the defect is an asymmetric ellipse with one border longer than the other. Closure of these wounds is done in a way commonly referred to as cheating. The excess tissue is gradually worked toward the midline of the wound, with the lateral parts kept as even as possible. This can be done temporarily with skin staples or directly with subcutaneous interrupted stitches. In this way, the excess tissue is evenly distributed along the wound. Small folds perpendicular to the wound axis may form, but these are more easily managed with suturing and very likely to disappear with time. If at the end of the procedure there is a significant amount of extra tissue at the midline, this can be excised perpendicular to the axis of the wound, thus creating a T-shaped scar. For smaller wounds, an effective way of eliminating length discrepancy is placing uneven dermal stitches by passing the needle horizontally in the long border (to capture more tissue) and vertically in the short one. Another similar way to correct uneven borders is with the subcuticular suture by taking longer bites on the long edge so that the excess skin is segmentally puckered to the length of the short edge.

Problem: Dog-ears.

Solution: Dog-ears are a very common "problem" in wound closure and a relatively frequent secondary procedure once complete healing and scar maturation from previous surgeries has occurred. They appear in situations such as the one described above or more commonly when one is attempting to close round defects. For this reason, as a first measure to avoid dog-ears, all excisions involving the skin should be elliptical in order to obtain a flat linear scar as described later in this chapter. In addition, it must be noted that dog-ears are sometimes produced by not only "excess" skin but also excess subcutaneous tissue. In these situations, skin excision and defatting must be performed. In any case, removal of dog-ears is easy and can sometimes make a difference in the final scar appearance and overall patient satisfaction. Their removal, though, usually implies lengthening of the scar (▶ Fig. 12.8).

Problem: Borders of unequal thickness.

Solution: Wounds with one edge thicker than the other can result in a step-off and a conspicuous scar if they are closed in a standard fashion. Correct apposition of the edges in these cases can be accomplished by using half-buried dermal sutures or stitches with bites of different thickness: thin bites in the thick border and thick bites in the thin border. Both of these techniques will bring the thin wound edge up to the level of the thick one (▶ Fig. 12.9).

Problem: Beveled edges.

Solution: On occasions, traumatic wounds (or incorrectly performed surgical incisions) result in beveled edges, which, if repaired in a standard fashion, can lead to step-offs and trapdooring. In order to obtain a linear and even scar, these wounds should be closed by taking a wider bite on the larger edge (▶ Fig. 12.10).

Problem: Corners, tips, and T's.

Solution: Sharp corners and flap tips are sometimes seen in traumatic wounds and, more commonly, in flaps or incisions with a certain configuration, such as V-Y flap, z-plasty, Brunner incisions, and the like. Placing a normal interrupted stitch at the tip may compromise survival and lead to dehiscence. A commonly used technique for corners is the corner stitch (also referred to as Gillies's stitch) (▶ Fig. 12.11). The same can be applied in T-shaped wounds to avoid ischemia at the critical point of intersection between the vertical and horizontal limbs.

12.5 The Unfavorable Scar: Prevention and Treatment

Even though scars are part of the everyday practice for all surgical specialists, in the case of plastic surgeons, they acquire certain relevance due to the common thought that plastic surgeons leave minimal scars. Not surprisingly, patients often seek consultation with a plastic surgeon to correct unsightly or function-limiting scars from previous procedures. There are a number of alternatives available to treat scars, both surgical and nonsurgical. However, before committing to any one technique, it is important to consider two fundamental aspects of scar revision:

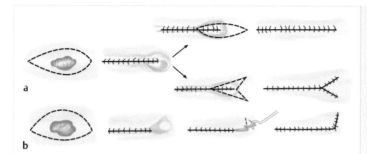

Fig. 12.8 Methods of dog-ear excision. **(a)** When a short ellipse is designed there is redundancy on both edges, which can be managed by lengthening the ellipse or converting it to a Y. **(b)** When an ellipse with borders of unequal length is designed, skin excess occurs at the longer border, which can be managed by converting it to an L.

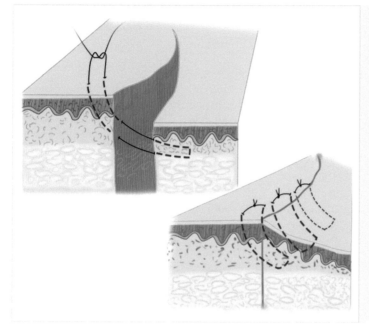

Fig. 12.9 Wounds with edges of unequal thickness are best managed with half-buried mattress sutures.

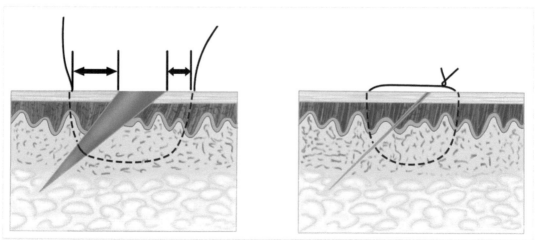

Fig. 12.10 Technique to close a wound with beveled edges. A wider bite is taken on the larger wound edge.

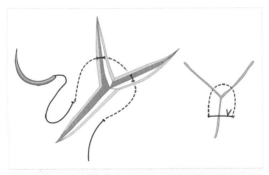

Fig. 12.11 Corner stitch. The needle enters on one side of the wound, passes through the dermis of the pointed flap, and then exits the skin at the other side.

expectations and timing. In the first place, as mentioned earlier in this chapter, scars cannot be erased. They can be improved, attenuated, or hidden, but they will always be there. This must be discussed with the patient to set a common ground on achievable goals and realistic expectations of scar revision. Secondly, there is the issue of timing and scar maturation. Wound healing is a dynamic process that goes well beyond suture removal, lasting approximately 12 months. Therefore any surgical attempt to revise a scar should preferably be done a year after wounding for two main reasons: first because the scar's appearance may change and what seems highly conspicuous to the patient at the time of consultation may well become less noticeable months later; and second because operating on a scar that is still in the process of maturing and remodeling may potentially reduce the benefits of the procedure.

Scars may be of varying sizes, depths, and shapes. For example, acne scars in the cheek are quite different from a widened and retracted appendectomy scar or a contractured burn scar in the neck. Moreover, a similar scar may be perceived differently depending on the patient. Hence, when it comes to revising a scar, an individual plan according to the scar characteristics and the patient's concerns should be tailored.

> **Reminder**   **M!**
>
> Scar revision should be performed once the scar is fully or near-fully mature. Performing it earlier can increase the risk of complications and reduce the potential benefit of revision.

12.5.1 Prevention

The first step in treating abnormal scars is prevention. Preventive measures start with gentle handling of tissues and proper wound closure followed by adequate wound care and timely suture removal. For a healed wound, the most popular approach to prevent excessive scarring is the use of silicone sheets. Silicone sheeting is both a first-line prophylactic and a therapeutic measure for abnormal scarring. Sheets are applied over the scar after sutures have been removed and should be worn daily for 1–3 months. The mechanism by which the application of silicone sheets reduces scarring is not entirely clear, although the following mechanisms have been suggested:

- Increasing temperature, which enhances the breakdown of collagen by collagenases.
- Increasing hydration, which has been postulated to decrease collagen deposition by inhibiting fibroblast proliferation and decreasing capillary activity.
- Increasing oxygen tension, which would reduce hypoxia-stimulated angiogenesis and tissue growth.
- Direct action of silicone oil released from the sheet into the wound.
- Polarization of scar tissue by a negative static electric charge elicited by the silicone sheet, which leads to scar reduction.
- Immunological effects, including a decrease in the number of mast cells, downregulation of profibrotic cytokines (e.g., transforming growth factor-$\beta2$), among others.

Silicone sheets can be difficult to wear in some areas, and some patients might find them uncomfortable and abandon their use. An alternative in these cases is using silicone-based gels or creams. Wound taping with hypoallergenic skin tape can be used as well, although its effects may not be the same as with silicone sheets. For extensive scars, such as those seen in burned patients, compression garments form an integral part of the rehabilitation program and should be started as early as possible. Adequate hydration is also important and should be encouraged for every healed wound. Despite the large amount of commercially available alternatives, in practice, any moisturizing lotion will do. Sunblock is also part of the preventive protocol and should be used for at least 1 year after wound epithelialization to avoid pigmentation alterations.

12.5.2 Treatment

Scar revision techniques include a vast array of procedures that can be broadly divided into surgical and nonsurgical techniques. Chapter 2 discusses nonsurgical management of hypertrophic scars and keloids. The discussion here will focus mainly on surgical strategies that can be applied to virtually any type of scar for which revision is indicated.

In order to select the best technique for a specific scar, there are several questions that need to be addressed regarding the characteristics of the scar and surrounding tissues: Where is the scar located? How is the scar oriented? Is it producing any functional impairment (e.g., joint contracture, eyelid retraction)? What is lying under the scar? What is the quality and mobility of surrounding tissues? Has the patient undergone previous revision procedures?

Depending on the case, there are different alternatives available to improve a scar from both a functional and an aesthetic point of view. Scars can be excised, lengthened, reoriented, released, and filled. Correct identification of clinical issues inherent to the scar (e.g., inversion, depression, widening, orientation, etc.) as well as the specific patient's concerns are key in the selection of the procedure.

Scar Excision

The simplest way to treat an unsightly scar is by excision and direct closure. Once the scar has been excised, it is important to bring deep tissues to the midline before skin closure so that the resulting scar lies flat and even with the surrounding tissues. For depressed scars, full-thickness excision may lead to a more marked depression; thus these scars are sometimes better treated by excising only the superficial part, leaving the deep component in situ as a filler over which the skin edges are sutured together (▶Fig. 12.12). If the subcutaneous portion has to be excised (e.g., due to retraction or functional impairment), then subcutaneous flaps need to be developed and sutured at the midline to fill the defect. In cases in which it is anticipated that direct tension-free closure will not be possible after scar excision, several techniques may be employed, including skin grafting, flap closure, serial excision, and tissue expansion. *Serial excision* involves excising a portion of the scar that allows direct closure without tension. The procedure is then repeated at suitable intervals until the scar is completely removed and the healthy tissue at both sides is finally brought together. It is important to assess the elasticity of surrounding skin as well as to perform wide undermining. Likewise, the different stages should be done at intervals that allow

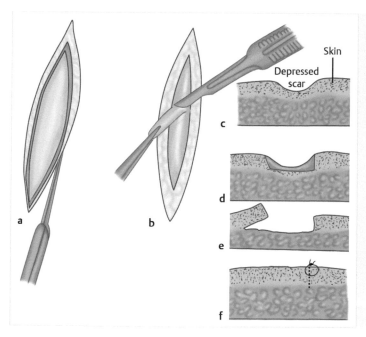

Fig. 12.12 (a-f) Partial-thickness excision of a scar. The base of the scar tissue is left in situ and the wound edges advanced and sutured over it.

the tissue to become loose again. *Tissue expansion* is a more straightforward technique than serial excision and is described in detail in Chapter 17. Both of these techniques have the great advantage of replacing missing tissue with their surrounding exact match, making them very useful for reconstruction of areas such as the scalp. Large, congenital, melanocytic nevi can also be effectively treated by serial excision or tissue expansion.

Scar Lengthening

Scars that produce deformity or functional impairment from contraction can be effectively treated by lengthening procedures. Because scar-lengthening procedures are all based in bringing tissue into the scarred area, the presence of healthy and mobile surrounding skin is an absolute requirement for success. The main representative of this group of techniques is the z-plasty and its variations including the plannimetric z-plasty, the four-flap z-plasty, five-flap z-plasty (also referred to as "jumping man flap"), double opposing z-plasty and multiple z-plasty.

Z-plasty: The z-plasty is composed of two triangular transposition flaps that interpose themselves along a longitudinal axis. Even though the z-plasty is mostly known as a method of scar lengthening, it actually has other important functions including breaking up a straight line, mobilizing tissue and obliteration or creation of a web or cleft. The z-plasty is composed of a central limb with a length x, which is designed over the line of contracture, and two lateral limbs of equal length (i.e. x) extending from each of the central limb's extremes. Once the scar is released and the flaps incised, the tissue itself should "automatically" make the flaps go into their new position (▶Fig. 12.13). By transposing the flaps, adjacent tissue is brought into the region where the scar originally laid, thus changing the orientation of the central limb to a position roughly perpendicular to its original axis, although this depends on the design. The angle at which the lateral limbs are designed dictates both the amount of tissue that will be recruited, and hence the percentage of scar lengthening, as well as the degree of transposition (▶Table 12.5). In this sense, the greater the angle, the more tissue is recruited, but at the expense of less (or a more difficult) transposition. The standard design is made with triangular flaps of 60°, which provides a 75% elongation without excessive tension. Z-plasty can be made in either a single or a multiple configuration. While the degree of scar lengthening is similar for both patterns, multiple z-plasties avoid excessive transverse shortening and are thus preferred in cases in which surrounding tissue is deemed insufficient to be transposed as one large single z-plasty. The double opposing z-plasty is a variation in which two z-plasty are designed opposite one another with their corresponding central limbs drawn along the line of contracture.

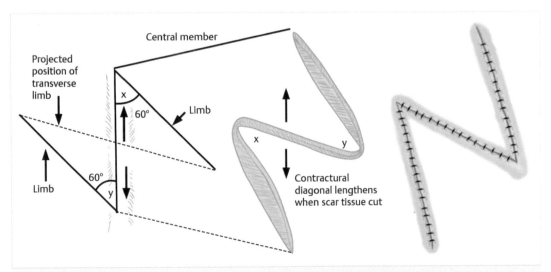

Fig. 12.13 The z-plasty. (Reproduced from Janis, Essentials of Plastic Surgery, 2nd edition, ©2014, Thieme Publishers, New York.)

Table 12.5 Z-plasty angles and scar elongation

Z-plasty angle	Degree of scar lengthening
30°	25%
45°	50%
60°	75%
90°	100%

Four-flap z-plasty: This technique is also a method of scar contracture release and uses the same basic principles of the z-plasty mentioned above. Even though it can be designed with different angles, the basic design is made as a 120° angle z-plasty in which the angles are bisected, thus creating four triangular flaps each of them of 60°. Alternatively, if the initial design is made as a 90° angle z-plasty, then four 45° triangular flaps are created (▶Fig. 12.14). The flaps are then transposed so that the inner ones fall on the outer edges with the external ones falling in the middle. This procedure is useful for scar contracture release of the thumb-index web space and axilla.

Five-flap z-plasty: Due to its appearance, the five-flap z-plasty is also referred to as the jumping man flap. Its design is similar to that of the double opposing z-plasty but adding a Y-V advancement flap in the middle (▶Fig. 12.14). After making all incisions, the corresponding flaps of each z-plasty are transposed and the central flap is advanced bringing tissue between the z-plasties. This method is very effective for medial canthal release or epicanthus correction as well as for finger web space contractures.

Reorientation

As mentioned earlier in this chapter, one of the factors affecting the final appearance of a scar is its orientation. Surgical incisions can be planned, but traumatic wounds are random and unfortunately in most cases do not follow RSTLs or do not fall between aesthetic subunits. The z-plasty, apart from being a scar-lengthening procedure, is also very effective for changing a scar's orientation so that it lies within a natural fold or wrinkle or at the border of an aesthetic subunit (▶Fig. 12.15). Careful

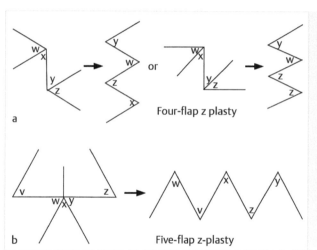

Fig. 12.14 Variations of the z-plasty. **(a)** Four-flap z-plasty. **(b)** Five-flap z-plasty (jumping man flap).

Four-flap z plasty

Five-flap z-plasty

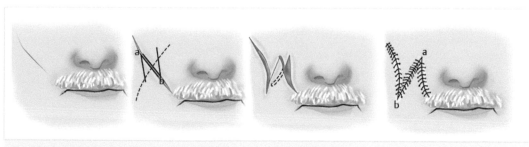

Fig. 12.15 Reorientation of a scar using a z-plasty.

planning and meticulous execution are essential to obtaining a pleasant result. It is important to note and inform the patient that, with a z-plasty, the main scar is reoriented but at the expense of adding more scars. The w-plasty is a method by which a linear scar is broken into multiple small triangles, which improves appearance and contour, but because there is no transposition of tissue, it neither changes the scar's orientation nor alters anatomical landmarks. (▶ Fig. 12.16)

Scar Release

Scars running perpendicularly across a joint or close to a critically mobile area, such as the eyelid, can become contracted and lead to severe functional impairment. Depending on the area and the degree of restriction, these scars should be treated as soon as possible to prevent ongoing deformity and irreversible damage (e.g., a stiff flexion contracture of the elbow or ectropion with severe corneal ulceration). Because the main problem with these scars is lack of soft tissue plus or minus structural support, surgical release is usually only the first part of the operation, followed by replacement of missing skin and subcutaneous tissue. Furthermore,

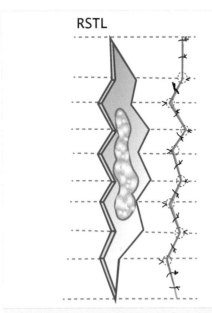

RSTL

Fig. 12.16 The w-plasty. (Reproduced from Weerda, Reconstructive Facial Plastic Surgery: A Problem Solving Manual, 2nd edition, ©2015, Thieme Publishers, New York.)

depending on the area and the nature and extent of the initial injury, scar release can be as simple as excising the scar, after which the cutaneous defect becomes immediately evident, or a challenging procedure involving isolation vessels and nerves trapped within the scar. Once the defect is created it should be resurfaced with the most appropriate coverage, which can include skin grafts; local, regional, or free flaps; dermal substitutes, and combinations of them. As stated previously, some of these defects may also require structural support, in which case a bony or cartilaginous framework is added to the reconstruction. In addition, injury to deep soft tissues, with or without cutaneous loss of continuity, can also result in a retracted scar that creates a contour deformity and/or a functional disability.

Scar Filling

For some depressed scars and skin-grafted areas in which there is a lack of subcutaneous tissue that produces hollowness, a simple way of getting the scar to the level of the surrounding healthy skin is by fat grafting. The principles of fat grafting are described with further detail in Chapter 14. If filling of a skin-grafted area is contemplated, it is important to make sure that what worries the patient most is actually the tissue deficit and not the external appearance of the scar, because, although it might improve partially with fat, it will never look like the surrounding healthy skin. The only way to significantly improve the external aspect in these cases is to replace the area with a flap or dermal substitutes.

Dermabrasion

Dermabrasion consists of the mechanical removal of the superficial layers of the skin using a diamond fraise or wire brush attached to a motorized hand piece. The basic principle of dermabrasion is that skin is removed as deep as it can heal by epithelialization from surrounding skin; therefore it is important to remain superficial to the reticular dermis in order to avoid further scarring. Dermabrasion may be applied for traumatic wounds as well as for surgical scars to make them more inconspicuous. During the procedure, the scar and surrounding skin must be stretched to provide a flat surface for the fraise to move evenly and smoothly along the scar.

12.6 Common Surgical Procedures

12.6.1 Oval Excision

If closed directly, a round excision of a skin lesion inevitably results in dog-ear formation. Such excess of tissue may be managed using the techniques described previously or, better yet, avoided from the beginning by performing an oval excision. Conversely, a circular excision is best closed with a purse-string suture, a skin graft, or a flap. Depending on the size and depth of the lesion, the ellipse should be designed with a length approximately three to four times its width and its ends having a maximum angle of 30 degrees to prevent dog-ears (▶ Fig. 12.17). Also, as long as the orientation of the lesion allows, the oval should be oriented with its long axis parallel to the relaxed skin tension lines. Always confirm that direct closure of the oval is possible before cutting. Finally, it is important to keep in mind that, for any skin lesion excised in this way, it is better to incise the borders of the whole ellipse to the desired depth first and then cut through the deep aspect with a knife, scissors, or electrocautery because this will allow an even resection of the entire lesion.

12.6.2 Epidermal Cyst Excision

Epidermal cysts are slow-growing benign skin tumors appearing in the deep layers of the skin. Surgical excision of an epidermal cyst is done by first incising a small ellipse centered on the punctum. Dissection then proceeds bluntly on the plane just above the cyst's capsule and all around it, avoiding damaging the wall and spilling the contents into the wound. Once the cyst has been completely removed, the wound should be washed and closed directly, making sure that all dead spaces are obliterated. Likewise, any skin redundancy is resected. Not

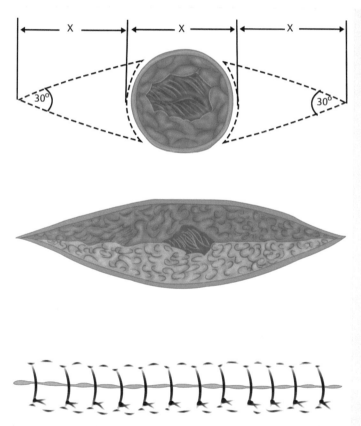

Fig. 12.17 Oval excision to achieve linear closure. The ellipse should be 3–4 times the diameter of the excised specimen and its angles not more than 30 degrees to avoid dog-ear formation.

infrequently, epidermal cysts become infected, and patients often seek consultation after several inflammatory/infectious episodes. Infected cysts should be drained and left open with frequent antiseptic dressings, along with a course of oral antibiotics. Once infection has resolved, surgical excision of any remnants of the cyst or capsule should be performed.

12.6.3 Lipoma Excision

Excision of one or multiple lipomas is generally indicated when they are large, painful, and unsightly. Additionally, in some cases, lipomas may cause compression of neighboring neurovascular structures, in which case their removal is also recommended. Most lipomas can be excised under local anesthesia. Surgical excision starts with a properly oriented incision and sharp dissection until the lesion, which is often encased by a thin, flimsy layer of connective tissue, is reached. Often, the fat contained in the lipoma can be distinguished from normal surrounding tissues by its slightly different color and larger lobules. Once identified, the lipoma can be "enucleated" or circumferentially dissected. Although enucleation is a very effective, fast, and straightforward technique for nonadherent and noninfiltrating lesions, it is not a good method when adhesions are present. In these cases, the lipoma must be released around its entire circumference by a mixture of blunt and sharp dissection, making sure to keep on the right plane so that no abnormal fat is left behind and avoiding damage to any associated neurovascular structures. After removal, a relatively large dead space is usually left behind that needs to be obliterated. It is important to keep in mind that some lipomas, especially those in the back of the neck, trapezium, and scapular areas, may infiltrate the underlying muscle, which makes their removal more challenging for the surgeon and painful for the patient (if under local anesthesia). Muscle infiltration can usually be determined by clinical examination; alternatively an ultrasound can be performed. Finally, do not forget to send the specimen for histopathological examination, both to confirm diagnosis and to rule out malignancy.

12.7 Conclusions

Suturing techniques are an essential part of every surgeon's practice, regardless of specialty and scope of work. A good suturing technique, including proper selection of the suturing material, can have a significant impact on the final appearance of a scar; hence it forms an important part of the overall surgical procedure, especially when operating on aesthetically sensible areas. There are also a number of factors that influence both wound healing and the resultant scar, and they should be managed accordingly.

12.8 Key Points

- Suturing a wound and obtaining the best scar possible should not be considered a trivial matter in plastic surgery or any other surgical specialty.
- The selection of suture material is influenced by a number of factors, including wound characteristics, systemic conditions, and surgeon's preference.
- Even though the final appearance of a scar is determined by a number of elements, the one factor that as surgeons we can fully control is surgical technique.
- An unsightly scar is a common consultation for any plastic surgeon. Although a number of techniques are available to improve scars, it is of utmost importance to set realistic expectations as to the potential of improvement to avoid unsatisfied patients afterward.

Recommended Readings

Berman B, Perez OA, Konda S, et al. A review of the biologic effects, clinical efficacy, and safety of silicone elastomer sheeting for hypertrophic and keloid scar treatment and management. Dermatol Surg. 2007; 33(11):1291–1302, discussion 1302–1303

Borges AF, Alexander JE. Relaxed skin tension lines, Z-plasties on scars, and fusiform excision of lesions. Br J Plast Surg. 1962; 15:242–254

Hsiao WC, Young KC, Wang ST, Lin PW. Incisional hernia after laparotomy: prospective randomized comparison between early-absorbable and late-absorbable suture materials World J Surg. 2000; 24(6):747–751

Monstrey S, Middelkoop E, Vranckx JJ, et al. Updated scar management practical guidelines: non-invasive and invasive measures. J Plast Reconstr Aesthet Surg. 2014; 67(8):1017–1025

Wilhelmi BJ, Blackwell SJ, Phillips LG. Langer's lines: to use or not to use. Plast Reconstr Surg. 1999; 104(1):208–214

13 Grafts: Skin, Fascia, Nerve, Tendon, Cartilage, and Bone

Álvaro Cabello, Aránzazu Menéndez, Diego Marré, Bernardo Hontanilla

Abstract

A graft is a segment of tissue of any kind that is transferred from one area to the other without maintaining its vascular supply, being therefore completely dependent on the wound bed for survival. Any tissue can potentially be transferred as a graft provided it is placed on the right environment. As with virtually any procedure in reconstructive surgery, the critical issue with grafting is vascularization, which in the case of grafts is governed by a balance between the thickness of the graft, its tolerance to ischemia, and the characteristics of the recipient bed, so that the thicker the graft or the poorer the bed, the lesser the chances of "take" and incorporation. In addition, because they lack their own blood supply, grafts are very vulnerable to contamination/infection. This chapter describes the basic principles of grafting of skin, fascia, nerve, tendon, cartilage, and bone together with the basic surgical technique of harvest for each of them.

Keywords: graft, wound bed, inosculation, nerve injury, tendon repair

13.1 Introduction

The use of skin grafts can be traced as far back as 3,000 years ago in ancient India. Grafts are one of the most commonly performed procedures in plastic surgery today, allowing like-with-like reconstruction of a wide range of defects. Any tissue, from skin to bone, can be grafted, including dermis, fat, fascia, cartilage, and nerve.

A graft is essentially a segment of tissue that is transferred from one area (donor site) to another (recipient site) without a blood supply of its own, thus depending on diffusion from the wound bed to survive until it becomes revascularized. Because of their lack of blood supply, the critical issue with grafts is related to the quality of the wound bed in terms of its vascularization and degree of contamination.

13.2 Skin Grafts

13.2.1 Basic Science

Skin grafting represents one of the simplest and most straightforward methods in the reconstructive ladder, only above secondary intention healing and primary closure. Compared with healing by secondary intention, skin grafting helps to accelerate healing, decrease fluid loss, reduce scar contracture, and improve overall appearance of the healed wound.

According to their thickness, skin grafts can be classified as full-thickness skin grafts (FTSGs) or split-thickness skin grafts (STSGs). FTSGs are composed of epidermis and the entire thickness of dermis, including adnexal structures, such as hair follicles and sweat glands, whereas STSGs include the epidermis and only a portion of the dermis (▶Fig. 13.1). Depending on the amount of dermis included STSGs can be further subdivided into thin (0.15–0.3 mm), intermediate (0.3–0.45 mm), and thick (0.45–0.75 mm). Inclusion of only a portion of the dermis in STSGs allows for spontaneous healing of the donor site through reepithelialization from residual dermal appendages and wound edges. Conversely, FTSG donor sites need to be closed with sutures because the removal of the full dermis leaves no potential for spontaneous reepithelialization.

Mechanism of Graft Take

The process of graft take is divided into three overlapping phases: plasmatic imbibition, inosculation, and revascularization.

1. *Plasmatic imbibition (0–2 days):* Following placement, the graft adheres to the wound bed by means of fibrin bonds and is kept alive by diffusion of nutrients from the bed. During this phase the graft appears edematous and may increase its volume by 40% because of fluid absorption.

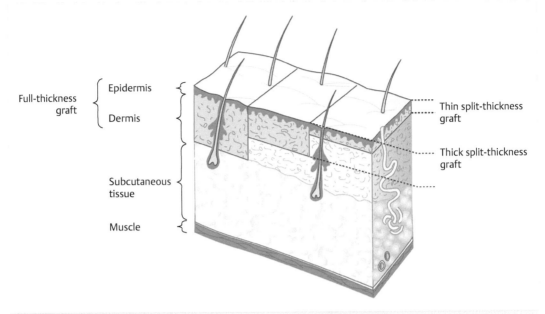

Fig. 13.1 Composition of skin grafts depending on the amount of dermis taken with the graft. (Reproduced from Weerda, Reconstructive Facial Plastic Surgery, ©2001, Thieme Publishers, Stuttgart.)

2. *Inosculation (2–4 days):* At this stage capillary buds in the recipient bed start to proliferate and connect with open vessels on the undersurface of the graft, establishing a fine vascular network that gives the graft a pink coloration. These vessels, however, are immature, and their flow is low. In addition, proliferation of fibroblasts and collagen deposition replace the fibrin network, keeping the skin graft adhered to the bed.

3. *Revascularization (5–7 days):* Approximately 5 days after grafting, the vascular connections become mature and fully functional, restoring blood flow through the graft. Angiogenesis, which is the development of new blood vessels from preexisting ones, further enhances graft vascularization.

Note

Graft adherence to the wound bed is most critical during the first 72 hours after grafting.

Successful take of a skin graft is dependent, partly, on its thickness. The dermis is less vascularized in its deeper surface, and the number of cut capillary ends exposed in a thick graft is smaller than in a thin graft, which is why thinner grafts exhibit faster and more reliable "take" than thick or full-thickness grafts. Lymphatic circulation resumes within the first week, concomitantly with the revascularization process. Reinnervation starts approximately 1 month after grafting and may take several months to years to be completed, occurring faster in STSGs but to a higher extent in FTSGs. Pain is recovered first, followed by touch and finally temperature, with all three assuming the characteristics of the recipient site. Cutaneous appendages, due to their localization within the dermis, have a higher chance of regenerating in thicker grafts. Once reinnervated, sweat glands behave like those at the recipient site, whereas sebaceous glands retain the original characteristics of the donor skin. Likewise, hair, which has the potential to grow in FTSGs only, maintains donor-site characteristics (▶ Table 13.1).

Graft Contracture: Primary versus Secondary

All skin grafts undergo two processes of contracture: primary and secondary. Primary contracture occurs immediately after harvest and is mediated by contraction of elastic fibers. Because elastin is predominantly found in the dermis, the thicker the graft, the greater its primary contraction, which for

Table 13.1 Summary of characteristics of skin grafts

	Split thickness	Full thickness
Composition	Epidermis and partial dermis • Thin: 0.15–0.3 mm • Intermediate: 0.3–0.45 mm • Thick: 0.45–0.75 mm	Dermis and full epidermis
Take	Easier and more predictable	Less robust and more dependent on wound bed conditions
Availability	High	Low
Donor site morbidity	Low—heals by reepithelialization, slower in thick grafts	Variable—leaves scar in donor site that needs to be concealed
Contracture	Primary < secondary	Primary > secondary
Reinnervation	Faster	Slower but better
Regeneration of skin appendages	Absent in thin grafts; variable in thick grafts	More likely
Hair growth	Absent	Possible, assuming donor-site characteristics
Graft growth	Very little	Graft grows with child development
Pigmentation	Unpredictable	More predictable
Cosmetic appearance	Poor; not to be used in cosmetically or functionally sensitive areas Meshed grafts usually worst In some situation grafted muscle flaps can yield good aesthetic outcome (e.g., scalp reconstruction in bald patients)	Very good; possibility of replacing like with like

FTSGs can be up to 40% of the original surface versus 10–20% for STSGs. Secondary contracture occurs as a consequence of scarring and is mediated by the contracting effect of myofibroblasts at the recipient site. The dermis in the graft exerts an inhibitory effect over these myofibroblasts; therefore, the thinner the graft, the greater its secondary contracture. Whereas (secondary) contracture may be beneficial in some situations to keep the skin graft as small as possible, in others it may lead to severe functional impairment or disfigurement, such as in the face or near joints.

13.2.2 Indications and Contraindications for Skin Grafting

In the broad sense, the main indication for skin grafting is any clean wound sufficiently vascularized to support the graft it is intended to be covered with. Conversely, the main contraindications would be infection, the presence of a poorly vascularized bed, and exposed structures, such as vessels, nerves, and bone. Likewise, skin grafts should be avoided in irradiated wounds. Full-thickness grafts are preferable for small defects in cosmetic or functional areas, where color match and absence of secondary contracture are a priority. Additionally, FTSGs are especially indicated for small wounds in the pediatric population because they retain the ability to grow with the developing child, thus reducing potential scar contracture. Finally, it is important to note that, in many cases, "graftable" defects are in fact much better reconstructed with flaps than with grafts.

13.2.3 Donor Sites for Skin Grafts

STSGs can be taken virtually from any area of the body, including the scalp and scrotum, a fact of special interest in burned patients with limited availability of healthy skin. By definition, donor sites of STSGs heal spontaneously in a period ranging from 7 to 21 days, depending on the thickness of the graft and the patient's health status. Importantly, once healed, donor sites may be reused or, alternatively, they may be expanded prior to harvest in order to increase their available surface. Conversely, donor sites of FTSGs are limited by the fact that their harvest inevitably results in a linear scar. Ideally, these grafts should be obtained from inconspicuous areas that best match the characteristics of the skin at the recipient site. Facial defects may be reconstructed with skin grafts from the preauricular, postauricular, nasolabial fold, glabellar, and supraclavicular areas. Redundant skin from the upper eyelid provides an excellent match for eyelid reconstruction. Wounds in the hand and fingers are usually resurfaced with FTSGs from the hypothenar eminence, volar wrist crease, and volar aspect of the forearm. Skin from the abdomen and thigh may be used as FTSGs as well.

13.2.4 Wound Bed Preparation

The quality of the wound bed is critical to ensure a successful graft take, with FTSGS generally needing better vascularized beds to survive due to their thickness. All necrotic tissue must be removed, and there should be no signs of infection. Serial debridements and/or negative pressure wound therapy is sometimes needed to prepare the wound to receive a skin graft. As discussed in Chapter 4, negative pressure wound therapy reduces edema, improves perfusion, and decreases bacterial colonization and wound exudate, all of which favor formation of well-vascularized "graftable" granulation tissue, which should be flat and beefy red. Considering that one of the most common causes of failure is hematoma, good hemostasis cannot be overemphasized. Although the graft itself does have some hemostatic properties, coagulation of bleeding points is mandatory. Also, before placing the graft, wound margins must be sharply excised to allow good adherence of the graft to the edges.

Apart from ensuring the best possible local environment, the patient's systemic conditions should also be addressed and optimized prior to skin grafting. Poorly controlled diabetes, malnutrition, vasculitis, chronic steroidal therapy, smoking, anticoagulant treatment, vascular insufficiency, history of radiotherapy, and ongoing chemotherapy can all impair the graft's survival. Finally, whenever possible, donor site characteristics as to color, texture, and thickness should be considered and should ideally match those of the recipient site to obtain the best possible cosmetic outcome.

Note

The deleterious effects of chronic steroids on wound healing can reversed by the administration of vitamin A 25,000 IU/d orally for 3–5 days or 200,000 IU topically three times a day.

13.2.5 Harvest Technique

Split-Thickness Skin Grafts

STSGs are harvested using dermatomes. Over the history of plastic surgery, a number of dermatomes have been introduced, a summary of which has been exhaustively elaborated by Ameer et al. Dermatomes can be broadly classified into freehand knives, drum dermatomes, and powered dermatomes (electric or air driven), with most units today using powered ones, due to their ease of use and consistency of results. The Zimmer air dermatome is one such example, which is powered by compressed water–pumped dry nitrogen (99.7% pure) operated at 100 psi (▶Fig. 13.2). This instrument is less technique dependent than freehand knives, and the harvested grafts are usually more uniform, with predefined width and thickness. Still, some surgeons prefer to use freehand knives, such as the Humby or Watson dermatome, which, when used correctly, can yield uniform grafts as well.

Surgical Technique

The donor site is shaved as necessary and properly prepared and draped. To reduce bleeding and postoperative pain, infiltration with an adrenaline-containing local anesthetic can be performed. The dermatome is placed on the skin at a 30- to 45-degree angle and advanced over the skin, applying uniform pressure until the end of the graft is reached and the dermatome is gently curved upward to cut the graft. Freehand knives involve a back-and-forth motion at the same time that the instrument is advanced on the skin until the desired graft size is obtained. For either procedure, the assistant's role is crucial in

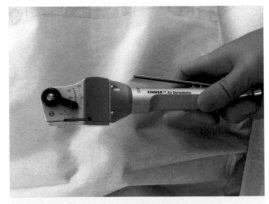

Fig. 13.2 The Zimmer air dermatome.

maintaining an even and taut surface during harvesting to prevent step-offs and tears (▶Fig. 13.3).

Once obtained, the graft is carefully handled with nontoothed forceps and applied to the wound with its dermal surface facing down. The shiny appearance of the dermis helps to distinguish it from the epidermis, which is duller. Also, the borders of the graft will usually roll toward the dermal side (▶Fig. 13.4). Finally the graft is fixed with sutures, staples, or glue as needed, and a dressing is applied on top.

Meshed Skin Grafts

STSGs can be meshed to expand their surface, which is very useful in situations when the availability of healthy skin is limited in relation to the surface needing coverage. In addition, meshing allows harvesting a graft smaller than the wound, thereby minimizing morbidity at the recipient site. The mesher is a device that creates pie cuts on the graft as it is passed through (▶Fig. 13.5), allowing expansion of 1.5:1, 2:1, 3:1 or larger. A ratio of 1.5:1 is usually used for small defects, whereas larger defects may require 3:1. Grafts may also be meshed manually using a no. 11 scalpel blade. Besides increasing the graft's surface, meshing als o makes it more "flexible" and therefore more easily adaptable to irregular and concave surfaces. Furthermore, fluid drainage through the slits prevents hematoma or seroma formation beneath the graft. On the contrary, disadvantages of meshed grafts include increased fragility and twisting—identification of the dermal side may be more difficult in these cases. Also, gap epithelialization takes longer in highly meshed grafts, and secondary contracture is directly proportional to the ratio of meshing. The cosmetic appearance of meshed grafts is also inferior compared to that of nonmeshed grafts.

Full-Thickness Skin Grafts

Harvesting of an FTSG is performed with a scalpel in the shape of an ellipse to allow linear closure of the donor site. In general, these grafts are harvested in a plane just deep to the dermis, trying to include as little fat as possible because this may compromise graft take. Remnants of fat should be trimmed off the graft with scissors. FTSGs are never meshed, though few incisions can be made to prevent hematoma formation. Finally, because harvesting of FTSG leaves behind a full-thickness wound incapable of reepithelializing, the donor site must be closed using standard suturing techniques (▶Fig. 13.6).

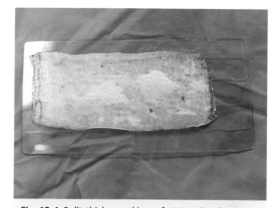

Fig. 13.4 Split-thickness skin graft. Note the shiny appearance of the dermis facing up and edges of the graft rolling toward the dermal side.

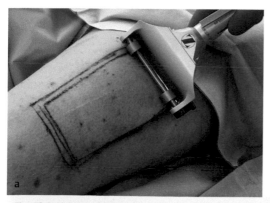
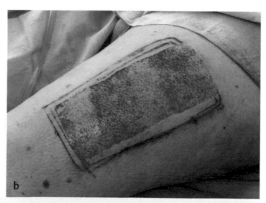

Fig. 13.3 Harvest of split-thickness skin graft with the Zimmer air dermatome. **(a)** The dermatome is held against the skin at a 45-degree angle and run evenly and at constant pressure against the skin surface. **(b)** Donor site after harvesting.

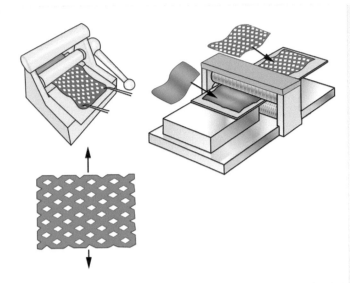

Fig. 13.5 Illustration of a skin graft mesher.

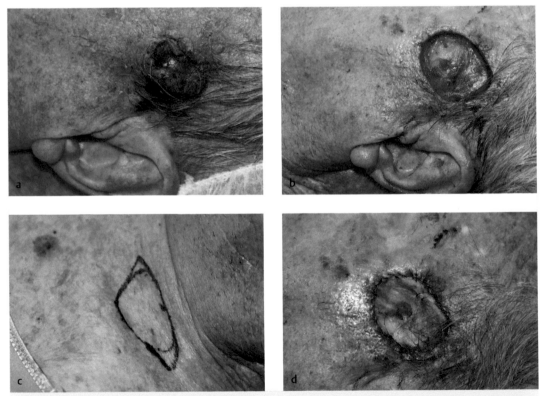

Fig. 13.6 Full-thickness skin grafting. **(a)** A 68-year-old patient presented with a squamous cell carcinoma on the left temple. **(b)** After excision. **(c)** Marking for harvest of a left supraclavicular full-thickness skin graft. **(d)** The wound was covered with the full-thickness skin graft.

13.2.6 Skin Graft Dressing

Grafts can be fixed in place using sutures, staples, or glue. Dressing then starts with a layer of nonadhesive gauze, such as Xeroform (Covidien) or Jelonet gauze (Smith & Nephew). A small amount of antibiotic ointment may be included in this layer. The nonadherent layer prevents the graft from adhering to the overlying sponge or gauze, which would cause the graft to be partially pulled away from the wound at the time of dressing change. The wound is then covered with a bulky dressing made of gauze or sponge (scrub or prep sponges are usually quite handy for this purpose), which is fixed to the surrounding skin with staples or sutured as a tie-over bolster dressing (▶Fig. 13.7). Ensuring adequate compression of the graft against the wound is critical to prevent shear and formation of hematoma as well as to maximize contact to allow inosculation and revascularization. Considering the natural evolution of graft take, the dressing should not be removed for at least 5–7 days, provided that no signs of infection, hematoma, or other complications are seen. Negative pressure wound therapy can be used as an effective dressing, especially for medium to large defects, those over mobile areas, or when bed vascularization is not optimal, such as in patients with diabetes or peripheral vascular disease. Apart from effectively immobilizing the graft, negative pressure wound therapy increases the quantity and quality of take of STSGs when compared to tie-over dressings.

13.2.7 Donor-Site Management

By definition, donor sites of STSGs heal by reepithelialization from the wound edges and remaining adnexal structures in a period ranging from 7 to 21 days, depending on graft thickness and the size of the donor area. Importantly, it is the epidermis and not the dermis that regenerates. The management of the donor area varies greatly among units, which shows that STSG donor sites will heal regardless of the dressing used, as long as they are kept clean and moist. These are simple superficial wounds, similar to an abrasion, that in most instances do not need much more than basic wound care. That said, patient comfort, frequency of change, and other logistical factors are important when choosing the best dressing. A large number of dressings are available for donor site management. Typically a layer of nonadherent Xeroform gauze is applied in direct contact with the wound, covered with gauze and a bandage and left to dry and adhere to the healing skin until it detaches once reepithelialization is complete. Artificial semipermeable transparent dressings (e.g., Opsite [Smith & Nephew], Biobrane [Smith & Nephew], or Tegaderm [3M]) promote exudate accumulation, which requires drainage with a syringe or through perforations made prior to application. By being transparent, these dressings allow continuous inspection of the wound without the need to remove them. Several other dressings have been studied, including biological (e.g., cadaveric skin, sterile irradiated allograft, pig skin, amniotic membrane, cultured keratinocyte grafts), alginates, or silver-base dressings. Finally, spare graft provides an excellent dressing and should be applied if present. Donor sites of FTSGs are managed as any primarily closed wound.

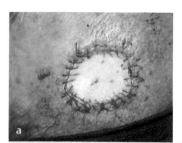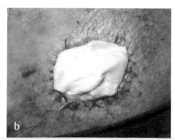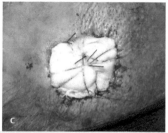

Fig. 13.7 Diagram of a bolster dressing. (a) A full-thickness skin graft was used to cover a wound on the forehead. (b) The graft is then dressed with a pack of nonadherent gauze (in this case Xeroform). (c) The dressing is then secured with tie-over sutures, which ensures adherence of the graft to the wound bed, prevents shear, and reduces the risk of fluid accumulation under the graft.

13.2.8 Postoperative Care

The postoperative management is critical to ensure complete graft survival. As mentioned earlier, during the first 48–72 hours adherence of the graft to the bed is based on fibrin bonds, which can be easily disrupted by shear or fluid accumulation. Slight limb elevation and immobilization are therefore important in grafted extremities. Depending on the thickness of the graft and the quality of the wound bed, the dressing is left in place for at least 5–7 days or longer in cases in which a "slow take" is anticipated. After this period of time, even though the graft is adhered and alive, it is still fragile and with the process of revascularization and maturation still active, so dressing removal should be done with care to avoid pulling the graft away from the wound. A protective dressing is then recommended, generally consisting of nonadherent gauze, with or without antibacterial ointment, changed every 2–3 days for approximately 2 weeks. Once the graft has healed completely, application of moisturizing lotion is usually recommended to keep it hydrated and healthy.

13.2.9 Complications and Main Causes of Failure

There are four main reasons for partial or complete graft failure: poorly vascularized beds, fluid accumulation, shear, and infection. The importance of proper wound bed preparation, including optimization of local and systemic conditions, cannot be overemphasized. Fluid (seroma or hematoma) accumulating between the graft and its bed acts as a barrier for adherence and revascularization and is best avoided by small drainage incisions in the graft (or meshing) and application of a tie-over or compressive dressing. Patients on anticoagulants are at higher risk of developing hematomas and should be closely monitored. If promptly identified, hematomas can be drained manually by removing a couple of stitches, allowing the still-viable graft to be repositioned on the wound bed. Shearing forces also impede adherence and disrupt the growing vascular connections between the graft and the underlying bed. A correctly placed dressing and immobilization should minimize shear, especially in situations where gliding structures, such as tendons, are lying directly underneath the graft. Finally, infection is highly detrimental

to skin graft survival. For cases at high risk of infection, a layer of silver-impregnated gauze can be incorporated into the dressing.

Long-term complications of skin grafts are mostly related to skin quality, pigmentation, and hypertrophic scarring. STSGs may sometimes become unstable and require repeated visits to a wound care specialist, which is bothersome for the patient and eventually expensive for the health care system. An unsuitable wound bed, chronic trauma, or pressure and contamination are the most frequent causes for graft instability. These situations should be tackled promptly by considering continued dressings versus regrafting or flap coverage. Skin grafts that are exposed to sunlight early during their evolution are at high risk of hyperpigmentation. Finally, scarring may also develop in skin-grafted areas, worsening their cosmetic appearance and potentially aggravating any functional impairment from contracture and retraction.

13.3 Fascia Grafts

The use of autologous fascial grafts in reconstructive surgery was introduced in the early 1900s when McArthur repaired inguinal hernias with pedicled strips of external oblique aponeurosis interlinked between conjoint tendon. Later on, Kirschner in 1909 reported the use of strips of autologous fascia lata to correct facial asymmetry secondary to facial nerve palsy. Following Blair's refinements and popularization of the technique, the use of fascia grafts became an important tool in the armamentarium of reconstructive surgery and has remained valid ever since.

Fascia is composed mainly of a dense collagen network that provides great mechanical strength— when stressed along the axis of its fibers, fascia lata exhibits remarkable tensile strength, which remains constant 1 year after transfer. Furthermore, the autologous nature of fascia grafts allows them to be readily incorporated with the tissues, making them highly superior to nonbiological substitutes, which are frequently complicated by infection, severe foreign body reaction, and extrusion. Fascia grafts are currently used for a number of reconstructive purposes requiring either strong support, such as facial slings, or reconstruction of missing layers, such as dura and abdominal wall.

Fascia lata slings are usually harvested using a fascia stripper. With the thigh in flexion and adduction, a small incision is made distally on the lateral aspect and the fascia lata identified. A small flap of fascia is cut, passed through the end of the fascia stripper, and held securely with mosquito forceps while the stripper is advanced proximally. Once the desired length is reached, the graft is cut using the guillotine-like system at the tip of the fascia stripper, and the graft is pulled through the incision. If a fascia stripper is not available, the grafts can be harvested through serial incisions.

In cases where tissue from the thigh is being used for reconstruction (e.g., anterolateral thigh flap), harvest of fascia lata is done under direct vision, either including it in the flap as a vascularized layer or harvesting it separately as a graft.

13.4 Tendon Grafts

Tendons are shiny white cord, straplike, or flat structures that connect muscles to bones. They transmit the force created in muscle to bone to generate joint motion. Tendons are made of hierarchically organized fibers, starting with tropocollagen, that sequentially organize into fibrils, fibers (primary bundles), fascicles (secondary bundles), tertiary bundles, and the tendon itself. The main cellular component of tendons includes well differentiated and metabolically active spindle-shaped fibroblasts (tenocytes) in charge of synthetizing all components of the extracellular matrix (ECM), and tenoblasts, which are undifferentiated cells residing in the epitenon and the main orchestrators of tendon healing. Other cells found in tendons are chondrocytes at bone insertion sites, synovial cells, and capillary endothelial cells. The ECM is made up mainly of type I collagen and other constituents, namely elastin, fibronectin, and proteoglycans (decorin and aggrecan). Tendons are covered by *epitenon*, a fine, loose connective tissue sheath containing the vascular, lymphatic, and nerve supply. The *endotenon* consists of epitenon extensions into the substance of the tendon, between tertiary bundles. Finally, a fine layer of loose areolar connective tissue called *paratenon*, which consists of type I and III collagen, elastic fibrils, and an inner lining of synovial cells, surrounds the tendon. In areas of increased mechanical stress, such as the finger joints, tendons are further encased in a two-layer synovial sheath comprising an outer fibrotic layer and an inner synovial layer. The latter is further composed of a parietal and a visceral sheet.

Tendons receive their blood supply from different sources depending on their location. Those within sheaths (intrasynovial) are supplied by vessels branching from regional arteries (e.g., digital arteries in the hand) that reach the tendon through the vincula or mesotenon. In the tendon, these vessels arborize to form a plexus at the level of the visceral portion of the synovial sheet and also penetrate the tendon's substance to run in the endotenon septae. Intrasynovial tendons also receive nutrients from the synovial fluid. A vascular network running in the paratenon with vessels penetrating through the epitenon and into the endotenon septae supplies extrasynovial tendons.

13.4.1 Tendon Healing

There has been much research and controversy as to the exact mechanisms by which tendons heal. As already mentioned, although resident tenocytes do play a role, tenoblasts in the epitenon are responsible for most of the processes involved in tendon healing, which is known to occur in three overlapping phases: inflammation, proliferation, and remodeling. Immediately after injury, the inflammatory phase begins with vasodilation, increased vascular permeability, release of proinflammatory cytokines, and recruitment of macrophages to the site of injury. Secretion of angiogenic factors is also observed as well as proliferation of tenocytes, which start to synthesize type III collagen. A few days later, inflammation gives way to the proliferative phase characterized by a peak in collagen III production and further synthesis of ECM. During the later stages of the proliferative phase (5–6 weeks after injury) cell proliferation and inflammation decrease, while production of collagen I is considerably enhanced. Finally, 6 weeks after injury, the tendon enters its remodeling phase, during which production of collagen I continues while cellularity and synthesis of ECM components decline. Strength is progressively gained by fibrosis, alignment of fibers in the direction of mechanical stress, and cross linking of collagen fibers.

Depending on whether it occurs from cells present in the tendon or from the surrounding tissues, tendon healing has been classified as intrinsic or extrinsic, respectively. In *intrinsic healing*, which occurs in intrasynovial tendons, residing tenocytes and tenoblasts orchestrate the reparative process with little contribution from external cell sources. Due to its intrinsic nature, this type of healing minimizes the formation of adhesions to surrounding tissues. Clean lacerations with minimal disruption of the tendon's blood supply are likely to heal mainly by intrinsic mechanisms. In *extrinsic healing*, cells from surrounding tissues command the repair, which generates adhesions that may jeopardize the functional outcome. This type of healing usually predominates in situations in which the vascularity of the tendon is compromised, as in severe hand trauma.

13.4.2 Tendon Repair

The goals of any tendon repair, either direct or through an interposition tendon graft, are to achieve gapless healing that provides sufficient strength to allow proper movement and/or support. Tendons are repaired using core and epitendinous sutures. Core sutures, which run in the substance of the tendon, are responsible for holding the edges together and providing mechanical strength to the repair, whereas peripheral epitendinous sutures add strength to the repair and close any remaining gaps, which reduces exposure to surrounding tissue and the possibility of extrinsic healing. A number of different techniques have been described for tendon repair, the full review of which goes beyond the scope of this chapter. Likewise, a considerable amount of literature has been published comparing different methods. In general terms, according to the number of strands, core sutures are classified as two-strand (conventional) or multistrand (e.g., four, six, or eight strands). The strength of any repair is usually proportionate to the number of strands, so that two strands < four strands < six strands (▶ Fig. 13.8). Additionally, depending on the tendon–suture junction configuration, core sutures can be either grasping or locking. Nonabsorbable sutures (e.g., Ethibond [Ethicon], Ticron [Covidien], or Prolene [Ethicon]) are most commonly used to repair tendons.

13.4.3 Common Donor Sites

Tendon grafts can be obtained from different areas, with their selection depending on the requirements of the reconstruction and availability. The main donor tendons include palmaris longus, plantaris, and second to fourth toe extensor.

Palmaris longus tendon: Located roughly along the midline of the volar aspect of the forearm, this tendon can be easily harvested through a single incision parallel to a flexion crease in the wrist and traced proximally with the use of a tendon stripper. The ease of harvest and lack of functional morbidity are important advantages of the palmaris

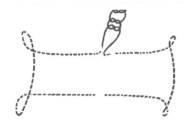

a   Modified kessler technique

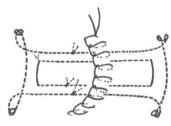

b   Indiana technique

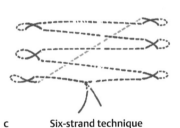

c   Six-strand technique

Fig. 13.8 Schematic illustration of two-strand, four-strand, and six-strand repair of tendon.

longus, whereas its main drawback is its absence in approximately 15% of patients. Preoperatively, the presence of one or both palmaris longus tendons can be determined by asking the patient to oppose the thumb against the little finger and flex the wrist against resistance (▶ Fig. 13.9).

Plantaris muscle: This muscle originates from the lateral femoral condyle and has a short muscle belly that ends in a long tendon running between the soleus and the gastrocnemius. Distally, the plantaris tendon runs medial to the Achilles tendon to insert on the calcaneus or, more rarely, to fuse with the Achilles tendon. It is harvested through a small incision on the medial aspect of the calcaneal tendon and traced proximally with a tendon stripper. The plantaris tendon provides enough length and caliber for a number of reconstructive needs because it can be used as a single thread, divided, or braided as required. It is absent in approximately 20% of the population and when absent on one side, two-thirds of patients will not have it on the other side—unfortunately there is no test to determine its presence preoperatively. As with the palmaris longus tendon, sacrifice of the plantaris tendon produces no functional morbidity.

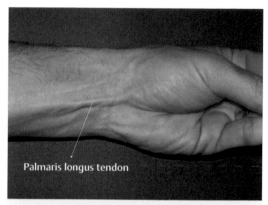

Fig. 13.9 The presence of the palmaris longus can be confirmed preoperatively by asking the patient to oppose the thumb against the little finger and flex the wrist against resistance.

Toe extensor tendons: Extensor tendons from the second, third, and fourth toes can be harvested as grafts. Their presence is constant and can provide long, robust grafts. Their sacrifice, however, may lead to flexion deformity of the toes. They are harvested through small serial transverse incisions on the dorsal aspect of the foot. A tendon stripper may be useful to avoid disruption of the extensor retinaculum.

13.5 Nerve Repair and Grafting

13.5.1 Basic Science

Nerve Anatomy

Nerves are formed by numerous individual axons, each of them surrounded by a fine layer of connective tissue called *endoneurium*. Several axons group together to form fascicles, which are encircled by *perineurium*. Depending on the fascicular pattern, nerves are classified as monofascicular, oligofascicular, and polyfascicular. The substance between fascicles is the (internal) *epineurium*, and the epineural sheath (or external epineurium) surrounds all fascicles and anatomically defines the nerve (▶ Fig. 13.10). Additionally, some authors have described yet another, more

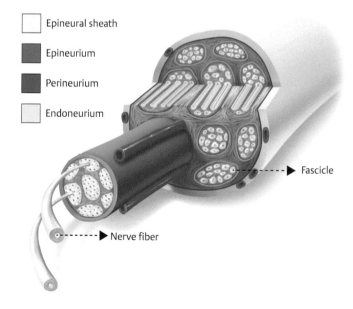

Epineural sheath

Epineurium

Perineurium

Endoneurium

Fascicle

Nerve fiber

Fig. 13.10 Schematic anatomical illustration of a peripheral nerve. (Modified from Slutsky, The Art of Microsurgical Hand Reconstruction, ©2013, Thieme Publishers, New York.)

external, connective tissue layer called the *meso-neurium* or adventitia, which allows the entrance of blood vessels into the nerve and also contributes to nerve gliding.

The vascular supply to nerves (e.g., vasa nervorum) comes from two interconnected systems, intrinsic and extrinsic. Blood vessels piercing the mesoneurium and ramifying into longitudinal branches along the epineurium and perineurium make up the extrinsic vascular system, from which multiple capillaries branch off in all directions through the endoneurium, forming the intrinsic vascular system.

Physiopathology of Nerve Injury

Following injury, a cascade of events occurs at both the proximal and the distal stumps in an attempt to restore nerve continuity and impulse conduction. The distal stump undergoes a process called Wallerian degeneration, by which the disconnected axons and myelin sheath follow a cell death pathway called chromatolysis, and the resultant debris is then cleared by Schwann cells and macrophages. Macrophages also release growth factors that stimulate Schwann cell proliferation. Proliferating Schwann cells fill the empty endoneurial space and form cylindrical structures called bands of Büngner, which are essential in guiding nerve regrowth. The proximal stump undergoes degeneration that is limited to the first adjacent node of Ranvier, and from this point, each axon sends numerous sprouts to reach the bands of Büngner in response to neurotrophic factors. Once one of these sprouts reaches a sensory receptor or a motor end plate, the remaining ones prune.

Neurotrophism refers to the capacity of certain molecules (e.g., neurotrophins) to stimulate the growth and maturation of nerve fibers. *Neurotropism*, in turn, describes the phenomenon by which regenerating fibers grow in the direction of their target organ.

> **Note**
>
> Nerve growth occurs at a rate of approximately 1 mm/d.

The progression of nerve regeneration can be clinically assessed by Tinel's sign, where tapping on the distal end of the regenerating axons produces tingling over the distribution of the growing nerve.

Depending on the extent of damage, nerve injury was originally classified by Seddon in 1947 as neurapraxia, axonotmesis, and neurotmesis. Sunderland later expanded Seddon's classification into five different degrees, and finally Mackinnon added a sixth degree, which describes a mixed injury where different degrees are seen within the same injury. This classification has important clinical utility because it predicts the outcome of reinnervation and the need for surgical repair versus conservative management (▶ Fig. 13.11 and ▶ Table 13.2).

13.5.2 Principles of Nerve Repair

Nerve repair requires the use of meticulous microsurgical techniques and adequate magnification systems, instruments, and sutures. Gentle dissection is required to avoid devascularization and scarring. In addition, unlike a microvascular anastomosis where

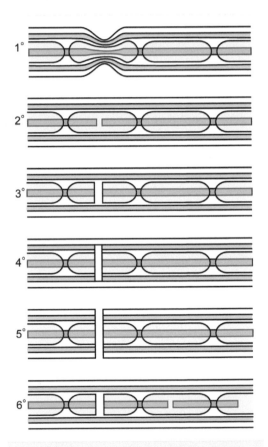

Fig. 13.11 Schematic illustration of the different degrees of injury. (Reproduced from Bullocks et al, Plastic Surgery Emergencies, ©2017, Thieme Publishers, New York.)

Table 13.2 Classification of nerve injury

Seddon	Sunderland	Features	Return of function	Treatment
Neurapraxia	Type I	Disruption of myelin sheath	Complete	None
Axonotmesis	Type II Type III Type IV	Disruption of axons Disruption of axons and endoneurium Disruption of axon and endoneurium and perineurium	Complete Incomplete None	None Variable Surgical repair/nerve transfer
Neurotmesis	Type V	Disruption of all layers, including epineurium	None	Surgical repair/nerve transfer
	Type VI (MacKinnon)	Mixed degrees within the same injury	Variable depending on the injury and combination of degrees	Variable

watertight repair is crucial, nerves are repaired using the least number of stitches to minimize scarring at the coaptation site. It should be noted that approximately 25% of axons are lost when trying to cross a coaptation site.

When repairing a nerve, it is crucial to properly align the fascicles, especially in mixed (e.g., sensory and motor) nerves. In this regard, thorough knowledge of the internal topography of the injured nerve cannot be overemphasized. This topography is generally more discernible distally, where the groups of axons have already adopted their position within the nerve. To achieve correct alignment of fascicles it is sometimes useful to align the vasa nervorum as well as to join fascicles with a similar caliber on each stump. Additionally, as a general rule, tension at the site of coaptation should not be tolerated and there should be a low threshold to use a graft in these situations because tension leads to ischemia, which has deleterious effects on nerve regeneration. It has been suggested that 15% elongation reduces blood flow in approximately 80% resulting in minimal recovery. Another important aspect to consider in nerve repair is level of injury, as proximal injuries have a worse functional prognosis due to irreversible changes occurring in the denervated muscle while the axons reach the motor end plate. At 12 months fibrosis, scarring and adipose infiltration of the muscle are seen, with changes being irreversible at 2 years. Repair of sensory nerves, however, is not affected by time because the target zones do not degenerate, allowing reconstruction at any time after injury. Finally, there are several patient factors that can affect the outcome of peripheral nerve repair, including age (young patients having significantly better recovery), smoking, diabetes, hypothyroidism, and peripheral vascular disease.

> **Note**
>
> Approximately 25% of axons are lost during nerve regeneration through a surgical coaptation site.

The vast majority of nerve repairs are done in an end-to-end fashion, aligning the nerve stumps at the level of the epineurium (e.g., epineural repair) or at the level of the fascicles (e.g., fascicular repair) as shown in ▶ Fig. 13.12. Even though robust evidence showing superiority of one technique over the other is lacking, in general terms, epineural repair is preferred if technically possible, taking care to precisely align the corresponding fascicles to achieve target-specific reinnervation, especially in nerves with a sensory and motor component. On the other hand, fascicular repair achieves better specificity but at the expense of more intraneural dissection, which carries an inherent degree of damage and devascularization.

End-to-side repair has been advocated when traditional techniques are not feasible, such as when there is no proximal stump. Different configurations of end-to-side repair have been described. In this case, the distal nerve stump of the recipient nerve is plugged onto an epineural window made at the side of an uninjured donor nerve from where sprouting occurs (▶ Fig. 13.13). The main

Epineurial nerve repair   Fascicular nerve repair

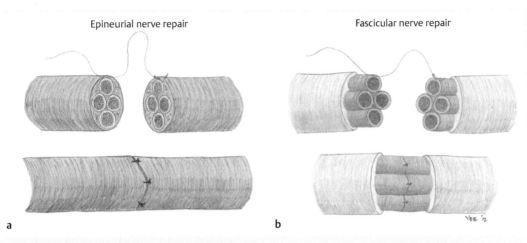

a   b

Fig. 13.12 (a,b) End-to-end epineural and fascicular nerve repair. (Reproduced from MacKinnon, Nerve Surgery, ©2015, Thieme Publishers, New York.)

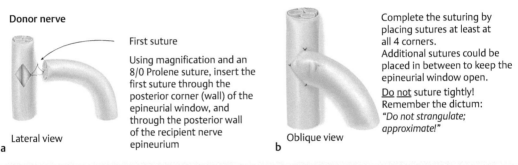

Donor nerve

First suture

Using magnification and an 8/0 Prolene suture, insert the first suture through the posterior corner (wall) of the epineurial window, and through the posterior wall of the recipient nerve epineurium

Lateral view

a

Complete the suturing by placing sutures at least at all 4 corners.
Additional sutures could be placed in between to keep the epineurial window open.
Do not suture tightly! Remember the dictum: *"Do not strangulate; approximate!"*

Oblique view

b

Fig. 13.13 (a,b) End-to-side nerve repair through the epineural window on the donor nerve. (Reproduced from Slutsky, The Art of Microsurgical Hand Reconstruction, ©2013, Thieme Publishers, New York.)

advantages of end-to-side repair include preservation of the architecture of the donor nerve (as it is not transected), the absence of morbidity from nerve graft harvesting, and the possibility to re-innervate closer to the target, thus optimizing the chances of recovery.

Timing is another important factor to consider in nerve repair and is broadly divided into primary, delayed, and secondary repair, with selection of timing depending on the type of nerve injury, conditions of the wound, and the vascular environment of the nerve bed. *Primary* repair is ideally done within the first 72 hours following injury and is generally advocated for sharp transections with little crushing component, in clean well vascularized wounds (▶Fig. 13.14). Within 72 hours, stimulation of the distal stump of an

injured motor nerve will elicit movement of the target muscle due to the presence of remaining neurotransmitters at the neuromuscular junction, thus facilitating proper identification of the stump and alignment of the fascicles. In addition, early repair avoids problems from scarring and retraction of the nerve ends, making direct end-to-end repair feasible. *Delayed* repair is done within 3 to 7 days postinjury and is recommended for contaminated wounds needing serial washouts or debridements. *Secondary* repair is indicated for cases with significant crush injury, avulsion injuries, gunshot injuries, or heavily contaminated or infected wounds. The patient should be followed for signs of recovery clinically and electrophysiologically. If no improvement is seen after approximately 3 months, then

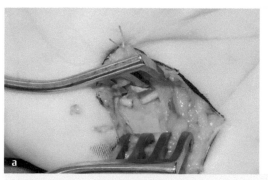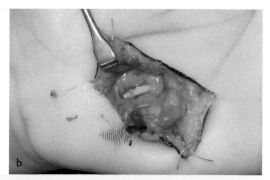

Fig. 13.14 (a,b) Direct immediate repair of a common digital nerve in a patient who sustained a glass injury. A clean wound and flush cut facilitate direct repair without tension.

a surgical exploration and repair is warranted. In these cases, because of significant retraction and scarring of the nerve stumps, direct repair is usually not possible, and nerve grafts are needed to bridge the gap.

13.5.3 Nerve Grafts and Conduits

Autologous nerve grafting is the gold standard technique to bridge nerve gaps (▶Fig. 13.15). In some instances in which a gap exists, neurolysis and nerve mobilization together with splinting in a certain posture may help to bring the ends together and avoid the need for a graft; however, if tension-free coaptation cannot be achieved, as is the case, for example, with defects greater than 1 cm in a digital nerve or 5 cm in the upper limb nerve, an interpositional graft is very likely to be required. As mentioned earlier, when the regenerating fibers cross a suture line, a portion of the axons are lost, which in the case of grafts is double due to the presence of two coaptation sites. Importantly, long nerve grafts should be reversed (e.g., distal stump of graft coapted to proximal stump of injured nerve) so that the regenerating fibers do not escape the main trunk through side branches, a problem not seen with short grafts. Vascularization is also critical for successful nerve grafting. Nerve grafts, as any graft, survive initially by diffusion and inosculation from the surrounding tissues (lateral inosculation) and also from the nerve stumps (longitudinal inosculation). Lateral inosculation is essential in long grafts in which longitudinal supply is not sufficient. The success of nerve grafting is inversely proportional to graft length and diameter because the longer and thicker the graft, the poorer its vascular supply.

Depending on the reconstructive need, there are a number of potential donor sites for nerve grafts, including the greater auricular nerve, the medial antebrachial cutaneous nerve, the posterior interosseous nerve at the level of the wrist, the dorsal branch of the ulnar nerve, the superficial branch of the radial nerve, the intercostal nerves, and the sural nerve (▶Fig. 13.16 and ▶Fig. 13.17). In general, sensory nerves are sacrificed and used as donors because sensory loss is much more acceptable and better tolerated than motor deficit. In addition, use of autologous nerve graft implies new incisions and the risk of neuroma formation at the donor site.

An alternative to autologous nerve graft is cadaveric allografts, which provide an excellent scaffold and source of biochemical signaling that stimulates the growth of axons through it. In general, allografts are used for defects less than 7 cm in length—beyond that length autografts show better results. Also, allografts carry the disadvantage of temporal immunosuppression therapy until adequate host Schwann cells have repopulated the graft.

Artificial conduits are another alternative to autografts, providing a scaffold, cells, and signaling molecules that promote the regeneration process; however, their use is limited to defects of less than 4 cm. Lastly, veins may also be used to bridge nerve defects, but their use is recommended for defects of not more than 2 cm due to the collapsibility of their walls.

13.6 Cartilage Grafts

Cartilage is composed of chondrocytes and matrix components, including collagen and elastic fibers,

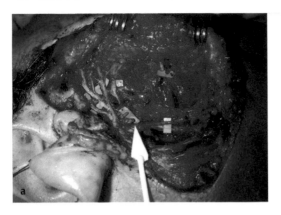
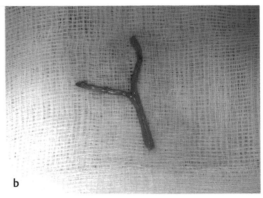
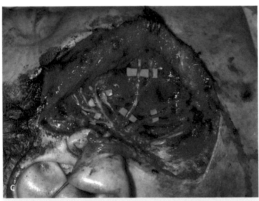

Fig. 13.15 Nerve grafting. (a) A patient showing a long defect of the buccal branch of the right facial nerve after parotidectomy. (b) A nerve graft was obtained from the sural nerve and split to reconstruct the two distal stumps. (c) Intraoperative view after interpositional nerve grafting.

all embedded in a firm gel-like matrix rich in mucopolysaccharides and water. Cartilage is flexible and has memory that allows it to return to its original shape after bending or deformation. In addition, the matrix acts as an immunological barrier, which makes cartilage a uniquely low immunogenic tissue. However, if the matrix is damaged, then chondrocytes become exposed and an immunogenic reaction can ensue.

Cartilage has very low metabolic requirements and can thus survive under low oxygen conditions. In fact, cartilage does not have any blood or lymphatic vessels, but depends on a diffusion mechanism from the perichondrium for nutrition and survival. This property allows cartilage to remain relatively unaltered after grafting, provided it is placed in a well vascularized, clean environment. Warping and curling may however occur following cartilage grafting.

Depending on the predominant type of matrix fibers, cartilage can be divided into three types:

1. *Hyaline cartilage:* Composed mainly of collagen II fibers, this subtype constitutes the base of the articular cartilage in long bones.
2. *Fibrous cartilage:* Composed mainly of collagen I fibers, this subtype is present in areas like the pubic symphysis, sternoclavicular joint, intervertebral disks, temporomandibular joint, and menisci.
3. *Elastic cartilage:* Composed mainly of elastic fibers, this subtype is present mainly in the pinna and larynx.

Cartilage grafts are normally used to provide support for a wide range of reconstructive as well as some aesthetic procedures. Auricular cartilage may be used to replace the tarsus in eyelid reconstruction or to restore contour and provide structural support in nasal reconstruction. In addition, the cartilaginous framework in total ear reconstruction is usually built using rib cartilage. Cartilage grafts from the nasal septum are also routinely

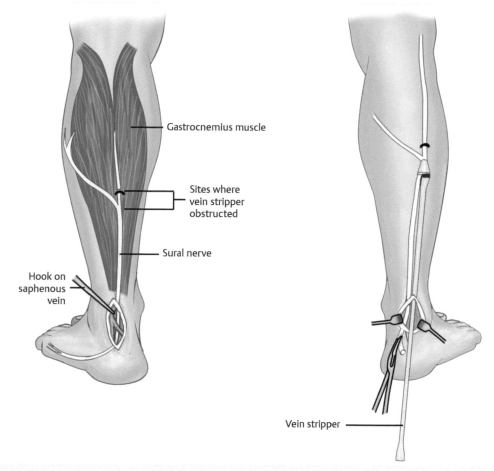

Gastrocnemius muscle

Sites where vein stripper obstructed

Sural nerve

Hook on saphenous vein

Vein stripper

Fig. 13.16 Schematic illustration of sural nerve harvest using a vein stripper through a small incision just posterior to the lateral malleolus.

used in aesthetic rhinoplasty for different purposes, including nasal dorsum augmentation and nasal valve opening (spreader grafts).

Donor sites for cartilage grafts include mainly auricular cartilage, the nasal septum, the hard palate, and the ribs, each with its unique properties as mentioned earlier. The ear (e.g., conchal cartilage) is one of the most frequent sites due to its ease of harvest, low morbidity, and the amount of cartilage that can be taken. Conchal cartilage is usually harvested through a postauricular incision, separating the cartilage from the anterior and posterior skin (▶Fig. 13.18). Composite grafts including cartilage and skin may also be harvested from the ear, particularly from the root of the helix and the conchal region as well.

13.7 Bone Grafts

Bone grafting is routinely performed in reconstructive surgery for a wide range of procedures, including extremity, hand, and head and neck reconstruction. Traditionally, and still today, bone grafts have been referred to as vascularized and nonvascularized; however, in the strict sense vascularized bone grafts should be referred to as bone flaps because they are transferred with preservation of their blood supply and do not depend on the wound bed for survival. Common indications for cancellous bone grafting include alveolar bone grafting, filling of defects following excision of bone cysts, or after osteosynthesis repair of hand fractures with bone loss, whereas cortical bone

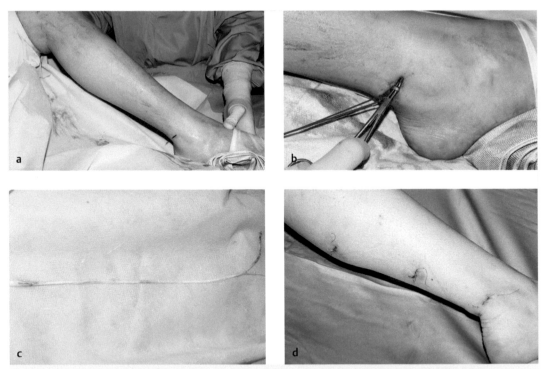

Fig. 13.17 Harvest of a sural nerve through serial small incisions on the posterolateral aspect of the leg. (a) Marking of the first incision posterior to the lateral malleolus. (b) Short saphenous vein retracted and sural nerve identified and isolated. (c) A long graft can be harvested depending on the reconstructive need. (d) Appearance of incisions at the end of the procedure.

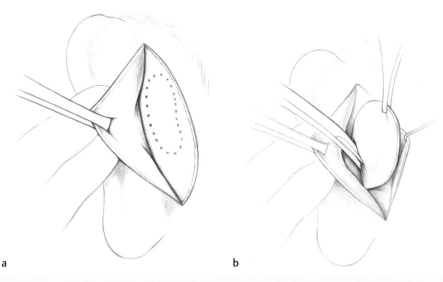

Fig. 13.18 (a,b) Schematic illustration of auricular cartilage graft harvest. An incision is made at the conchoscaphal angle and the cartilage dissected off the posterior and anterior skin. (Reproduced from Sherris and Larrabee, Principles of Facial Reconstruction, ©2010, Thieme Publishers, New York.)

graft is usually performed to reconstruct segmental bone defects after tumor excision or traumatic injuries of the extremities and the head and neck as well as to restore contour in patients with congenital hypoplasia of the craniofacial skeleton.

Bone grafts may be of allogenic or autologous origin. Whereas the use of allografts reduces morbidity and operative time from graft harvest, their osteogenic, osteoinductive, and osteoconductive potential is very limited compared to autografts. In addition, synthetic bone substitutes, such as hydroxyapatite, tricalcium phosphate, polymethyl methacrylate (PMMA), are also alternatives to autologous bone grafting.

As with any grafts, the success of bone grafting is based on placing the graft in a clean, well vascularized environment and proper immobilization to maximize incorporation to the host tissue. Incorporation of bone graft follows a process similar to that of normal bone healing and includes hematoma formation, inflammation, vascular invasion, focal resorption, and formation of new bone. The three main mechanisms underlying bone graft healing are osteoconduction, osteoinduction, and osteogenesis. In *osteoconduction*, the graft acts as a biological matrix allowing the invasion of blood vessels and osteoprogenitor cells, which gradually replace the graft with native bone, a process also known as *creeping substitution*. *Osteoinduction*, in turn, refers to the stimulation of local tissue to differentiate into mature bone cells and is largely orchestrated by a family of proteins called bone morphogenetic proteins (BMPs) within the graft. Finally, *osteogenesis* refers to the formation of new bone by surviving osteoblasts in the graft. The predominating mechanism will depend on the type of graft, with autologous cancellous grafts showing rapid vascularization within 2–4 weeks, as well as high osteoinductive and osteoconductive potential, which allows them to heal largely by osteogenesis, but at the expense of providing little to no strength initially. Cortical grafts, in turn, provide immediate structural support but are less biologically active than cancellous grafts and thus take longer to incorporate, doing so mainly by osteoconduction (creeping substitution). Finally, allografts and alloplasts are mainly osteoconductive.

Donor sites for cancellous bone graft include the distal radius, iliac crest, and tibia. Cortical bone graft is usually obtained from the radius, fibula, iliac crest, ribs, and calvarium. Calvarial bone grafts should include the outer table alone, leaving the inner table in situ (▶ Fig. 13.19). Alternatively, a full-thickness graft may be harvested, which is then split along the diploë in the back table, and the inner layer is replaced onto the calvarium.

13.8 Conclusions

Grafting of tissues represents one of the basic techniques in plastic surgery, being largely applied to a wide range of reconstructive and aesthetic procedures. Even though each type of tissue has its own tenets, they all share in common the basic principle of grafts that rely on the wound bed to survive. Wound bed preparation is therefore key for successful grafting, regardless if it is skin, fascia, nerve, cartilage, or bone. The importance of a clean, healthy, well-vascularized bed cannot be overemphasized, and if viability is questionable, then further preparation should be performed or alternatively other options of reconstruction, namely flaps, should be considered.

13.9 Key Points

- Grafts are segments of tissue transferred from a donor site to a recipient site without retaining their own vascularity and therefore rely on the wound bed to survive.
- A clean, well-vascularized bed is paramount to optimize graft take and incorporation.
- STSGs include epidermis and varying portions of dermis, whereas FTSGs include the whole dermis.
- The three phases of skin graft take are plasmatic imbibition, inosculation, and revascularization.
- The main complications responsible for graft loss are infection, hematoma, and shear.
- Following nerve injury, the distal stump undergoes Wallerian degeneration while the proximal stump sends sprouts for regeneration.
- Nerve repair under tension leads to ischemia and subsequent poor regeneration.
- Nerve regeneration occurs at a rate of ~ 1 mm/d.
- Nerve autografts are the gold standard to bridge nerve gaps.
- Tendon heals by a mixture of extrinsic and intrinsic healing, with the latter being preferable.
- Six-strand tendon repair provides the greatest strength, followed by four-strand and lastly two-strand repair.

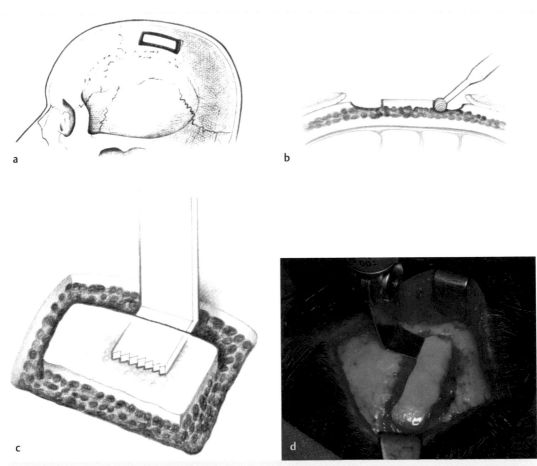

Fig. 13.19 Harvest of split calvarial bone graft. **(a)** The desired size of the graft is marked, preferably on the parietal skull. **(b)** The skull is burred around the planned graft to the level of the diploic space. **(c)** A saw blade is then inserted into the diploic space parallel to the inner table, and the graft is carefully lifted, taking care not to injure the inner table. **(d)** Intraoperative view of the procedure. (Reproduced from Sherris and Larrabee, Principles of Facial Reconstruction, ©2010, Thieme Publishers, New York.)

- Cartilage is largely avascular and therefore highly resistant to ischemic situations following grafting.
- Bone grafts heal by a combination of osseoconduction, osseoinduction, and osteogenesis, with the predominating mechanism depending on the type of graft.

Recommended Readings

Ameer F, Singh AK, Kumar S. Evolution of instruments for harvest of the skin grafts. Indian J Plast Surg. 2013; 46(1):28–35

Azzopardi EA, Boyce DE, Dickson WA, et al. Application of topical negative pressure (vacuum-assisted closure) to split-thickness skin grafts: a structured evidence-based review. Ann Plast Surg. 2013; 70(1):23–29

Blair VP. Notes on the operative corrections of facial palsy. South Med J. 1926; 19:116

Chan DB, Temple HT, Latta LL, Mahure S, Dennis J, Kaplan LD. A biomechanical comparison of fan-folded, single-looped fascia lata with other graft tissues as a suitable substitute for anterior cruciate ligament reconstruction. Arthroscopy. 2010; 26(12):1641–1647

Chuan HC, Wu YF, Tang JB. Molecular biology of tendon healing. In: Tang JB, Amadio PC, Guimberteau JC, Chang J, eds. Tendon Surgery of the Hand. Philadelphia, PA: Elsevier; 2012:e26–e33

Clark WL, Trumble TE, Swiontkowski MF, Tencer AF. Nerve tension and blood flow in a rat model of immediate and delayed repairs. J Hand Surg Am. 1992; 17(4):677–687

Corps BV. The effect of graft thickness, donor site and graft bed on graft shrinkage in the hooded rat. Br J Plast Surg. 1969; 22(2):125–133

Diao E, Hariharan JS, Soejima O, Lotz JC. Effect of peripheral suture depth on strength of tendon repairs. J Hand Surg Am. 1996; 21(2):234–239

Feldman DL. Which dressing for split-thickness skin graft donor sites? Ann Plast Surg. 1991; 27(3):288–291

Guimberteau JC, Delage JP, McGrouther DA, Wong JK. The microvacuolar system: how connective tissue sliding works. J Hand Surg Eur Vol. 2010; 35(8):614–622

Haas F, Seibert FJ, Koch H, et al. Reconstruction of combined defects of the Achilles tendon and the overlying soft tissue with a fascia lata graft and a free fasciocutaneous lateral arm flap. Ann Plast Surg. 2003; 51(4):376–382

Hardwicke JT, Tan JJ, Foster MA, Titley OG. A systematic review of 2-strand versus multistrand core suture techniques and functional outcome after digital flexor tendon repair. J Hand Surg Am. 2014; 39(4):686–695.e2

Harvey FJ, Chu G, Harvey PM. Surgical availability of the plantaris tendon. J Hand Surg Am. 1983; 8(3):243–247

Karaaltin MV, Orhan KS, Demirel T. Fascia lata graft for nasal dorsal contouring in rhinoplasty. J Plast Reconstr Aesthet Surg. 2009; 62(10):1255–1260

Kargi E, Yeşilli C, Akduman B, Babuççu O, Hoşnuter M, Mungan A. Fascia lata grafts for closure of secondary urethral fistulas. Urology. 2003; 62(5):928–931, discussion 931

Kelton PL. Skin grafts and skin substitutes. Selected readings. Plast Surg. 1999; 9:1–24

Kirschner M. Über freie Sehnen- und Faszientransplantation. Beitr Klin Chir. 1909; 65:472

Leckenby JI, Harrison DH, Grobbelaar AO. Static support in the facial palsy patient: a case series of 51 patients using tensor fascia lata slings as the sole treatment for correcting the position of the mouth. J Plast Reconstr Aesthet Surg. 2014; 67(3):350–357

Llanos S, Danilla S, Barraza C, et al. Effectiveness of negative pressure closure in the integration of split thickness skin grafts: a randomized, double-masked, controlled trial. Ann Surg. 2006; 244(5):700–705

MacKinnon SE, ed. Nerve Surgery. New York, NY: Thieme; 2015

Mackinnon SE. New directions in peripheral nerve surgery. Ann Plast Surg. 1989; 22(3):257–273

McArthur LL. Autoplastic sutures in hernia and other diseases: Preliminary report. JAMA. 1901; 37:1162

Mehling IM, Arsalan-Werner A, Sauerbier M. Evidence-based flexor tendon repair. Clin Plast Surg. 2014; 41(3):513–523

Nakano T, Yoshikawa K, Kunieda T, et al. Treatment for infection of artificial dura mater using free fascia lata. J Craniofac Surg 2014; 25(4):1252–1255

Rose EH. Autogenous fascia lata grafts: clinical applications in reanimation of the totally or partially paralyzed face. Plast Reconstr Surg. 2005; 116(1):20–32, discussion 33–35

Seddon H. Three types of nerve injury. Brain. 1943; 66:237

Sharma P, Maffulli N. Basic biology of tendon injury and healing. Surgeon. 2005; 3(5):309–316

Sharma P, Maffulli N. Biology of tendon injury: healing, modeling and remodeling. J Musculoskelet Neuronal Interact. 2006; 6(2):181–190

Silfverskiöld KL, May EJ. Flexor tendon repair in zone II with a new suture technique and an early mobilization program combining passive and active flexion. J Hand Surg Am. 1994; 19(1):53–60

Sunderland S. A classification of peripheral nerve injuries producing loss of function. Brain. 1951; 74(4):491–516

Tang JB, Xie RG. Biomechanics of core and peripheral tendon repairs. In: Tang JB, Amadio PC, Guimberteau JC, Chang J, eds. Tendon Surgery of the Hand. Philadelphia, PA: Elsevier; 2012:35–48

Tiengo C, Giatsidis G, Azzena B. Fascia lata allografts as biological mesh in abdominal wall repair: preliminary outcomes from a retrospective case series. Plast Reconstr Surg. 2013; 132(4):631e–639e

Van Wachem PB, van Gulik TM, van Luyn MJA, Bleichrodt RP. Collagen-based prostheses for hernia repair. In: Bendavid R, Abrahamson J, Arregui ME, Flament JB, Phillips EH, eds. Abdominal Wall Hernias: Principles and Management. New York, NY: Springer; 2001:250–257

Wan D, Potter JK. Biomaterials. In: Janis JE, ed. Essentials of Plastic Surgery, 2nd ed. New York, NY: Thieme; 2014:87–106

14 Fat Grafting

Stefan Danilla Enei, Ekaterina Troncoso Olchevskaia

Abstract

Fat grafting is an excellent approach as a natural filler in aesthetic and reconstructive surgery, with the advantage of producing a permanent, natural-looking result. The main downside of fat grafting however is the unpredictability of the final volume due to resorption of the fat graft. The surgical technique for fat harvesting, processing and injecting should be standardized as stated by Coleman, and the fat graft should be handled with delicacy at every step of the process in order to improve the final result. In reconstructive surgery, fat grafting has been used to improve contour and symmetry after trauma or tumor resection, among others, while in aesthetic surgery it has been widely used to correct the loss of facial volume due to aging as well as for breast and gluteal augmentation.

Keywords: Fat, grafting, lipofilling, lipografting, Coleman technique

14.1 Introduction

Autologous fat grafting is the transfer of adipose tissue to a recipient site without its vascular support. It is widely used as natural filler in both reconstructive and aesthetic surgery, due to its versatility, availability, and natural results, in contrast with alloplastic fillers. Autologous fat grafting has proven that is the best method with which to increase subcutaneous tissue and to permanently correct contour deformities. However, the main problem with this method is the variability of the results due to the unpredictable loss of graft volume.

Neuber described the first autologous fat graft in humans in 1893 when he first used it to reconstruct a tuberculous osteitis sequelae of the face with small grafts of subcutaneous tissue from the patient's upper arm. In 1895 Czerny reported the first case of breast reconstruction utilizing a fat graft. Thereafter, surgeons used autologous fat grafting for many purposes; however, because of the variability and unpredictability of the initial results, the technique was largely abandoned until Illouz introduced liposuction, which opened the gate to modern fat grafting. In the mid-1990s, and thanks to

the renewed interest in fat grafting, Coleman standardized the technique and proved the long-term stability of the graft. Recent advances in fat grafting indicate not only its capability for volume augmentation but also a potential regenerative effect due to the transfer of stem cells within the graft.

According to the American Society of Plastic Surgery's report in 2016 a total of 79.208 grafts were made in the United States, representing a 21% increase with respect to the year 2000.

14.2 Basic Science

Adipose tissue is composed of three main elements: (1) the adipose cell, or adipocyte; (2) its precursor, the preadipocyte; and (3) the stromal vascular cells, including fibroblasts, immune cells, collagen fibers, and blood vessels. The extracellular matrix forms the fat lobules in adipose tissue.

There are mainly two types of adipose tissue: brown fat and white fat. The fat in the adult human body is mainly white fat, which is the focus of this chapter.

Adipocytes are cells with a single large vacuole filled with lipids inside and a peripherally located nucleus. In contrast, preadipocytes resemble fibroblasts. As they differentiate into adipocytes, the expression of collagen I and III decreases, and the production of collagen IV, glycosaminoglycans, and other compounds increases.

As the harvested fat is transplanted to the recipient site, it survives by diffusion until approximately day 4, when the process of neovascularization begins. During the process, and because of mechanisms not fully elucidated, some adipocytes undergo apoptosis, which partly determines the unpredictable graft loss (▶ Fig. 14.1). In 1950, after a series of fat transplantations, Peer observed that the average loss of autografts is 45% of their original volume at 1-year follow-up. He also observed that the viable adipocytes at the time of transplantation determine the volume of the final fat graft.

Also, adipose tissue contains a reservoir of mesenchymal stem cells within the stroma of the tissue. These stem cells are transplanted to the recipient site along with the rest of the fat graft's cells. In 1997, Rigotti reported successful outcomes for managing radiodermatitis with fat grafting,

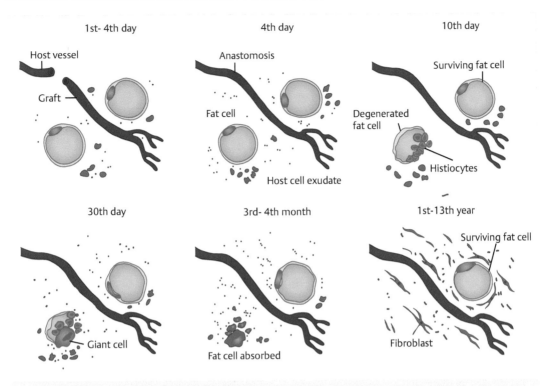

1st- 4th day

Host vessel

Graft

4th day

Anastomosis

Fat cell

Host cell exudate

10th day

Surviving fat cell

Degenerated fat cell

Histiocytes

30th day

Giant cell

3rd- 4th month

Fat cell absorbed

1st-13th year

Surviving fat cell

Fibroblast

Fig. 14.1 Evolution of two adipose cells after lipoinjection. For unknown reasons some fat cells activate an apoptotic mechanism and degenerate around the fourth day.

explained by the regenerative potential of the stem cell population contained within the transplanted adipose tissue.

14.3 Surgical Technique

14.3.1 Fat Harvesting

Common donor sites for fat harvesting include the abdomen, flanks, lumbar area, dorsum, and thighs. Because donor sites are similar to one another in terms of fat viability and long-term stability, donor site selection depends on accessibility, the patient's position on the operating table, the patient's fat deposits, and the patient's desires. Harvesting approaches include syringe aspiration and lipoaspiration. There is no difference in fat viability with either technique as reported in a recent literature review by Sinno et al.

In our practice, adipose tissue is harvested through small, easily concealed incisions. We use infiltration with a tumescent technique, with

1:1,000,000 epinephrine. If general anesthesia is used, we avoid adding lidocaine or other local anesthetic into the infiltration solution, mainly because of its marginal benefits in comparison to the risk of adverse effects. When harvesting fat for microinjection, we prefer low-pressure syringe aspiration as described by Coleman. Conversely, when macroinjection is needed, we use the traditional liposuction technique with a recollection recipient. It is of the utmost importance that a favorable body contour be achieved at the donor site, with careful attention paid to avoid wrinkling and contour deformities.

14.3.2 Fat Processing

Following harvest, the fat needs processing in order to separate the viable adipose cells from the oil, cell debris, blood, and infiltration solution, with three main techniques having been described for this purpose: centrifugation, washing, and sedimentation and straining. There is no evidence of superiority of any one technique, but the graft must be handled with the least possible trauma and ischemic time.

Centrifugation of the lipoaspirate is usually done in a centrifuge at 1,500–3,000 rpm for 2–3 minutes. This yields a three-layered solution composed of oil and cell debris on top, viable adipose cells in the middle, and blood and infiltration solution on the bottom.

Washing consists of mixing the harvested fat with washing solutions, such as normal saline, lactated Ringer solution, glucose 5% solution, or even sterile water. The mixture is then left to rest in order to separate the oil, debris, water, blood, and infiltration solution from the viable adipose cells. This method, nevertheless, may traumatize the adipose cells and reduce their viability.

Sedimentation is believed to be the least traumatic technique and is the authors' preferred method. The harvested fat is left still until the components separate into a three-layered product with the oil and debris on top, the viable cells in the middle, and the blood and infiltration solution at the bottom.

Lastly, straining involves rolling the fat gently through cotton gauze until the liquid component of the harvested tissue is filtered and separated from the stroma.

14.3.3 Fat Injection

Because initial survival of the fat graft is by diffusion, injection should maximize the surface area of contact with the surrounding tissue in order to optimize graft survival. Furthermore, small amounts of graft

should be injected in a multiplanar radially oriented fashion because injection of large volumes of fat graft can result in central ischemia and subsequent necrosis, leading to partial graft loss, loss of volume, and possible cyst formation. For microinjection the authors prefer a Coleman cannula with 1 mL syringes, whereas for macroinjection, a 3 mm blunt cannula is usually used with 50 mL syringes. To reduce the risk of vessel injection, the graft should be injected with low pressure and during withdrawal of the cannula. There is evidence that survival of macroinjected fat can be enhanced with the use of an external expansion device for several weeks preoperatively.

> **Note**
>
> We prefer harvesting the nearest available fat deposit with a blunt cannula technique followed by sedimentation and immediate injection of small amounts of fat in multiple passes.

14.4 Clinical Applications

14.4.1 Facial Lipoinjection

Facial lipoinjection is a versatile method to restore loss of volume resulting from normal aging as well as for reconstructive purposes. Aging produces volume loss by absorption of the fat pads and the bony structures of the face (▶ Fig. 14.2). In the authors' experience, better outcomes are obtained with fat grafting of the malar region and facial grooves. Results are less predictable with the temporal fossa, forehead, and lips. For lipoinjection of

Age: 35   Age: 45   Age: 55

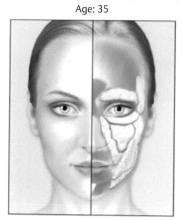 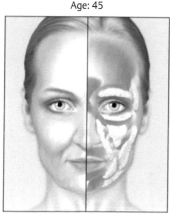 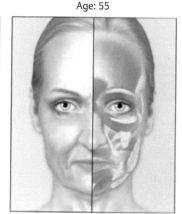

Fig. 14.2 Facial fat deflation due to aging.

the face careful harvesting of the fat by low-pressure syringe aspiration, fat decantation, or centrifugation and microinjection while withdrawing the Coleman cannula in multiple passages is recommended. The quantity of fat graft and areas to treat are depicted in ▶ Fig. 14.3. In reconstructive surgery larger amounts of fat may be needed to fill the defect and achieve symmetry (▶ Fig. 14.4).

14.4.2 Breast Lipoinjection

Breast augmentation with lipoinjection creates a natural look without the complications of a breast implant (▶ Fig. 14.5). The main disadvantage is the unpredictability of the results and the need for multiple sessions to obtain the desired volume. To optimize results, it is important to inject multiplanar, radially oriented small grafts. The authors recommend using syringes no larger than 10 mL for optimal outcomes. Evidence suggests that external tissue expansion can improve graft survival.

14.4.3 Gluteal Lipoinjection

Fat grafting of the buttocks is the first choice to improve gluteal contour, especially in a patient with enough fat deposits, having the advantage of

allowing remodeling of the area by liposuction and subsequent injection (▶ Fig. 14.6). However, the main problem with gluteal fat grafting is fat embolism due to intraluminal injection of the gluteal vessels, as reported by a number of authors worldwide. To prevent this complication, the authors recommend introducing the cannula parallel to the floor, using thick and blunt cannulas, avoiding intramuscular injection, aspirating during introduction of the cannula, and injecting small amounts of fat in a multiplanar manner during withdrawal. Although it is possible to achieve optimal results, the graft intake is unpredictable.

14.5 Conclusions

- Lipoinjection is the best method with which to permanently increase soft tissue volume.
- There are no differences between donor areas in terms of fat survival and long-term results.
- We recommend the less traumatic method for handling the fat graft, by using low-pressure syringes for harvest, decantation, and injection of small amounts of fat.
- Even though fat grafting is safe and easy to perform, there are complications associated with the procedure, some of which can be serious,

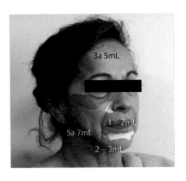

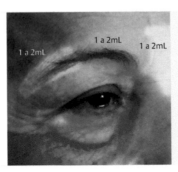

Fig. 14.3 The quantity of fat graft and areas to treat in facial lipoinjection.

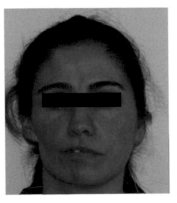

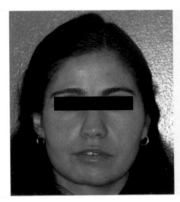

Fig. 14.4 Reconstructive lipoinjection of a patient with Parry–Romberg syndrome to improve face symmetry.

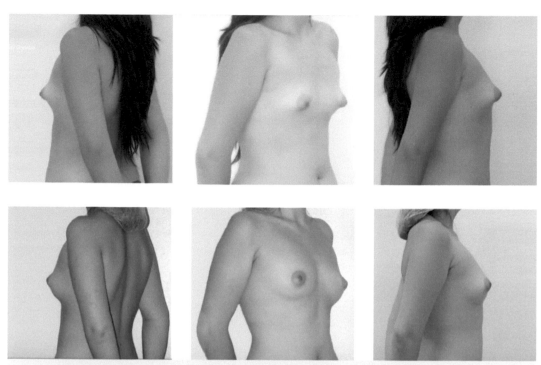

Fig. 14.5 Breast augmentation with lipoinjection for reconstruction of tuberous breasts.

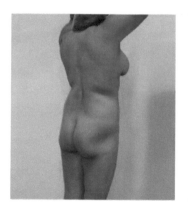

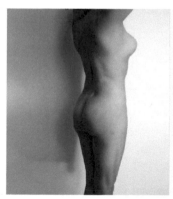

Fig. 14.6 Fat grafting of the buttocks. It has the advantage of allowing remodeling of the area by liposuction and subsequent lipoinjection.

especially in gluteal lipoinjection. The patient and family should be made aware of this.

14.6 Key Points

- For microinjection, use small-size syringes for fat harvest.
- For larger volumes, harvest is best done by routine liposuction using a sterile recipient to collect the lipoaspirate.

- Fat graft survival is maximized by avoiding excessive trauma to the harvested fat. In this sense, we recommend sedimentation as the best method for separating the adipose tissue from the other components.
- Multiplanar small grafts improve fat survival and avoid complications.
- To minimize the risk of fat embolism during gluteal lipoinjection we recommend using blunt cannulas parallel to the floor and avoiding intramuscular injection.

Recommended Readings

American Society of Plastic Surgeons. 2016 Plastic Surgery Statistics Report. Arlington Heights, IL: ASPS Public Relations; 2016

Billings E, Jr, May JW, Jr. Historical review and present status of free fat graft autotransplantation in plastic and reconstructive surgery. Plast Reconstr Surg. 1989; 83(2):368–381

Cárdenas-Camarena L, Bayter JE, Aguirre-Serrano H, Cuenca-Pardo J. Deaths Caused by Gluteal Lipoinjection: What Are We Doing Wrong? Plast Reconstr Surg. 2015; 136(1):58–66

Choi IH, Chung CY, Cho T-J, Yoo WJ. Angiogenesis and mineralization during distraction osteogenesis. J Korean Med Sci. 2002; 17(4):435–447

Coleman SR. Long-term survival of fat transplants: controlled demonstrations. Aesthetic Plast Surg. 1995; 19(5):421–425

Czerny V. Plastic replacement of the breast with a lipoma. Chir Kong Verhandl. 1895; 2:216

Danilla S, Fontbona M, de Valdés VD, et al. Analgesic efficacy of lidocaine for suction-assisted lipectomy with tumescent technique under general anesthesia: a randomized, double-masked, controlled trial. Plast Reconstr Surg. 2013; 132(2):327–332

Geneser F. Histología sobre bases biomoleculares. Madrid, Spain: Editorial Médica Panamericana; 2000:813

Gir P, Brown SA, Oni G, Kashefi N, Mojallal A, Rohrich RJ. Fat grafting: evidence-based review on autologous fat harvesting, processing, reinjection, and storage. Plast Reconstr Surg. 2012; 130(1):249–258

Khouri RK, Khouri RK, Jr, Rigotti G, et al. Aesthetic applications of Brava-assisted megavolume fat grafting to the breasts: a 9-year, 476-patient, multicenter experience. Plast Reconstr Surg. 2014; 133(4):796–807, discussion 808–809

Peer LA. Loss of weight and volume in human fat grafts: with postulation of a "cell survival theory." Plast Reconstr Surg. 1950; 5(3):45:217

Rigotti G, Marchi A, Stringhini P, et al. Determining the oncological risk of autologous lipoaspirate grafting for post-mastectomy breast reconstruction. Aesthetic Plast Surg. 2010; 34(4):475–480

Shim YH, Zhang RH. Literature Review to Optimize the Autologous Fat Transplantation Procedure and Recent Technologies to Improve Graft Viability and Overall Outcome: A Systematic and Retrospective Analytic Approach. Aesthetic Plast Surg. 2017; 41(4):815–831

Sinno S, Chang JB, Brownstone ND, Saadeh PB, Wall S, Jr. Determining the Safety and Efficacy of Gluteal Augmentation: A Systematic Review of Outcomes and Complications. Plast Reconstr Surg. 2016; 137(4): 1151–1156

Thorne CH. Grabb and Smith's Plastic Surgery. Philadelphia, PA: Wolters Kluwer Health; 2013:3536

Tuin AJ, Domerchie PN, Schepers RH, et al. What is the current optimal fat grafting processing technique? A systematic review. J Craniomaxillofac Surg. 2016; 44(1):45–55

15 Vascular Anatomy of the Skin and Muscles

Diego Marré, Michael Tecce, Alejandro Conejero

Abstract

The evolution of plastic surgery has been intimately related to the knowledge of the arterial and venous anatomy of skin, soft tissues, and bone because their transfer and complete survival depend on an adequate blood supply. The first anatomical works, though elegant and precise, were purely descriptive without incorporating a great deal of clinical and surgical correlations in their findings. However, as flap surgery began to rise, particularly during the World Wars, the intrinsic relationship between flap survival and blood supply became evident, prompting surgeons to reappraise the anatomical works of previous anatomists and later on to return to the dissection lab in the search of vascular sources that would provide a reliable supply to a block of tissue. The description of the blood supply to the fascia, the classification of muscles according to their blood supply, the angiosome concept, and more recently the perforasome concept, are all part of a fascinating evolving period that has led us to the current status of flap surgery and tissue transfer that we know today. Nevertheless, despite the great advances that have contributed to increase the safety and reliability of tissue transfer, we still see portions of flaps becoming congested or ischemic, which makes us wonder whether we should have taken that extra perforator or designed our flap differently. Ultimately, the exact territory supplied by a single (perforator) vessel remains a mystery. This chapter describes the different sources of blood supply to the skin and muscles together with an anatomical outline of the vascular sources most commonly used in flap surgery.

Keywords: angiosome, blood supply, direct cutaneous vessel, musculocutaneous perforator, perforasome, septocutaneous perforator, skin

Plastic surgery is a constant battle between blood supply and beauty.

— Sir Harold Gillies, 1957

15.1 Introduction

If a flap is defined as a block of tissue that is transferred from one area to another while maintaining its own blood supply, then it becomes clear that a thorough knowledge of the anatomy of the vascular network is one of plastic surgery's essential pillars. The knowledge and understanding of the blood supply to the skin and muscles has evolved gradually over the past 135 years. The initial works provided a detailed and exquisite anatomical description. Subsequent studies, inspired by the preceding ones, began to incorporate important clinical interpretations with the aim of offering a surgical solution to a clinical problem. However, the evolution from anatomical descriptions to (plastic) surgical applications was not as straightforward as one would imagine. Belatedness in scientific communication, language barriers, historical conflicts, egos, and personalities were likely responsible for the delay in the application of anatomical findings to reconstructive surgery. For example, because the works of Manchot and Salmon were written in French, those of Pieri in Italian, and those of Spalteholz and Esser in German, they all remained unknown to most of the (English speaking) surgical community until they were translated to English decades later. Another example is that, while Sir Harold Gillies reconstructed wounded British soldiers with his randomly based tubed flaps, Esser in Germany used "arterial" or "biological" flaps, which incorporated a known vascular axis on their base, hence ensuring a more reliable blood supply. Once it became evident that a block of tissue could be safely transferred based on a known vascular pedicle and that such pedicle had a relatively constant anatomy, surgeons were urged to return to the lab to perform anatomical dissections to reappraise the findings of their pioneers and put them in a clinical context. Thus, thanks to the invaluable and exhaustive work of many landmark plastic surgeons, anatomical research steadily met flap surgery until their separate histories converged into the completely interdependent and inseparable marriage we know today. In addition, the discovery of radiology and the development of sophisticated methods of vascular imaging have greatly enhanced the relationship between vascular anatomy and flap surgery as well as significantly aided in the preoperative planning and execution of a large number of flaps.

15.2 Basic Science

15.2.1 Blood Supply to the Skin

The skin is the body's largest organ, accounting for 8% of the total body mass, with a surface area of approximately 2 square meters. From a vascular point of view, the skin is supplied by a rich and fully interconnected network, hierarchically organized into layers with distinct anatomical features and physiological functions. The cutaneous circulation delivers nutrients and oxygen and removes waste metabolites, and it also orchestrates thermoregulation, one of the skin's main tasks. Even though skin has relatively low metabolic demands, it is endowed with a remarkable ability to increase or decrease its capacity by as much as 20-fold as part of its thermoregulatory function, dissipating or conserving heat as required. Moreover, in normal conditions, the blood supply to the skin far exceeds its nutritional requirements, a feature to consider when designing, executing, and monitoring skin flaps.

Cutaneous Vascular Plexuses

The skin is irrigated by cutaneous branches originating from underlying larger vessels. After piercing the deep fascia, cutaneous vessels begin to ramify to form five interconnected vascular plexuses, which are ultimately responsible for supplying the integument. These plexuses can be found in close association with the different layers of the skin. Three of them are found within the skin, irrigating its adnexal structures, whereas the other two are located deeper in the subcutaneous tissue and deep fascia. From superficial to deep, the cutaneous vascular plexuses are subpapillary, dermal, subdermal, subcutaneous, and fascial, which includes subfascial, intrafascial, and suprafascial (prefascial) components (▶ Fig. 15.1).

Subpapillary plexus: The subpapillary plexus, also called the subepidermal plexus, is located just below the dermal papillae, at the junction between the papillar and reticular dermis. Capillary loops emanate from this plexus into each dermal papilla to supply the overlying epidermis. Due to their terminal configuration, the vessels contained within the subpapillary plexus have no muscular layer and serve a primarily nutritional function.

Dermal plexus: The dermal plexus is located within the reticular dermis. It contains a rich venous network as well as arterioles with a discontinuous muscular wall. The main function of this plexus is thermoregulation. This particular function is possible due to the presence of glomera (plural for *glomus*), which consist of arteriovenous anastomoses surrounded by connective tissue and muscle fibers. Glomera control the flow of blood toward or away from the superficial plexuses in response to autonomic vasomotor control.

Subdermal plexus: Located between the dermis and the underlying subcutaneous fat, the subdermal plexus has long been considered the main vascular supply to the skin. The arteries running at this level have a continuous muscular layer, with their function being mainly the distribution of blood flow. From these arteries, branches are given off to both the overlying dermis and the underlying adipose tissue. Within the dermis, these branches join each other to form vascular arcades from which vessels forming more superficial plexuses originate.

Subcutaneous plexus: The subcutaneous plexus runs parallel to the skin and is located at the level of the superficial fascia (e.g., Scarpa's fascia in the trunk). This plexus is nourished by branches coming from direct and indirect vessels

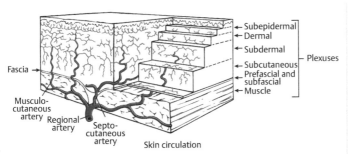

Fig. 15.1 Blood supply to the skin, including the subpapillary (subepidermal), mid-dermal (dermal), subdermal, subcutaneous, and fascial plexuses. (Reproduced from Zenn, Jones, Reconstructive Surgery Anatomy, Technique, and Clinical Applications, ©2012, Thieme Publishers, New York.)

(described below), and in turn it sends off branches to supply the overlying network.

Fascial plexus: As early as 1936, Michel Salmon noted that "the fascia is a very poorly vascularized structure and it is rare to encounter an arteriole within its substance." Later on Lang identified a fine intrafascial plexus running within the fascia, which was subsequently confirmed by Schafer and Batchelor et al, who concluded that the intrafascial plexus is supplied by the suprafascial and subfascial plexuses. Thus we know now that fascia contains three plexuses—suprafascial, intrafascial, and subfascial. The blood supply to these plexuses comes from branches of perforating vessels (described later in this chapter) and from *fascial feeders,* which are vessels that do not penetrate the fascia but take part in the subfascial plexus and have no accompanying vena comitantes (▶Fig. 15.2). It is important to note that, because the deep fascia varies in different areas of the body, so may its vascular supply.

Cutaneous Vessels: Direct and Indirect

The anatomical configuration of the cutaneous vascular supply has been a matter of debate, particularly regarding denomination and classification of vessels. In fact, systems classifying vessels into 2, 3, and up to 10 different types have been proposed, hampering communication and teaching. Moreover, because the classification of the skin's vasculature has direct implications in flap terminology and classification, several definitions and systems have also been proposed for perforator flaps.

Although there are some specific regional exceptions, the overall configuration of the skin's vascular supply is based on source vessels from which cutaneous vessels (perforators) stem to reach the skin. While source vessels are located deep to the deep fascia, perforators travel through different pathways to pierce the deep fascia and reach the skin. Cutaneous vessels can be broadly classified as direct or indirect, according to the route they make on their way to the skin (▶Fig. 15.3).

Direct vessels: These vessels travel between tissues to reach their main destination, which is the skin. In addition, direct vessels can be subclassified into direct cutaneous and septocutaneous. Direct cutaneous vessels, also known as axial vessels, pierce the deep fascia directly without previously passing through muscle or an intermuscular septum. Once above the fascia, these vessels travel parallel to the skin in the subcutaneous plane, giving off branches that supply the overlying plexuses. Direct cutaneous vessels form the vascular basis of axial flaps; the dorsalis pedis, supratrochlear, and superficial circumflex iliac arteries are good examples of direct cutaneous vessels supplying the well-known dorsalis pedis, forehead, and groin axial flaps, respectively. Direct septocutaneous vessels (also called septocutaneous perforators) travel within an intermuscular septum before piercing the deep fascia and reaching the skin

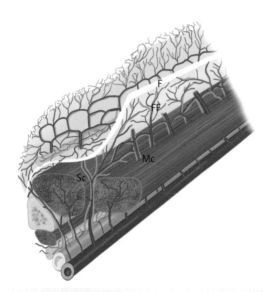

Fig. 15.2 Diagram showing the vessels nourishing the fascia and its associated vascular plexuses (subfascial, intrafascial, and suprafascial). Mc, musculocutaneous perforator; Sc, septocutaneous perforator; F, fascia; Ff, fascial feeder.

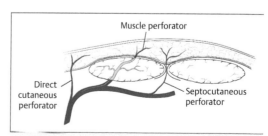

Fig. 15.3 Basic configuration of vessels supplying the skin. (Reproduced from Zenn, Jones, Reconstructive Surgery Anatomy, Technique, and Clinical Applications, ©2012, Thieme Publishers, New York.)

without experiencing a significant change in caliber. Examples of septocutaneous vessels include perforators from the descending branch of the lateral circumflex femoral artery running between the rectus femoris and the vastus lateralis to supply the anterolateral thigh flap or perforators from the peroneal artery traveling in the posterior intermuscular septum to supply the skin paddle of a fibular osteocutaneous flap. It is important from a semantic and clinical point of view not to confuse or interchangeably use the terms *septocutaneous* and *fasciocutaneous*. As we have illustrated here, *septocutaneous* describes the anatomical course of a blood vessel on its way to the skin, whereas *fasciocutaneous* refers to a particular type of skin flap that includes the deep fascia for a specific reconstructive purpose or to enhance vascularization.

Indirect vessels: These vessels originate from source vessels and reach the skin secondarily after traveling through muscle, which they supply through numerous side branches. A good example of indirect vessels includes the deep inferior epigastric artery perforator (DIEP) flap supplying the abdominal wall. From a surgical point of view, the importance in differentiating indirect vessels with direct ones is that, in general, flaps based on the former are more technically demanding because the perforator needs to be dissected off its whole intramuscular course all the way down to its source vessel.

It can be seen that different terms have been used to name the same structure. This is not an unusual situation when describing the vessels supplying the integument. ▶ Table 15.1 illustrates the equivalence of these terms.

Six Types of Vascular Input to the Skin

The simplest way to understand how cutaneous vessels are classified is to appreciate that they are named based on one main concept—the pathway they take to get to the skin upon branching from their source vessel. As already described, direct

cutaneous, direct septocutaneous, and indirect vessels supply the integument. Notwithstanding the anatomical accuracy of such a description, from a surgical standpoint it may be considered too broad and simplistic because, as noted by Nakajima et al, cutaneous vessels may actually follow six different pathways on their way to the skin (▶ Fig. 15.4). The first type is the direct cutaneous vessel, which, after branching off the source artery, bypasses all structures en route to its final destination to the skin. These vessels are typically found around the joints and areas of loose skin because these areas lack muscle and provide space for vessels to directly contact the skin. Direct septocutaneous vessels provide direct blood supply to the skin, but their pathway to get there is slightly different because it traverses through the intermuscular septum of the extremity muscles before reaching the skin. Importantly, even though these vessels travel between muscles, they do not supply them. The third type corresponds to direct cutaneous branches of muscular vessels. As their name implies, the main destination of these vessels is the skin; however, before reaching it they travel through intermuscular spaces. Additionally, in the strict sense, unlike the previous two, direct cutaneous branches of muscular vessels do not stem from the source vessel directly but from one of its muscular branches. Despite their anatomical differences, the three types of vessels discussed so far share in common being direct suppliers to the

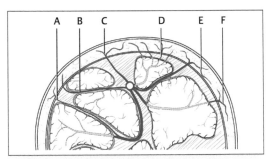

Fig. 15.4 The classification of cutaneous vessels according to Nakajima. Type A, direct cutaneous branch of muscular vessel; Type B, septocutaneous perforator; Type C, direct cutaneous; Type D, musculocutaneous perforator; Type E, direct septocutaneous; Type F, perforating cutaneous branch of a muscular vessel. (Reproduced from Zenn, Jones, Reconstructive Surgery Anatomy, Technique, and Clinical Applications, ©2012, Thieme Publishers, New York.)

Table 15.1 Terms' equivalence of cutaneous blood vessels

Direct cutaneous	→ Axial vessel
Direct septocutaneous	→ Septocutaneous perforator
Indirect vessel	→ Musculocutaneous perforator

skin; that is, they do not branch to any other structure along their course, in contrast to the following three, which do supply other tissues (mainly muscles) apart from skin. Perforating cutaneous branches of a muscular vessel branch from the source artery and travel through and supply a muscular structure before reaching the skin. Septocutaneous perforators course in the intermuscular septum; however, in doing so, they give off branches to supply the fascial plexus as well muscle in some cases. Lastly, musculocutaneous perforators are branches from a muscular artery located within the muscle that emerge above the deep fascia and arborize to form the fascial plexus.

15.2.2 Angiosome Concept

Over the last 35 years, Ian Taylor and his large number of contributors and colleagues have provided some remarkable foundations to the current knowledge and understanding of the vascular supply to the skin. Inspired mainly by the works of Manchot and Salmon (▶Fig. 15.5 and ▶Fig. 15.6), Taylor and his colleagues have undertaken an

impressive amount of anatomical research with a strong clinical perspective providing several key concepts for flap surgery. A detailed description of these works is beyond the scope of this chapter—for a full review on the topic the reader is referred to Taylor's numerous articles and seminal work *The Angiosome Concept and Tissue Transfer*.

An angiosome (from the Greek *angiome* [vessel] and *somite* [segment or sector of the body]) is a three-dimensional block of tissue supplied by one source artery and its accompanying veins. An angiosome usually spans all the way from skin to bone, though in some cases it can be restricted to the deeper layers. Similarly, the representation of an angiosome is not always the same in the deep tissues and the skin—in some areas an angiosome may include a wide portion of deep tissues but a comparatively small skin territory, and vice versa. In their initial work, Taylor and Palmer described 40 different vascular territories (angiosomes), each of them based on a different source artery (▶Fig. 15.7). These authors also observed that contiguous angiosomes were interconnected by vessels without a change in caliber (true anastomoses)

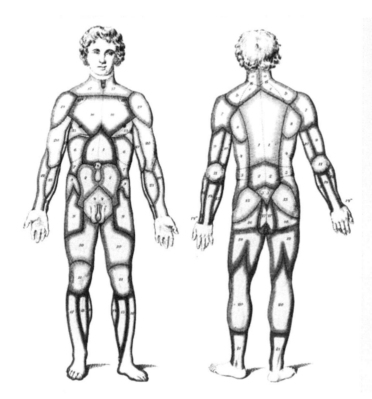

Fig. 15.5 Illustration of the territories supplied by cutaneous arteries according to Carl Manchot, 1889. (Reproduced from Zenn, Jones, Reconstructive Surgery Anatomy, Technique, and Clinical Applications, ©2012, Thieme Publishers, New York.)

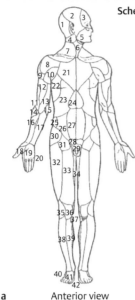

Schematic summary of the cutaneous arterial territory of the ventral surface of the body.

1. Occipital artery
2. Superficial temporal artery
3. Ophthalmic artery
4. Sternocleidomastoid artery
5. Facial artery
6. Thyroid arteries
7. Transverse cervical and suprascapular arteries
8. Deltoid branch of the acromiothoracic trunk
9. Circumflex humeral arteries
10. Small thoracic branches of the acromiothoracic trunk
11. Profunda brachii artery
12. Brachial artery (muscular branches)
13. Brachial artery (direct branches)
14. Epicondylar arteries
15. Epitrochlear arteries
16. Radial artery
17. Ulnar artery
18. Deep palmar arch
19. Superficial palmar arch
20. Anterior interosseous artery
21. Internal mammary artery
22. External mammary (lateral thoracic) and subscapular arteries
23. Intercostal arteries
24. Superficial superior epigastric artery
25. Lumbar arteries
26. Inferior superficial epigastic artery
27. Deep epigastric artery
28. External superior pudendal artery
29. External inferior pudendal artery
30. Superficial circumflex iliac artery
31. Femoral artery
32. Artery to the vastus lateralis muscle
33. Superficial femoral artery
34. Artery to the adductor muscles
35. Lateral articular branches
36. Medial articular branches
37. Genus descendens artery
38. Anterior tibial artery
39. Posterior tibial artery
40. Peroneal artery
41. Dorsalis pedis artery
42. Medial plantar artery

a   Anterior view

Schematic summary of the cutaneous arterial territories of the dorsal surface of the body.

1. Superficial temporal artery
2. Occipital artery
3. Posterior auricular artery
4. Deep cervical artery
5. Sternocleidomastoid artery
6. Deep branch of the transverse cervical artery
7. Suprascapular artery
8. Dorsospinal branch of the intercostal artery
9. Subscapular artery
10. Posterior circumflex humeral artery
11. Brachial artery (medial collateral branches)
12. Profunda brachii artery
13. Posterior recurrent ulnar artery
14. Radial recurrent artery
15. Ulnar artery
16. Posterior interosseous artery
17. Anterior interosseous artery
18. Dorsal branch of the ulnar artery
19. Dorsal carpal artery
20. Posterior interosseous arteries
21. Deep palmar arch
22. Digital arteries
23. Intercostal arteries (perforating branches)
24. Lumbar arteries (dorsospinal branches)
25. Lumbar arteries (perforating branches)
26. Superficial circumflex iliac artery
27. Superior gluteal artery
28. Internal pudendal artery
29. Inferior gluteal artery
30. Artery to the adductors
31. Artery accompanying the sciatic nerve
32 and 33. Perforating arteries
34. Popliteal artery
35. Gastrocnemius arteries
36. Small saphenous artery
37. Posterior tibial artery
38. Peroneal artery
39. Dorsalis pedis artery
40. Medial plantar artery

b   Posterior view

Fig. 15.6 (a,b) The vascular territories of the human body according to Michel Salmon, Artères de la Peau, 1936. (Reproduced from Zenn, Jones, Reconstructive Surgery Anatomy, Technique, and Clinical Applications, ©2012, Thieme Publishers, New York.)

or, more commonly, by vessels of reduced caliber, which they named choke vessels. These choke vessels have the capacity to dilate in response to metabolic and oxygen requirements. This increase in diameter (and hence improvement of blood supply) is maximal at 48–72 hours after surgery and once established is permanent and irreversible. One of the most important clinical applications derived from the angiosome concept was the fact that, when harvesting a flap, it is

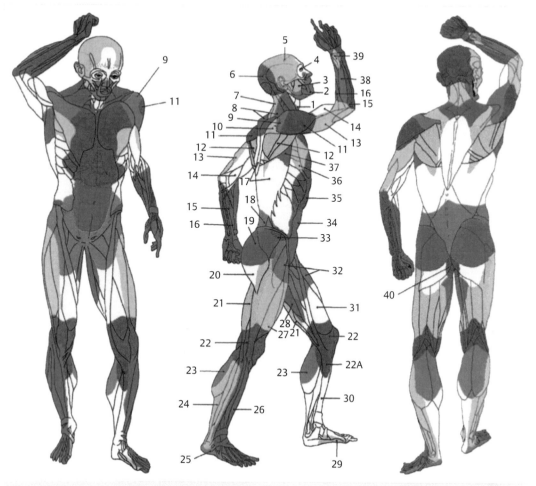

Fig. 15.7 The vascular territories (angiosomes) described by Taylor. Vascular territories of the integument of the skin are delineated according to the source vessel of the perforator. 1, thyroid; 2, facial; 3, buccal internal maxillary; 4, ophthalmic; 5, superficial temporal; 6, occipital; 7, deep cervical; 8, transverse cervical; 9, acromiothoracic; 10, suprascapular; 11, posterior circumflex humeral; 12, circumflex scapular; 13, profunda brachii; 14, brachial; 15, ulnar; 16, radial; 17, posterior intercostals; 18, lumbar; 19, superior gluteal; 20, inferior gluteal; 21, profunda femoris; 22, popliteal; 22A, descending geniculate saphenous; 23, sural; 24, peroneal; 25, lateral plantar; 26, anterior tibial; 27, lateral femoral circumflex; 28, adductor profunda; 29, medial plantar; 30, posterior tibial; 31, superficial femoral; 32, common femoral; 33, deep circumflex iliac; 34, deep inferior epigastric; 35, internal thoracic; 36, lateral thoracic; 37, thoracodorsal; 38, posterior interosseous; 39, anterior interosseous; 40, internal pudendal. (Reproduced from Zenn, Jones, Reconstructive Surgery Anatomy, Technique, and Clinical Applications, ©2012, Thieme Publishers, New York.)

possible to safely include tissues from an immediately adjacent angiosome; however, capturing the one beyond may lead to necrosis of the distal portion unless the different angiosomes are linked by "true" anastomoses or a delay procedure is performed prior to flap transfer.

The perforators originating from an angiosome's source artery supply the cutaneous territory of that angiosome. According to Taylor, each perforator has its own territory, which connects radially with its neighbors via true anastomoses or choke vessels, so that all perforators together make up for the angiosome's cutaneous territory. The same author has noted that the territory irrigated by a single perforator is influenced by its size and the density of perforators in the same area. Thus, in regions like the head and neck, torso, and proximal limbs, where perforators are large and low in number, one can anticipate that a single perforator supplies a large area; conversely, in the presence of small and numerous perforators, the territory of each is likely small, as is usually the case in distal limbs, hands, and feet. Again, as before, the territory beyond the one adjacent to the selected perforator is at higher risk of necrosis (▶Fig. 15.8). These findings and others have provided remarkable insights not only to the design and harvest of flaps but also to the understanding of ischemic complications seen in flap surgery.

Remember M!

An angiosome is a three-dimensional block of tissue supplied by one source artery and its accompanying veins. Adjacent angiosomes are linked by true anastomoses or choke vessels.

15.2.3 Anatomic, Dynamic, and Potential Territories and the Delay Procedure

Cormack and Lamberty in their work *The Arterial Anatomy of Skin Flaps* describe three different types of cutaneous vascular territories, namely, anatomical, dynamic, and potential (▶Fig. 15.9).

The *anatomical territory* of a vessel refers to the area irrigated by that vessel before anastomosing with any of its neighbors. This is analogous to Taylor's cutaneous territory of a single perforator. The observation that whenever a cutaneous vessel is occluded the adjacent one supplies its territory, led to the denomination of the *dynamic territory*. Dynamic territories are therefore developed following flap elevation where a cutaneous vessel is divided and nevertheless the area it used to irrigate remains viable thanks to a rearrangement of the local blood flow that allows an adjacent vessel to "invade" that territory. This concept correlates with Taylor's observation that the safe area of a single cutaneous perforator is formed by its own territory and those immediately adjacent to it. The *potential territory* of a cutaneous vessel includes areas beyond its dynamic territories and can only be captured following a delay procedure.

Bearing the concepts of angiosome and cutaneous vascular territories in mind, the understanding of the *delay procedure* becomes easier. Flap delay consists in the segmental interruption of blood supply to a piece of tissue (most commonly skin, but can be muscle as well) in a staged manner so that the vascular inflow from the main pedicle gradually extends to the distal portion of the flap, which would otherwise not survive if raised in one

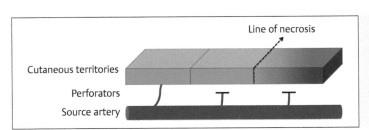

Fig. 15.8 The vessel supplying one territory is able to supply the adjacent one. However, capturing one territory beyond usually leads to necrosis of the distal portion.

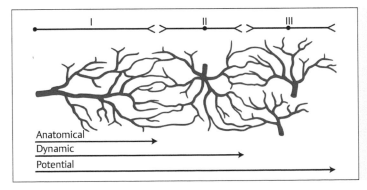

Fig. 15.9 The anatomical, dynamic, and potential territories of cutaneous vessels. Although anatomical and dynamic territories can be safely harvested based on a single vessel, potential territories will not be adequately perfused unless a delay procedure is performed. (Reproduced from Zenn, Jones, Reconstructive Surgery Anatomy, Technique, and Clinical Applications, ©2012, Thieme Publishers, New York.)

stage. The opening of choke vessels and the subsequent capture of potential territories form the basic anatomical and physiologic basis of the delay phenomenon (▶Fig. 15.10). An important aspect in flap delay is the fact that after partial elevation, the flap is sutured back at the donor site so that it can adapt to the new vascular situation without the "stress" elicited by complete elevation and transfer. Chapter 16 provides a more detailed explanation of the surgical steps and the physiologic changes of flap delay.

15.2.4 Perforasome Concept

Earlier concepts introduced by Taylor and Nakajima as already discussed helped to formulate the work of Saint-Cyr, who described the perforasome theory in 2009. In this work, the authors used dye injections followed by tomographic angiography to assess vascular anatomy and flow characteristics for the unique vascular arterial territory of a given perforator—termed a perforasome. The theory blends classic concepts of vascular anatomy and introduces four principles that define the perforasome.

First principle: Each perforasome is linked with neighboring perforasomes via linking vessels that can vary in size. The larger vessels directly link one perforator to the next and as such are termed direct vessels. Conversely, indirect vessels are smaller in size, located in the subdermal plexus, and represent recurrent flow to adjacent perforator branches. The principle in this theory further postulates that these two distinct and different flow patterns are protective mechanisms that help to ensure blood flow throughout the perforasome in the event of vascular injury.

Second principle: Flap design should be based on the direction of linking vessels. The reason for this is because the orientation of linking vessels corresponds to maximal blood flow. In the extremities, this blood flow follows the axial direction of the involved limb, whereas the direction of flow in the trunk is perpendicular to the midline. Larger perforasomes typically contain more linking vessels and have more variability. Therefore, perforators with a very large perforasome will have a higher degree of freedom in flap design and orientation.

Third principle: The filling of vessels from the source artery begins with perforators of that same source artery and then continues to include perforators of adjacent source arteries. Only after the source artery fully perfuses the vessels within its own perforasome do the linking vessels perfuse adjacent perforasomes.

Fourth principle: Source vessels found near joints and articulations have branching vessels that preferentially lead away from the articulation. In contrast, perforators located at a midpoint between two articulations have flow in many directions.

The perforasome theory helps to explain the mechanism by which large perforator flaps can be harvested based on a single perforator. Linking vessels of different sizes enable shared perfusion of adjacent perforasomes and act as a protective feature to ensure collateral blood flow in the event of disruption.

15.3 Blood Supply to the Muscles

The use of muscle (flaps) to reconstruct defects of varying nature brought forward a whole new perspective as to the possibilities of reconstructive surgery, which until then were "limited" to employing skin flaps only. Their bulk, reliable blood supply, and, for most, consistent anatomy, were

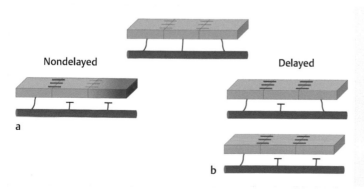

Nondelayed

Delayed

a

b

Fig. 15.10 Schematic diagram of the changes occurring in vessels connecting adjacent territories during a delay procedure. (a) If the flap is raised completely based on a single vessel, necrosis of the distal portion will likely occur. (b) If the blood supply is interrupted in a segmental fashion, dilation of choke vessels allows the interrupted area to be supplied by its neighbors so that eventually all territories are adequately connected and perfused.

seen as major advantages, as was also the fact that they were based on sizeable vascular pedicles. Later on, when it became evident that a muscle was able to support an overlying skin paddle or that they could be used to provide functional restoration of a paralyzed segment, muscle flaps became a fundamental tool in the plastic surgeon's armamentarium.

15.3.1 Vascular Patterns of Muscles—the Mathes–Nahai Classification

The vascular anatomy of muscles is, luckily, far less variable than that of skin, the proof being that there is only one classification system that has stood the test of time and remained unchanged since Stephen Mathes and Foad Nahai described it 35 years ago. Through anatomical, injection, and radiographic studies, these surgeons described five different patterns of circulation based on the following anatomical features: (1) the regional source of the pedicle entering the muscle; (2) the number and (3) size of the pedicle; (4) the location of the pedicle in relation to the muscle's origin and insertion; and (5) the angiographic patterns of the intramuscular vessels (►Fig. 15.11 and ►Table 15.2).

Type I: One Vascular Pedicle

These muscles are supplied by a single vascular pedicle. The gastrocnemius, rectus femoris, and tensor fascia lata are examples of muscles with a type I vascular pattern.

Type II: One Dominant Vascular Pedicle and Several Minor Vascular Pedicles

Type II muscles are supplied by one or more large pedicles plus a series of minor ones. Usually, the large (dominant) pedicle enters the muscle at either its origin or its insertion, whereas the minor pedicles are distributed along the muscle belly. The most important clinical aspect of this group of muscles is that they can be reliably harvested based on their dominant pedicle alone, but not on the minor pedicles, unless a delay procedure is performed prior to transfer. The vast majority of muscles in the body have a type II vascular pattern.

Type III: Two Dominant Pedicles

Muscles in this group have two different large pedicles, each arising from a different regional source, and each of them capable of supplying the whole

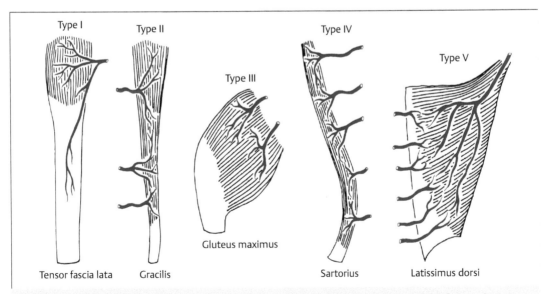

Fig. 15.11 Mathes–Nahai classification of muscles. (Reproduced from Zenn, Jones, Reconstructive Surgery Anatomy, Technique, and Clinical Applications, ©2012, Thieme Publishers, New York.)

Table 15.2 Mathes–Nahai classification of muscles

Type I	Type II	Type III	Type IV	Type V
Genioglossus	Sternocleidomastoid	Temporalis	External oblique	Pectoralis major
Hyoglossus	Trapezius	Orbicularis oris	Sartorius	Latissimus dorsi
Longitudinalis linguae	Platysma	Pectoralis minor	Tibialis anterior	Internal oblique
Transversus and verticalis linguae	Triceps	Serratus anterior	Extensor digitorum longus	
Styloglossus	Coracobrachialis	Intercostal	Extensor hallucis longus	
Anconeus	Brachioradialis	Rectus abdominis	Flexor digitorum longus	
Abductor pollicis brevis	Flexor carpi ulnaris	Gluteus maximus	Flexor hallucis longus	
Abductor digiti minimi (hand)	Gracilis			
First dorsal interosseous	Biceps femoris			
Tensor fascia lata	Rectus femoris			
Vastus lateralis	Vastus medialis			
Gastrocnemius medial and lateral	Soleus			
	Peroneus longus			
	Peroneous brevis			
	Flexor digitorum brevis			
	Abductor hallucis			
	Abductor digiti minimi			

muscle for transfer. Gluteus maximus and rectus abdominis muscles are examples of muscles with a type III irrigation pattern.

Type IV: Several Segmental Vascular Pedicles

These muscles do not have a large dominant pedicle, but instead are supplied by a number of vessels of similar diameter, each one supplying a confined segment. Due to this segmentary distribution, division of two or three pedicles usually results in necrosis of the distal portion. The sartorius is a good example of a type IV muscle.

Type V: One Dominant Pedicle and Secondary Segmental Vascular Pedicles

Type V muscles have a dual supply provided by a dominant pedicle near the muscle's insertion site and several secondary segmental pedicles at the origin. Most importantly, muscles with a type V vascular pattern can be safely harvested based on either their dominant pedicle or the group of segmental pedicles. This feature greatly expands the versatility of these flaps by conferring on them two different arcs of rotation, each based on one of the vascular inputs. The latissimus dorsi and pectoralis major are the main exponents of this group.

15.3.2 Innervation Patterns of Muscles—the Taylor's Classification

From a reconstructive point of view, it is fundamental to know not only how a muscle is vascularized but also its innervation pattern. Such knowledge will help in selecting the most suitable muscle for a functional reconstruction, as well as in leaving a functional remnant when only a segment of the muscle is needed. To address these and other important issues regarding free vascularized muscle transfer, Taylor et al. described four different patterns of innervation (▶Fig. 15.12 and ▶Table 15.3).

Type I: One Motor Nerve

These muscles are innervated by a single motor nerve that divides after entering the muscle. The latissimus dorsi, innervated by the thoracodorsal nerve, is an example of a type I muscle.

Type II: One Motor Nerve That Divides

Type II muscles are supplied by one motor nerve that divides before entering the muscle. The gluteus maximus muscle innervated by the inferior gluteal nerve is an example of a type II muscle.

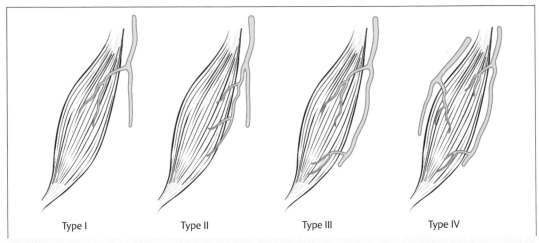

Type I   Type II   Type III   Type IV

Fig. 15.12 Taylor's classification of muscles. (Reproduced from Zenn, Jones, Reconstructive Surgery Anatomy, Technique, and Clinical Applications, ©2012, Thieme Publishers, New York.)

Table 15.3 Taylor classification of muscles

Type I	Type II	Type III	Type IV
Latissimus dorsi	Deltoid	Subscapularis	Digastric
Teres minor	Trapezius	Teres major	Erector spinae group
Extensor indicis	Serratus anterior	Flexor digitorum	Levator scapulae
Extensor pollicis longus	Biceps brachii	superficialis	Internal oblique
Abductor pollicis longus	Brachialis	Extensor carpi ulnaris	Rectus abdominis
Palmaris longus	Flexor pollicis longus	Extensor digitorum longus	
Popliteus	Pectineus	Gluteus medius	
Plantaris	Adductor longus	Gluteus minimus	
Extensor hallucis longus	Adductor brevis	Sartorius	
	Flexor hallucis longus	Vastus medialis	
	Flexor digitorum longus	Vastus intermedius	
		Peroneus longus	
		Soleus	
		Tibialis posterior	

Type III: Multiple Motor Branches from a Common Trunk

Multiple motor branches originating from a common trunk supply these muscles. This feature allows them to be divided into separate functional subunits for transfer. The gastrocnemius and semimembranosus are some of the several muscles with a type III innervation pattern.

Type IV: Multiple Motor Nerves from Different Origins

This last group of muscles are supplied by multiple motor nerves from different origins. The rectus abdominis muscle, which is segmentally innervated by

motor branches of the 7th through 12th intercostal nerve, is an example of a type IV innervation muscle.

> **Note**
>
> The Mathes–Nahai classification categorizes muscles into five different types according to their pattern of vascularization, whereas in Taylor's system, muscles are grouped in four kinds depending on their pattern of motor innervation.

15.4 Regional Blood Supply

The previous sections of this chapter have been devoted to the overall configuration of the blood supply to the skin with a special emphasis on plexuses, vessels, and vascular territories. Herein, an anatomical description of blood vessels supplying skin flaps commonly used in reconstructive surgery is provided. Throughout this section, some flap terminology will be used sporadically; for those not yet familiarized with these terms, we recommend reading first the section "Classification of Flaps" in Chapter 16 to better understand the "flap–applied" anatomical descriptions given here.

15.4.1 Head and Neck

Knowledge of the anatomy and territories of the main arteries supplying the integument of the scalp and face is essential for the design of flaps, replantation of parts, and exposure of recipient vessels for microsurgical tissue transfer (▶Fig. 15.13).

Scalp

The scalp is richly vascularized by five sources: supratrochlear, supraorbital, superficial temporal, posterior auricular, and occipital arteries. These vessels course superficial to the galea aponeurotica—although small to medium random flaps can be safely raised in the scalp without including the galea, larger flaps should be raised in the subgaleal plane to make sure the pedicle is included in the flap.

Supraorbital and supratrochlear arteries: These vessels are branches of the ophthalmic artery, thus representing terminal elements of the internal carotid artery. The supraorbital vessel exits the skull through the supraorbital foramen and divides into a superficial and a deep branch. Together with the supraorbital nerve, it courses upward to reach the

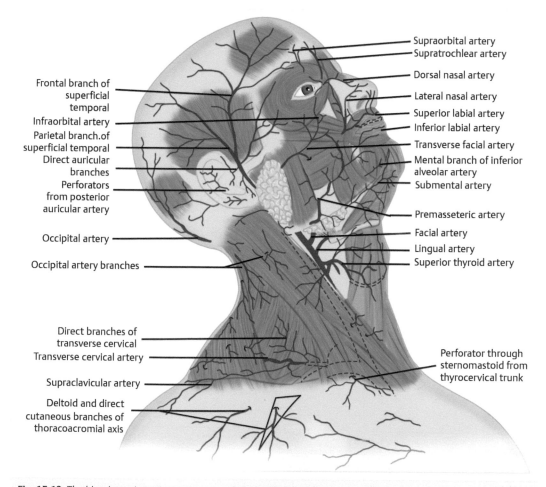

Fig. 15.13 The blood supply to the integument of the head and neck.

anterior scalp. The supratrochlear artery emerges through the frontal notch and courses medial and parallel to the supraorbital artery in association with the supratrochlear nerve. Together these arteries supply the upper eyelid, forehead, and anterior scalp. They anastomose with each other, their contralateral homologues, and the frontal branch of the superficial temporal artery. The supratrochlear artery forms the pedicle of the axial forehead flap, commonly used for nasal reconstruction.

Superficial temporal artery: The superficial temporal artery (STA) is one of the most important vascular elements of the scalp. It arises as a terminal branch of the external carotid artery within the parotid gland and then courses upward to become more superficial at the level of the zygomatic process of the temporal bone. The superficial temporal vein is located anterior and superficial to the artery, whereas the auriculotemporal nerve can be found just posterior to it. Above the zygomatic arch, the STA gives off the middle temporal artery, which supplies the temporalis muscle. It then continues on the superficial temporal fascia and divides into a frontal and a parietal branch. The frontal branch supplies the anterior scalp and forehead and is found in association with the frontal branch of the facial nerve. The parietal branch supplies the parietal scalp up to the vertex and extends posteriorly to anastomose with the occipital artery. The STA is the main pedicle supplying a number of flaps, including the superficial temporal fascia flap, the large hair-bearing temporoparietooccipital (Juri's) flap, and the transverse forehead (McGregor's) flap. The STA is also a reliable recipient for microsurgical reconstruction of the scalp. Additionally, it has been noted that the whole scalp can survive based on one STA following scalp replantation.

Occipital artery: The occipital artery arises from the posterior aspect of the external carotid artery in the neck. It travels in the occipital groove of the temporal bone, medial to the mastoid process. It pierces the deep cervical fascia together with the greater occipital nerve at the point where the cranial insertions of the trapezius and sternocleidomastoid muscles connect, and then runs upward and anteriorly on the surface of the occipitalis muscle. It anastomoses with its contralateral fellow and supplies the posterior scalp all the way to the vertex, where it links with the posterior auricular and superficial temporal arteries. Each occipital artery alone can supply a large posteriorly based flap for scalp reconstruction.

Face

The face is a richly vascularized area supplied mainly by the facial artery. It also receives important contributions from the superficial temporal and ophthalmic arteries in the upper third and from branches of the superficial temporal and maxillary artery in its lower two-thirds (▶ Table 15.4 and ▶ Fig. 15.13).

Facial artery: The facial artery arises from the external carotid artery and runs deep to the platysma before curving up the inferior border of the mandible and entering the face approximately 3–4 cm anterior to the mandibular angle. At this point the facial artery and vein are found in close association, with the vein lying posterior to the artery; however, further along their course in the face, the two vessels separate apart. In the face, the artery has a tortuous course in a plane between muscles, namely deep to the zygomaticus major, risorius, and orbicularis and superficial to the buccinators and levator anguli oris. Branches from the facial artery include the superior and inferior labial branches, which run between the mucosa and muscle of the corresponding lip. These arteries form the vascular basis of Abbé's and Estlander's flaps used in lip reconstruction. The facial artery then continues its course upward toward the nose, giving off the lateral nasal artery, which supplies the nasal ala and dorsum, to end up as the angular artery, which is found rather superficial just beneath the skin anastomosing with the infraorbital artery and supplying the nasal dorsum and medial cheek. The angular artery is the main pedicle to the nasolabial flap. In addition the facial artery supplies the facial artery myomucosal flap used for intraoral reconstruction.

Table 15.4 Vascular supply of the face

Upper third	Middle and lower thirds
Ophthalmic artery	Facial artery
• Supraorbital	• Premasseteric
• Supratrochlear	• Superior labial
• Lacrimal	• Inferior labial
• Medial palpebral	• Lateral nasal
• External nasal	• Angular (terminal
Superficial temporal artery	branch)
• Transverse facial	Maxillary artery
• Auricular	• Inferior alveolar
• Zygomatic–orbital	• Mental branch
• Frontal (anterior)	• Infraorbital

Neck

The vascular supply to the neck comes from trunks and branches originating from the subclavian and external carotid arteries (▶Table 15.5). From a reconstructive point of view, the vessels in the neck are more commonly used as recipients in microsurgical head and neck reconstructions rather than as pedicles of skin flaps. Some exceptions to this include the submental and supraclavicular arteries, which supply equally named flaps.

Submental artery: Just before curving up the mandibular border, the facial artery gives off its major branch, the submental artery, which courses toward the midline running under the inferior border of the mandible on the surface of the mylohyoid supplying the submandibular gland and adjacent muscles. In most cases the artery passes under the anterior belly of the digastric muscle to end up on the surface of the chin, where it anastomoses with its contralateral fellow and the mental and inferior labial arteries. The submental artery forms the vascular basis of the submental flap.

Supraclavicular artery: Though not commonly described in anatomy textbooks, the supraclavicular artery is found in the vast majority of patients and has a relatively constant anatomy. Most commonly it arises from the transverse cervical artery in the triangle formed by the sternocleidomastoid muscle anteriorly, the trapezius muscle posteriorly, and the clavicle inferiorly (▶Fig. 15.13). It pierces the deep fascia anterior to the trapezius and runs laterally in the subcutaneous plane toward the lateral end of the clavicle. This artery is the vascular basis of the supraclavicular axial flap, which can be harvested from the neck all the way to the mid-deltoid region.

15.4.2 Torso

The trunk is irrigated by a large number of arteries, which are summarized in ▶Table 15.6. According to Cormack and Lamberty, from a vascular point of view, the torso can be divided into anterior, dorsal, dorsolateral, and lateral. To avoid exhaustive information, only those vessels supplying commonly used skin flaps will be described.

Internal mammary artery: The internal mammary artery (IMA), also known as internal thoracic artery (ITA), arises from the first part of the subclavian artery and descends into the chest behind the costal cartilages 1–1.5 cm lateral to the sternal border (▶Fig. 15.14). Along its course it gives off

Table 15.5 Branches of external carotid and subclavian arteries

Subclavian artery	External carotid artery
Vertebral artery	Superior thyroid artery
Internal mammary artery	Ascending pharyngeal artery
Thyrocervical trunk	Lingual artery
• Inferior thyroid artery	Facial artery (submental)
• Transverse cervical artery (supraclavicular)	Occipital artery
• Suprascapular artery	Posterior auricular artery
Costocervical trunk	Maxillary artery
• Deep cervical artery	Superficial temporal artery
• Superior intercostal artery	

Table 15.6 Blood supply to the trunk

Anterior	Dorsal	Dorsolateral	Lateral
Thoracoacromial trunk	Superficial and dorsal scapular branches of transverse cervical artery	Superficial branch of transverse cervical artery	Thoracodorsal artery
• Acromial branch		Intercostal arteries	Lateral thoracic artery
• Clavicular branch	Intercostal arteries	Circumflex scapular artery	Superficial thoracic artery
• Deltoid branch	Lumbar arteries	Thoracodorsal artery	Intercostal arteries
• Pectoral branch	Lateral sacral arteries		
Lateral thoracic artery			
Internal mammary artery			
Deep superior epigastric artery			
Deep inferior epigastric artery			
Superficial inferior epigastric artery			
Deep circumflex iliac artery			
Superficial circumflex iliac artery			

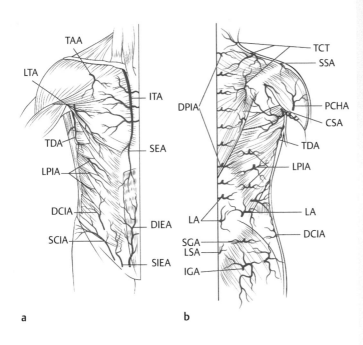

Fig. 15.14 The blood supply to the trunk. (a) Anterior trunk. DCIA, deep circumflex iliac artery; DIEA, deep inferior epigastric artery; ITA, internal thoracic (mammary) artery; LPIA, lateral branches of posterior intercostal arteries; LTA, lateral thoracic artery; SCIA, superficial circumflex iliac artery; SEA, superior epigastric artery; SIEA, superficial inferior epigastric artery; TAA, thoracoacromial artery; TDA, thoracodorsal artery. (b) Posterior trunk. CSA, circumflex scapular artery; DCIA, deep circumflex iliac artery; DPIA, dorsal branches of posterior intercostal arteries; IGA, inferior gluteal artery; LA, lumbar arteries; LPIA, lateral branches of posterior intercostal arteries; LSA, lateral sacral arteries; PCHA, posterior circumflex humeral artery; SGA, superior gluteal artery; SSA, suprascapular artery; TCT, thyrocervical trunk; TDA, thoracodorsal artery. (Reproduced from Blondeel et al, Perforator Flaps: Anatomy, Technique and Clinical Applications, 2nd edition, ©2013, Thieme Publishers, New York.)

perforators at the first five or six intercostal spaces, which pierce (and supply) the pectoralis major and its fascia to reach the skin. The perforator from the second intercostal space is usually the largest, although in women perforators at the third and fourth may also be substantial due to their role in supplying the breast tissue, especially during lactation. The artery has a diameter of approximately 2 mm and is accompanied usually by two venae comitantes of varying size. At the third intercostal space, the two veins join together into a single vessel located medial to the artery. At the level of the sixth intercostal space, the IMA divides into the musculophrenic artery that runs obliquely inferolaterally, and the superior epigastric artery, which courses downward behind the rectus abdominis. The IMA, through its second and third perforating branches, supplies the deltopectoral axial flap with its skin paddle extending from the sternum to the deltopectoral groove. The skin over the deltoid muscle may also be recruited following a delay procedure. Furthermore, isolation of the perforators and harvest of the internal mammary vessels allows elevation of an internal mammary artery perforator flap, which provides greater versatility in design, a larger arc of rotation, and the possibility

of transferring it as a free flap. Finally, the IMA is routinely used as a recipient in microsurgical breast and chest reconstruction.

Deep superior epigastric artery: As mentioned earlier, the deep superior epigastric artery (DSEA) is a terminal branch (or continuation) of the IMA (▶ Fig. 15.14). It passes between the costal and xiphoid origins of the diaphragm to run on the surface of the transversus thoracis and the transversus abdominis. It then enters the rectus sheath coursing inferiorly on the posterior aspect of the rectus abdominis, sending off musculocutaneous perforators that supply the muscle and overlying skin. A study by Hamdi et al showed a mean of 4 perforators per midline, with the largest ones located in an area between 1.5 and 6.5 cm from the x-axis on both sides and between 3 and 16 cm below the y-axis. A skin flap based on such perforators can be harvested and used for locoregional reconstruction, including the anterior chest and abdominal wall. The DSEA anastomoses with the deep inferior epigastric artery at the midpoint between the umbilicus and the xiphoid.

Deep inferior epigastric artery: After leaving the external iliac artery just above the inguinal ligament, the deep inferior epigastric artery (DIEA) runs upward obliquely and pierces the transversalis fascia to then ascend between the fascia and rectus abdominis. Above the arcuate line, the DIEA continues in the plane between the posterior rectus sheath and the muscle (▶ Fig. 15.14). Two veins usually accompany the artery. Along its course, the DIEA may run as a single vessel dividing into a medial and a lateral branch (most common pattern) or divide in three (less common). Perforators from the DIEA's medial and lateral branches penetrate through the rectus abdominis and pierce the anterior sheath to reach the skin. Occasionally, medial perforators may travel along the medial border of the muscle without going through it. A recent systematic review of anatomical and clinical studies showed that the vast majority of perforators from the DIEA are found within a circle of a 5 cm radius centered on the umbilicus. In 1989, Koshima and Soeda described a skin flap based on the perforators from the DIEA without sacrificing the muscle. This flap soon became known as the DIEP flap and is regarded by many as the gold standard in autologous breast reconstruction.

Superficial inferior epigastric artery: The superficial inferior epigastric artery (SIEA) is a direct cutaneous vessel arising either directly from the femoral artery or from a common trunk with the superficial circumflex iliac artery (SCIA) below the inguinal ligament. After piercing the cribriform fascia in the femoral triangle, the artery runs upward into the abdomen in the subcutaneous plane deep to Scarpa's fascia. It anastomoses with perforators from the DIEA medially and branches from the intercostal arteries laterally. Two small venae comitantes travel with the artery. The superficial inferior epigastric vein (SIEV) is found more medial and superficial in relation to the artery. Clinically, the SIEA forms the vascular basis of the SIEA flap used mainly for breast reconstruction. However, because of the inconsistency of the vessel, the flap is not routinely used. A study by Spiegel and Khan revealed that only 31% of their patients had an SIEA of sufficient size to be used in a free flap.

Superficial circumflex iliac artery: After originating from the femoral artery (alone or form a common trunk with the SIEA) approximately 3 cm below the inguinal ligament, the SCIA travels laterally parallel to and roughly two fingerbreadths below the inguinal ligament. At the medial border of the sartorius muscle, the artery divides into a superficial branch, which runs laterally in the subcutaneous plane approximately 1.5 cm below the inguinal ligament, and a deep branch, which travels deep to the fascia,

sometimes penetrating through the sartorius. Below the anterior superior iliac spine, the deep branch then pierces the deep fascia to return to the subcutaneous plane. The SCIA supplies the groin axial flap, which can be used either as a pedicled or a free flap. This flap can be reliably based on either branch of the SCIA. However, because of the small diameter and short length of its pedicle (average diameter of 1.5 mm and 1.5 cm in length) the use of the groin flap as a free flap is more challenging in comparison to other flaps. Nevertheless, it does provide a large and relatively thin skin paddle particularly useful for soft tissue reconstruction of the hand.

Circumflex scapular artery: The subscapular artery arises from the third portion of the axillary artery and divides into the circumflex scapular artery (CSA) and thoracodorsal artery approximately 3–4 cm from its origin. The CSA then curves backward around the lateral border of the scapula, passing through the triangular space bordered by the subscapularis above, the teres major below, and the long head of the triceps laterally. From a posterior view, the upper border of the triangle is formed by the teres minor muscle (▶ Fig. 15.15a). The SCA then gives off two major cutaneous branches, transverse and descending, which pierce the deep fascia and run in the subcutaneous plane. A third ascending branch is also described. The transverse branch runs in a medial direction parallel to the scapular spine, whereas the descending branch courses inferomedially parallel to the lateral border of the scapula (▶ Fig. 15.15b). These branches supply two named fasciocutaneous flaps: the scapular flap, based on the transverse branch, and the parascapular flap, based on the descending branch. These may be used as pedicled flaps, for example, for axillary or upper arm reconstruction, particularly the parascapular, or as free flaps.

15.4.3 Buttock and Thigh

Branches from the internal iliac and femoral arteries supply the gluteal region and thigh (▶ Table 15.7). The full description of each of these vessels is beyond the scope of this chapter; instead a brief anatomical description of those supplying commonly used flaps, namely the superior gluteal, inferior gluteal, and lateral circumflex femoral arteries, is provided. The named flaps are further described in the "Perforator Flaps" section of Chapter 16.

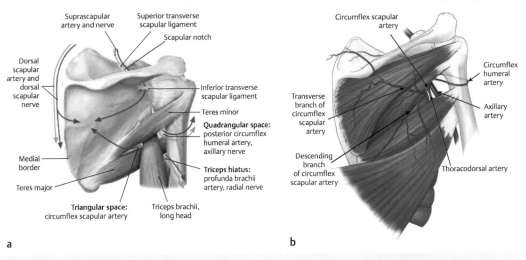

a

b

Fig. 15.15 (a) The muscular spaces of the scapular region and their associated neurovascular structures. (Reproduced from Schuenke, Schulte, and Schumacher, Atlas of Anatomy, ©2010, Thieme Publishers, New York. Illustration by Karl Wesker/Markus Voll.); **(b)** The circumflex scapular artery and its main cutaneous transverse and descending branches. Note that the long head of the triceps has been removed for illustration purposes. (Reproduced from Zenn, Jones, Reconstructive Surgery Anatomy, Technique, and Clinical Applications, ©2012, Thieme Publishers, New York.)

Table 15.7 Blood supply to the buttock and thigh

Buttock Internal iliac artery	Thigh Femoral artery
Iliolumbar artery	Superficial inferior epigas-
• Iliac branch	tric artery
• Lumbar branch	Superficial circumflex iliac
Lateral sacral arteries	artery
Obturator artery	External pudendal artery
• Pubic branch	• Anterior scrotal/labial
• Anterior branch	branch
• Posterior branch	• Inguinal branch
Superior gluteal artery	Descending genicular
• Superficial branch	artery
• Deep branch	• Saphenous branch
Inferior gluteal artery	• Articular branch
• Medial branch	Lateral circumflex femoral
• Lateral branch	artery
• Descending branch	• Ascending branch
Internal pudendal artery	• Transverse branch
• Perineal artery	• Descending branch
• Scrotal/posterior labial	Medial circumflex femoral
branch	artery
• Dorsal penile/clitoral	• Deep branch
artery	• Ascending branch
	• Descending branch
	Perforating arteries (4)

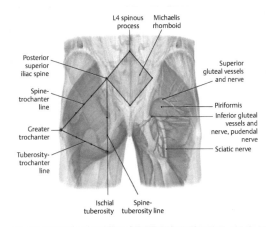

Fig. 15.16 Reference lines used to locate the neurovascular structures in the gluteal region. (Reproduced from Schuenke, Schulte, and Schumacher, Atlas of Anatomy, ©2010, Thieme Publishers, New York. Illustration by Karl Wesker/Markus Voll.)

Superior gluteal artery: After arising as a continuation of the posterior trunk of the internal iliac artery or from a common trunk with the inferior gluteal vessels, the superior gluteal artery (SGA)

enters the buttock together with the superior gluteal nerve through the greater sciatic foramen above the piriformis muscle. The point of entry can be mapped out on the skin at the junction of the medial third with the lateral two-thirds of a line going from the posterior superior iliac spine to the greater trochanter (▶ Fig. 15.16). The SGA then divides into a superficial branch, which enters the gluteus maximus, and a deep branch that runs between the gluteus medius and minimus. Musculocutaneous perforators supply the overlying skin and form the vascular basis of the SGA perforator flap.

Inferior gluteal artery: The inferior gluteal artery (IGA) is a terminal branch of the anterior trunk of the internal iliac artery and enters the buttock below the piriformis muscle together with the inferior gluteal nerve and in close association with the sciatic nerve, which is located lateral to the vessels. The point of entry of the IGA into the buttock lies approximately at half the distance of a line going from the posterior superior iliac spine and the ischial tuberosity (▶Fig. 15.16). Musculocutaneous perforators that penetrate through the gluteus maximus to reach the skin supply the IGA perforator flap. The IGA also gives a descending branch, which courses downward in the company of the posterior cutaneous nerve of the thigh and forms the vascular axis of the posterior gluteal thigh fasciocutaneous flap.

Lateral circumflex femoral artery: The lateral circumflex femoral artery (LCFA) arises most commonly from the deep femoral artery (75%) and from the (superficial) femoral artery in the remainder. It runs laterally behind the sartorius and rectus femoris and divides into three major branches: ascending, transverse, and descending (▶Fig. 15.17). The ascending branch enters the tensor fascia lata and sends off sizeable perforators to the overlying skin. The descending branch runs downward behind the rectus femoris and on the surface of the vastus intermedius, giving off perforators that supply the skin on the anterolateral aspect of the thigh. Most of these perforators are musculocutaneous, penetrating the vastus lateralis, although on the proximal third septocutaneous perforators can be found traveling in the intermuscular septum between the rectus femoris and the vastus lateralis. Commonly used flaps based on the LCFA system include the tensor fascia lata fasciocutaneous flap based on perforators from the ascending branch, and the anterolateral thigh (ALT) flap, which is supplied by perforators from the descending branch. Either pedicled or free, the ALT is considered a workhorse flap for a number of reconstructions.

15.4.4 Leg and Foot

After coursing downward on the adductor canal, the superficial femoral artery enters the popliteal

fossa through the adductor hiatus to become the popliteal artery. After giving off genicular and sural arteries, the popliteal artery divides into the three major vascular axes of the leg: the anterior tibial artery, posterior tibial artery, and peroneal artery (▶Table 15.8 and ▶Fig. 15.18). Through its various branches and perforators, these vessels supply the leg and foot from where a number of skin flaps can be harvested. In addition, any one of these vessels can be used as a recipient in microsurgical reconstructions, in which case it is important to ensure permeability of the remainder so that adequate distal perfusion is maintained. Alternatively, end-to-side anastomosis or flow-through flaps may be employed for the same purpose. In some cases of critical distal limb perfusion, a revascularization procedure may be indicated before tissue transfer.

Anterior tibial artery: The anterior tibial artery (ATA) stems off the popliteal artery in the posterior compartment of the leg passing through an opening in the interosseous membrane to reach the anterior compartment. Here it runs downwards on the interosseous membrane in company of the deep peroneal nerve. In the proximal third of the leg, the ATA is found between tibialis anterior (TA) and extensor digitorum longus (EDL) muscles, whereas in the distal two-thirds it lies between the TA and

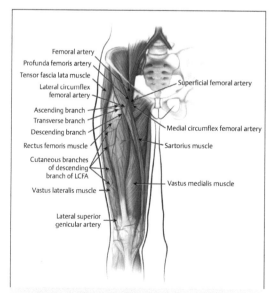

Fig. 15.17 The blood supply of the thigh, anterior view. LCFA, lateral circumflex femoral artery. (Reproduced from Zenn, Jones, Reconstructive Surgery Anatomy, Technique, and Clinical Applications, ©2012, Thieme Publishers, New York.)

Table 15.8 Blood supply to the leg and foot

Popliteal artery	Anterior tibial artery	Posterior tibial artery	Peroneal artery

Medial and lateral superior genicular aa.
Medial and lateral inferior genicular aa.
Medial, lateral, and median superficial sural aa.
	• Anterior lateral malleolar a.
	• Anterior medial malleolar a.
	• Dorsal pedal a.
	  ° Lateral and medial tarsal a.
	  ° Arcuate a.
	  ° Deep plantar a.
	  ° Dorsal metatarsal aa.
	  ° Dorsal digital aa.
		• Medial malleolar bb.
		• Medial calcaneal br.
		• Medial plantar a.
		  ° Superficial br.
		  ° Deep br.
		• Lateral plantar a.
		  ° Deep plantar arch
		  ° Plantar metatarsal aa.
		  ° Common plantar digital aa.
		  ° Proper plantar digital aa.
			• Communicating br.
			• Perforating br.
			• Lateral malleolar bb.
			Lateral calcaneal br.

Abbreviations: a, artery; aa, arteries; br, branch; bb, branches.

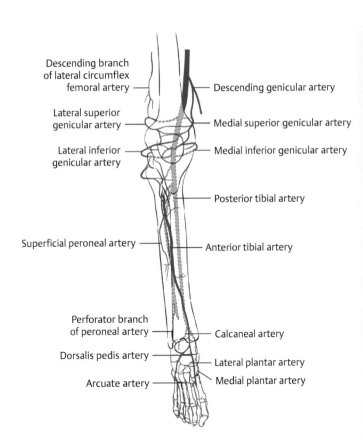

Descending branch of lateral circumflex femoral artery

Lateral superior genicular artery

Lateral inferior genicular artery

Superficial peroneal artery

Perforator branch of peroneal artery

Dorsalis pedis artery

Arcuate artery

Descending genicular artery

Medial superior genicular artery

Medial inferior genicular artery

Posterior tibial artery

Anterior tibial artery

Calcaneal artery

Lateral plantar artery

Medial plantar artery

Fig. 15.18 The vessels of the leg. (Reproduced from Blondeel et al, Perforator Flaps: Anatomy, Technique and Clinical Applications, 2nd edition, ©2013, Thieme Publishers, New York.)

the extensor hallucis longus (EHL) (▶ Fig. 15.19). A number of studies have looked into the distribution of cutaneous perforators in the leg. According to Martin et al, clusters of perforators from the ATA can be found in the proximal, middle, and distal thirds of the leg emerging between the tibia and the TA; the TA and the EDL; and the EDL and the peroneus longus. Distal to the extensor retinaculum, the ATA becomes the dorsal pedal artery, which runs between the tendons of the EDL and the EHL. This artery supplies the dorsalis pedis axial flap.

Posterior tibial artery: Distal to the origin of the ATA, the popliteal artery continues as the tibiofibular trunk, which then divides into the posterior tibial artery (PTA) and the peroneal artery (PA). The PTA runs with the tibial nerve in the deep posterior compartment of the leg behind the tibialis posterior muscle (▶Fig. 15.20). It supplies the muscles of the posterior compartment and the overlying skin. According to Schaverien and Saint-Cyr, the perforators from the PTA are the largest in the leg and are found in its proximal, middle, and distal thirds. Although some of these perforators are musculocutaneous vessels traveling through the soleus muscle, most of them run in the septum between the soleus and the flexor digitorum

longus. After passing behind the medial malleolus, the PTA divides into medial and lateral plantar arteries. The former supplies the medial plantar artery fasciocutaneous flap, commonly used for reconstruction of the heel and sole of the foot.

Peroneal artery: After originating from the tibiofibular trunk approximately 2.5 cm distal to the popliteus muscle, the peroneal artery (PA) descends along the medial crest of the fibula between the tibialis posterior and the flexor hallucis longus (FHL) (▶Fig. 15.20). Less commonly, the

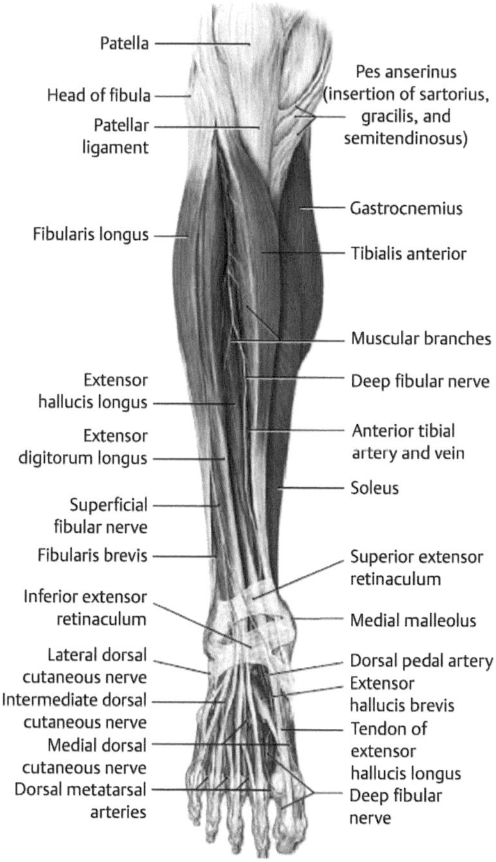

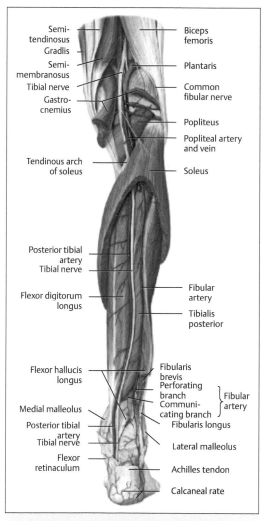

Fig. 15.19 Anatomical relationships of the anterior tibial artery. (Reproduced from Schuenke, Schulte, and Schumacher, Atlas of Anatomy, ©2010, Thieme Publishers, New York. Illustration by Karl Wesker/Markus Voll.)

Fig. 15.20 Anatomical relationships of the posterior tibial and peroneal arteries. (Reproduced from Schuenke, Schulte, and Schumacher, Atlas of Anatomy, ©2010, Thieme Publishers, New York. Illustration by Karl Wesker/Markus Voll.)

artery and its venae comitantes travel within the substance of the FHL. Along its course, the PTA gives off a nutrient artery to the fibula, which enters the bone on its posteromedial aspect approximately 15 cm below the apex. Perforators from the PTA are concentrated on the middle and distal thirds of the leg and usually travel within the posterior intermuscular septum between the soleus and peroneous longus muscles to reach the skin. More proximal perforators may penetrate directly through the soleus muscle. Perforators from the PA can supply local perforator flaps and more commonly the skin paddle of a fibular osteocutaneous flap. Additionally, the most distal perforators form the vascular basis of the reverse sural flap used for soft tissue reconstruction of the lower third of the leg and foot.

15.4.5 Upper Extremity

At the lower border of the teres major muscle, the axillary artery becomes the brachial artery, which supplies the entire upper limb through its different branches and progressive divisions (▶Table 15.9 and ▶Fig. 15.21).

Deep brachial artery: The deep brachial artery (DBA) arises from the posteromedial aspect of the brachial artery and runs in company of the radial nerve in the spiral groove of the humerus covered by the lateral head of the triceps. After sending branches to the deltoid, the three heads of the triceps, and the nutrient artery to the humerus, the DBA divides into the radial collateral and middle collateral (also called posterior radial collateral) arteries. The posterior radial collateral

artery (PRCA) descends on the posterior aspect of the lateral intermuscular septum between the brachialis muscle and the lateral head of the triceps, giving off 4–5 septocutaneous perforators to supply the overlying skin. Distally, the PRCA may pierce the deep fascia and become a cutaneous vessel or continue deep to the fascia to anastomose with the recurrent interosseous artery at the elbow joint. The PRCA forms the vascular basis of the lateral arm fasciocutaneous flap.

Radial artery: Approximately 1 cm distal to the flexion crease of the elbow, the brachial artery divides into the two main arteries of the forearm and hand: the radial and ulnar arteries. The radial artery (RA) descends along the lateral side of the forearm accompanied by two venae comitantes. Proximally the RA lies between the pronator teres and the brachioradialis, being covered by the latter along part of its course. In its distal two-thirds, the RA lies beneath the skin and deep fascia between the tendons of the flexor carpi radialis and the brachioradialis (▶Fig. 15.22). Through numerous perforators along its course, the radial artery supplies the skin over the anterolateral aspect of the forearm, including a small portion of dorsal skin. The radial artery fasciocutaneous flap is a very reliable pedicled or free flap. It is commonly used for a number of reconstructive purposes, especially in the upper limb and head and neck, including tongue, intraoral, lip, and nose reconstruction, among others.

Ulnar artery: After the brachial artery divides, the ulnar artery, the largest of the two, obliquely inferomedially under the pronator teres, flexor carpi radialis, palmaris longus, and flexor digitorum

Table 15.9 Blood supply to the upper extremity

Brachial artery	Radial artery	Ulnar artery
Deep brachial artery • Posterior descending branch: middle collateral (also called posterior radial collateral) • Anterior descending branch: radial collateral Superior ulnar collateral artery Inferior ulnar collateral artery	Radial recurrent artery Palmar carpal branch Superficial palmar branch Dorsal carpal branch (forms dorsal carpal arch with branch from ulnar artery) • Dorsal metacarpal arteries • Dorsal digital branches First dorsal metacarpal artery Princeps pollicis artery Radialis indicis artery Deep palmar arch • Palmar metacarpal arteries • Perforating branches	Anterior and posterior ulnar recurrent arteries Common interosseous artery • Anterior interosseous • Posterior interosseous • Recurrent interosseous Dorsal cutaneous branch Palmar carpal branch Dorsal carpal branch (forms dorsal carpal arch with branch from radial artery) Deep palmar branch Superficial palmar arch • Common palmar digital arteries • Proper palmar digital arteries

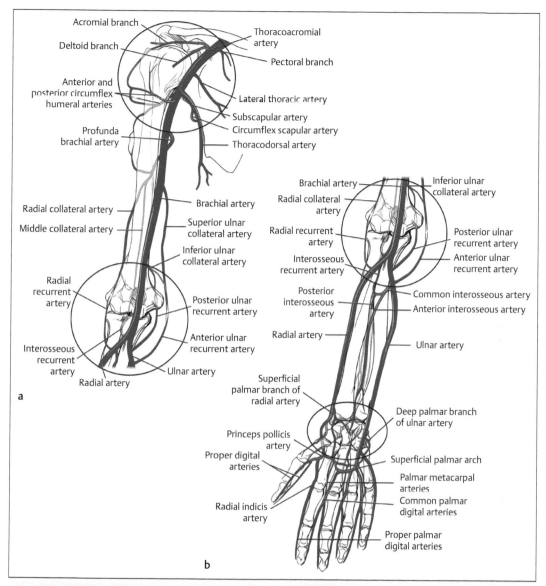

Fig. 15.21 (a,b) The vessels of the upper limb. (Reproduced from Blondeel et al, Perforator Flaps: Anatomy, Technique and Clinical Applications, 2nd edition, ©2013, Thieme Publishers, New York.)

superficialis. The common interosseous artery arises from the proximal portion of the ulnar artery and soon divides into anterior and posterior branches. Subsequently, the ulnar artery and its two venae comitantes run downward in the medial side of the forearm, on the surface of the flexor digitorum profundus and between the flexor carpi ulnaris (FCU) and the flexor digitorum superficialis (FDS). Distally, the ulnar artery is covered only by skin and deep fascia (▶Fig. 15.22). Along its

course, the ulnar artery supplies the overlying skin through a series of five septocutaneous perforators, which travel in the septum between the FCU and the FDS. In the distal two-thirds of the forearm, the ulnar artery is found in close association with the ulnar nerve, which runs lateral to the artery. Similar to the radial artery flap, a fasciocutaneous flap can be raised based on the ulnar artery and used as a pedicled or free flap. Also, a fasciocutaneous flap based on the posterior interosseous

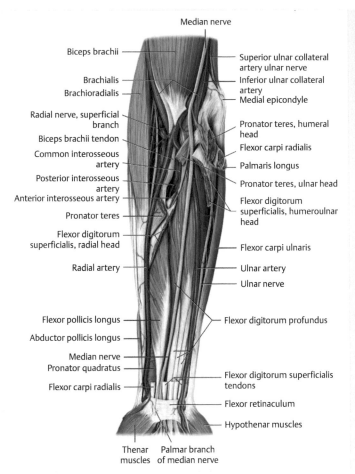

Median nerve

Biceps brachii

Brachialis
Brachioradialis

Radial nerve, superficial branch
Biceps brachii tendon
Common interosseous artery
Posterior interosseous artery
Anterior interosseous artery
Pronator teres
Flexor digitorum superficialis, radial head
Radial artery

Flexor pollicis longus
Abductor pollicis longus
Median nerve
Pronator quadratus
Flexor carpi radialis

Thenar muscles
Palmar branch of median nerve

Superior ulnar collateral artery ulnar nerve
Inferior ulnar collateral artery
Medial epicondyle
Pronator teres, humeral head
Flexor carpi radialis
Palmaris longus
Pronator teres, ulnar head
Flexor digitorum superficialis, humeroulnar head
Flexor carpi ulnaris
Ulnar artery
Ulnar nerve

Flexor digitorum profundus

Flexor digitorum superficialis tendons
Flexor retinaculum
Hypothenar muscles

Fig. 15.22 Anatomical relationships of the vessels in the forearm. (Reproduced from Schuenke, Schulte, and Schumacher, Atlas of Anatomy, ©2010, Thieme Publishers, New York. Illustration by Karl Wesker/Markus Voll.)

artery can be harvested as a pedicled flap for soft tissue coverage of the distal forearm and hand.

Note

The Allen Test
Before sacrificing the radial or ulnar artery for reconstruction, it is important to confirm the presence of sufficient interconnections between them to ensure that the remaining vessel will be able to supply the distal hand. This is assessed by the Allen test in which the patient is asked to elevate the hand and make a fist to drain blood from it. The examiner then occludes both arteries at the wrist and releases them in turns, observing return of normal coloration—the test is positive when the hand regains its color in 5–15 seconds.

15.5 Conclusions

In 1957, Sir Harold Gillies wrote, "Plastic surgery is a constant battle between blood supply and beauty." Sixty years have passed since and numerous advances have been made in all areas of plastic surgery; however, the statement and its essence remain the same—blood supply is the cornerstone of tissue transfer. Through the work of anatomists and surgeons, and more recently with the aid of sophisticated imaging techniques, we have come to understand in considerable detail the intricacies of the cutaneous vascular network. Although this knowledge is fascinating on its own, it has also brought key insights into the design and execution of flaps, at times making the procedure more predictable and expeditious, ultimately leading to improved patient outcomes.

15.6 Key Points

- The skin is supplied by five different plexuses: subepidermal, dermal, subdermal, subcutaneous, and fascial.
- Blood vessels supplying the skin can be broadly classified as direct and indirect.
- Adjacent angiosomes are connected by either true or choke anastomoses.
- During flap transfer, one source vessel can reliably supply its angiosome and the adjacent one. Capturing the one beyond usually leads to necrosis of the distal portion.
- There are five different patterns of blood supply to the muscles according to the Mathes–Nahai classification.
- The main difference between a type 2 and type 5 muscle is that type 5 muscles can survive based on either their dominant pedicle or their segmental pedicles, whereas type 2 muscles can do so based only on their dominant pedicle.
- Taylor classifies muscles into four different types according to their pattern of motor innervation.

Recommended Readings

Batchelor JS, Moss AL. The relationship between fasciocutaneous perforators and their fascial branches: an anatomical study in human cadaver lower legs. Plast Reconstr Surg. 1995; 95(4):629–633

Boyd JB, Taylor GI, Corlett R. The vascular territories of the superior epigastric and the deep inferior epigastric systems. Plast Reconstr Surg. 1984; 73(1):1–16

Cormack GC, Lamberty BG. The Arterial Anatomy of Skin Flaps. 2nd ed. New York, NY: Churchill Livingstone: 1994

Esser JFS. Artery flaps. Antwerp: De Vos-van Kleef; 1929

Hamdi M, Craggs B, Stoel AM, Hendrickx B, Zeltzer A. Superior epigastric artery perforator flap: anatomy, clinical applications, and review of literature. J Reconstr Microsurg. 2014; 30(7):475–482

Hamdi M, Van Landuyt K, Ulens S, Van Hedent E, Roche N, Monstrey S. Clinical applications of the superior epigastric artery perforator (SEAP) flap: anatomical studies and preoperative perforator mapping with multidetector CT. J Plast Reconstr Aesthet Surg. 2009; 62(9):1127–1134

Ireton JE, Lakhiani C, Saint-Cyr M. Vascular anatomy of the deep inferior epigastric artery perforator flap: a systematic review. Plast Reconstr Surg. 2014; 134(5):810e–821e

Koshima I, Soeda S. Inferior epigastric artery skin flaps without rectus abdominis muscle. Br J Plast Surg. 1989; 42(6):645–648

Lang J. On the texture and vascularization of fascia [in German]. Acta Anat (Basel). 1962; 48:61–94

Martin AL, Bissell MB, Al-Dhamin A, Morris SF. Computed tomographic angiography for localization of the cutaneous perforators of the leg. Plast Reconstr Surg. 2013; 131(4):792–800

Mathes SJ, Nahai F. Classification of the vascular anatomy of muscles: experimental and clinical correlation. Plast Reconstr Surg. 1981; 67(2):177–187

Nakajima H, Fujino T, Adachi S. A new concept of vascular supply to the skin and classification of skin flaps according to their vascularization. Ann Plast Surg. 1986; 16(1):1–19

Niranjan NS. Invited commentary. J Plast Reconstr Aesthet Surg. 2011; 64(9):1214–1215

Niranjan NS, Price RD, Govilkar P. Fascial feeder and perforator-based V-Y advancement flaps in the reconstruction of lower limb defects. Br J Plast Surg. 2000; 53(8):679–689

Saint-Cyr M, Wong C, Schaverien M, Mojallal A, Rohrich RJ. The perforasome theory: vascular anatomy and clinical implications. Plast Reconstr Surg. 2009; 124(5):1529–1544

Sch, ä, fer K. Studies on angioarchitecture of the fascia (lower extremity) [in German]. Z Anat Entwicklungsgesch. 1972; 139(1):21–54

Schaverien M, Saint-Cyr M. Perforators of the lower leg: analysis of perforator locations and clinical application for pedicled perforator flaps. Plast Reconstr Surg. 2008; 122(1):161–170

Skin and its appendages. In: Standring S, ed. Gray's Anatomy: The Anatomical Basis of Clinical Practice. 40th ed. London: Churchill Livingstone, Elsevier; 2008:145–164

Spiegel AJ, Khan FN. An Intraoperative algorithm for use of the SIEA flap for breast reconstruction. Plast Reconstr Surg. 2007; 120(6):1450–1459

Taylor GI, Corlett RJ, Ashton MW. The blood supply of the skin and skin flaps. In: Thorne C, Chung K, Gosain AK, et al., eds. Grabb and Smith's Plastic Surgery. 7th ed. Philadelphia, PA: Lippincott Williams & Wilkins; 2014:29–42

Taylor GI, Gianoutsos MP, Morris SF. The neurovascular territories of the skin and muscles: anatomic study and clinical implications. Plast Reconstr Surg. 1994; 94(1):1–36

Taylor GI, Palmer JH. The vascular territories (angiosomes) of the body: experimental study and clinical applications. Br J Plast Surg. 1987; 40(2):113–141

Taylor GI, Tempest M. Salmon's Arteries of the Skin. Edinburgh: Churchilll-Livingstone; 1988

The angiosome concept. In: Taylor GI, Pan WR, eds. The Angiosome Concept and Tissue Transfer. New York, NY: Thieme Publishers; 2014:173–393

16 Flaps

Diego Marré, Leigh Jansen, Sandhya Deo

Abstract

A flap is a unit of tissue transferred from a donor to a recipient while retaining its own blood supply. Their composition, vascularity, and method of transfer constitute the main features by which flaps are classified and named, ranging from small local rotation flaps to large composite free flaps. Nevertheless, regardless of their complexity, all flaps are governed by the same principles, including thorough preoperative planning of the procedure and possible lifeboats, replacement of like with like, meticulous surgical technique, and mindful consideration of the donor area. In flap surgery there is always a trade-off, namely, morbidity of the donor site, that needs to be proportionate to the benefit gained from the reconstruction, and which may range from a small scar to a graft, a noncritical sensory loss, or a mild functional deficit. Finally, the understanding of the blood supply to the skin together with the evolution and refinements in surgical technique have led to the description and development of perforator flaps, which constitute an important part of the armamentarium in reconstructive surgery.

This chapter describes the main aspects of flap surgery, including the physiological events that take place after transfer and the main factors affecting flap survival, followed by a thorough description of flap classification and refinements. Lastly, a section on perforator flaps is provided.

Keywords: fasciocutaneous flaps, flap, local flaps, perforator flaps, tissue transfer

16.1 Introduction

The term *flap* originates from the 16th-century Dutch word *flappe*, which means something that hangs broad and loose, fastened only by one side. The roots of flap surgery can be traced back to 600 BC when Sushruta Samhita described a technique for nasal reconstruction using a cheek flap. Later Greek, Hellenistic, and Roman physicians described reconstructive procedures mirroring the Indian methods.

In the 16th century, during the Renaissance period, the transfer of tissue to a distant site using tubed and pedicled flaps was reported in Italian literature. One particular application of this technique—reconstructing a nose from a forearm skin flap—was popularized by Tagliacozzi.

Despite these early descriptions, flap surgery did not gain wide acceptance during this time. Two centuries passed before skin grafts and flaps reemerged in Europe. During this time there were descriptions of the transportation of skin to an adjacent area through rotation or transposition. The French were the first to describe advancement flaps, but this was done in isolation of any knowledge regarding blood supply, rendering these flaps random pattern.

The evolution of flap surgery continued through the First and Second World Wars, when pedicled flaps were used extensively. Despite the meticulous planning that was involved, it is likely that these flaps were designed without an appreciation for their axial vascular supply. These so-called random flaps were designed with a strict length to width ratio under the assumption that the flap would only survive in its entire length if its base were wide enough to allow proper blood supply. Esser, however, in Germany, did note the importance of incorporating a vascular pedicle within the flap; he named his flaps biological or arterial flaps. In the 1960s, Stuart Milton demonstrated that the reliability of a skin flap depended on its vascularization. This led to the work of Ian McGregor and Gwyn Morgan, who made a distinction between axial and random pattern skin flaps in the early 1970s.

Also in the 1970s came the introduction of muscle and musculocutaneous flaps. As the use of these flaps gained momentum, the understanding of flap surgery increased, and this eventually led to the birth of free tissue transfer. In 1973, Rollin Daniel and Ian Taylor reported the first cutaneous free microvascular transfer—a groin flap used for lower extremity reconstruction. The ability to perform safe, reproducible, and reliable microvascular procedures dramatically expanded the surgeon's options to close, replace, or augment areas of deficit and deformity.

In the 1980s the tissue types used within flaps increased significantly. Fasciocutaneous flaps, osseous flaps, and osteocutaneous flap were all described during this time. Further advancement came in the 1990s with the introduction of perforator flaps. With this development came mapping of the perforator vessels throughout the body, allowing the design of countless potential flaps.

Today free flaps and perforator flaps are a routine part of our armamentarium as reconstructive surgeons. Further innovations and advancements will be influenced by our knowledge of perforator anatomy and by the growth of supermicrosurgery.

16.2 Basic Science

A flap is a unit of tissue that maintains its own blood supply while being transferred from a donor site to a recipient site. Unlike grafts, flaps are not dependent on the recipient bed for vascularization. Therefore the volume of tissue that can be transferred is significantly greater than that of a graft and can contain multiple types of tissue, including skin, muscle, fascia, nerve, and bone.

The term *reconstructive ladder* has been coined by plastic surgeons to describe the options for management of wounds, starting from the most simple and ascending in complexity. The lowest rung of the ladder is healing by secondary intention. ▶Fig. 16.1 demonstrates the rungs increasing in complexity until the top of the ladder—free flaps—is reached.

Typically a surgeon would consider options for wound closure in a systematic way so that with any given wound they would work up the ladder until they reached the *simplest* option that would facilitate closure of the wound in question. This method, though safe and systematic does not necessarily provide the best solution. Nowadays, with the technical advancements and increasing experience in complex reconstructive methods, including microsurgery and free tissue transfer, the reconstructive ladder has been gradually displaced by the "reconstructive elevator," where the *best* option is chosen—which may or may not be the simplest. This approach allows the reconstructive surgeon to move up and down freely and select the most appropriate option for any given defect.

16.2.1 Flap Physiology

Flaps rely on the maintenance of adequate perfusion for their survival. An understanding of the physiology as it relates to the metabolic demands of the mobilized tissue allows the surgeon to best plan flaps. In addition, the understanding of flap physiology relies on a detailed knowledge of the normal blood supply to the skin.

Cutaneous blood supply provides thermoregulation and nutritional support. Nutritional support is

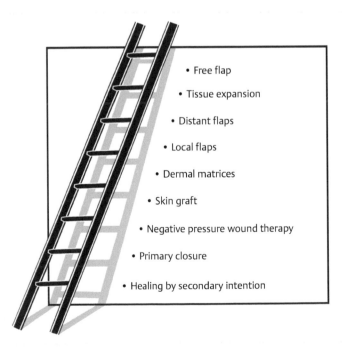

- Free flap
- Tissue expansion
- Distant flaps
- Local flaps
- Dermal matrices
- Skin graft
- Negative pressure wound therapy
- Primary closure
- Healing by secondary intention

Fig. 16.1 The reconstructive ladder. (Reproduced from Janis, Essentials of Plastic Surgery, 2nd edition, ©2014, Thieme Publishers, New York.)

regulated largely by the capillary network, whereas thermoregulation is controlled by arteriovenous shunts, which are mainly located in the dermal vascular plexus within the reticular dermis. A number of factors in the microcirculation contribute to the regulation of blood flow, and these can be broken down into local and systemic factors.

Local control, or autoregulation, includes the following:

- *Metabolic factors:* These primarily act as vasodilators and include hypercapnea, hypoxia, acidosis, and hyperkalemia. These factors are more significant in muscle compared with skin because muscle has a higher metabolic requirement.
- *Myogenic reflex:* This reflex triggers vasoconstriction in response to distension of isolated cutaneous vessels, thereby maintaining capillary flow at a constant level independent of arterial pressure.
- *Local hypothermia:* This acts directly on vascular smooth muscle, which causes vasoconstriction.
- *Increased blood viscosity:* This is less significant but may also decrease cutaneous blood flow.

Systemic control is facilitated by the following:

- *Neural regulation:* This is the most important system of control in cutaneous blood supply. It acts through sympathetic adrenergic fibers—vasoconstriction is induced by α-adrenergic receptors and vasodilation by β-adrenergic receptors. These act together to maintain vascular smooth muscle control at the microcirculatory level.
- *Humoral regulation:* The cutaneous circulation is extremely sensitive to circulating adrenaline and noradrenaline, which cause vasoconstriction through their action on α-adrenergic receptors. Serotonin and thromboxane A_2 may also produce vasoconstriction, whereas histamine and bradykinin cause vasodilation.

Another important concept in cutaneous blood supply is the angiosome as described in Chapter 15. Taylor and Palmer coined the term *angiosome* to refer to the tissue supplied by a named artery and observed that adjacent angiosomes are in communication with one another via choke vessels. This relationship is important when designing flaps. When raising a flap on an axial blood vessel the angiosome supplied by that vessel and the adjacent angiosome can be supported. Incorporating tissue distant to this invites vascular compromise and flap failure.

The elevation of a skin flap elicits a number of changes that disrupts the delicate balance in cutaneous blood flow. Success of a flap relies on physiological changes that allow adequate perfusion to be maintained and restored. Initially there is a reduction in arterial blood supply and ischemia. This leads to a dilatation of the arterioles and capillaries with resultant congestion and edema. At ~ 72 hours there is a progressive increase in circulatory efficiency—vascular anastomoses develop between the flap and the recipient bed, the size and number of functioning vessels increase, and functioning vessels are reoriented along the long axis of the flap. These changes plateau about 7 days after flap elevation.

Flap failure can be caused by arterial or venous insufficiency. Inadequate arterial inflow causes ischemia and inflammation, with increased edema. The microcirculation narrows, blood flow slows, and clot forms within the micro- and macrocirculation. Initially these changes are reversible, if the arterial inflow is restored, but as time goes on the changes become irreversible. Inadequate venous outflow can also result in flap necrosis, independent of arterial supply. If both arterial and venous circulation are inadequate the risk of flap failure increases exponentially.

16.2.2 Risk Factors for Flap Survival

The success of tissue transfer depends on several factors, which must be considered by the surgeon and optimized as needed before embarking on a flap reconstruction procedure. Systemic conditions, such as diabetes mellitus, immunosuppression, malnutrition, connective tissue disorders, and peripheral vascular disease, can compromise flap vascularity and result in delayed healing or total flap failure. These conditions should ideally be medically optimized prior to undertaking flap surgery.

Smoking is associated with an increased risk of flap necrosis. Nicotine has a number of negative effects—it causes direct endothelial damage and systemic vasoconstriction. These effects significantly decrease capillary blood flow and limit oxygen delivery. Distal perfusion and flap survival are affected by nicotine in a dose- and time-dependent fashion. Smoking also generally impairs healing due to vasoconstriction, decreased neutrophil function, and decreased collagen synthesis.

Irradiation has short- and long-term effects on both the macro- and microvasculature. Radiation causes decreased oxygenation and decreased blood supply, leading to altered wound healing. These changes are proportional to the radiation dose and fractionation. Where possible, flap surgery should be performed several months after irradiation in order for the short-term changes to resolve.

16.3 Principles of Flap Surgery

Successful flap surgery is based on five key principles:

1. Replace like with like. When reconstructing a defect, where possible replace like with like. If this cannot be achieved, use the next most similar tissue substitute available. This assists in producing the most natural result for the patient.
2. Think of reconstruction in terms of units. According to Millard, the body can be divided into seven main areas—the head, neck, trunk and four extremities. Each of these areas can further be separated into units and subunits. Each of these subunits should be considered separately when establishing a reconstructive plan.
3. Always have a plan, a pattern, and a lifeboat. When considering a defect, utilize the reconstructive elevator to establish viable options and compare the advantages and disadvantages of each of these. Sometimes the simplest plan is the safest, but on some occasions a more complex option may provide the best overall result. One should always aim to restore form and function to the best of their ability. In the operating room design the flap and check the markings before starting. The old adage "measure twice, cut once" should hold true no matter how experienced the surgeon. Additionally, anticipate potential difficulties and have a backup plan in mind should the original option fail—"hope for the best but plan for the worst."
4. Rob Peter to pay Paul. Using the "Robin Hood" principle—rob Peter to pay Paul—but only if Peter can afford it. Everything comes at a price, and with flap surgery we must consider where the tissue is coming from and the potential negative consequences of borrowing that tissue. This goes hand in hand with the fifth and final principle.
5. Never forget the donor area. Both the primary defect and the secondary donor site must be considered equally. We need to ensure that the resultant scars, deformity, and/or disability created by utilizing the donor tissue can be justified.

16.4 Flap Classification

By definition, a flap is a segment of tissue of whatever composition that is transferred from one area to another while maintaining its own vascular supply. This fundamental characteristic is what differentiates a flap from a graft, which depends on vascularization from the wound bed to survive. Any given flap can be classified according to different aspects, though these different classifications are complementary, not mutually exclusive. As a medical student or early surgical trainee, one starts to read and hear about flaps, later participating in flap surgeries, and all these classifications, patterns, and geometrical terms become mixed in a seemingly random manner. Given the different flap classifications, each with its own subcategories, the combinations are multiple, and not all classifications are applicable to all flaps. The problem usually isn't names and terminology, but instead it is trying to memorize everything instead of acquiring the basic concepts and principles. By incorporating the latter, it will be quite easy to name any flap just by looking at it for a few seconds. However, it is important to note that knowing the "full name" of a flap does not mean that we use the full name every time.

Learning the different classifications of flaps is useful for nomenclature and communication purposes among plastic surgeons and other colleagues. Furthermore, knowing a flap's potential components, its vascularization, and how it can be transferred to the defect has significant clinical implications in preoperative planning, the surgical procedure itself, the management of postoperative complications, and the execution of secondary procedures.

Flaps are classified mainly according to their composition, their vascularization pattern, and their method of mobilization. But before going into each classification in detail, the first thing to address is the difference between a pedicled and a free flap. Of course they are both flaps in the sense that they carry their own vascular supply; however, they do so in different ways. *Pedicled* flaps are those that, in the process of transfer, always remain attached to the body at the point from which they receive their vascular supply. This point can be a broad bridge of skin, a known vascular axis, or even a small, 2 mm perforator vessel. *Free flaps*, in turn, are those in which the tissue and accompanying vascular pedicle are completely disconnected from the body and transferred to the defect, where the vessels in the flap (donor vessels) are anastomosed to recipient vessels at the recipient site using microsurgical techniques.

16.4.1 Classification According to Composition

A flap may be composed of one or several kinds of tissue depending on the reconstructive needs. Furthermore, the various tissue types may be combined in different ways to suit the defect that is being reconstructed. The vast majority of flaps used in reconstructive surgery will include one of the tissues illustrated in ▶ Fig. 16.2.

If a flap contains only one of these components, then it will usually be named as appears in the figure (i.e., skin flap, fascial flap, fat flap, muscle flap, and bone flap). However, when combined, these components are usually referred to by the following combining forms:
- Skin: -cutaneous
- Fat: adipo-
- Muscle: myo-
- Fascia: fascio-
- Bone: osteo-

- Nerve: neuro-
- Cartilage: chondro-

In general, the components are named from deep to superficial. Thus examples of correct terminology regarding flap composition would be myocutaneous flap (muscle and skin), fasciocutaneous (fascia and skin), osteomyocutaneous (bone, muscle, and skin).

16.4.2 Classification According to Vascularization

Flaps receive their blood supply through either a random or an axial pattern.

Random Flaps

These flaps are generally composed of skin and fat and are named because they are based mainly on the subpapillary, dermal reticular, and subdermal plexuses without an identifiable source vessel (▶ Fig. 16.3). This fact poses some restrictions on flap design and elevation, such as a limited arc of rotation and the need for proximity to the defect. Also, given that their blood supply comes from their base, it has been a traditional belief that, in order to survive, random flaps should adhere to relatively rigorous length to width ratios of around 2:1 (or 3:1 on the face given its rich vascularization). Although this has been challenged and is no longer a strict rule to follow, it does

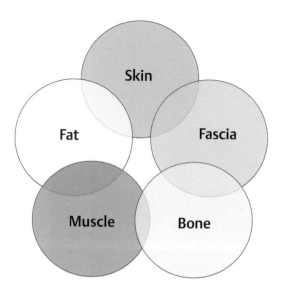

Fig. 16.2 The main components of flaps. Any given flap may include one or more of these tissues.

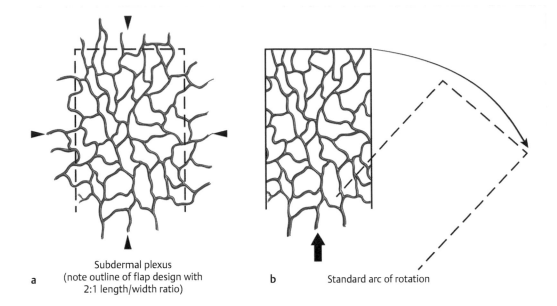

a — Subdermal plexus (note outline of flap design with 2:1 length/width ratio)

b — Standard arc of rotation

Fig. 16.3 (a,b) Vascular basis of random flaps. (Reproduced from Zenn, Jones, Reconstructive Surgery Anatomy, Technique, and Clinical Applications, ©2012, Thieme Publishers, New York.)

illustrate the principle that random flaps do need to have an adequate width to ensure sufficient vascularization.

Axial Pattern Flaps

Axial flaps incorporate an identified vessel along their longitudinal axis, usually coursing in the subcutaneous plane. This fact makes these flaps much more reliable from a vascular point of view, and of course less subject to the restrictions already mentioned, thereby allowing larger arcs of rotation and greater versatility in design. However, the need to have a known blood vessel within these flaps poses certain anatomical limitations, as opposed to random flaps, which can be elevated virtually anywhere in the body. Commonly used axial flaps and their vascular source are listed in ▶ Table 16.1.

Because the axial vessel often runs in the subcutaneous plane, these flaps are usually composed of skin and fat. However, for either reconstructive purposes or to enhance their vascularization, the underlying fascia (with its vascular plexuses) can also be included, thus forming an axial fasciocutaneous flap. Fasciocutaneous flaps have their own systems of classification, which are described later in this chapter.

Table 16.1 Examples of axial pattern flaps

Flap	Axial vessels
Forehead	Supratrochlear
Retroauricular	Retroauricular
Deltopectoral	Second and third intercostal perforators from internal mammary artery
Groin	Superficial circumflex iliac
Dorsalis pedis	Dorsalis pedis

16.4.3 Classification According to Method of Movement

In order to reach the defect, the flap must be mobilized in a certain direction. The basic principle of flap mobilization rests on taking tissue from a mobile area and bringing it into the defect without undue tension. Whenever possible, the donor site is closed directly; otherwise a skin graft can be used. There are four basic ways to mobilize a flap into a defect: *rotation*, *advancement*, *transposition*, and *interpolation*. The method of mobilization depends on a number of factors, including the area of the body where the flap is to be raised; the condition, laxity, and neurovascular supply of the neighboring tissues; and the dimensions and shape of the defect, although the latter can be adapted for the flap to fit properly, even if this means sometimes removing healthy tissue. Rotation, transposition, and interpolation flaps all have a *pivot point*, around which the flap rotates to reach the defect, and an *arc of rotation*, which is the area that can be effectively covered by the flap. In addition, the *line of maximal tension* is a line that runs from the pivot point to the point of the flap that will be furthest away from it after inset (▶ Fig. 16.4). It should be noted that, when a flap is progressively turned through its arc of rotation, its effective length decreases accordingly (▶ Fig. 16.5). Therefore, careful planning of these flaps keeping these features in mind and making the flap longer than the defect is crucial. Before making any incisions, a good recommendation is to simulate the movement of the proposed flap into the defect by using a piece of cloth or gauze held firmly at the pivot point. This gives a good estimate of the actual reach of the flap and allows redesign if necessary. It is generally better to err on the side of excess, provided that there are no issues with the donor site. A flap that outreaches the defect can be easily trimmed; a flap that does not reach the defect, or does so with excessive tension, is a disaster.

Rotation Flaps

These flaps are one of the most utilized resources in reconstructive surgery. They can be used virtually anywhere on the body, from the scalp to the sole of the foot, with varying dimensions and composition. The defect is tailored to an isosceles triangle that represents the edge of a semicircle, which corresponds to the flap. The circumference of the flap should generally be four to six times the diameter of the defect to allow adequate mobilization onto the defect. Once elevated, the flap is rotated over the defect to cover it (▶ Fig. 16.4). To facilitate rotation, either a **back cut** or a **Burow's** triangle excision can be performed at the pivot point (▶ Fig. 16.4). Since the back cut is made toward the center of the semicircle, care must be taken to ensure that the flap's vascularization is not compromised. A Burow's triangle incision, in contrast, is made away from the pedicle and hence has no influence on the flap's blood supply. The donor area can usually be closed primarily, although a skin graft might be necessary in some instances.

Transposition Flaps

Transposition flaps resemble rotational flaps in that they too rotate about a pivot point to reach

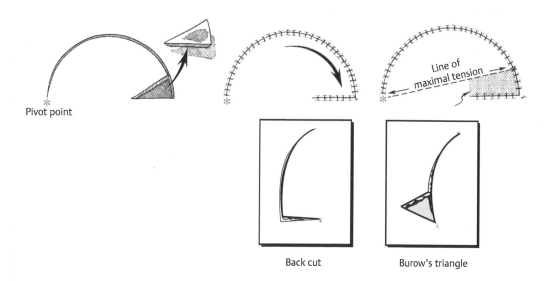

Pivot point

Line of maximal tension

Back cut

Burow's triangle

Fig. 16.4 Rotational flap illustrating the position of the pivot point and direction of line of maximal tension. Back cut or excision of Burow's triangle can be done to increase mobilization. (Reproduced from Janis, Essentials of Plastic Surgery, 2nd edition, ©2014, Thieme Publishers, New York.)

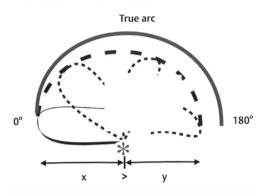

Fig. 16.5 Effective length of a flap. Note the decrease in length (*dotted line*) as the flap is turned around its pivot point(*). (Reproduced from Janis, Essentials of Plastic Surgery, 2nd edition, ©2014, Thieme Publishers, New York.)

the defect; however, whereas rotational flaps are semicircular in shape, transposition flaps generally have a more linear configuration (e.g., rectangular, rhombic). Transposition flaps are based at the edge of the defect and designed anywhere from right next to the defect to 90 degrees from it (▶Fig. 16.6). Hence, in most instances, a transposition flap must jump over a segment of healthy tissue to reach the wound. When designing a transposition flap, it must be considered that, as the angle of the flap's axis in relation to the defect is increased, the flap's effective length decreases (▶Fig. 16.5). Closure of the donor site is done either by direct closure or by skin grafting. Rhombic flaps and the z-plasty are common examples of transposition flaps.

Advancement Flaps

These flaps are designed with their leading edge on one of the borders of the defect, which they close by sliding over it (▶Fig. 16.7). Advancement flaps may have different configurations, but the gliding movement remains the same. As can be inferred, advancement flaps must be designed and used in areas with sufficient skin laxity that allows for adequate mobilization. Common advancement flaps include the rectangular and V-Y flaps.

Interpolation Flaps

By definition these flaps do not share a border with the defect; hence their transfer implies crossing over healthy intervening tissue. They are a useful tool to reconstruct full-thickness wounds with nearby like tissue when adjacent skin is not available or is insufficient. Once the portion of the flap covering the defect becomes vascularized from the wound bed (approximately 2–3 weeks after transfer), a second operation is needed to cut the pedicle and fully inset the flap. Alternatively, interpolation flaps may be tunneled through the subcutaneous tissue to reach the defect, in which case a second procedure would not be needed. The forehead flap for nasal reconstruction, and the heterodigital neurovascular island flap (i.e., Littler's flap), are good examples of interpolation flaps (▶Fig. 16.8).

Hinge Flaps

Because of the way by which these flaps are mobilized into the defect, hinge flaps are also named turnover flaps. They are tailored right next to the defect with their pedicle based at the flap–defect interface. The flap is then elevated in the subcutaneous plane and turned over the wound like a page in a book. This movement results in the superficialmost surface of the flap facing downward on the wound. These flaps can be raised with or without skin; in the former case, the skin can be used for internal epithelial lining. Additionally, because the flap's raw surface becomes exposed after hinging, either a second flap or a skin graft is necessary to resurface the wound.

16.4.4 Classification According to Proximity

Based on their spatial relationship with the defect, flaps can be broadly grouped into local, regional, and distant. Minding some inevitable exce ptions, local and regional flaps are almost always pedicled flaps, whereas distant flaps are usually transferred as microvascular free flaps.

Local Flaps

As their name implies, local flaps are obtained from tissues in the immediate vicinity of a defect, providing a relatively simple, straightforward, and reliable solution to coverage of a number of wounds. Nevertheless, in many cases local tissues are either insufficient or inadequate to be used for reconstruction (e.g., due to scarring from previous surgeries or stiffness and poor vascularity

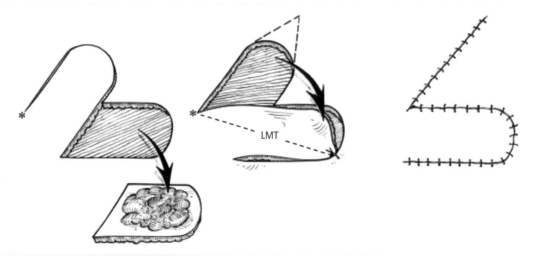

Fig. 16.6 Transposition flap. *, pivot point; LMT, line of maximal tension. (Modified from Zenn, Jones, Reconstructive Surgery Anatomy, Technique, and Clinical Applications, ©2012, Thieme Publishers, New York.)

Fig. 16.7 Rectangular advancement flap with excision of Burow's triangles at the base to increase mobilization. (Reproduced from Janis, Essentials of Plastic Surgery, 2nd edition, ©2014, Thieme Publishers, New York.)

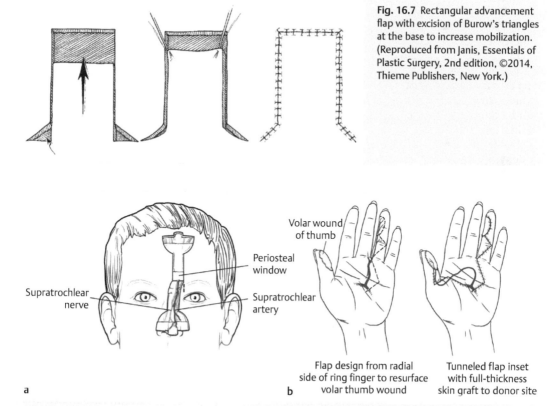

Fig. 16.8 Examples of interpolation flaps. **(a)** The forehead flap for nasal reconstruction. **(b)** The heterodigital neurovascular island from the ring finger to resurface a defect in the thumb. (Reproduced from Zenn, Jones, Reconstructive Surgery Anatomy, Technique, and Clinical Applications, ©2012, Thieme Publishers, New York.)

269

from previous radiation). In these cases, regional or distant options must be contemplated to achieve successful coverage and proper wound healing. It is important to note that, although local flaps may comprise one or more of the components listed earlier in this chapter, this does not alter in any way their "local" denomination. In this sense, a small rhomboid skin transposition flap for a defect in the temple area, an advancement pectoralis major muscle flap for a sternal wound, and a large rotational fasciocutaneous flap to resurface a sacral pressure sore are all examples of local (and of course pedicled) flaps, even though their size and composition are quite different.

Regional Flaps

These flaps are harvested from an area near the primary defect, usually from the same anatomical region, and therefore generally provide a good match with the tissue at the recipient area. The transfer of these flaps involves passing their vascular pedicle over healthy skin (i.e., interpolation flap) or subcutaneously (i.e., island flap). Regional flaps provide a good alternative for defects not amenable to reconstruction with local tissue; however, they have the shortcoming of not always being able to provide all tissues needed (e.g., robust bone, muscle, and skin for complex head and neck reconstruction), and their donor-site morbidity can sometimes be much more conspicuous and limiting than that of a distant free flap. Some examples of commonly used regional flaps include the forehead flap for nasal reconstruction, the submental flap for facial reconstruction, the temporalis muscle flap for facial reanimation, the deltopectoral fasciocutaneous or pectoralis major muscle/musculocutaneous flap for head and neck reconstruction, the posterior interosseous flap for hand reconstruction, and the sural neurocutaneous flap for distal leg reconstruction.

Distant Flaps

As stated earlier, distant flaps are usually transferred as microvascular free flaps, although this isn't always the case (e.g., groin flap for hand reconstruction). Distant flaps offer surgeons a wide range of tissue component options and greater design versatility so as to optimize the reconstructive outcome and at the same time reduce donor site morbidity. The relative downsides of free flaps

are their more technically challenging nature, the learning curve of microsurgery, and the need for some basic infrastructure with regard to magnification systems and surgical instruments.

16.5 Putting It All Together: Examples of Commonly Used Local Flaps

Having understood the basic principles of flap composition, vascularity, mobilization, and contiguity to the defect, we can now move on to describe some of the more commonly used local flaps. Local flaps are governed by certain key geometrical principles that apply regardless of the anatomical area or the flap's composition. In contrast, the use of regional and distant flaps is dictated to a greater extent by anatomical and technical aspects specific to the individual flap. Such detailed description goes beyond the scope of this chapter.

16.5.1 Rhomboid Flaps

These are one of the most commonly used and more illustrative examples of transposition flaps. Even though the principle is the same, there are two kinds of rhombic flaps, namely Limberg and Dufourmental flaps. For the Limberg flap, the defect is first tailored into a rhomboid with 60- and 120-degree angles. A line with a length equal to the rhomboid's short axis is extended laterally from one of the 120-degree angles. At the extreme end of this line, another one of equal length and parallel to either side of the rhomboid is delineated (▶Fig. 16.9). Thus, for any given rhomboidal defect, four possible flaps can be designed, but care should be taken to design and elevate the flap with the most appropriate donor site (e.g., from the zone with greatest laxity that allows for primary closure) (▶Fig. 16.10). Accordingly, the design must consider leaving the donor site scar parallel to the relaxed skin tension lines when possible. The Dufourmental flap follows the same principle as the Limberg but with a slightly different design. The angles of the rhomboid of a Dufourmental flap are usually of 30 and 150 degrees, although angles up to 90 degrees are possible (which technically creates a square rather than a rhombus). The first incision is made at the line bisecting the angle formed by the lateral extension of the short axis and either side of the rhomboid. The second

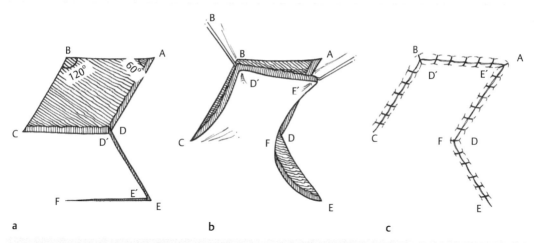

Fig. 16.9 (a-c) Limberg's rhomboid flap. (Reproduced from Janis, Essentials of Plastic Surgery, 2nd edition, ©2014, Thieme Publishers, New York.)

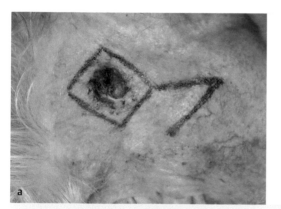
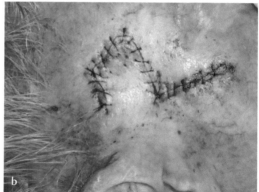

Fig. 16.10 (a) Basal cell carcinoma on the right temple and design of a rhomboid flap over area with greater laxity. (b) Result after excision and flap transposition.

incision is made at the extreme end of the previous one and is parallel to the rhomboid's long axis. Through this design, the Dufourmental flap has a narrower tip and a decreased arc of rotation compared with the Limberg, but direct closure of the donor site is usually easier. Depending on the reconstructive needs, rhomboid flaps can be performed either individually or in a double or triple configuration.

16.5.2 Bilobed Flap

Originally described by Esser and later modified by Zitelli, the bilobed flap is an ingenious transposition flap composed of two adjacent flaps in which the first flap covers the original defect, and the second flap is made to cover the secondary defect that has been created after mobilization of the primary flap. This design is useful in situations where skin immediately adjacent to the defect does not allow for primary closure after flap transposition. The secondary flap must, however, lie in an area of laxity and positioned parallel to the relaxed skin tension lines so that direct closure is possible. The primary flap is designed immediately adjacent to the defect, with an equal diameter. The second flap is delineated at the opposite edge of the primary flap and is narrower in width. When the first flap is transposed onto the primary defect, the second flap is pulled over to cover the secondary wound (▶Fig. 16.11). The total arc of rotation of a bilobed flap is the sum of the arcs of each flap. So if each flap rotates 45–50 degrees to reach its corresponding defect, the whole flap's arc would be 90–100 degrees. The degree of rotation will depend on the wound and local tissue characteristics; however, it should be kept in mind that too much rotation makes flap inset and closure difficult and should therefore be avoided.

16.5.3 Rectangular Advancement Flap

In this procedure a rectangle of mobile skin is tailored immediately adjacent to the defect and glided over it (▶Fig. 16.7). As with all advancement flaps, this requires adequate tissue surrounding the defect to allow proper advancement and closure with the least possible tension. If sufficient advancement is not achieved initially, or if evident dog-ears form at the base of the flaps after mobilization, excision of Burow's triangles is a good solution. Furthermore, if prior to flap design and elevation one deems the tissues not mobile enough to cover the whole defect, consideration can be given to performing an "H" flap, which consists of two opposing rectangles at either side of the defect that meet in the midline. With this, each flap covers only half the defect, and thus closure without tension is more achievable.

16.5.4 V-Y Advancement Flap

Together with rotation flaps, the V-Y advancement flap is probably one of the most used resources in flap surgery. Following the principle of sliding movement described earlier, this flap is designed as a **V** with its leading edge on one of the borders of the defect. The width of the flap equals the width of the defect, and its length is two to three times that of the wound. The flap is incised and completely islanded, releasing attachments at the base and advancing edge to allow adequate mobilization. Once adequate advancement is obtained, the donor site is closed directly, thus turning the original **V** design into a **Y** scar (▶Fig. 16.12). Given the fact that this flap is supplied from its deep aspect, the design and execution must anticipate proper vascularization, either through fascial plexuses, a known vascular axis, or a Dopplered perforator.

16.5.5 A-to-T Advancement Flap

This technique begins by shaping the wound to a triangle (i.e., an **A**). Then incisions are extended from the base of the triangle on both sides, undermining the tissue to create the flaps, which are advanced toward the midline, transforming the **A**-shaped defect to a **T** scar (▶Fig. 16.13). In some instances, excision of Burow's triangles is necessary to enhance mobilization or eliminate dog-ears.

16.5.6 O-to-Z Flap

This is another method of flap closure for circular defects around which two opposing rotation flaps are designed and elevated. Each flap covers half the wound; hence, when they meet in the middle, the **O**-shaped original wound is converted to a **Z**-shaped scar (▶Fig. 16.14).

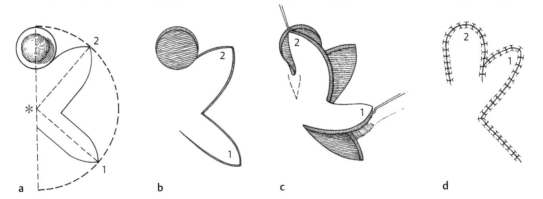

Fig. 16.11 (a-d) The bilobed flap. *, pivot point. (Reproduced from Janis, Essentials of Plastic Surgery, 2nd edition, ©2014, Thieme Publishers, New York.)

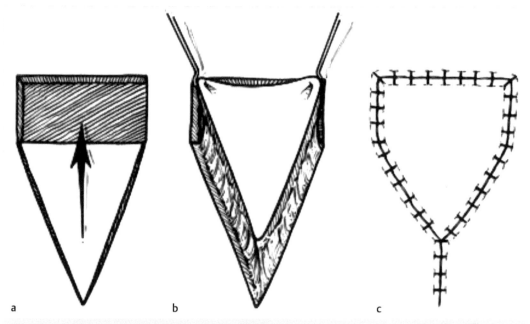

a   b   c

Fig. 16.12 (a-c) The V-Y advancement flap. (Reproduced from Zenn, Jones, Reconstructive Surgery Anatomy, Technique, and Clinical Applications, ©2012, Thieme Publishers, New York.)

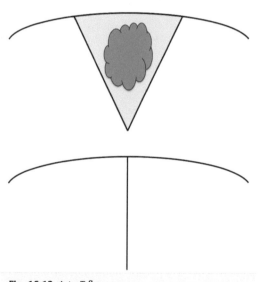

Fig. 16.13 A-to-T flap.

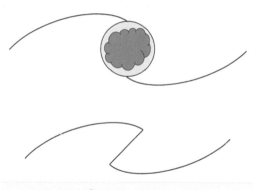

Fig. 16.14 O-to-Z flap.

16.5.7 Bipedicled Flap

The bipedicled flap consists of a segment of undermined tissue adjacent to the defect that is advanced onto it in a direction perpendicular to the flap's longitudinal axis while still being attached on both ends.

This characteristic improves blood supply compared to a single pedicle flap, but it reduces mobility. Furthermore, in a number of cases the secondary defect must be covered with a skin graft, which adds to the disadvantages of the procedures. Bilateral bipedicled flaps can be used in situations in which a single flap cannot resurface the whole wound (▶Fig. 16.15).

16.5.8 Keystone Flap

Described by Felix Behan, the keystone flap has an ingenious yet simple design that allows coverage

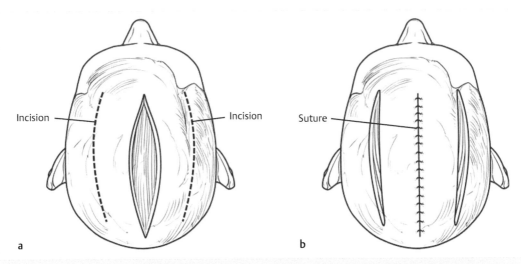

Incision — Incision Suture —

a b

Fig. 16.15 (a, b) Diagram of a double bipedicled flap to cover a defect on the scalp. (Reproduced from Zenn, Jones, Reconstructive Surgery Anatomy, Technique, and Clinical Applications, ©2012, Thieme Publishers, New York.)

of defects of varying sizes and in virtually any area of the body. It is designed in a trapezoidal curvilinear shape immediately adjacent to the defect and within the dermatomal segments so as to incorporate longitudinal running structures, such as cutaneous nerves and superficial veins. As with any other flap, the keystone should be tailored over an area of redundant tissue that allows adequate mobilization and primary closure of the donor site. In essence, the keystone flap is composed of two V-Y advancement flaps end-to-side. Once incised, the surrounding soft tissues are bluntly dissected without any flap undermining in order to preserve blood supply. If needed, the fascia on the outer curvilinear margin can be incised. The flap is then advanced to cover the defect and each end of the flap is closed in a V-Y configuration (▶Fig. 16.16).

16.6 Fasciocutaneous Flaps

Fasciocutaneous flaps were first described by Bengt Pontén in 1981 for lower extremity reconstruction and later reported by Tolhurst, Haeseker, and Zeeman. In essence, fasciocutaneous flaps are flaps raised below the level of the deep fascia but sparing the underlying muscle. Fascia itself is a relatively avascular tissue, so its inclusion does not per se enhance flap vascularity, but a robust

blood supply can usually be obtained by including the associated subfascial and prefascial (or suprafascial) plexuses. Although the former is comparatively minor, the latter comprises a rich network supplied by branches from perforating vessels traveling between muscle compartments, between muscle bellies, or through muscles. Additionally, "fascial feeders" are branches stemming from source arteries that do not reach the skin, but rather terminate at the level of the fascia (see Chapter 15). Raising a flap below the level of the deep fascia may also ensure better vascularity by avoiding injury to an axial vessel traveling within the subcutaneous plane. Finally, incorporation of fascia might add an extra layer of tissue for any given reconstructive need. Fasciocutaneous flaps can be classified according to two systems:

1. *Mathes–Nahai classification:* This system recognizes three types of flaps based on the course of the vascular pedicle through the underlying tissues before it pierces the fascia and reaches the skin (▶Fig. 16.17 and ▶Table 16.2).
   - *Type A:* Direct cutaneous vessel. The vascular pedicle branches off a regional source vessel and courses initially deep to the fascia to then continue superficial to it within the subcutaneous plane giving off small perforators that supply the skin.

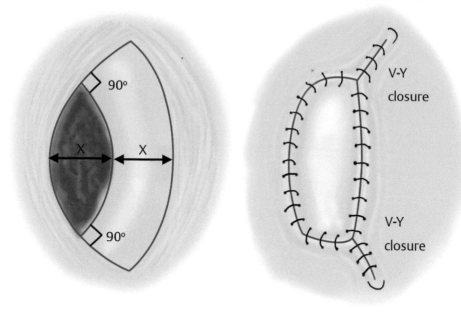

Fig. 16.16 The keystone flap.

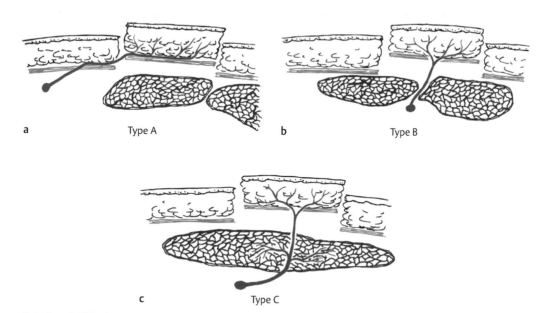

Fig. 16.17 (a-c) Mathes and Nahai classification of fasciocutaneous flaps. (Reproduced from Zenn, Jones, Reconstructive Surgery Anatomy, Technique, and Clinical Applications, ©2012, Thieme Publishers, New York.)

Table 16.2 Mathes–Nahai classification of fasciocutaneous flaps

Type A	Type B	Type C
Deep external pudendal artery	Anterior lateral thigh	Anterior lateral thigh
Digital artery	Anterior tibial artery	Deltopectoral
Dorsal metacarpal artery	Deltoid	Nasolabial
Gluteal thigh	Dorsalis pedis	Thoracoepigastric (transverse abdominal)
Great toe (hallux)	Inferior cubital artery (antecubital)	Transverse back
Groin	Lateral arm	
Lateral thoracic (axillary)	Lateral plantar artery	
Pudendal-thigh	Lateral thigh	
Saphenous	Medial arm	
Scalp	Medial plantar artery	
Second toe	Medial thigh	
Standard forehead	Peroneal artery	
Superficial external pudendal artery	Posterior interosseous	
Superficial inferior epigastric artery	Posterior tibial artery	
Sural artery	Radial forearm	
Temporoparietal fascia	Radial recurrent	
	Scapular	
	Ulnar recurrent	

- *Type B:* Septocutaneous vessel. The vascular pedicle courses through the intermuscular septum between adjacent muscles or muscle compartments before piercing the deep fascia and reaching the skin.
- *Type C:* Musculocutaneous vessel. In type C flaps, the vascular pedicle originates from a source vessel and travels through muscular structures, supplying them, before piercing the deep fascia and reaching the overlying skin.

This classification, apart from its anatomic features, has other important implications. From a technical point of view, dissection of the vascular pedicle all the way to its origin on the source vessel is increasingly difficult as one goes from type A to type C. In general terms, dissecting a direct cutaneous vessel is less complicated than dissecting a musculocutaneous pedicle in which muscle fibers must be gently separated from the vessel and ligation of tiny muscular branches is necessary to skeletonize the pedicle.

2. *Cormack and Lamberty classification:* Through extensive research on cutaneous blood supply

with an emphasis on flap surgery, Cormack and Lamberty also classified fasciocutaneous flaps according to their vascular anatomy. However, while the Mathes–Nahai system focuses on the anatomical course of the pedicle through underlying tissues, this system describes the vascular pattern of the flap itself (▶ Fig. 16.18).

- *Type A:* These flaps do not rely on one single pedicle but are rather supplied by several fasciocutaneous perforators located at the base of the flap and oriented along its longitudinal axis. Hence, in a way, these flaps are reminiscent of random pattern skin flaps. Type A flaps can be based either proximally or distally. Alternatively the skin island of these flaps can be completely incised, thus creating an island flap.
- *Type B:* Type B flaps are based on one single, moderately sized, and fairly consistent fasciocutaneous perforator. If the vessel is of good size, these flaps can be used as free flaps. Alternatively, these flaps may also be transferred as free flaps by incorporating the segment of the source vessel from which the supplying perforator branches branch off (B-modified).
- *Type C:* The vascular supply to these flaps comes from multiple perforators sequentially emanating from an underlying major vessel. These small perforators travel within a fascial septum to reach the skin. Because they are usually not sizeable enough to supply the whole flap, the source vessel must be included. These flaps can be used as either proximally or distally based pedicled flaps or as free flaps. One of the most illustrative examples of a type C flap is the radial forearm flap.
- *Type D:* Type D flaps are really composite flaps, which include bone, muscle, fascia, and skin (thus named osteomusculofasciocutaneous). Their vascular configuration is similar to that of type C flaps.

16.7 Flap Modifications

Over the past decades a number of modifications have been introduced to either improve flap viability or suit a specific reconstructive need. Most of these modifications have arisen as a result of meticulous anatomical dissections, studies on the physiology of cutaneous blood supply, and remarkable technical advancements. These variations have allowed reconstructive surgeons to manage a wide rage of defects

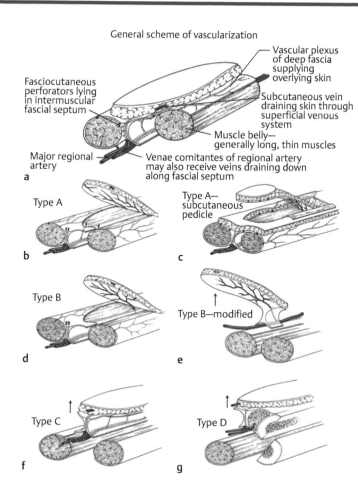

General scheme of vascularization

Fasciocutaneous perforators lying in intermuscular fascial septum

Vascular plexus of deep fascia supplying overlying skin

Subcutaneous vein draining skin through superficial venous system

Muscle belly— generally long, thin muscles

Major regional artery

Venae comitantes of regional artery may also receive veins draining down along fascial septum

a

Type A

b

Type A— subcutaneous pedicle

c

Type B

d

Type B—modified

e

Type C

f

Type D

g

Fig. 16.18 (a–g) Cormack and Lamberty's classification of fasciocutaneous flaps. (Reproduced from Zenn, Jones, Reconstructive Surgery Anatomy, Technique, and Clinical Applications, ©2012, Thieme Publishers, New York.)

of varying dimensions in different areas of the body. Furthermore, the use of these "tricks" in many instances allows the undertaking of a very precise and elegant reconstruction with a clearly superior functional and aesthetic outcome compared to what would be obtained by simply "filling the hole."

16.7.1 Flap Delay

The term *delay* in flap surgery refers to partial interruption of a flap's blood supply with the purpose of (paradoxically) enhancing flap vascularity and increasing its viable area. These maneuvers are performed prior to transfer with the flap still at the donor site and include at least one and sometimes two or three procedures. Two methods of delay have been described: surgical delay and vascular delay.

Surgical delay is done by first incising the borders of the planned flap along its longitudinal axis and

undermining it so that a bipedicled flap is created. The wounds are sutured, and the flap is left to rest at the donor site. After a period ranging from 10 days to 3 weeks, the distal portion is incised and the flap is transferred. If the flap is too long or there is doubt about distal tip viability, distal division may be done in two stages and/or the flap can be transferred a few days after. Surgical delay may also be performed by completely raising the flap in one procedure, and then suturing it back on the donor site and transferring it 2–3 weeks later.

Vascular delay consists of selectively ligating one or more pedicles (or perforators) supplying a flap, leaving it nourished only by a dominant one at its base. Eventually, 2–4 weeks after this procedure, the remaining pedicle will supply the whole flap more reliably than it would have if the flap had been harvested and transferred based on that same pedicle in a single stage. This technique has been used extensively in superiorly based transverse rectus abdominis myocutaneous (TRAM) flaps. Here, the deep inferior epigastric vessels are ligated so that the planned TRAM is supplied by its superior epigastric pedicle only. Flap transfer is then performed 2–4 weeks later. It is important to note that in a healthy patient this would not be needed; however, in patients with comorbidities (e.g., smokers), in which complete flap survival based on the superior epigastric is uncertain, a delay procedure can be a safe and reliable strategy to improve flap survival. Despite the unquestionable effectiveness of delay, there is still some debate around the exact mechanisms that lead to improved survival. Reported findings on this matter include changes in the vascular tree within the flap, ischemic conditioning, stimulation of angiogenesis, a sympathectomy effect, and reduction of vasoconstrictors and prothrombotic agents.

Through work in rabbits, pigs, and dogs, Taylor and colleagues demonstrated that the partial interruption of a flap's blood supply produces an initial reduction and subsequent gradual increase in the caliber of choke vessels connecting two adjacent vascular territories and the one beyond. They observed that this effect was maximal at 48–72 hours post delay, and that, once established, it was permanent and irreversible. This opening of choke vessels is one of the main mechanisms through which vascularity is boosted in delayed flaps (▶ Fig. 16.19). It has also

been suggested that, by rendering a flap partially ischemic, it eventually adapts to the hypoxic state in situ and is therefore better able to withstand the insult from mobilization. In addition, the production of vasoconstrictors and prothrombotic agents that occurs with any surgical procedure, and has a direct effect on the flap's blood supply, might be reduced if the flap is raised in a staged manner. Furthermore, it has been postulated that the ischemic environment elicits an angiogenic response within the flap, leading to improved survival upon definitive transfer. Finally, by incising a flap's borders, sympathetic nerve fibers are severed, which theoretically reduces the adrenergic stimulus to the flap and leads to vessel dilatation.

16.7.2 Flap Prefabrication and Prelamination

Prefabrication refers to the transposition of a sizeable vascular pedicle into the subcutaneous plane at another nearby location. Following implantation, significant capillary sprouting occurs from the transposed vessels to the overlying tissue such that after approximately 6–8 weeks that segment of tissue is supplied by the aforementioned vessels and can thus be transferred as either a pedicled or a free flap. This technique is useful in situations in which tissues from established donor sites are

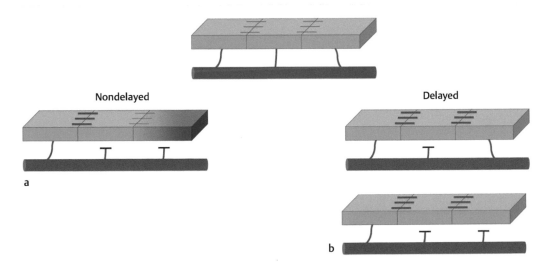

Fig. 16.19 Diagram depicting the opening of choke vessels in flap delay. **(a)** Full elevation in one stage leads to vascular compromise of the distal portion. **(b)** Partial elevation and selective division of blood supply allows opening of choke vessels and survival of the distal segment.

unusable (e.g., burned or scarred) but the underlying pedicle remains intact. Additionally, prefabrication can be combined with tissue expansion, which adds further versatility and allows creation of a larger flap. Flap prefabrication, however, requires at least two procedures for transfer, and the vascular supply from the "neopedicle" is not always reliable, especially its venous drainage. These limitations, together with the vast array of flaps that are currently available, have relegated this technique to a far second or third choice of reconstruction.

In *prelamination* the flap is elevated and tailored according to the reconstructive need on a known vascular pedicle at the recipient site. This may involve flap shaping and suturing only, or the addition of other types of tissues, such as skin or cartilage, which are grafted within the flap. Once the prelaminated construct is healed, it is transferred to the defect. By allowing everything to heal prior to transfer, prelamination in theory reduces the chances of complications in complex three-dimensional reconstructions requiring layers of different tissues. However, it can be impractical due to the need for staged procedures, and the additional stages can result in excessive scarring. Flap prelamination has been used with success for total nasal reconstruction and other complex defects in the head and neck.

16.7.3 Reverse Flow Flaps

Reverse flow flaps are perfused through the distal end of their corresponding source vessel, which has been divided proximally, thus relying on arcades and connections between two neighboring source arteries. The venous drainage of these flaps is also retrograde, so alternative pathways are required to bypass the valves. As investigated by Piñal and Taylor, this is accomplished by the presence of "macrovenous" connections between the *venae comitantes*, a rich microvenous plexus surrounding the artery (i.e., *venae arteriosa*), and the anatomical variability of venous valves. The reverse flow radial forearm flap is a good example, in which the radial artery is divided proximally, and the flap then becomes vascularized in a reversed manner through the ulnar artery (▸Fig. 16.20). Reverse flow flaps should not be confused with flaps based on secondary pedicles in which the main dominant pedicle has been divided. In this case, despite division of the main blood supply, arterial supply to the flap remains antegrade, and the direction of venous drainage follows the direction of the valves. Even though these flaps are often called reverse flaps, they are named so after the way they reach the defect rather than the direction of their blood supply. The "reverse" pectoralis major muscle flap supplied by its secondary pedicles from the internal mammary artery is an example of such a flap (▸Fig. 16.21).

16.7.4 Compound Flaps

Over the years, there has been some confusion surrounding the classification and terminology of compound flaps. Apart from being useful for communication, knowing the different types of compound flaps has important clinical implications, because these flaps can provide an elegant alternative to a number of complex reconstructions. In the most simplistic way, *compound flaps* are defined as flaps that incorporate different tissues in a single flap unit. According to their vascular configuration, compound flaps are further divided and subdivided as shown in ▸Fig. 16.22.

16.7.5 Vascular Augmentation: Supercharged and Turbocharged Flaps

In most instances, pedicled or free flaps can be reliably transferred based on their dominant

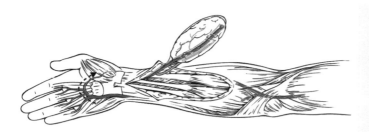

Fig. 16.20 Reverse flow radial forearm flap. Note division of radial artery proximally at the cubital fossa and reverse flow through ulnar artery (*dotted arrow*). (Modified from Zenn, Jones, Reconstructive Surgery Anatomy, Technique, and Clinical Applications, ©2012, Thieme Publishers, New York.)

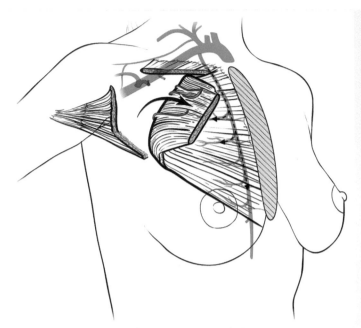

Fig. 16.21 "Reverse" pectoralis major muscle flap. Note division of main pedicle from thoracoacromial trunk and antegrade perfusion by internal mammary perforators *(dotted arrows)*. (Modified from Zenn, Jones, Reconstructive Surgery Anatomy, Technique, and Clinical Applications, ©2012, Thieme Publishers, New York.)

pedicle. Moreover, anastomosing both venae comitantes in a free flap can improve venous drainage. Extra sources of arterial inflow or venous outflow are often needed, which can only be created using microsurgical techniques. *Supercharged* flaps are those in which an external vascular source (arterial and/or venous) is brought to the flap and anastomosed to any given vessel stump. *Turbocharged* flaps, in turn, are created by artificially linking vessels within the flap, thus enhancing the flap's potential without external sources. The deep inferior epigastric perforator (DIEP) flap provides a good example to illustrate these concepts. A (venous) supercharged DIEP could be created by anastomosing the flap's superficial inferior epigastric vein to the cephalic vein at the recipient site in addition to the main anastomoses between the deep inferior epigastric and internal mammary vessels. However, if the same superficial inferior epigastric was connected to the proximal stump of the deep inferior epigastric vein (i.e., intraflap vascular connections), then the flap would be classified as a (venous) turbocharged flap. Although the example given here is with a free flap, supercharging and turbocharging are also applicable to pedicled flaps. Both of these techniques provide useful lifeboats to enhance flap perfusion or drainage and therefore have an important role in flap salvaging.

16.7.6 Flow-through Flaps

Flow-through flaps can theoretically be applied to reconstruction in any area; however, they have their prime indication in upper and lower limb defects in which one or more vascular axes have been damaged from trausma, or resected as part of an oncological ablative procedure. In either case, distal limb perfusion may be compromised; therefore, the reconstruction must not only consider restoration of soft tissues and wound coverage, but also reestablishment of blood flow. A flow-through flap is a free flap harvested together with its source vessel, which is anastomosed to the recipient artery and vein proximally and distally in order to restore distal perfusion.

16.7.7 Venous Flaps

A venous flap is a block of tissue (most commonly skin and subcutaneous) that is both nourished and drained by a single vein and its intraflap network. From a vascular standpoint, these flaps have been established to be intermediate between full-thickness grafts and normal free flaps. Given their suboptimal vascularization, venous flaps are generally limited in size and therefore best indicated for small, relatively shallow defects, such as in hand

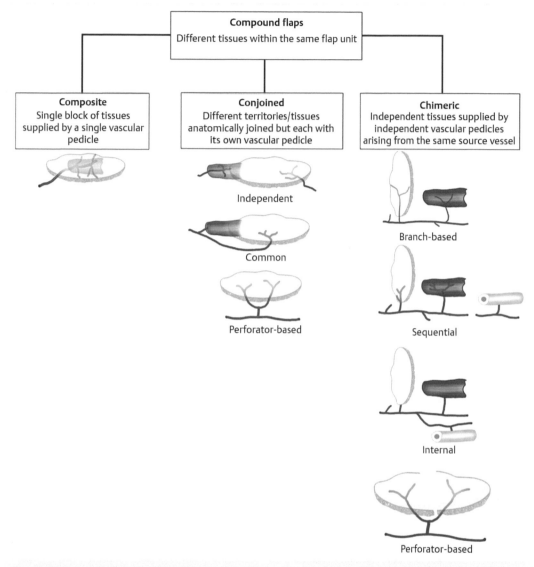

Fig. 16.22 Compound flaps are flaps that incorporate different tissues into a single unit and can be further subdivided into composite, conjoined, and chimeric.

reconstruction, where they can be used as either pedicled (proximally or distally based) or free flaps. During the early postoperative period these flaps generally have a dusky appearance and may present with significant swelling, congestion, and even some degree of epidermolysis. These changes tend to fade gradually, and the flap reaches a normal coloration 2–3 weeks after transfer. Three types of venous flaps have been described according to their vascular configuration (▶Fig. 16.23).

16.8 Perforator Flaps

As described in Chapter 16, the integument is supplied by more than 300 individual perforating vessels (i.e., perforators) arising from underlying source vessels, with each perforator supplying a circumscribed territory called the *perforasome* (▶Fig. 16.24). After branching from their parent vessel, perforators may reach the skin directly (direct cutaneous perforator), course through intermuscular septa (septocutaneous perforator), or course through muscle (musculocutaneous perforator). A perforator flap is in essence a block of skin and/or subcutaneous fat supplied by isolated perforators, which travel through or between tissues (mostly muscle) en route to their target cutaneous territory. Over the years there has been some controversy regarding what constitutes a true perforator, with some postulating that the only true perforators are those piercing through muscle on their route to the skin. From a surgical point of view, dissection of musculocutaneous perforators is more challenging, takes longer, and carries a higher risk of injury compared to dissection of direct cutaneous and septocutaneous perforators; therefore a distinction should be made. Despite these anatomical and surgical differences, current classification systems still consider all three kinds as perforators.

By sparing the underlying muscle, perforator flaps generally carry less donor site morbidity and faster recovery times when compared to their musculocutaneous counterpart. In addition, given the abundance of perforators throughout the body, the availability of perforator flaps is considerably higher than that of muscle flaps because, in theory, a perforator flap can be raised from virtually any area with a sizeable perforator. Other main advantages of perforator flaps are listed in ▶ Table 16.3. Taken altogether, these advantages allow the surgeon to elegantly tailor the flap to the defect, thus optimizing the reconstructive outcome.

16.8.1 Classification

Since the beginning of the "perforator flap era," there has been some confusion as to the proper naming and classification of perforator flaps. During the early 1990s different surgeons around the world would be performing the same flap but giving it different names. For example, abdominal perforator flaps based on the deep inferior epigastric artery would be referred to as *paraumbilical perforator flaps* or *DIEP flaps*, and flaps based on the thoracodorsal system would be named *thoracodorsal artery perforator flaps, latissimus dorsi perforator flaps*, or *thoracodorsal perforator-based cutaneous island flaps*. Since then different systems of classification have been proposed, with

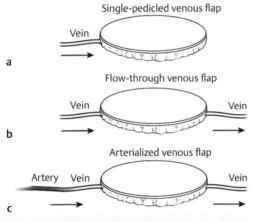

Fig. 16.23 Venous flaps. **(a)** Type I is an unipedicled flap with a single vein at its cephalad edge as the only vascular source. **(b)** Type II or "flow-through," with one afferent and one efferent vein flowing from toward the cephalad portion of the flap. **(c)** Type II or arterialized, involves an arteriovenous microsurgical anastomosis proximally and a draining vein distally. (Reproduced from Janis, Essentials of Plastic Surgery, 2nd edition, ©2014, Thieme Publishers, New York.)

Table 16.3 Advantages of perforator flaps

Availability
Reduced donor site morbidity
Versatility in design
Malleability (depending on thickness of flap)
Size (large flaps may be harvested by including more than one perforator)
Possibility of thinning
Possibility to include sensory nerve for sensate flap

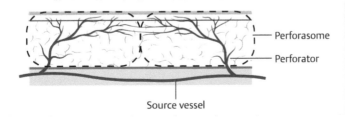

Source vessel

Fig. 16.24 The perforasome concept. (Reproduced from Janis, Essentials of Plastic Surgery, 2nd edition, ©2014, Thieme Publishers, New York.)

the Gent Consensus and the Canadian System being the most widely used.

The Gent Consensus names flaps after the nutrient source vessel, adding the word *perforator* at the end, such as DIEP flap. Now, in cases in which the nutrient vessel supplies more then one flap, these would be named after the associated muscle or the anatomical region. For example flaps supplied by the lateral circumflex femoral system could be named tensor fascia lata perforator flaps (if the perforator traveled through tensor fascia lata), or anterior lateral thigh perforator flaps.

The Canadian System names all flaps based on their nutrient vessel, adding the word *artery* (deep inferior epigastric *artery* perforator [DIEAP] flap). However, unlike the Gent Consensus, in cases where one parent vessel supplies different flaps, a suffix with an abbreviation of the muscle involved is added (▶ Fig. 16.25). In addition, if the perforator is septocutaneous, then an *-s* suffix is added; for example, LCFA-*s* would denominate a flap based on a septocutaneous perforator from the lateral circumflex femoral artery (e.g., ALT).

16.8.2 Preoperative Vascular Mapping

The preoperative planning of a perforator flap is based on two main aspects: the availability and quality of tissue in the planned donor area, including the presence of previous scars, radiotherapy changes or trauma, and the presence of a reliable perforator in a favorable location. In addition, when planning to do a free perforator flap other important factors come into play, such as pedicle length and caliber, presence of a sensory nerve in situations where a sensate flap is desired, patient positioning, among others.

Along with the evolution and technical refinements of perforator flaps, methods of perforator mapping have been developed to assist in the preoperative planning of these flaps.

The handheld Doppler is a simple yet useful method to look for perforators in any area of the body. Although simple, fast, inexpensive, noninvasive, and easy to perform at the bedside or intraoperatively, this method is only able to provide limited information, namely the presence and approximate location of perforators, which serves as an aid in flap design. Limitations on the handheld Doppler are that it does not give any information on size (e.g., the audible signal correlates poorly with the vessel's caliber) or anatomical course (e.g., septocutaneous or musculocutaneous), and in some cases, especially in thin patients, it may be misleading because it can capture the signal of an underlying source vessel and not necessarily a perforator.

Color Doppler ultrasonography is able to provide far more information than the handheld Doppler because it is able to precisely identify the presence of perforators, their size above the deep fascia, their location, the point where they pierce the deep fascia, and their anatomical course. Color Doppler also gives valuable information on the underlying source vessel and can be used to assess recipient vessels as well as to detect any vascular abnormalities or disease. The method is, however, operator dependent, time consuming, and more expensive.

Multidetector-row computed tomography (MDCT) angiography, commonly known as computed tomographic angiography (CTA or CT-angio), is currently the gold standard method of preoperative perforator mapping because it provides highly precise information on the position, size, and anatomical course of perforators, characteristics of the source vessel, and characteristics of the deep and superficial systems at the same time (e.g., deep inferior and superficial inferior epigastric systems) (▶ Fig. 16.26). Furthermore, different potential donor sites and recipient vessels can be evaluated simultaneously with CT-angio and, unlike color Doppler, where usually only representative photos

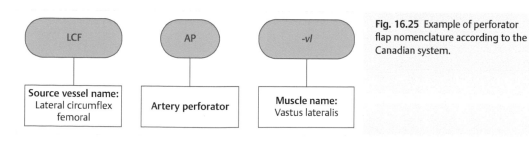

Fig. 16.25 Example of perforator flap nomenclature according to the Canadian system.

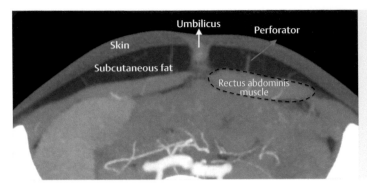

Fig. 16.26 Abdominal computed tomographic angiogram showing perforators from the deep inferior epigastric artery during the preoperative planning of a deep inferior epigastric artery perforator flap.

are taken, the surgeon can scroll up and down the images to explore the anatomy, choose the best perforator(s), and precisely delineate it (them). Finally, the procedure is fast (e.g., less than 10 minutes) and usually well tolerated by patients. Disadvantages of CT-angio include the need for contrast with its inherent risk of anaphylaxis, the delivery of radiation, and cost.

Magnetic resonance angiography (MRA) is another method of perforator mapping, which, like the CT-angio, provides extremely precise information without the need for radiation. However, its cost and the fact that it is not available in many institutions have impeded MRA from becoming a widespread method of perforator mapping.

Preoperative vascular mapping has not only proven to be a useful tool in flap planning, but, more importantly, it has had a substantial impact in the actual surgical procedure inasmuch as it has shown to significantly reduce operative time. Before these methods became widespread, surgeons would go and "hunt" for the best perforator with very little information, apart from a potential location detected with the handheld Doppler. Thus the whole decision-making process was done intraoperatively. What is more, sometimes these decisions were made with limited vision because the sparing of the initial perforators encountered during the dissection prevented adequate visualization of other perforators beyond that point. Moreover, once the best perforator was selected, its anatomical course would remain a mystery until it was completely dissected. Preoperative mapping allows surgeons to select the best perforator, and therefore go directly toward it during flap harvest, as well as providing a very clear picture of

what to expect with respect to the vessel's anatomical course.

> **Note**
>
> Choosing the best perforator is not only about size. Location in relation to the planned skin paddle (e.g., trying to have the perforator as close to the center as possible) and the anatomical course are also key factors to consider.

16.8.3 Surgical Technique and Common Perforator Flaps

Even though differences exist when harvesting perforator flaps from different anatomical regions, some basic principles apply to all of them regardless of their location. Elevation of a perforator flap is a procedure with varying degrees of complexity, which can be broken down to four main steps: (suprafascial) approach to the perforator; opening of the deep fascia; perforator dissection; and dissection of the nutrient vessel. Once the skin paddle is designed around the selected perforator (e.g., preoperative mapping), incisions are made down to fascia, and dissection proceeds in the suprafascial plane toward the perforator. This dissection is usually straightforward and can be done with monopolar cautery. As the perforator is approached, dissection proceeds more carefully with monopolar turned down to a lower setting, bipolar, or, alternatively, with tenotomy scissors. If no method other than handheld Doppler has been used preoperatively, then some exploration needs to be done to select the most adequate perforator. In general terms, a diameter greater than 1 mm and a visible pulse are good indicators of a good-quality perforator. Once identified, the perforator is dissected free from surrounding fat and

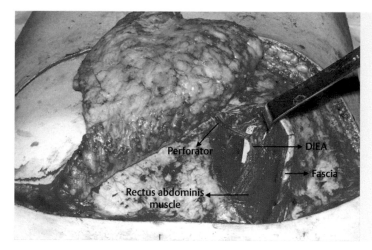

Fig. 16.27 Intraoperative view of a perforator dissected to its origin from the deep inferior epigastric artery.

areolar tissue, but full skeletonization is unnecessary and risky and therefore discouraged. The next step is to open the deep fascia. In cases in which the point where the perforator pierces the deep fascia is big enough, the fascia can be opened through this interval with little risk of damaging the vessels; however, if this is not possible, it is safer to cut a cuff of fascia around the perforator. In addition, one should be cognizant that perforators may travel under the deep fascia for a variable distance before entering the muscle, putting them at risk of injury during splitting of this layer. With the fascia fully divided and the muscle exposed, the pattern of the perforator (i.e., septocutaneous or musculocutaneous) is revealed and its dissection begins. Dissection of a septocutaneous perforator is relatively straightforward and safe, as opposed to intramuscular dissection, which is more tedious. Side branches are ligated to maintain a bloodless operative field. The perforator should be fully released from its four aspects (e.g., roof, floor, and both sides) all the way until the source vessel is reached (▶Fig. 16.27). To avoid injury and bleeding, it is best to dissect the perforator in the loose areolar plane around it. Leaving a small cuff of muscle around as a means to "protect" the vessel often results in capillary oozing and obscuring of the surgical field. Once the nutrient vessel is reached, dissection continues until adequate length and caliber are obtained, making sure to ligate side branches, some of which can be quite sizeable. During the whole procedure it is imperative to maintain a bloodless field and ensure wide surgical exposure, either with the help of an assistant or by the use of strategically placed self-retaining retractors.

Although these steps are common to most perforator flaps, each flap has its own tenets regarding perforator location, design, incisions, and dissection/elevation. A full description of these is beyond the scope of this chapter. Herein we summarize the main anatomical landmarks, location of perforators, uses, advantages, and disadvantages of three commonly used perforator flaps, namely the DIEP, anterolateral thigh flap (ALT), and thoracodorsal artery perforator flap (TDAP) (▶Fig. 16.28, ▶Fig. 16.29, and ▶Fig. 16.30).

Remember	M!

Harvest of a perforator flap involves four main steps:
1. Suprafascial approach to the perforator
2. Opening of the deep fascia
3. Perforator dissection (deroofing)
4. Dissection of the nutrient vessel

16.9 Propeller Flaps

As mentioned earlier, theoretically any area where a suitable perforator is identified can potentially become a donor site for a perforator flap, a concept elegantly illustrated with *propeller flaps*. Propeller flaps are completely islanded fasciocutaneous or skin (e.g., skin and subcutaneous tissue) flaps based on a single perforator around which they rotate to reach the defect. Rotation can be up to 180 degrees; if more is needed then the flap is rotated in the opposite direction. Although such twisting

Source vessel: deep inferior epigastric artery

Associated muscle: rectus abdominis

Location of perforators: medial and lateral rows, most periumbilical within a circle of 5 cm radius centered on the umbilicus

Size of skin paddle: 20 × 45 cm

Length of pedicle: 8 – 10 cm

Diameter of pedicle: 1.0 – 2.5 mm

Common regional uses: abdominal, genital and groin reconstruction.

Common free uses: breast reconstruction, soft tissue defects elsewhere in the body

Main advantages: large skin paddle, good match with breast tissue, long and sizeable pedicle, reduced donor site morbidity by sparing muscle and fascia, can be converted to musculocutaneous flap if needed, presence of superficial system (SIEA-V) allows vascular augmentation if necessary.

Main disadvantages: variable perforator anatomy, perforator dissection difficult if long intramuscular course, learning curve

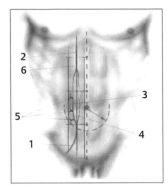

Fig. 16.28 Summary of the deep inferior epigastric artery perforator flap. 1, deep inferior epigastric artery; 2, deep superior epigastric artery; 3, lateral branch of DIEAP; 4, medial branch of DIEAP; 5, paraumbilical perforators; 6, rectus abdominis muscle; 7, sheath of rectus; 10, branches of 10th and 11th intercostal nerves. (Reproduced from Straucj, Yu, Atlas of Microvascular Surgery Anatomy, Technique, and Clinical Applications, ©2012, Thieme Publishers, New York.)

Source vessel: descending branch of lateral circumflex femoral artery

Associated muscle: vastus lateralis, tensor fascia lata

Location of perforators: within a circle of 3 cm radius at the midpoint between the ASIS and superolateral border of patella

Size of skin paddle: 25 cm long and up to 8 – 10 cm wide to allow primary closure

Length of pedicle: 10 – 12 cm

Diameter of pedicle: 2.0 mm

Common regional uses: abdominal, groin, lower thigh and knee reconstruction

Common free uses: head and neck and lower extremity reconstruction, soft tissue defects elsewhere in the body

Main advantages: large skin paddle, long pedicle, acceptable donor morbidity (direct closure), ease of dissection (septocutaneous perforators), can be made chimeric, can incorporate sensory nerve for sensate flap, can be harvested with fascia lata for tendon reconstruction or with vastus lateralis for bulk.

Main disadvantages: unsightly donor site if skin grafted, musculocutaneous perforators may be difficult to dissect, not ideal in obese patients

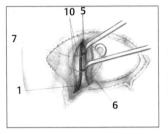

Fig. 16.29 Summary of the anterior lateral thigh flap. 1, descending branch of lateral circumflex femoral artery; 2, perforator (musculocutaneous above right and septocutaneous below right); 3, rectus femoris muscle; 4, vastus lateralis muscle; 5, muscular branch of femoral nerve; 6, LCFA; 7, ascending and transverse branch of LCFA (ligated); 8, vastus intermedius muscle. (Reproduced from Straucj, Yu, Atlas of Microvascular Surgery Anatomy, Technique, and Clinical Applications, ©2012, Thieme Publishers, New York.)

Source vessel: thoracodorsal artery

Associated muscle: latissimus dorsi

Location of perforators: along a line parallel to the lateral border of latissimus dorsi and 2 cm medial to it. Proximal perforator is usually dominant and located 8 cm below the posterior axillary fold

Size of skin paddle: 14 x 25 cm

Length of pedicle: 14 – 18 cm

Diameter of pedicle: 1.5 – 3.0 mm

Common regional uses: breast, chest, shoulder, upper arm, back

Common free uses: lower extremity reconstruction, soft tissue defects elsewhere in the body

Main advantages: long pedicle, possibility of incorporating different tissues (skin, muscle and bone) based on the thoracodorsal system, usually straightforward dissection of perforator

Main disadvantages: difficult to identify suitable perforators preoperatively, usually few perforators and therefore narrow margin for error

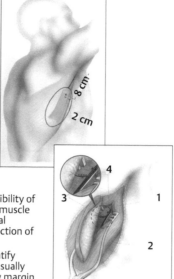

Fig. 16.30 Summary of the thoracodorsal artery perforator flap. 1, latissimus dorsi muscle; 2, serratus anterior muscle; 3, musculocutaneous perforator; 4, thoracodorsal artery, vein, and nerve. (Reproduced from Straucj, Yu, Atlas of Microvascular Surgery Anatomy, Technique, and Clinical Applications, ©2012, Thieme Publishers, New York.)

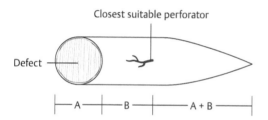

Fig. 16.31 Propeller flap. In order to reach the defect, the portion of the flap proximal to the perforator should be equal to the diameter of the defect plus the distance from the defect to the perforator. (Reproduced from Janis, Essentials of Plastic Surgery, 2nd edition, ©2014, Thieme Publishers, New York.)

of the pedicle may be detrimental to flap perfusion and, particularly, venous drainage, complete skeletonization of the perforator and thorough release of the fascial attachments avoids this problem. The design of propeller flaps is dependent on the position of the perforator—the farther away from the defect the larger the flap because it has to cover the defect plus the distance between it and the perforator (▶Fig. 16.31). Direct closure of the donor site is desirable and should be attempted whenever possible, keeping in mind that too tight a closure may compress the pedicle and render the flap ischemic, or more commonly, congested,

in which case it is preferable to cover the donor area with a skin graft. Finally, because propeller flaps use local neighboring tissues, a proper assessment of the quality of the surrounding skin is paramount to achieving wound coverage with healthy, well-vascularized tissue (▶Fig. 16.32). In some cases radiotherapy changes or the extent of trauma may extend well beyond the defect, making local tissue unusable.

16.10 Conclusions

The history of plastic surgery has been inherently related to the development of flaps and will continue to be as they form a fundamental pillar of our specialty. Flaps represent an ingenious and effective way of covering a wide range of defects, from small to large, and including different components, though always at the expense of some morbidity at the donor site, usually in the form of a scar or a graft. Flaps then require careful planning, meticulous execution, and proper postoperative care to optimize outcomes. Technical advancements and refinements in reconstructive surgery have greatly contributed to the development of flaps, leading to the gradual expansion of the armamentarium of possible alternatives for reconstruction. In this regard, perforator flaps have brought a whole new set of tools offering elegantly tailored reconstruction with

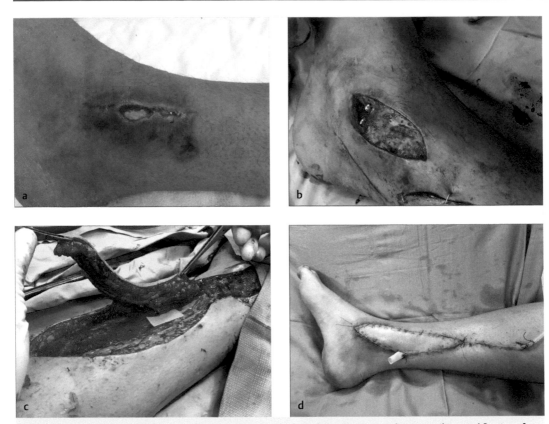

Fig. 16.32 Case example of a propeller flap. **(a)** Wound breakdown following open reduction and internal fixation of a fracture to the medial malleolus. **(b)** After debridement, there is exposed bone and metal hardware. **(c)** A propeller flap was raised based on a perforator from the posterior tibial artery. **(d)** The flap was turned 180 degrees to reach the defect, and the donor site was closed directly. (This case is provided courtesy of Dr. Álvaro Cabello.)

either local or distant tissues with the great advantage of reduced donor site morbidity in most cases.

16.11 Key Points

- The reconstructive ladder concept has been replaced by the reconstructive elevator, where surgeons can move freely between the different options of reconstruction, skipping simpler techniques and going primarily to more complex procedures to obtain a better result.
- Flaps are blocks of tissue with their own vascular supply. They may include one or more of several tissues, such as skin, subcutaneous fat, fascia, muscle, bone, mucosa, nerve, and cartilage.
- Flaps can be classified according to different parameters, including vascularization (e.g., random or axial), method of movement (e.g.,

advancement, rotation, transposition, and interpolation), and proximity to defect (e.g., local, regional, distant).
- Fasciocutaneous flaps are composed of skin and deep fascia and are classified into three types according to Mathes and Nahai and five types according to Cormack and Lamberty.
- There are two ways to delay a flap: vascular delay, which consists of selective ligation of vascular pedicles to enhance perfusion from the remaining ones; and surgical delay, which is based on raising parts of the flap in a staged manner prior to transfer.
- Perforator flaps are flaps made of skin and/ or subcutaneous fat supplied by isolated perforators, which travel through or between tissues (mostly muscle) en route to their target cutaneous territory (e.g., perforasome).

- There are two main systems for naming perforator flaps: the Gent Consensus and the Canadian System.
- Methods of perforator mapping include handheld Doppler, color Doppler ultrasonography, CT angiography, and MRA.
- Raising of perforator flaps usually involves four basic steps: suprafascial approach to the perforator; division of deep fascia; perforator dissection; and nutrient vessel dissection.
- Propeller flaps are completely islanded pedicled flaps, which rotate around an off-center perforator that acts as the pivot point.

Recommended Readings

Blondeel PN, Van Landuyt KH, Monstrey SJ, et al. The "Gent" consensus on perforator flap terminology: preliminary definitions. Plast Reconstr Surg. 2003; 112(5):1378–1383, quiz 1383, 1516, discussion 1384–1387

Blondeel PN. Technical aspects of perforator flap dissection. In: Blondeel PN, Morris SF, Hallock GC, Neligan PC, eds. Perforator Flaps: Anatomy, Techniques and Clinical Applications. 2nd ed. New York, NY: Thieme Medical; 2013:137–162

Cormack GC, Lamberty BGH. The arterial anatomy of skin flaps. edinburgh: Churchill Livingston; 1989

Geddes CR, Morris SF, Neligan PC. Perforator flaps: evolution, classification, and applications. Ann Plast Surg. 2003; 50(1):90–99

Guo L, Pribaz JJ. Clinical flap prefabrication. Plast Reconstr Surg. 2009; 124(6, Suppl):e340–e350

Hallock GG. Further clarification of the nomenclature for compound flaps. Plast Reconstr Surg. 2006; 117(7):151e–160e

Ireton JE, Lakhiani C, Saint-Cyr M. Vascular anatomy of the deep inferior epigastric artery perforator flap: a systematic review. Plast Reconstr Surg. 2014; 134(5):810e–821e

Kayser MR. Surgical Flaps. In: Barton FE Jr, ed. Selected Readings in Plastic Surgery. 1999; 9(2):1–63

Masia J, Navarro C, Clavero JA, Alomar X. Noncontrast magnetic resonance imaging for preoperative perforator mapping. Clin Plast Surg. 2011; 38(2):253–261

Pelissier P, Gardet H, Pinsolle V, Santoul M, Behan FC. The keystone design perforator island flap. Part II: clinical applications. J Plast Reconstr Aesthet Surg. 2007; 60(8):888–891

Pontén B. The fasciocutaneous flap: its use in soft tissue defects of the lower leg. Br J Plast Surg. 1981; 34(2):215–220

Rozen WM, Garcia-Tutor E, Alonso-Burgos A, et al. Planning and optimising DIEP flaps with virtual surgery: the Navarra experience. J Plast Reconstr Aesthet Surg. 2010; 63(2):289–297

Semple JL. Retrograde microvascular augmentation (turbocharging) of a single-pedicle TRAM flap through a deep inferior epigastric arterial and venous loop. Plast Reconstr Surg. 1994; 93(1):109–117

Taylor GI, Palmer JH. The vascular territories (angiosomes) of the body: experimental study and clinical applications. Br J Plast Surg. 1987; 40(2):113–141

Taylor GI, Pan WR. The Angiosome Concept and Tissue Transfer. New York, NY: Thieme Medical; 2013

Teo TC. The propeller flap concept. Clin Plast Surg. 2010; 37(4):615–626, vi

Thomas BP, Geddes CR, Tang M, Williams J, Morris SF. The vascular basis of the thoracodorsal artery perforator flap. Plast Reconstr Surg. 2005; 116(3):818–822

Vedder NB. Flap physiology. In: Mathes SJ, ed. Plastic Surgery. Vol. 1, Principles. 2nd ed. Philadephia, PA: Saunders, Elsevier; 2006:483–506

Wei FC, Jain V, Celik N, Chen HC, Chuang DC, Lin CH. Have we found an ideal soft-tissue flap? An experience with 672 anterolateral thigh flaps. Plast Reconstr Surg. 2002; 109(7):2219–2226, discussion 2227–2230

17 Tissue Expansion

Álvaro Cuadra, Bruno Dagnino

Abstract

Reconstruction of soft tissue defects may be achieved by different methods. Skin grafts and flaps, either local, regional, or free, are all valid alternatives, depending on the case. However, they all produce varying degrees of morbidity on the donor area, may lead to a poor functional or cosmetic result in the case of skin grafts, and may be technically demanding. Also, in some cases, even these techniques may not provide enough healthy tissue for coverage. Tissue expansion is based on the use of a silicone device that is placed under the skin and gradually inflated with saline, thus causing stretching of the overlying tissue (skin, subcutaneous fat, fascia, muscle). Such forces favor cell proliferation and angiogenesis as well as the recruitment of neighboring skin so that at the end of the expansion process newly generated, well-vascularized tissue is available for reconstruction. Tissue expansion presents a spectrum of treatment options, including expansion of a skin graft donor site, expansion of neighboring skin to be used as a local flap, and expansion of distant skin to be used as a free flap. Regarding its clinical applications, tissue expansion may be used to treat soft tissue defects secondary to trauma, burns, oncologic resection, and congenital conditions, with postmastectomy breast reconstruction being one the most frequent indications. This chapter describes the main aspects of tissue expansion with regard to changes in tissues, surgical technique, potential complications, and clinical applications.

Keywords: biological creep, implant, infection, stress relaxation, tissue expansion

17.1 Introduction

The capacity of tissues to stretch and expand gradually over time has been observed in physiologic and pathological circumstances, as well as being part of cultural ornaments. Some examples of physiologic changes of the skin and soft tissues may be seen during pregnancy, massive weight loss, and cranial development during the first years of life. Skin and soft tissues may also experience stretching and expansion as a consequence of pathological growth from underlying tumors, as may happen with soft tissue sarcomas and benign tumors from the skin or subcutaneous tissue. Classical examples of tissue expansion as cultural ornaments are seen in the Chad tribes, where people undergo lip stretching, or the Padaung tribe from Burma, famous for their elongated necks from the use of metallic rings.

The history of tissue expansion did not begin with skin or soft tissue, but with the expansion of bones. In 1905 Codevilla and then Magnuson described bone lengthening using traction devices. In 1921, Putti, in Italy, demonstrated that sustained traction for a period of several months could lead to bone lengthening and also stretching of surrounding noble structures, such as nerves and blood vessels, preceding the method later described by Ilizarov.

In 1957 Neumann used a rubber ball placed underneath the skin to obtain skin for cutaneous coverage of a subtotal ear amputation. Nevertheless, his results did not have much impact at that time. Two decades later, in 1976 and 1978, Radovan reported the use of a subcutaneous tissue expander that could be inflated percutaneously with normal saline through a remote valve. In 1979 and 1982, Austad and Rose described the use of a device that employed the osmotic gradient of sodium chloride for its inflation, which avoided the need for repeated injections. Despite this advantage, the long periods of expansion and the risks related to exposure of surrounding tissues to hypertonic solutions in case of rupture, made Radovan's the preferred method for tissue expansion, which has remained to our days.

Since its description, tissue expansion (TE) has had a significant impact on reconstructive surgery. The main advantages of TE include its capacity to provide additional tissue, with excellent blood supply due to increased blood flow, and to provide like-quality tissue in terms of contour, texture, and color match. Its chief uses include soft tissue coverage of traumatic and postoncologic defects as well as burn reconstruction, among others. Currently tissue expansion also has a major role in modern breast reconstruction and even microsurgery, where it has been applied for preexpansion of free flaps.

Radovan (1976) first reported on the use of silicone subcutaneous skin expanders. To date this is the most frequently used method of tissue expansion.

17.2 Basic Science

The skin has viscoelastic properties, which determine that, in response to a stretching force, both the elastic and viscous components are affected. Collagen types I and III are produced by fibroblasts and represent the predominant proteins found in the dermis. In their natural state they are arranged as a triple helix, but under shear stress these fibers stretch to take a parallel disposition, resuming their original helical configuration once strain subsides. The biomechanical properties of the skin change with increasing age or under repeated stress. These properties determine the skin's response to tissue expansion and are measured considering shear stress, elasticity, creep, and stress relaxation. Shear stress can be defined as the product of force and cross-sectional area, whereas strain (elongation) corresponds to the change in length in comparison with the original dimension. The relationship between stress and length can be represented as a stress–strain curve (▶ Fig. 17.1).

During the initial phases of strain the material becomes deformed in direct relation to stress until it reaches a point known as Young's modulus or elastic modulus (E). Materials with higher values of E are more rigid than those with lower values. The equation that represents this relation is known as Hooke's Law ($\sigma = Ee$) where σ is defined as stress and e as strain. Point A represents the elastic limit, so if a material is stretched beyond this point it will not be able to recover its original shape once stress is relieved, thus producing permanent deformity. As stress is reduced the elastic portion recovers, following a line that is parallel to the original curve

The stress–strain relationship

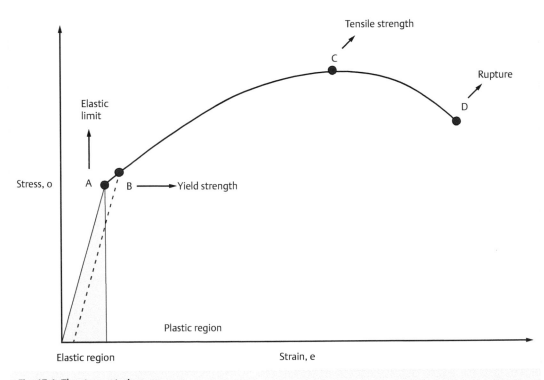

Fig. 17.1 The stress–strain curve.

and leaving a permanent deformity (▶Fig. 17.1 dotted line). The limit of an elastic behavior is known as point B, or yield strength. If stress is applied between the limits of the plastic region, an increase in stress will produce a nonlinear increase in the stretching of the material (▶Fig. 17.1 points B, C). In case stress is sustained it will reach a point (▶Fig. 17.1 point C) in which the tensile strength of the material is exceeded, followed by accelerated stretching and rupture.

> **Remember** M!
>
> Dermis collagen types I and III consist of a triple helix structure. During expansion these fibers adopt an increasingly parallel alignment.

During tissue expansion the surgeon tries to optimize stress in order to produce the maximum stretching that the skin can tolerate. Accordingly the region under the curve between B and C must be considered, without exceeding the tensile strength of the skin, which would lead to its rupture, represented by area C, D of the curve.

Skin can be stretched because of its inherent elasticity and as a result of biological and mechanical creep. Mechanical creep occurs when skin is stretched at a constant force, leading to extrusion of fluids from the interstitium of the collagen chain and subsequent skin stretching beyond its inherent elasticity. Apparently blood supply is not compromised during this process. A consequence of this phenomenon is stress relaxation, produced by the fact that if skin is stretched at a constant length the force required to maintain this state gradually reduces. On the other hand, biological creep is the slow and gradually expansion seen during pregnancy, weight increase, or tissue expansion, in which continuous stretching and tissue thinning stimulate production of new epithelium, collagen, elastic fibers, and neovasculogenesis as a means to reduce stress (stress relaxation).

> **Remember** M!
>
> Mechanical creep phenomenon occurs when tissue is acutely stretched beyond its inherent elasticity, whereas biological creep occurs during slow expansion (e.g., pregnancy, weight gain), where the stretching induces tissue regeneration.

17.2.1 Tissue Changes during Expansion

Upon expansion, different tissues (e.g., skin, muscle, bone, and the vascular network) experience a number of changes, which are summarized as follows:

- Epidermal thickening and dermal thinning.
- Formation of a capsule around the expander.
- Muscle thinning and reduction in mass.
- Bone thinning and new bone formation peripherally.
- Mechanical strain triggering DNA synthesis and cellular proliferation.
- Increased vascularity.

The epidermis becomes thicker during tissue expansion. Initially this occurs as a consequence of tissue edema, which lasts for approximately 4 weeks; nevertheless, even after edema subsides, the epidermis remains thickened for several months. Conversely, the dermis becomes thinner, and changes in the dermal thickness last for at least 36 weeks after expansion has ceased.

Total skin area increases from recruitment of adjacent skin and an increase in the mitotic rate. Hair follicles and appendages may become compressed but do not degenerate, and there is an increase in melanocytic activity, which reverts once the expander is removed.

Following expander placement, a dense fibrous capsule is formed around the device, which shows increased vascularity and reduced cellularity as expansion progresses.

Muscle always atrophies regardless of whether the tissue expander is placed above or below. Animal studies have shown that expansion induces growth of muscle cells and an increase in the total number of sarcomeres for each fiber of striated muscle. Once the expander is removed, muscle recovers its normal architecture, blood supply, and function.

Bone density is not compromised; however, a decrease in its thickness is seen as a consequence of osteoplastic resorption, whereas peripheral bone may become thicker due to periosteal reaction. Bone density is not compromised. Cranial vault hollowing is frequent in children under 1 year of age, but it tends to recover after expansion has ceased. Long bones begin remodeling during the first 5 days after the expander is removed, reaching normalcy after approximately 2 months.

17.2.2 Cellular Changes and the Effect of Tissue Expansion on Blood Supply

Applying a mechanical stress on living cells affects a series of cellular structures and signaling pathways that lead to cell proliferation, growth, and tissue regeneration, which explains the formation of new tissue during the process of expansion. Mechanical deformation triggers a series of cellular responses involving the cytoskeleton, extracellular matrix, enzymatic activity, second messengers, and ionic channels. The cytoskeleton plays a major role in transforming extracellular forces into intracellular events, which are also transmitted to neighbor cells.

Several growth factors essential for normal cell growth also appear to be involved in cell proliferation induced by stretching. These include epidermal growth factor (EGF), basic fibroblast growth factor (bFGF), transforming growth factor (TGF) family, platelet-derived growth factors (PDGFs), and angiotensin II. Activation of EGF receptors (EGFRs) generates an ionic influx that induces membrane ruffling, a phenomenon commonly seen previous to cellular division. TGF increases fibroblast growth and stimulates extracellular matrix production. In the absence of exogenous proteins, mechanical stretching by itself induces upregulation of growth factors, such as PDGF and angiotensin II, suggesting that tissue elongation may have an autocrine function too.

The extracellular matrix is also essential for cell proliferation. Under mechanical forces there is an increase in DNA and collagen synthesis. In addition, the mechanical stress deforms the matrix, altering the configuration of adhesion proteins (e.g., integrins), which act as mechanochemical transducers, transmitting this extracellular signal to the intracellular environment by producing changes in the cytoskeleton. Several cellular morphological changes also occur as a result of rearrangement of actin filaments induced by mechanical stress. Actin also plays a key role in cell to cell signaling. Other families of transmembrane proteins, such as protein G, are also relevant for mechanotransduction in that their strain-induced conformational changes are supposed to initiate second-messengers signaling cascades and cellular growth.

Ionic channels sensitive to mechanical stimulus favor the passage of several cations as Na^+, K^+, and Ca^{++} in response to strain, which promotes a diversity of secondary chemical reactions that determine cellular responses, including depolarization, cellular contraction, and generation of myogenic tone.

Protein kinases, especially protein kinase C, are strong transducers of cellular signaling also favoring membrane ruffling.

Some second-messenger systems, such as cyclic adenosine monophosphate (cAMP) take part in cell growth, differentiation, and protein synthesis. During mechanical stress the rate of protein synthesis is inverse to the concentration of cAMP, suggesting that this substance is consumed during such synthesis. In all, mechanical stress induces several cellular signaling pathways that lead to the expression of genes and proteins regulating cell proliferation (▶ Fig. 17.2 and ▶ Fig. 17.3).

> **Remember**   M!
>
> Mechanotransduction is the phenomenon by which cells convert mechanical stimuli into electrochemical signals; it plays a major role in the generation of new tissue during expansion.

Vascularization is significantly enhanced by tissue expansion and is determined by an increase in the number and size of blood vessels. Angiogenesis, which is the generation of new blood vessels from preexisting ones, involves the microcirculation and occurs in response to tissue ischemia. Vascular endothelial growth factor (VEGF) is a known family of angiogenic factors and has been found to be elevated in expanded tissue following cyclic dermal stretching.

From a clinical standpoint tissue expansion behaves similarly to flap delay because flaps raised on expanded tissue exhibit increased vascularity and higher survival rates and are usually of greater dimensions. Animal studies have shown a survival increase of 117% expanded versus nonexpanded flaps. However, it should be stated that fast expansion during the first 48 hours may compromise flap survival, and the rate of expansion should be guided by patient discomfort.

17.3 Types of Expanders

There is a wide variety of tissue expanders, and their choice depends on the needs of each particular case. Originally, Radovan's expander consisted of one silicone prosthesis with two valves connected to the main reservoir by silicone tubes, where one valve was employed for

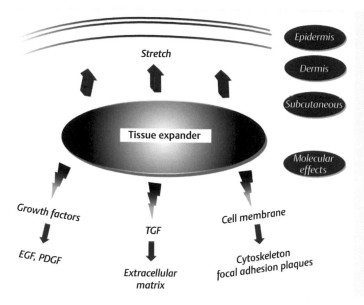

Fig. 17.2 Effects of tissue expansion on surrounding tissues. Stretching of surrounding tissues induces growth factors, which mediate cell proliferation and increased angiogenesis. Factors such as transforming growth factor-β influence extracellular matrix production, whereas membrane-bound protein kinases, focal adhesion points, and cytoskeleton influence intracellular signaling cascades. EGF, epidermal growth factor; PDGF, platelet-derived growth factor; TGF, transforming growth factor. (Adapted from Takei T, Mills I, Arai K, Sumpio BE. Molecular basis for tissue expansion: clinical implications for the surgeon. Plast Reconstr Surg 1998;102:247–258. With permission from Wolters Kluwer Health, Inc.)

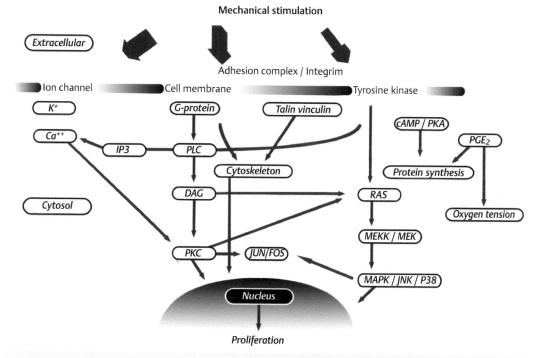

Fig. 17.3 Schematic of possible signal transduction pathways induced by mechanical strain. A wide variety of strain-induced signals triggers sequential activation of transduction pathways and transmits signals through appropriate membrane receptor or ion channels. Terminal enzymes that are activated by these intracellular cascades transduce these signals into the nucleus. cAMP, cyclic adenosine monophosphate; EGF, epidermal growth factor; TGF-α and -β, transforming growth factor-α and -β; PDGF, platelet-derived growth factor; CTGF, connective tissue growth factor; IGF, insulin-like growth factor; PLC, phospholipase C; IP3, inositol-phosphate 3; PKA, protein kinase A; PKC, protein kinase C; DAG, diacylglycerol; MAPK, mitogen-activated kinases; MEKK, MEK kinase; MEK, MAPK kinase; JNK, c-jun amino terminal kinase. (Adapted from Takei T, Mills I, Arai K, Sumpio BE. Molecular basis for tissue expansion: Clinical implications for the surgeon. Plast Reconstr Surg 1998;102:247–258. With permission from Wolters Kluwer Health, Inc.)

fluid injection and the other for fluid removal. There are now tissue expanders with integrated valves and remote valves, as well as self-inflating expanders, each with its own advantages and disadvantages. The basic design includes an empty reservoir made of silicone elastomer that is filled with fluid through an integrated or remote valve.

Expanders with remote valves reduce the risk of accidental puncture during expansion because the valve is placed far from the reservoir, which is useful in cases of thin and tight skin coverage. Nevertheless, there is a risk of migration, obstruction, and kinking of the injection port. The port can also be placed outside the skin, but this has a risk of colonization and infection.

Expanders with integrated valves minimize the risk associated with the remote injection port and connection tubing, but in turn have a risk of puncture of the reservoir during injection when the integrated port is not adequately located. However, this has been simplified by incorporating metallic ports that can be readily identified by ultrasound or magnetic devices, the latter being very common in breast reconstruction.

In 1982 Austad and Rose created a self-inflating device consisting of a silicone balloon filled with hypertonic sodium chloride (NaCl), creating an osmotic gradient that would allow its filling without the disadvantages associated with injection ports. These devices are now infrequently used because they require long periods of inflation between 8 and 14 weeks and have high rates of early rupture and tissue necrosis. K. Günter Wiese and then Shaheel Chummun developed expanders using an osmotically active hydrogel with the capacity to expand more than 10 times its original size. They consist of a polymeric matrix and an aqueous component, which absorbs fluid from the extracellular space causing edema of the hydrogel. They have the advantage of requiring fewer visits to the office, reduced pain, and faster expansion. However, their main downside is that expansion cannot be stopped in case of complications or doubts about tissue vitality.

Expanders come in many shapes and sizes, which are determined by the characteristics of the defect and its location. Round expanders are frequently used for breast reconstruction, and crescent or rectangular expanders for the scalp or lower limbs. In addition, in some cases expanders

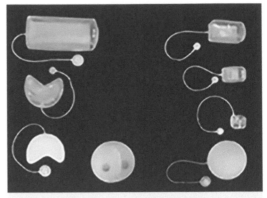

Fig. 17.4 Types of tissue expanders.

may be custom made specifically for one patient/defect. There are also textured expanders as a means to reduce shifting and capsular contracture (▶Fig. 17.4).

17.4 Preoperative Planning and Surgical Technique

The main factors to consider during the preoperative planning of tissue expansion include the type, shape, and size of the expander, as well as the expected volume of expansion.

Almost any kind of tissue is susceptible to expansion, but those with underlying bone tissue will have better results due to the transmission of the tensile strength of the expansion, preferably to the more compliant overlying skin, and not to the rigid bone.

The presence of active infection, heavy smoking, and a previous history of radiotherapy are contraindications to tissue expansion given the unacceptable risk of complications. In addition, children under 7 years of age, expanders in the extremities, and integrated valve expanders in children have been identified as risk factors for complications; hence close surveillance during the expansion process is recommended in these cases. The use of expansion in trauma cases is advocated as a delayed rather than an immediate method of reconstruction.

Careful preoperative planning is key for a successful tissue expansion, analyzing the location and size of the defect to be restored as well as the conditions of the surrounding tissues. For any given defect, it is generally better to use two medium-sized expanders rather than a single large one, as more tissue can be recruited using two devices. The base diameter of the expander should be approximately 2–2.5 times the diameter of the defect to be resurfaced. Additionally, a good estimate of the amount of tissue that can be advanced at the end of the expansion process may be calculated by subtracting the length of the base to the length of the circumference of the expander (▶Fig. 17.5). In terms of shape, certain expanders are more suitable for specific areas, such as round or anatomically shaped devices used for breast reconstruction, and rectangular and crescent-shaped devices used in the scalp and extremities. Routine antibiotic prophylaxis is recommended to minimize the risk of infection.

Surgical incisions should preferably be made at the margin between the defect and healthy skin to be expanded and, in the face, with attention to the aesthetic units and subunits. Closure should be performed without tension and in a layered fashion, including as many layers as possible (e.g., muscle, fascia, subcutaneous tissue) to prevent extrusion. Tension at the suture line may be reduced by placing the incisions radial or perpendicular to the long axis of the expander, though this is not always feasible. Careful hemostasis and the use of drains when necessary are paramount to reduce the risk of hematoma and seroma. Intraoperative expansion also serves as an aid to collapse small blood vessels.

Selection of the type of valve (remote or built-in) depends on the surgeon's preferences and each particular case. Remote valves should be placed far from the expander to avoid superposition of both during the expansion process. Also, they should ideally be superficial enough to allow easy identification, over a hard non-weight-bearing surface and fixed with sutures to avoid migration and kinking. Of note, bacterial colonization of the capsule has been reported in up to 82% of expanders with remote valves. Following insertion, intraoperative inflation up to 10–15% of the total volume may be performed, which helps to fill dead space and reduce risk of hematoma/seroma. Two to 3 weeks after placement and provided that all wounds are healed, expansion can begin on a weekly basis (or twice weekly in children with less volume infiltrated on each session), injecting approximately 10–15% of the total volume on each session. During expansion, it is important to pay attention to the development of pain and skin blanching because these are hallmarks of ischemia. Overexpansion up to 25% of the device's volume is usually possible and may be performed to obtain enough skin coverage. Once the desired volume is reached, the second stage is planned, during which the expander is removed and the flap advanced into the defect. At this stage, scoring of the capsule can be done to allow improved mobilization of the flap.

> ### Remember M!
>
> - Careful planning is key for a successful tissue expansion.
> - Incisions must be placed close to the defect, not the expander, and as perpendicular as possible to the long axis of the expander.
> - During expansion, infiltration should be stopped before pain appears.
> - Over expansion is possible in case extra skin is needed.
> - Scoring of the capsule allows improved advancement of the flap.

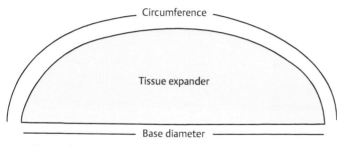

Fig. 17.5 Formula to calculate amount of skin that can be advanced with a tissue expander.

Tissue advancement (cm) = dome circumference - base diameter

17.5 Complications

Depending on whether the expansion process is interrupted or not, complications can be divided into minor (no interruption) and major (expansion interrupted or ceased).

17.5.1 Minor Complications

- *Pain:* This may reflect nerve compression or skin overstretching. There is also the possibility of subsequent ischemia.
- *Neurapraxia:* This may last from minutes to long-standing symptoms. It reflects stretching or compression of a nerve and may be an indication to deflate the expander and reposition it if it doesn't recover with deflation alone.
- *Scar widening:* This is seen in the majority of cases as an almost inevitable consequence of the expansion process. The widened scar can easily be removed during skin advancement at the second stage.
- *Body contour distortion:* This is an inevitable effect of tissue expansion, often temporary and reversible following expander removal in the second stage. Permanent deformity may be seen on the deep surface on which the expander sits (e.g., thoracic wall).

17.5.2 Major Complications

- Infection
- Hematoma
- Wound dehiscence and expander exposure (▶ Fig. 17.6)

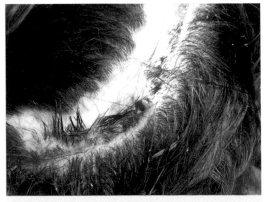

Fig. 17.6 Exposed tissue expander.

- Expander deflation or rupture
- Skin necrosis

Except for some cases of mild infection, all other major complications require surgical revision.

Traditionally, the reported overall complication rate in tissue expanders is 10–39%. In the first place, adequate patient selection is crucial to reduce complication rates; the expansion process needs full cooperation and care from the patient. In terms of the surgical procedure itself, careful planning, adequate size of the pocket, placement of the expander as far as possible from the incision, and layered closure without any tension must be ensured. Complications may also be related to the orientation of the skin incision whereby wounds parallel to the long axis of the expander are submitted to more tension than radial or perpendicular ones. During the expansion process, a nontraumatic and sterile filling technique is paramount. One of the most common complications associated with tissue expanders is infection, which can be secondary to direct inoculation of skin flora at the moment of insertion or due to exposure. A nonsterile infiltration technique may also contribute to expander infection. Furthermore, translocation of bacteria from distant sites has also been advocated as a mechanism of infection. Mild cases of infection can be treated conservatively with deflation and antibiotics. If infection persists, the expander may be salvageable by surgical washout and intravenous antibiotics; however, if this is not successful, expander removal and intravenous antibiotics are indicated.

Some risk factors for high complication rates have been identified, such as extreme ages, use of expanders in extremities (higher rate in lower extremity), tissue expansion in irradiated tissue, and burn reconstruction, although in the last 2 decades this complication profile seems to be changing. Wang et al. have recently shown that the number of expanders per region has direct correlation with the overall complication rate. Furthermore, some locations in the head and neck have been related to specific complications (e.g., hematoma in the cheek and wound dehiscence in the scalp). A meta-analysis by Huang spanning a period of 20 years up to 2010, found a 17.4% overall complication rate for tissue expansion, confirmed infection as the main complication, and established the lower limb and the trunk as the sites with the highest and lower complication rates, respectively (odds ratio 2.80 and 0.78 respectively, 95% CI). They also found that expander site, smoking habit, and radiation therapy are specific risk factors for complications. In addition, a significant association between previous radiation therapy and expander complications, including skin necrosis, has been demonstrated experimentally in rabbits. In one study, the surgeon's experience level did not prove to be a significant risk factor for complications, although more experienced surgeons did have fewer major complications than less experienced ones.

17.6 Clinical Applications

17.6.1 Head and Neck

The scalp tissue is usually rigid and noncompliant with long rotation or advancement with direct closure of the donor site; therefore, it is one of the most frequent areas where tissue expansion is used, and one with a low complication rate as well. Traumatic alopecia, burn sequelae, congenital nevi, and androgenic baldness are some of the many indications for tissue expansion of the scalp (▶ Fig. 17.7). When used for baldness reconstruction, tissue expansion has the advantage of re-creating the anterior hairline, even though new follicles cannot be generated. Moreover, the expander should be placed in the subgaleal plane to avoid hair follicle ischemia and subsequent

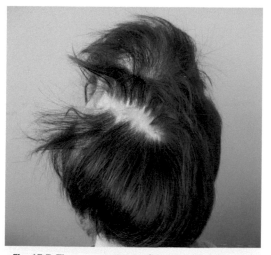

Fig. 17.7 Tissue expansion in alopecia. (This figure is provided courtesy of Dr. Silvana Acosta, Pontifical Catholic University of Chile.)

secondary alopecia. Transient alopecia may occur during the first weeks of expansion and last for a few months to then recover spontaneously. Placing the expander under the main vessels of the scalp, such as the superficial temporal or occipital arteries, is recommended because this may improve the blood supply to the expanded flap. The expander should be placed in a way that, once the flap is rotated or advanced, the hair orientation is preserved and in harmony with the surrounding scalp.

Losses involving more than 50% of the total scalp area are bad candidates for expander reconstruction because excessive capillary thinning may be produced. Tissue expansion for patch alopecia is also not recommended.

Tissue expansion has a major role in the management of auricular defects, both acquired and congenital, where it is used to obtain thin, pliable, non-hair-bearing skin to cover the cartilage framework of the auricular reconstruction. Customized expanders with special shapes and sizes have been created and used for this purpose. In these cases, the expander is placed beneath the superficial temporal fascia and inflated over a period ranging from 4 to 12 weeks. During the second stage, the capsule may be removed in order to achieve better definition and increased skin mobilization.

In the forehead, a submuscular (e.g., under the frontalis muscle) plane is recommended (which corresponds to the subgaleal plane of the parieto-occipital scalp) and, when possible, should be placed above the eyebrows. Forehead expansion can be used to treat giant nevi and other large local lesions, as well as to increase the size of regional flaps, such as preexpanding a forehead flap to obtain full coverage in nasal reconstruction and direct closure of the donor site.

In the face, the unit/subunit principle should be applied when planning for tissue expansion because replacement of entire units with incisions placed on natural folds or creases (e.g., the nasolabial fold, periorbital ring) usually achieves a better functional and aesthetic result, even if this means resecting some remaining healthy tissue within the unit.

In the neck, the usual recommendation is to place the expander in the subcutaneous plane, over the platysma muscle, to avoid nerve injury and excessive bulk. The shape of the neck, the cervicomandibular angle, and the beard in male patients impose some limitations to the use and results of tissue expansion in this area. For the lower third of the face, flaps should be advanced in a caudo-cephalic direction and anchored to deep tissues to avoid gravitational pull and subsequent complications (e.g., orbicularis oris ectropion). Furthermore, rotation is preferred to advancement to allow better distribution of the tension in the cephalocaudal direction of the cheek and lower third of the face.

Finally, despite the presence of major vessels, vascular complications following expansion in this area are rare.

> **Remember** M!
>
> The plane of insertion is subgaleal in the scalp, submuscular in the forehead, and subcutaneous in the neck.

17.6.2 Upper and Lower Extremities

Congenital defects, scars, trauma sequelae, and tumor resections in the extremities can be treated with tissue expansion (▶ Fig. 17.8 and ▶ Fig. 17.9).

Although the principles remain the same as for other anatomical regions, the use of tissue expansion in the extremities is associated with an increased risk of complications, which is even higher in the lower extremity below the knee, with rates varying from 24% as reported by Zoltie et al, to 70% as described by Manders et al, with

an average of 38%. The upper part of the leg is easier to expand, given the thickness of the skin and subcutaneous tissue. A single large or multiple small expanders can be used. Major lymphatic and venous complications are most often reported under the knee.

Extremities present some anatomical and functional differences from other areas of the body, which may explain the higher rate of complications. Constant muscular activity and movement produce compressive, shearing, and disruptive forces. In addition, previous scars may limit tissue availability, and complex designs are sometimes needed to obtain proper orientation and flap advancement to cover convex and curved surfaces. Recommendations for the use of tissue expanders in extremities include the use of multiple, large expanders of low projection oriented parallel to the long axis of the extremity, and a minimal incision approach oriented perpendicular to the long axis of the expander to minimize the risk of wound breakdown. A suprafascial plane is preferred to prevent motor nerve compression, and, when using remote ports, these should be located close to the expander but far from joints and neurovascular structures. The expansion process must be gradual and slow to avoid transient nerve compression. During the second stage, the capsule may be used for tendon and joint coverage because it allows

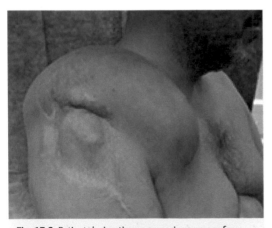

Fig. 17.8 Patient during tissue expansion process for replacement of a skin graft in the upper arm. (This figure is provided courtesy of Dr. Silvana Acosta, Pontificia Universidad Católica de Chile.)

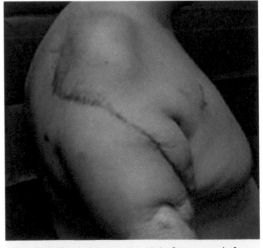

Fig. 17.9 The patient in ▶ Fig. 17.8 after removal of the tissue expander and replacement of the skin graft by a skin flap.

adequate gliding and may help to prevent tissue adhesions.

> **Remember**   **M!**
>
> Expanders in the extremities should be oriented parallel to the long axis of the limb, far from joints and in a suprafascial plane to avoid nerve compression.

17.6.3 Trunk

Tissue expansion of the trunk in adults is mainly used for breast and burn reconstruction, whereas in the pediatric population the list of indications also encompasses myelomeningocele, giant congenital nevi, and ectopia cordi, among others (▶Fig. 17.10). The trunk offers an extensive surface of donor tissue and an even, uniform surface, which allows high volumes of expansion. When used in the abdomen, the expander should ideally have a semi-rigid base to compensate for the softness of the muscular abdominal wall, which may hinder expansion due to transmission of the expanding force to the underlying wall instead of the overlying skin. Tissue expansion of the back can be challenging; a longer interval is usually needed between expanding sessions to prevent migration of the device within a large pocket expansion. The use of multiple expanders in this region can yield large dimensions of expanded tissue, minimizing anatomical distortion and allowing a faster expansion process. Expanders in the trunk can be placed supra- or subfascially, and some regional muscles, such as the latissimus dorsi and pectoralis major, may be expanded for reconstruction as well. In some cases the use of multiple expanders can be optimized by leaving the device in place after deflation and flap advancement are completed. Further expansion (e.g., reexpansion) may be resumed in a couple weeks.

> **Remember**   **M!**
>
> The trunk is a wide area of potential donor tissue, where skin, fascia, and muscle can be included in the expanding flap.

17.6.4 Breast

Tissue expansion for the breast was first introduced by Radovan in the 1980s as a means to provide implant coverage in mastectomy patients. The early results with skin expansion only were discouraging, due to the thinness of the expanded tissue, which yielded very rounded and firm reconstructed breasts. In addition, high complication rates were reported, especially in patients with subsequent radiation therapy. Changes to the technique, namely the change to a submuscular plane, offered an effective solution to the issue of thickness by providing a robust and well vascularized layer of tissue for coverage, all of which has made tissue expander implant reconstruction a reliable method of breast reconstruction, which is now the most widely performed method.

Expanders and implants have undergone important modifications during the last decades, which has improved results and predictability of the procedure, offering the possibility of achieving natural-looking breasts and reduced complications. Anatomically shaped expanders with greater lower pole projection and the introduction of a textured surface for less capsular contracture are the most important features in this regard. In addition, the complication rates have

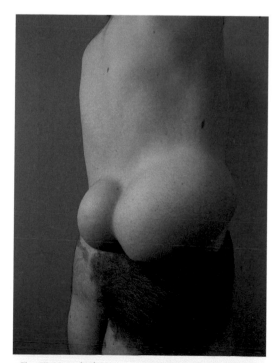

Fig. 17.10 Multiple tissue expanders in trunk congenital nevi. (This figure is provided courtesy of Dr. Silvana Acosta, Pontifical Catholic University of Chile.)

also been lowered since the introduction of integrated valve expanders.

Different factors should be considered when choosing tissue expansion as the method of breast reconstruction, including the patient's preference, availability of autologous donor areas, breast shape and size, and a previous history of radiotherapy. Patients lacking abdominal or gluteal donor tissue, who have small to midsized breasts (< 750 g) with minimal or no ptosis, good skin quality, and no prior or planned radiation therapy are the best candidates for this treatment modality.

The advantages of expander use in these cases are straightforward surgery with a low operative time, use of local tissue providing good match of color and texture, preservation of local sensate innervation, no donor site morbidity, less scarring, and faster recovery. Furthermore, placing an expander does not preclude the use of autologous tissue for definitive reconstruction once expansion has been completed.

The use of tissue expansion in breast reconstruction involves two operative times: in the first surgery the expander is placed beneath the pectoralis major, serratus anterior, and upper portions of the anterior rectus fascia; in a second procedure, once the desired volume is reached, the expander is removed and replaced by either a permanent implant or autologous tissue (e.g., a pedicled or free flap) (▶ Fig. 17.11). An alternative to this approach necessitating one surgery only, is the use of an expander-implant (Baker implant), which consists of a silicone-filled implant with an expansible portion similar to a standard breast expander. Once this portion is inflated to the final desired volume, the device is left in place.

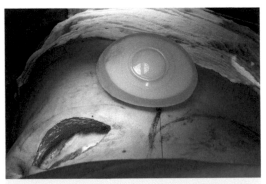

Fig. 17.11 Expander-based breast reconstruction. The expander was removed and the pocket filled with a free flap.

The use of acellular dermal matrices (ADMs) as an adjunct for expander/implant–based reconstruction was first introduced in 2005 and has since gained increasing popularity. These matrices are placed on the inferolateral portion of the pocket, where they act as a supportive sling, provide improved coverage, and allow better definition of the inframammary fold. In addition, the use of ADMs can spare the use of the serratus anterior (which is the muscle that covers the inferolateral portion in the standard technique), thus reducing morbidity of the procedure and allowing faster filling of the expander, requiring fewer visits to the office for expansion. Disadvantages of this method include the high cost of the matrix and the frequent seroma formation associated with its use.

Radiotherapy is another important factor to consider when planning breast reconstruction with an expander and implant because it has been proven to be a risk factor for complications, including infection, extrusion, wound breakdown, and capsular contracture, eventually leading to a poor aesthetic result. Consequently, most would consider radiotherapy to be a contraindication for tissue expansion. On the other hand, the delivery of radiotherapy to an already placed expander may follow different protocols. Whereas some prefer to completely deflate the device and reexpand once radiotherapy is finished, others advocate for keeping it inflated throughout radiation.

Other Anomalies of the Breast

Tissue expansion has also been used to correct congenital and acquired anomalies of the breast. The timing of reconstruction of these defects will depend on the age of the patient and the degree of development, delaying surgery preferably until breast growth is complete. Acquired defects consist mainly of burn sequelae, in which a submuscular plane and slow expansion are recommended because breast burns treated with skin grafts or healed by secondary intention often present scars that can restrict the skin's compliance and are prone to ulceration and expander extrusion.

Congenital or developmental abnormalities, such as hypoplasia, tuberous breast, and Poland's syndrome, are also amenable to treatment with tissue expansion, Just as for acquired defects, reconstruction of congenital anomalies should be performed once full breast development has occurred; however, in these cases a subglandular or submuscular plane can be used depending on the amount of gland present.

17.7 Reexpansion

Reexpansion was first described by Sellers in 1986 in a patient with extensive scar tissue from a skin graft on the thigh that was replaced by serial expansions and skin advancements. Subsequently, different authors began to use tissue reexpansion for defects of varying nature, including burn scars and congenital nevi, with satisfactory outcomes and demonstrating that reexpanded tissue has good viability and elasticity, allowing replacement of extensive areas of skin with good texture and color matching and no added scars. Experimental animal studies have shown that reexpansion produces mild cellular damage, and in response to that injury there is an increase of cellular proliferation and activation, with the consequent improvement in tissue quality. Surgical technique follows the same principles as previously described, using the same incision (located at the advancing edge of the flap) and plane (easily identifiable by the capsule) in each procedure. Moreover, by placing expanders of increasing size in each flap advancement surgery the whole process can be accelerated. Regarding timing, whereas some advocate waiting a period of 3–12 months before inserting a new expander, others have reported using the same device during flap advancement, in which case reexpansion is initiated 4–6 weeks later. This latter approach reduces the number of surgeries needed to fully cover the defect. Lastly, complication rates of reexpansion are similar to those reported in single expansion procedures.

17.8 Preexpanded Free Flaps

There are two methods that can provide large amounts of healthy, well-vascularized tissue for reconstruction: free flaps and tissue expansion. Originally, these techniques were used separately until 1986, when Leighton et al. showed experimentally that, by combining the two, a sizeable piece of thin and flexible skin with enhanced vascularity could be obtained. Since then, successful use of preexpanded free flaps has been reported in head and neck, thoracic, and abdominal reconstruction. As in reexpansion surgery, one of the main applications of preexpanded free tissue transfer is for patients with extensive scars or areas of contractures in whom neither local nor distant tissues are able to provide adequate coverage. In these cases, a preexpanded free flap is a reliable way of obtaining thin and pliable skin that adapts very well to the recipient area.

The surgical technique is the same as previously described. A correct design is paramount to maximize the area of expanded tissue for transfer, and once expansion is completed, it is best to wait some weeks before definitive transfer. At that moment, some authors advocate for the conservation of the expander capsule in the flap as a means to enhance its vascularity and viability; nevertheless, the capsule may be removed if better contact of the flap with the recipient area or a thinner flap is desired.

Important advantages of preexpanded free flaps include the ability to obtain large, thin, and flexible flaps with enhanced vascularity and enlarged perforators, resulting in a better contour of the reconstruction, avoiding the need for remodeling procedures, and reducing donor site morbidity by achieving direct closure. Conversely, disadvantages of this method are the need for an extra procedure (expander insertion) and its inherent costs and risks, potential complications related to the presence of an alloplastic material and the expansion process itself, the need for repeated visits to the office for expansion, and the possibility of increased technical difficulty in harvesting the free flap due to scarring from the previous surgery and the presence of the expander's capsule.

> **Remember**   M!
>
> Preexpansion allows obtaining thinner, pliable, and well vascularized free flaps.

17.9 Conclusions

Tissue expansion has an established role in reconstructive surgery, allowing soft tissue reconstruction of a wide range of defects using neighboring skin, which offers excellent match and contour without added scars. Preoperative planning is key for a successful tissue expansion, carefully assessing the characteristics of the defect as well as the conditions of surrounding skin. Radiated skin expands poorly and is prone to breakdown with subsequent expander exposure and infection; therefore, radiotherapy is currently considered one of the main contraindications to the use of this technique. Surgical pearls include orientation of incisions, plane of insertion, and layered closure as described previously in this chapter. The expansion process often requires several visits to the office for injection; patients should be made aware of this and be able to comply. The complication rate of tissue expansion varies in different areas of the body, with extrusion/infection being the most frequent, often requiring removal of the device, surgical washout, and long-term antibiotics, although more conservative approaches with expander preservation are possible in cases of mild infection. Finally, the surgeon should remember that tissue expansion represents a spectrum of possibilities; apart from the "traditional" use of tissue expansion (i.e., expanding adjacent skin), expansion can be used to increase the area of a skin graft donor site or to augment a free flap, and it may also be used repeatedly over the same region by reexpanding previously expanded tissues.

17.10 Key Points

- In 1976 Radovan reported the use of a silicone subcutaneous skin expander, which continues to be the most frequent type of expansion device used.
- Mechanical creep occurs as a consequence of acute stretch by the realignment of collagen fibers and recruitment of adjacent tissue.
- Biological creep occurs in chronically stretched tissue and is secondary to cellular growth and tissue regeneration.
- Histological changes of the expanded tissue normalize after expander removal.
- Mechanical forces on the skin induce several cellular changes that lead to tissue proliferation, mediated by growth factors, extracellular matrix proteins, and multiple molecular cascades.
- Muscle or fascia can be expanded in the trunk and thus incorporated in the expanded flap.
- Expanders must be placed entirely in the submuscular plane in postmastectomy breast reconstruction. Consideration should be given to the use of ADMs for inferolateral pole coverage.
- Radiotherapy is considered by many a contraindication for expander/implant breast reconstruction.
- Reconstruction of congenital or acquired anomalies should be delayed until full development and growth occur.

- Reexpansion allows serial expansion and greater advancement of neighboring skin.
- Preexpansion allows obtaining thin, pliable, and well-vascularized free flaps from areas distant to the defect.

Recommended Readings

American Society of Plastic Surgeons. 2007 Reconstructive Surgery Procedures. Arlington Heights, IL: American Society of Plastic Surgeons; 2008

Antonyshyn O, Gruss JS, Mackinnon SE, Zuker R. Complications of soft tissue expansion. Br J Plast Surg. 1988; 41(3):239–250

Argenta LC, VanderKolk C, Friedman RJ, Marks M. Refinements in reconstruction of congenital breast deformities. Plast Reconstr Surg. 1985; 76(1):73–82

Austad ED, Pasyk KA, McClatchey KD, Cherry GW. Histomorphologic evaluation of guinea pig skin and soft tissue after controlled tissue expansion. Plast Reconstr Surg. 1982; 70(6):704–710

Austad ED, Rose GL. A self-inflating tissue expander. Plast Reconstr Surg. 1982; 70(5):588–594

Barone FE, Perry L, Keller T, Maxwell GP. The biomechanical and histopathologic effects of surface texturing with silicone and polyurethane in tissue implantation and expansion. Plast Reconstr Surg. 1992; 90(1):77–86

Bauer BS. The role of tissue expansion in reconstruction of the ear. Clin Plast Surg. 1990; 17(2):319–325

Bauer BS. Tissue expansion. In: Thorne CH, ed., Grabb and Smith's Plastic Surgery. 6th ed. Philadelphia, PA: Lippincott Williams & Wilkins; 2007:84–90

Bauer BS, Few JW, Chavez CD, Galiano RD. The role of tissue expansion in the management of large congenital pigmented nevi of the forehead in the pediatric patient. Plast Reconstr Surg. 2001; 107(3):668–675

Bauer BS, Vicari FA, Richard ME. The role of tissue expansion in pediatric plastic surgery. Clin Plast Surg. 1990; 17(1):101–112

Baumeister S, Follmar KE, Erdmann D, Baccarani A, Levin LS. Tissue expansion of free and pedicled flaps after transfer: possibilities and indications. J Reconstr Microsurg. 2007; 23(2):63–68

Becker H. Breast reconstruction using an inflatable breast implant with detachable reservoir. Plast Reconstr Surg. 1984; 73(4):678–683

Beier JP, Horch RE, Kneser U. Bilateral pre-expanded free TFL flaps for reconstruction of severe thoracic scar contractures in an 8-year-old girl. J Plast Reconstr Aesthet Surg. 2013; 66(12):1766–1769

Breuing KH, Warren SM. Immediate bilateral breast reconstruction with implants and inferolateral AlloDerm slings. Ann Plast Surg. 2005; 55(3):232–239

Brobmann GF, Huber J. Effects of different-shaped tissue expanders on transluminal pressure, oxygen tension, histopathologic changes, and skin expansion in pigs. Plast Reconstr Surg. 1985; 76(5):731–736

Brody GS. Safety and efficacy of breast implants. In: Spear SL, ed., Surgery of the Breast: Principles and Art. Philadelphia, PA: Lippincot-Raven; 1998:335–345

Canter HI, Igde M, Vargel I, Ozgur F. Repeated tissue expansions on split-thickness skin graft in a patient with neurocutaneous syndrome. J Craniofac Surg. 2007; 18(3):699–703

Carneiro R, Dichiara J. A protocol for tissue expansion in upper extremity reconstruction. J Hand Surg [Br]. 1991; 16:147–151

Casanova D, Bali D, Bardot J, Legre R, Magalon G. Tissue expansion of the lower limb: complications in a cohort of 103 cases. Br J Plast Surg. 2001; 54(4):310–316

Cheng A, Saint-Cyr M. Use of a pre-expanded "propeller" deep inferior epigastric perforator (DIEP) flap for a large abdominal wall defect. J Plast Reconstr Aesthet Surg. 2013; 66(6):851–854

Cherry GW, Austad E, Pasyk K, McClatchey K, Rohrich RJ. Increased survival and vascularity of random-pattern skin flaps elevated in controlled, expanded skin. Plast Reconstr Surg. 1983; 72(5):680–687

Chummun S, Addison P, Stewart KJ. The osmotic tissue expander: a 5-year experience. J Plast Reconstr Aesthet Surg. 2010; 63(12):2128–2132

Chun YS, Verma K, Rosen H, et al. Implant-based breast reconstruction using acellular dermal matrix and the risk of postoperative complications. Plast Reconstr Surg. 2010; 125(2):429–436

Cloutier M, Maltais F, Piedboeuf B. Increased distension stimulates distal capillary growth as well as expression of specific angiogenesis genes in fetal mouse lungs. Exp Lung Res. 2008; 34(3):101–113

Codivilla A. On the means of lengthening the lower limb, the muscles and tissues which are shortened through deformity. Am J Orthop Surg. 1905; 2:353–369

De Filippo RE, Atala A. Stretch and growth: the molecular and physiologic influences of tissue expansion. Plast Reconstr Surg. 2002; 109(7):2450–2462

Dunn MG, Silver FH. Viscoelastic behavior of human connective tissues: relative contribution of viscous and elastic components. Connect Tissue Res. 1983; 12(1):59–70

Farzaneh FC, Kaldari S, Becker M, Wikström SO. Tissue expansion 1984–1999: a 15-year review. Scand J Plast Reconstr Surg Hand Surg. 2006; 40(2):89–92

Friedman RM, Ingram AE, Jr, Rohrich RJ, et al. Risk factors for complications in pediatric tissue expansion. Plast Reconstr Surg. 1996; 98(7):1242–1246

Gibson T. The physical properties of skin. In: Converse JM, ed. Reconstructive Plastic Surgery. Vol 1. Philadelphia, PA: WB Saunders; 1977:70–77

Goodman T, White S, Shenaq SM. Tissue expansion. A new modality in reconstructive surgery. AORN J. 1987; 46(2):198–201, 204–205, 208–209 passim

Gutierrez JA, Perr HA. Mechanical stretch modulates TGF-beta1 and alpha1(I) collagen expression in fetal human intestinal smooth muscle cells. Am J Physiol. 1999; 277(5 Pt 1):G1074–G1080

Hocaoğlu E, Arıncı A, Berköz Ö, Özkan T. Free pre-expanded lateral circumflex femoral artery perforator flap for extensive resurfacing and reconstruction of the hand. J Plast Reconstr Aesthet Surg. 2013; 66(12):1788–1791

Hocaoğlu E, Emekli U, Çızmecı O, Uçar A. Suprafascial preexpansion of perforator flaps and the effect of pre-expansion on perforator artery diameter. Microsurgery. 2014; 34(3):188–196

Huang X, Qu X, Li Q. Risk factors for complications of tissue expansion: a 20-year systematic review and meta-analysis. Plast Reconstr Surg. 2011; 128(3):787–797

Hudson DA, Arasteh E. Serial tissue expansion for reconstruction of burns of the head and neck. Burns. 2001; 27(5):481–487

Hudson DA, Lazarus D, Silfen R. The use of serial tissue expansion in pediatric plastic surgery. Ann Plast Surg. 2000; 45(6):589–593, discussion 593–594

Johnson PE, Kernahan DA, Bauer BS. Dermal and epidermal response to soft-tissue expansion in the pig. Plast Reconstr Surg. 1988; 81(3):390–397

Johnson TM, Brown MD, Sullivan MJ, Swanson NA. Immediate intraoperative tissue expansion. J Am Acad Dermatol. 1990; 22(2 Pt 1):283–287

Kane WJ, McCaffrey TV, Wang TD, Koval TM. The effect of tissue expansion on previously irradiated skin. Arch Otolaryngol Head Neck Surg. 1992; 118(4):419–426

Kawashima T, Yamada A, Ueda K, Asato H, Harii K. Tissue expansion in facial reconstruction. Plast Reconstr Surg. 1994; 94(7):944–950

Kim KH, Hong C, Futrell JW. Histomorphologic changes in expanded skeletal muscle in rats. Plast Reconstr Surg. 1993; 92(4):710–716

Kronowitz SJ, Robb GL. Radiation therapy and breast reconstruction: a critical review of the literature. Plast Reconstr Surg. 2009; 124(2):395–408

Lantieri LA, Martin-Garcia N, Wechsler J, Mitrofanoff M, Raulo Y, Baruch JP. Vascular endothelial growth factor expression in expanded tissue: a possible mechanism of angiogenesis in tissue expansion. Plast Reconstr Surg. 1998; 101(2):392–398

Leighton WD, Russell RC, Feller AM, Eriksson E, Mathur A, Zook EG. Experimental pretransfer expansion of free-flap donor sites: II. Physiology, histology, and clinical correlation. Plast Reconstr Surg. 1988; 82(1):76–87

Leighton WD, Russell RC, Marcus DE, Eriksson E, Suchy H, Zook EG. Experimental pretransfer expansion of free-flap donor sites: I. Flap viability and expansion characteristics. Plast Reconstr Surg. 1988; 82(1):69–75

Lemmon JA. Tissue expansion. In: Janis JE, ed., Essentials of Plastic Surgery: A UT Southwestern Medical Center Handbook. St Louis, MO: Quality Medical Publishing; 2007

Li J, Hampton T, Morgan JP, Simons M. Stretch-induced VEGF expression in the heart. J Clin Invest. 1997; 100(1):18–24

LoGiudice J, Gosain AK. Pediatric tissue expansion: indications and complications. J Craniofac Surg. 2003; 14(6):866–872

Lozano S, Drucker M. Use of tissue expanders with external ports. Ann Plast Surg. 2000; 44(1):14–17

MacLennan SE, Corcoran JF, Neale HW. Tissue expansion in head and neck burn reconstruction. Clin Plast Surg. 2000; 27(1):121–132

Magnuson PB. Lengthening shortened bones of the leg by operation. Ivory screws with removable heads as a means of holding the two bone fragments. Surg Gynecol Obstet. 1913:17–63

Manders EK, Graham WP, III, Schenden MJ, Davis TS. Skin expansion to eliminate large scalp defects. Ann Plast Surg. 1984; 12(4):305–312

Manders EK, Oaks TE, Au VK, et al. Soft-tissue expansion in the lower extremities. Plast Reconstr Surg. 1988; 81(2):208–219

Manders EK, Schenden MJ, Furrey JA, Hetzler PT, Davis TS, Graham WP, III. Soft-tissue expansion: concepts and complications. Plast Reconstr Surg. 1984; 74(4):493–507

Marcus J, Horan DB, Robinson JK. Tissue expansion: past, present, and future. J Am Acad Dermatol. 1990; 23(5 Pt 1):813–825

Marks MW, Argenta LC, Thornton JW. Burn management: the role of tissue expansion. Clin Plast Surg. 1987; 14(3):543–548

Marks MW, Mackenzie JR, Burney RE, Knight PR, Anderson SH. Response of random skin flaps to rapid expansion. J Trauma. 1985; 25(10):947–952

Marks R. Mechanical properties of the skin. In: Goldsmith LA, ed. Biochemistry and Physiology of the Skin. New York, NY: Oxford University Press; 1983:1237–1254

Mason AC, Davison SP, Manders EK. Tissue expander infections in children: look beyond the expander pocket. Ann Plast Surg. 1999; 43(5):539–541

McCauley RL, Oliphant JR, Robson MC. Tissue expansion in the correction of burn alopecia: classification and methods of correction. Ann Plast Surg. 1990; 25(2):103–115

Neale HW, High RM, Billmire DA, Carey JP, Smith D, Warden G. Complications of controlled tissue expansion in the pediatric burn patient. Plast Reconstr Surg. 1988; 82(5):840–848

Pandya AN, Vadodaria S, Coleman DJ. Tissue expansion in the limbs: a comparative analysis of limb and non-limb sites. Br J Plast Surg. 2002; 55(4):302–306

Pitanguy I, Carreirão S, Iglesias MCS, Mendia JGQ. Repeat expansion of the skin. Rev Soc Bras Cir Plast Est Reconst. 1994; 9:10–22

Pitanguy I, Gontijo de Amorim NF, Radwanski HN, Lintz JE. Repeated expansion in burn sequela. Burns. 2002; 28(5):494–499

Pusic A, Thompson TA, Kerrigan CL, et al. Surgical options for the early-stage breast cancer: factors associated with patient choice and postoperative quality of life. Plast Reconstr Surg. 1999; 104(5):1325–1333

Putti V. The operative lengthening of the femur. JAMA. 1921; 77:934

Radovan C. Breast reconstruction after mastectomy using the temporary expander. Plast Reconstr Surg. 1982; 69(2):195–208

Radovan C. Tissue expansion in soft-tissue reconstruction. Plast Reconstr Surg. 1984; 74(4):482–492

Ramon Y, Ullmann Y, Moscona R, et al. Aesthetic results and patient satisfaction with immediate breast reconstruction using tissue expansion: a follow-up study. Plast Reconstr Surg. 1997; 99(3):686–691

Refojo MF. Vapor pressure and swelling pressure of hydrogels. In: Andrade JD, ed., Hydrogels for Medical and Related Application. Washington, DC: American Chemical Society; 1976

Riser BL, Cortes P, Yee J. Modelling the effects of vascular stress in mesangial cells. Curr Opin Nephrol Hypertens. 2000; 9(1):43–47

Rohrich RJ, Lowe JB, Hackney FL, Bowman JL, Hobar PC. An algorithm for abdominal wall reconstruction. Plast Reconstr Surg. 2000; 105(1):202–216, quiz 217

Ronert MA, Hofheinz H, Manassa E, Asgarouladi H, Olbrisch RR. The beginning of a new era in tissue expansion: self-filling osmotic tissue expander—four-year clinical experience. Plast Reconstr Surg. 2004; 114(5):1025–1031

Santanelli F, Grippaudo FR, Ziccardi P, Onesti MG. The role of pre-expanded free flaps in revision of burn scarring. Burns. 1997; 23(7–8):620–625

Sasaki GH. Tissue Expansion in Reconstructive and Aesthetic Surgery. St Louis, MO: CV Mosby; 1998

Seko Y, Seko Y, Takahashi N, Shibuya M, Yazaki Y. Pulsatile stretch stimulates vascular endothelial growth factor (VEGF) secretion by cultured rat cardiac myocytes. Biochem Biophys Res Commun. 1999; 254(2):462–465

Sellers DS, Miller SH, Demuth RJ, Klabacha ME. Repeated skin expansion to resurface a massive thigh wound. Plast Reconstr Surg. 1986; 77(4):654–659

Serra JM, Mesa F, Paloma V, Ballesteros A. Use of a calf prosthesis and tissue expansion in aesthetic reconstruction of the leg. Plast Reconstr Surg. 1992; 89(4):684–688

Silver FH. Biological Materials: Structure, Mechanical Properties and Modeling of Soft Tissues. New York, NY: New York University Press; 1987:75–79, 164–195

Silver FH, Kato YP, Ohno M, Wasserman AJ. Analysis of mammalian connective tissue: relationship between hierarchical structures and mechanical properties. J Long Term Eff Med Implants. 1992; 2(2–3):165–198

Song B, Xiao B, Liu C, et al. Neck burn reconstruction with pre-expanded scapular free flaps. Burns. 2015; 41(3):624–630

Spear SL, Majidian A. Immediate breast reconstruction in two stages using textured, integrated-valve tissue expanders and breast implants: a retrospective review of 171 consecutive breast reconstructions from 1989 to 1996. Plast Reconstr Surg. 1998; 101(1):53–63

Spear SL, Parikh PM, Reisin E, Menon NG. Acellular dermis-assisted breast reconstruction. Aesthetic Plast Surg. 2008; 32(3):418–425

Spear SL, Spittler CJ. Breast reconstruction with implants and expanders. Plast Reconstr Surg. 2001; 107(1):177–187, quiz 188

Takei T, Mills I, Arai K, Sumpio BE. Molecular basis for tissue expansion: clinical implications for the surgeon. Plast Reconstr Surg. 1998; 102(1):247–258

Vergnes P, Taieb A, Maleville J, Larrègue M, Bondonny JM. Repeated skin expansion for excision of congenital giant nevi in infancy and childhood. Plast Reconstr Surg. 1993; 91(3):450–455

Wagh MS, Dixit V. Tissue expansion: Concepts, techniques and unfavourable results. Indian J Plast Surg. 2013; 46(2):333–348

Wang J, Huang X, Liu K, Gu B, Li Q. Complications in tissue expansion: an updated retrospective analysis of risk factors. Handchir Mikrochir Plast Chir. 2014; 46(2):74–79

Wang Y, Huo R, Hao HB, Yang B, Li SB, Yu QP. Microscopic study on skin and soft tissue after repeated expansion[in Chinese]. Zhonghua Zheng Xing Wai Ke Za Zhi. 2006; 22(4):294–297

Wieslander JB. Tissue expansion in the head and neck. A 6-year review. Scand J Plast Reconstr Surg Hand Surg. 1991; 25(1):47–56

Wilson E, Mai Q, Sudhir K, Weiss RH, Ives HE. Mechanical strain induces growth of vascular smooth muscle cells via autocrine action of PDGF. J Cell Biol. 1993; 123(3):741–747

Woo SH, Seul JH. Pre-expanded arterialised venous free flaps for burn contracture of the cervicofacial region. Br J Plast Surg. 2001; 54(5):390–395

Workman P. Inhibiting the phosphoinositide 3-kinase pathway for cancer treatment. Biochem Soc Trans. 2004; 32 (Pt 2):393–396

Yang M, Li S, Xu J. Clinical application of repeated tissue expansion [in Chinese]. Zhonghua Zheng Xing Shao Shang Wai Ke Za Zhi. 1996; 12(5):364–366

Yanko-Arzi R, Gur E, Margulis A, et al. The role of free tissue transfer in posterior neck reconstruction. J Reconstr Microsurg. 2014; 30(5):305–312

Zan T, Li H, Du Z, et al. Reconstruction of the face and neck with different types of pre-expanded anterior chest flaps: a comprehensive strategy for multiple techniques. J Plast Reconstr Aesthet Surg. 2013; 66(8):1074–1081

Zoltie N, Chapman P, Joss G. Tissue expansion: a unit review of non-scalp, non-breast expansion. Br J Plast Surg. 1990; 43(3):325–327

18 Burns

José Manuel Collado Delfa

Abstract

Burns are one of the most devastating traumatic injuries, mainly affecting the most vulnerable population groups (children, women, and elderly) living in the poorest social conditions. Thermal injuries occur by an increase in temperature able to cause tissue damage. The most frequent etiologic agent is fire/flames, closely followed by scalds. Aside from local destruction (coagulative necrosis), when burn injuries involve > 20% of the total body surface area the systemic inflammatory response puts life at risk: the shock in the acute phase and the sepsis for the rest of the evolution are the leading causes of death. Inhalation injury in the context of a fire/flame burn dramatically worsens the prognosis. Primary assessment of the burned patient must follow the Advanced Trauma Life Support guidelines, and major burns demand transfer to a burn unit. Accurate diagnosis of burn depth is the main challenge because early and definitive coverage with skin grafts remains the gold standard definitive treatment.

Other traumatic agents, such as electricity, chemicals, and cold, can also cause tissue damage that resembles a thermal injury. Although an increase in temperature may coexist in some circumstances, the main injurious mechanisms of these other agents are different, and they are classified as nonthermal injuries.

Keywords: burn, chemical injury, cold injury, electrical injury, nonthermal injury, thermal injury

18.1 Introduction

Thermal injury can be defined as a traumatic injury caused by a temperature increase beyond a threshold able to cause tissue damage. Etiologic factors are contact with hot elements (solids, liquids or scalds, gases), thermal radiation (fire/flames, sun, infrared lamps, etc.), and mechanical friction.

Other nonthermal traumatic agents, such as electricity, chemicals, and cold, can also cause tissue damage with an appearance and behavior reminiscent of a burn injury; however, they have a singular pathophysiology, clinical presentation, and treatment.

18.2 Epidemiology

According to the latest estimates, 973 million people suffered some kind of traumatic injury that required medical care in 2013. Of these, 31 million were injured by fire/flames, heat, and hot substances (337 injured/100,000 inhabitants), resulting in 12.3 million years of disability-adjusted life years (DALYs). Even though the global rate of DALYs has fallen by 33% since 1990, in regions like sub-Saharan Africa, Oceania, eastern Europe, and the Caribbean this figure remains relatively unchanged.

The population distribution of thermal injuries is one of the most unjust among traumatic injuries, with the most vulnerable population groups being children, the elderly, and women. Over 95% of deaths from fire/flames burns are concentrated in low- and middle-income countries, and in high-income countries, they affect the poorest social sectors.

According to the 2015 National Burn Repository of the American Burn Association the most frequent etiologic burn agent is fire/flames (43%), followed by scalds (34%), contact with hot objects (9%), electrical injuries (4%), and chemical injuries (3%). While electrical and chemical etiologies occur mainly in work-related industrial settings, the rest of the agents are more common outside the workplace. Of note, high-voltage electrical injuries have been related to illegal sales of copper in times of economic crisis.

Most adults suffer burns by fire/flames followed by scalds, men commonly at the workplace and in outdoor accidents, whereas women and the elderly usually at home. Children sustain burns mainly by scalds at home, followed by contact with hot objects in younger than 2 years and fire/flames in older than 2 years.

Described risk factors for burns are poverty, unemployment, illiteracy, overcrowding, nonwhite race, toxic habits (tobacco, alcohol, and drugs), epilepsy, sensory deficits (blindness, deafness, neuropathy), motor deficits (arthritis, paraplegia), and mental and psychiatric deficits. Particular risk factors in children include the presence of preexisting impairments, lapses in child supervision, storage of flammable substances at home, and low maternal education level.

Cold injuries are a well-documented problem in countries with extreme temperatures and frequent among military personnel during wartime, alpinists, and the homeless, and following occupational accidents with refrigerants and propellants (Freon gas, liquid nitrogen, carbon dioxide).

About 3–10% of burn injuries are intentional in the context of suicide and aggression. Suicide has an overall mortality rate of 65% worldwide, with flame and chemicals being the most frequent causal agents. Risk factors include psychiatric conditions, drug addictions, and gender violence. Children < 2 years are at greater risk of aggression, mainly by immersion in hot liquids and contact with cigarettes or hot objects.

Total days of acute hospital stay approximately equals the burn size expressed as the percent of total body surface area (TBSA), except in the group with burns 50–80% TBSA where hospital stay increases. Fire/flame burns have the highest complication and mortality rates, followed by electrical injuries. Regardless of the cause, the maximal rate of complications occurs in infants and the elderly and increases progressively with age. Associated inhalation injury increases mortality, though it is less evident for burns > 60% TBSA because these already bear a poor prognosis.

Although most burn injuries are not fatal, those who survive do so with varying functional and aesthetic sequelae, which may cause psychological distress and generate a cascade of personal, family, social, and labor repercussions.

Finally, prevention through strategies like regulation of electrical systems, smoke detectors, temperature limiters in running water heaters, and use of fireproof clothes and construction materials have proven effective in reducing morbidity, mortality, and the economic burden of burns in developed countries.

> **Remember**   **M!**
>
> Burns mainly affect the poorest and the most vulnerable people.

18.3 Thermal Injury

18.3.1 Basic Science

Temperature is a measurement of the average kinetic energy resulting from the random movement of molecules constituting a physical element. In theory, temperature can range from absolute zero (no molecular movement) to infinite.

A rise in tissue temperature occurs when energy is transferred. Conceptually, the energy that originates from a thermal source is called heat, and the energy that originates from a nonthermal source is called work.

Heat can be transferred by conduction, convection, or radiation, with the first two involving direct physical contact with the energy source. In conduction, the energy source remains static, as when one is touching an incandescent material or dipping a hand in a bowl of hot water. In convection, the contact is established with a fluid in motion as with running water or steam causing a continuous turnover of molecules at the source–tissue interface, which prevents the system from reaching thermal equilibrium. Radiation requires no contact and can be emitted by any physical element with temperature other than absolute zero in the form of electromagnetic waves (0.1–100 μm). Examples include sunlight and infrared lamps. The surface of living organisms behaves as a dark body that easily absorbs radiation.

Work implies not only a physical force that causes displacement but also opposition forces that interfere with it. Friction is the opposition force involved in burns.

Energy transferred as heat or generating friction increases random molecular movement in tissue at the interaction point, elevating its temperature. The energy is then transmitted from the surface to the deep tissues by conduction. Biological tissues are poor conductors of heat; the less their water content, the poorer their conduction capacity.

The effects of temperature in living tissues are conditioned by the value of maximum temperature reached and the length of exposure. When exposed to high temperatures, tissues undergo several changes in their physical properties, including tissue dilation, increased pressure, and decreased electrical resistance. In addition, biological effects are possible (▶Table 18.1).

Moderately high temperatures have beneficial effects and are used as thermotherapy in physical rehabilitation within a narrow temperature range (40–45°C) for short periods of time (5–30 minutes). Beyond that range injury becomes a possibility. Due to skin's resilience to temperature increase and its poor conductivity, it takes a considerable amount of time both to heat it up and to cool it down, which

Table 18.1 Biological effects of temperature on living tissues

Temperature (°C)	Biological effects
40–45	Analgesic, anti-inflammatory, antispasmodic, sedative Improves elongation of collagen fibers
45–60	Pain Protein denaturation
60	Protein coagulation and cell death
100	Tissue vaporization and thermal ablation
200	Tissue carbonization
300	Tissue fusion (solid to liquid physical state)

is why burn management requires not only the removal of the energy source but also cooling down the skin surface to prevent progression of injury.

The first signs of cellular injury begin to appear at temperatures > 45°C when proteins and nucleic acids denature, leading to metabolic and structural dysfunction. The most remarkable histological feature is cell edema due to failure of the sodium-potassium adenosine triphosphatase (Na^+/K^+-ATPase) pump. Denaturation may be slowly reversed by cooling down. With temperatures > 60 °C, proteins and nucleic acids precipitate and cells die. It is an irreversible phenomenon whose histological expression is the coagulative necrosis. Macroscopically, tissues appear desiccated and mummified with a yellow-gray or blackish hue (eschar tissue), whereas microscopically the original histological architecture remains identifiable. Burns destroy skin and its appendages, dermal vascular plexus, and sensitive cutaneous nerves impairing its protective function as a physical and biological barrier, as well as its other functions, such as thermoregulation, synthesis of vitamin D, and sensation, all of which are essential for our adaptation to the external environment and social interaction. Cell destruction releases electrolytes, enzymes, and other cytoplasmic proteins that serve as injury markers (K^+, myoglobin, creatine phosphokinase [CPK], L-lactate dehydrogenase).

18.3.2 Histological Zones of Thermal Injury

Jackson identified three zones of thermal injury: coagulation, stasis, and hyperemia. In the coagulation zone, injury is maximal and irreversible, featuring coagulative necrosis. The stasis zone surrounds the area of coagulation and is characterized by protein denaturation, cell dysfunction, and blood stasis. The outermost is the hyperemia zone, which shows minimal cell injury and intense local vasodilation. It is important to note that final extension of the necrosis zone depends on the evolution over time of the other two zones. Additional cell death can be explained by the onset of immediate autophagy and delayed cellular apoptosis as well as by the addition of factors that hinder healing in the areas of stasis and hyperemia, such as hypoxemia, deficient blood supply, interstitial edema, desiccation, and local infection.

> **Remember**   **M!**
>
> Coagulative necrosis is the histological lesion of a thermal injury.

18.3.3 Physiopathology

Local Changes

The repair of any wound, including burn wounds, comprises three successive and partially overlapping phases.

The inflammatory phase takes place during the first week and begins with the release of primary mediators of cellular origin (histamine, serotonin, platelet-activating factor, and arachidonic acid metabolites) and plasmatic origin (coagulation factors, complement and kynin pathways components). They cause changes in the local microcirculation with primary vasoconstriction followed by vasodilation, increased endothelial permeability with interstitial edema, circulatory stasis, and microthrombosis. These mediators also stimulate the homing of other inflammatory cells in charge of removing debris and releasing cytokines that modulate and amplify the inflammatory response as secondary mediators.

The proliferative phase starts approximately 4 days after injury and lasts 3 weeks. Key features of this phase include a high rate of collagen production by fibroblasts, formation of new blood vessels from preexisting ones (angiogenesis), and the start of epithelialization.

The remodeling phase starts at week 3 and lasts up to a year. During this phase equilibrium between collagen synthesis and breakdown is reached, the normal 4:1 ratio of collagen I to collagen III is restored, and the wound gradually regains its tensile strength to a maximum of 80% of unwounded skin.

Systemic Changes

When burn injuries involve > 20% TBSA, the inflammatory response mediated by cytokines becomes systemic and may last for several months.

Acute Phase

The most prominent features of the acute phase are the abrupt increase in endothelial and cell membrane permeability and cellular dysfunction. The increase in permeability causes a rapid shift of protein-rich fluid into the interstitial space and subsequent interstitial and cellular edema. As a response to the hypovolemic shock, peripheral and splanchnic vasoconstriction occurs to ensure perfusion of vital organs.

The origin of cellular dysfunction is multifactorial and not only explained by tissue hypoxia. There is a tendency toward hypothermia, and basal metabolism is depressed in the acute phase. In addition, there is low cardiac output secondary to a reduced preload and the negative effect of cytokines in heart contractility, with a characteristic poor response to vasoactive drugs (cardiogenic shock). Renal function is affected by reduced blood volume, and there is renal tubular dysfunction due to hypoperfusion and tubular obstruction by cell debris. Mesenteric hypoperfusion causes mucosal edema and paralytic ileus. Leukocytosis with neutrophilia is prominent due to intravascular displacement and depletion of bone marrow reserves. In addition, destruction of red blood cells within the cutaneous vascular plexus leads to anemia and coagulation. Coagulation is affected by the loss of coagulation factors to the interstitial space, direct platelet destruction by temperature, and consumption of both from intravascular thrombosis.

> **Remember**   M!
>
> The burn shock is primarily hypovolemic but also distributive and cardiogenic.

Subacute Phase (> 48–72 Hours)

Restoration of permeability follows a downward-sloping exponential curve. It is already evident at 8–12 hours and normalizes from 48 hours onward, allowing reversal of the hypovolemic shock and edema reabsorption with transient polyuria.

During this phase, the stress state from burn injury generates a nonspecific clinical picture known as the systemic inflammatory response syndrome (SIRS), which sets in motion a hypermetabolic, hyperdynamic, and inflammatory response.

The *hypermetabolic response* is aimed at generating enough energy to withstand the inflammatory response and cope with subsequent tissue repair. It correlates with burn size, doubling the basal metabolism with burns > 40% TBSA, and may take up to 2 years to return to preinjury values. Thyroid function is inhibited, and basal metabolism becomes regulated by stress response hormones (cortisol, catecholamines, and glucagon). Because the use of sugars and fats is partially blocked, proteins represent the primary source of energy in this phase. Although gluconeogenesis is stimulated and the release of insulin is increased, there is peripheral insulin resistance that limits cellular intake of glucose, leading to hyperglycemia. Fortunately, uptake of sugar by the central nervous system, red blood cells, and wound bed works independently of the action of insulin. Hyperinsulinism blocks ketogenesis from fatty acids, and hyperglycemia promotes their hepatic reesterification back into triglycerides. Because the synthesis of transport lipoproteins is also insufficient, triglycerides cannot return to the fatty tissue and thus remain in the liver (steatosis), producing hepatomegaly.

The generation of energy from protein breakdown has a severe impact, with skeletal muscle being the most affected tissue because of its high protein content. Additionally, there is a rearrangement of liver protein synthesis, with acute phase proteins taking over visceral ones. The net result is weight loss and reduction in lean body mass with weakened muscle (known as self-cannibalism), all of which compromise inflammatory response, wound healing, and growth of pediatric patients. Laboratory workup will show a low serum protein level, a negative nitrogen balance, increased blood and urine urea, elevated C-reactive protein, and reduction of protein synthesis markers (albumin, prealbumin, and transferrin).

In order to withstand the hypermetabolic response, a *hyperdynamic state* ensues, with increased cardiac output, tachycardia, tachypnea, and peripheral vasodilation, the latter being more evident after the first week.

The inflammatory response mediated by cytokines can affect the entire organism. Internal core temperature and basal metabolism are increased. Acute respiratory distress syndrome (ARDS) may develop, usually from day 5 postburn. The renal system is affected by elevated glomerular filtration rate but impaired tubular function. Splanchnic vasoconstriction and the increase in hydrochloric acid production can cause gastrointestinal ulcers (Curling's ulcer), typically multiple in the stomach and single in the duodenum. Malabsorption and bacterial translocation are possible. There is bone marrow suppression, and the use of iron is blocked, perpetuating anemia that responds only to blood transfusions. The risk of thrombosis is increased due to thrombocytosis and a deficit of anticoagulative factors, such as antithrombin III. Humoral and cellular immunity are depressed by the effects of cortisol and reduced antibody synthesis, with greater risk of infection. Bone and mineral metabolism are depressed with low levels of parathyroid hormone (associated with parathyroid hormone receptors' block), growth hormone, insulin-like growth factor-1, calcium, Pi, magnesium, and vitamin C synthesis, causing osteoporosis, loss of bone remodeling capacity, and, in children, delayed growth for years after burn injury. Lastly, stress blocks gonadal function causing reduced libido, impotence, and amenorrhea.

Although initially beneficial, a SIRS prolonged in time can overcome the compensatory mechanisms and cause multiple organ dysfunction syndrome (MODS) and death by exhaustion.

> **Remember** M!
>
> The leading causes of burn mortality are renal failure in the acute phase and sepsis and MODS in the subacute phase.

18.3.4 Classification of Burns

Skin burns are classified into three degrees according to the injured histological layer (▶Table 18.2 and ▶Fig. 18.1, ▶Fig. 18.2, ▶Fig. 18.3, ▶Fig. 18.4, ▶Fig. 18.5). The fourth degree involves subcutaneous and deeper injuries.

Given that energy transference is rarely homogeneous, different depths within the same lesion are frequently found. Occasionally a gradient of injury is clearly recognized (▶Fig. 18.6). On other occasions, a patchy geographic distribution may be seen.

Finally, because the zone of necrosis can progress depending on the evolution of stasis and hyperemic zones, it may take several days for the lesion to fully demarcate and an accurate diagnosis to be made.

> **Remember** M!
>
> Thermal damage is heterogeneous in its spatial distribution and can change over time due to necrosis progression into the stasis and hyperemic zones.

18.3.5 Inhalation Injury

Inhalation injury is the leading cause of death during a fire, and a significant worsening factor when associated with a burn injury.

Local effects of inhalation are irritant (physical stimulus of mechanical receptors by solid particles in suspension), thermal (hot gases that burn the mucosal layer), and, most important, toxic, which is dependent on the chemical nature of combustion products. Irritant and toxic effects can freely affect the entire airway, whereas burns rarely cause injury beyond the glottis because the upper airway absorbs most of the heat of inspired air. The reflex response is immediate and involves sneezing, mucous hypersecretion, cough with carbonaceous sputum, and laryngeal and bronchial spasms. The clinical features of mucosal injury present later following a typical temporal sequence and are secondary to inflammation, loss of cilia function and alveolar surfactant, and necrosis. Edema develops within the first hours after injury and may be silent or present with hoarseness, dysphonia, and glottis obstruction. ARDS and atelectasis usually appear on day 3–5, followed by lower airway infection after the first week.

Inhalation injury should be ruled out in cases in which there is a history of fire exposure, especially when it occurs in a closed space and if the victim is found unconscious; in the presence of the clinical features just described; and in burns affecting the face, neck, nasal, and oropharynx mucosa, particularly those showing adhered carbonaceous particles (▶Fig. 18.7).

Systemically, inhalation leads to hypoxia that can cause death in a few minutes. Hypoxia depends on oxygen consumption by the combustion and the eventual production of asphyxiant gases that interfere with cell respiration, namely carbon monoxide (CO) and hydrogen cyanide (HCN).

Table 18.2 Classification of skin burns

	Superficial burn First degree	Partial-thickness burn		Full-thickness burn Third degree
		Superficial second degree	Deep second degree	
	• Epidermal injury	• Papillary dermal injury	• Partial reticular dermal injury	• Total reticular dermal injury
Tissue lesion	• Epithelial desquamation • Non visible epithelial desquamation	• Blister	• Blister • Eschar	• Eschar
Color	• Pink • Blanches with pressure	• Bright red (only visible after blister removal) • Blanches with pressure	• Dark red • Yellowish white with red specks • Does not blanch with pressure	• Marble white, gray or black (carbonization) • Does not blanch with pressure
Appearance	• Dry • Normal elasticity • Mild edema	• Intensely wet • Normal elasticity • Severe edema	• Mildly wet • Decreased elasticity • Mild edema	• Dry (leathery) • Non elastic • Depressed • Thrombosed vessels
Sensitivity	• Pain (+)	• Pain (++)	• Hypoesthesia • Painless hair removal • Deep pressure (+)	• Anesthesia • Deep pressure (+/-)
Healing	4–5 days	< 21 days	> 21 days	> 21 days (possible chronic wound)
Scar	• No	• No • Pigmentary changes	• Yes • Pigmentary changes • Hypertrophic and retracted scar	• Yes • Pigmentary changes • Hypertrophic and retracted scar • Skin cancer (Marjolin's ulcer)
Treatment	• Topical hydration	• Dressings	• Surgery recommended	• Surgery mandatory

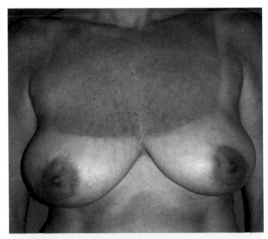

Fig. 18.1 First-degree burn (sunburn).

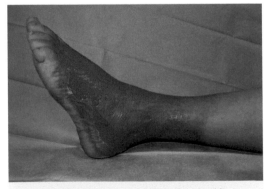

Fig. 18.2 Superficial second-degree burn (scald).

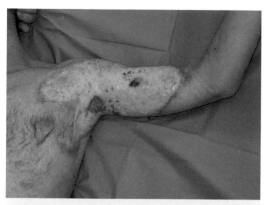

Fig. 18.3 Deep second-degree burn (flame).

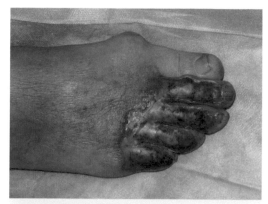

Fig. 18.4 Third-degree burn (hot solid contact).

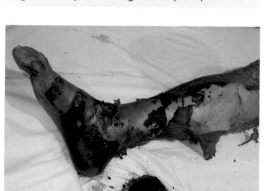

Fig. 18.5 Fourth-degree burn (flame).

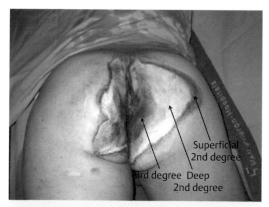

Superficial 2nd degree

3rd degree Deep 2nd degree

Fig. 18.6 Flame burn on buttocks with a clearly identifiable gradient of injury.

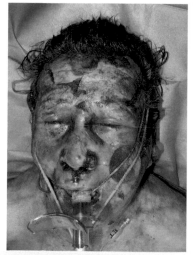

Fig. 18.7 Flame burn on face with adhered carbonaceous particles around nostrils suggesting inhalation injury.

CO results from incomplete combustion of carbon-based compounds. It is a colorless, odorless, insipid, and nonirritating gas, all of which make its inhalation unnoticeable. It can be eliminated only by respiration and has a half-life of 3–4 hours when one is breathing ambient air. It competes with O_2 for the heme groups in hemoglobin (whose affinity for CO is 240 times that of O_2), myoglobin (whose affinity for CO is 40 times that of O_2), and cytochrome C mitochondrial oxidase. It also shifts the hemoglobin (Hb) dissociation curve to the left, hindering the delivery of O_2 to tissues. Clinical presentation is nonspecific and conditioned by hypoxia and a direct toxic effect of CO. It has been related to the levels of carboxyhemoglobin (COHb) (▶Table 18.3). The first neurological sign is usually headache caused by vasodilation, followed by disorientation, irritability, weakness, as well as visual, hearing, and balance alterations,

Table 18.3 Clinical signs and symptoms related to carboxyhemoglobin levels

% COHb	Clinical finding
< 10%	Asymptomatic
10–20%	Headache, cutaneous vasodilatation, arterial hypotension Nausea and vomiting, especially in children
20–30%	Dyspnea, tachycardia, acute coronary syndrome
30–40%	Weakness, visual and hearing impairment, dizziness, drowsiness
40–50%	Cardiogenic shock
50–60%	Cheyne–Stokes breathing, seizures, coma
> 60%	Cardiorespiratory arrest, death

and ultimately obnubilation, seizures, and coma. CO depresses myocardial contractility (cardiogenic shock) and causes arrhythmias (the most common cause of death in CO intoxication). An acute coronary syndrome may develop from the combination of reduced perfusion and hypoxia. Respiratory features include dyspnea, tachypnea, Cheyne–Stokes breathing caused by lactic acidosis, ARDS, and pulmonary hemorrhage in severe cases. Skin may show a cherry red hue secondary to vasodilation and high O_2 content of venous blood. Children usually present gastrointestinal symptoms, such as nausea, vomiting, and diarrhea. Surviving patients may experience a late-onset syndrome featuring neurologic, cognitive, and psychiatric alterations, which is why follow-up is recommended. Of note, in pregnant patients CO intoxication is always worse in the fetus than in the mother.

HCN in its pure state is a colorless liquid or gas. Its gaseous form is generated in large quantities by the combustion of nitrogen materials of domestic (plastic, wool, silk, polyurethane) or industrial origin. Its absorption is immediate and travels mainly bound to plasma proteins with a half-life of 4–8 hours. Most of it is cleared renally after being transformed into thiocyanide in the liver. HCN inhibits different metabolic pathways, such as the cytochrome C mitochondrial oxidase pathway. Its clinical features are also nonspecific, derived from cellular hypoxia, and include peripheral vasodilation, low blood pressure, and neurologic symptoms, such as headache, lethargy, and coma. Survivors may show permanent neurologic

disabilities. The smell of sour almonds is noticeable in < 40% of patients.

Clinical Workup and Treatment of Inhalation Injury

Low values of oxygen saturation (SaO_2) and oxygen partial pressure (pO_2) are always present in severe cases of inhalation injury but their normal values do not rule out it. Among asphyxiant gases only CO diminishes the capacity of blood to transport O_2 but the usual pulse oximeters do not differentiate between carboxyhemoglobin (COHb) and oxyhemoglobin (O_2Hb), displaying a mistaken normal SaO_2.

Direct visualization of the mucosa using indirect laryngoscopy and bronchoscopy helps to identify local airway injuries and confirm a diagnosis of inhalation; however, in cases of pure intoxication with asphyxiant gases, the airway might be normal. Chest X-ray is of little use initially and only shows positive signs within a few days once respiratory complications appear. Chest computed tomography, radionuclide imaging with 133-xenon, and pulmonary function testing are not routinely used.

Diagnosis of CO intoxication requires COHb > 10% (normal values are < 5% in nonsmokers and 5–10% in smokers); however, if enough time has elapsed or oxygen has been applied to favor CO clearance, normal values may be observed. HCN plasma levels can also be measured but this test is not readily available and is time consuming, making it of little value in common clinical practice. If an anoxic encephalopathy is suspected, a full neurologic assessment is mandatory, and as soon as the patient's state allows, a cranial computed tomographic (CT) scan should be performed.

Treatment should be aggressive and start immediately at the slightest suspicion. Although management of inhalation injury is mainly symptomatic, specific therapies exist for asphyxiant gas intoxication.

If CO intoxication is suspected, administering 100% O_2 reduces CO half-life to 80–100 minutes. In pregnant women O_2 therapy should continue for a period of time after COHb normalization due to the different fetal pathophysiology. Hyperbaric O_2 should be considered when COHb is > 20%, but its application in patients with severe burns is limited due to logistical difficulties.

When HCN intoxication is suspected, treatment should favor its metabolism. The first choice is intravenous hydroxycobalamin (70 mg/kg), which combines with HCN rending cyanocobalamin to be eliminated by secretions producing a reddish hue in the skin, mucosa, and urine for several days. Sodium thiosulfate (150 mg/kg) forms thiocyanide when combined with HCN, but it is a second choice because of its delayed onset of action. In severe cases, a slow perfusion of sodium nitrate (5 mg/kg) can be used, which generates methemoglobin (MHb) that binds to HCN to create cyano-MHb, favoring HCN transport to the liver for its final metabolism. Levels of MHb > 40% should be avoided in order to prevent further hypoxia.

18.3.6 Treatment

Every burned patient should be considered a trauma patient and treated accordingly until proven otherwise. The burn can be a distracting factor that diverts the attention from other coexisting injuries that might result to be more deleterious.

Prehospital Care

Primary Assessment and Intubation Criteria

Primary assessment must identify and treat immediate life-threatening injuries, following the ABCDE algorithm of the Advanced Trauma Life Support guidelines.

Airway: Burns can block airway due to edema and/or laryngeal spasm. Orotracheal intubation (OTI) should be performed whenever a patent upper airway cannot be secured.

Breathing: It may be impaired by burns restricting ventilation (deep circumferential burns affecting the thorax and abdomen) and by inhalation injury. As a general rule, high flow (15 L/min), 100% oxygen should be administered, ideally with a reservoir mask, to ensure maximum fraction of inspired oxygen. If intoxication by asphyxiant gases is suspected act accordingly. Failure to maintain respiratory function requires OTI and mechanical ventilation.

Prophylactic OTI use should be considered in cases where respiratory failure is foreseen (▶ Table 18.4). Its indication should be precise, weighing risks and benefits.

Circulation: A good cardiocirculatory function must be ensured. All traumatic patients require immediate fluid resuscitation using 0.9% normal saline (NS) or Ringer's lactate (RL). In stable patients, 500 mL of fluid (10 mL/kg in children) should be administered in 30 minutes,

Table 18.4 Indications for orotracheal intubation

Absolute	Prophylactic
• A (airway): a patent upper airway cannot be secured • B (breathing): acute respiratory insufficiency • C (circulation): refractory shock • D (disability): Glasgow Coma Scale score ≤ 8	• Extensive facial and cervical burns (especially in children) • Suspected inhalation • Incipient signs of upper airway compromise: dysphonia, hoarseness, laryngeal stridor • Transport related limitations: delayed evacuation, long-distance transfer, limited health care resources, helicopter transportation

whereas unstable patients require a bolus of 1,000 mL (20 mL/kg in children) and reassessment according to response. Intoxication by asphyxiant gases should be suspected in hemodynamically unstable patients who do not respond to adequate fluid resuscitation. OTI should be performed in cases of refractory shock.

Disability: A basic neurologic status assessment is performed including the Glasgow Coma Scale (GCS). Burn injuries rarely affect neurologic status, with the exception of asphyxiant gas intoxication. GCS ≤ 8 is an indication for OTI.

Exposure: All clothing and accessories should be removed. It allows primary assessment, eliminates any retained heat source, and prevents compartment syndrome as a consequence of subsequent edema. The patient should be covered immediately after to reduce the risk of hypothermia.

Secondary Assessment

Secondary assessment should be performed only on stable patients, with continuous monitoring of vital functions. The priority for unstable patients is their transport to a hospital facility.

Four questions characterize the accident: *when* ("hour 0"), *what* (the injurious agent), *how* (injury mechanisms and circumstances of the incident; accidental or intentional), and *where* (indoor or outdoor; domestic or work-related). A general physical examination must be performed quickly and in an orderly fashion from head to toe, always ruling out associated injuries. Physical examination of the burn injury should define its extent, location, and depth. The percentage of TBSA must not include first-degree injuries, because these are not considered when calculating fluid resuscitation. For extensive wounds, an approximate approach is Wallace's "rule of nines". In children percentages of head and lower legs must be adapted due to their different body proportions (▶ Fig. 18.8). Small

extensions should be calculated using the patient's hand and it is applicable for adults and children: the palm including all fingers represents approximately 1% TBSA. It is advisable to identify burns in areas of particular functional or aesthetic interest, such as the face (particularly the eyes), neck,

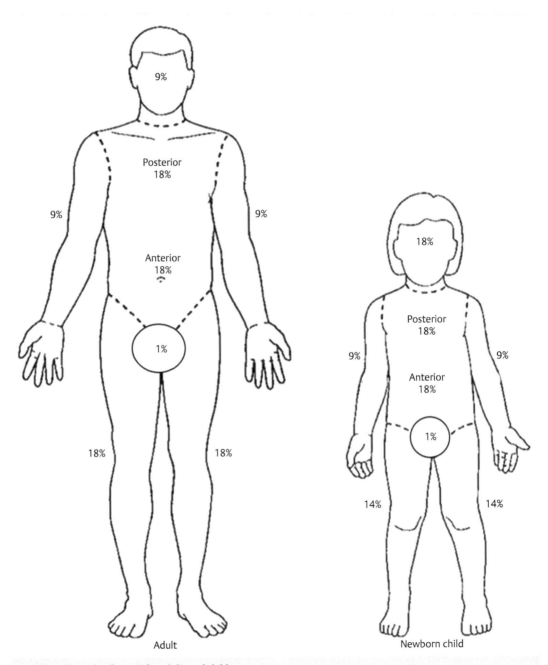

Fig. 18.8 The "rule of nines" for adults and children.

breasts, genitals, perineal area, hands and feet, major joints and flexure areas, and nasal and oropharyngeal mucosa. Deep circumferential burns affecting the neck, trunk, extremities, and penis should also be ruled out.

Initial Care

Burns should be cooled down by means of irrigation or immersion in tap water or 0.9% NS at room temperature (12–18°C) for 15–20 minutes, which also provides an analgesic effect, though it is discouraged for adult burns > 15% TBSA and for children burns due to the risk of hypothermia. An alternative is hydrogel dressings, which provide a refreshing sensation without increasing the risk of hypothermia. Debridement of blisters and applying wound dressing that might interfere with definitive hospital assessment should be postponed. Burns should be covered with sterile drapes or clean dry linen to avoid contamination and reduce painful stimuli. Finally the patient should be covered with a thermal blanket, keeping affected areas elevated.

Superficial second-degree burns are the most painful. Topical treatment provides some analgesic effects, but it is often insufficient and systemic analgesia is necessary. When conventional analgesia is inadequate, intravenous opioids are the treatment of choice.

A strict indication for nothing by mouth should be made before hospital admittance. If paralytic ileus is suspected, gastric decompression should be considered especially when the patient is to be transported by means of unpressurized air cabins (helicopter).

Early fluid resuscitation is indicated in adult burns > 15% TBSA and children burns > 10% TBSA. Multiple empirical formulas have been described to calculate fluid reposition (►Table 18.5), with Parkland's being the most widely accepted. Children's formulas are specific for them and their accuracy increases when body surface is used instead of weight, as Carvajal's formula. RL is the fluid of choice because it is an isotonic crystalloid with an electrolyte composition similar to plasma, and contains lactate, which counteracts the initial shock's metabolic acidosis. Hourly diuresis remains the single most useful indicator for tissue perfusion monitoring. The goal is 0.5 mL/kg/h in adults (1 mL/kg/h in children < 30 kg, and 2 mL/kg/h in lactants). Except in cases where rapid hospital arrival is secured, a permanent urinary catheter must be placed for precise quantification.

Table 18.5 Fluid resuscitation formulas for adult burn patients[a]

Name	First 24 hours	Next 24 hours
Evans[b]	NS: 1 mL/kg/%TBSA burn C: 1 ml /kg/%TBSA burn D5W: 2,000 mL	NS: 0.5 mL/kg/%TBSA burn C: 0.5 mL/kg/%TBSA burn D5W: 2,000 mL
Brooke[b]	RL: 1.5 mL/kg/%TBSA burn C: 0.5 mL/kg/%TBSA burn D5W: 2,000 mL	RL: 0.5 mL/kg/%TBSA burn C: 0.25 mL/kg/%TBSA burn D5W: 2,000 mL
Parkland	RL: 4 mL/kg/%TBSA burn C: No D5W: No	RL: No C: 20–60% of estimated plasma volume D5W: to maintain diuresis
Modified Brooke	RL: 2 mL/kg/%TBSA burn C: No D5W: No	RL: No C: 0.3–0.5mL/kg/%TBSA burn D5W: to maintain diuresis
Modified Parkland	RL: 4 mL/kg/%TBSA burn C: No D5W: No	RL: No C: 0.3–1 mL Alb 5%/kg/%TBSA burn/16 per hour D5W: to maintain diuresis

Abbreviations: Alb, human albumin; C, colloid solution; D5W, 5% dextrose in water; NS, 0.9% normal saline; RL, Ringer's lactate; TBSA, total body surface area.
[a] Perfusion rate: 50% first 8 hours and 50% next 16 hours (starting from "hour 0").
[b] Use 50% when burn ≥ 50% TBSA.

Remember M!

Resuscitation formulas are only an initial guide. The goal is 0.5 mL/kg/h in adult patients, that is, 30–50 mL/h (no more, no less).

Referral Criteria

Referral criteria are established based on burn injury categorization (►Table 18.6). First- and superficial second-degree burns < 5% TBSA, without affecting compromised areas or aggravating factors can be referred to primary care facilities

Table 18.6 Burn injury categorization

Burn severity	Aggravating factors

• Extension (% TBSA)
• Deep:
  ° First-degree
  ° Superficial second-degree
  ° Deep second-degree
  ° Third-degree
• Location:
  ° Uncompromised areas
  ° Compromised areas
	• Trauma related:
	  ° Inhalation injury
	  ° Other associated injuries
	  ° Suspected aggression
	• Patient related:
	  ° Illnesses prone to worsen with stress caused by burn injury
	  ° Pregnancy
	  ° Unfavorable social conditions

and derived to a specialist only if healing is not achieved in a period of 15 days. Major burns, including burns > 15% TBSA (> 10% TBSA in children and elderly patients), third-degree burns ≥ 5% TBSA, and burns affecting compromised areas or with aggravating factors should always be referred to a hospital facility and the more complex ones taken directly to a burn care unit.

Hospital Care

Initial Assessment

On arrival to the burn unit, the ABCDE algorithm is reassessed and continuing monitoring of vital signs is maintained. Intubation criteria should be reviewed and indirect laryngoscopy or bronchoscopy performed if airway injury is suspected.

Burns are then washed with 0.9% NS and neutral soap or diluted chlorhexidine soapy solution, debriding all blisters, although small ones in painful areas such as the palms can be initially preserved. Location and depth of lesions is reassessed, and extension is calculated using the Lund and Browder's chart (▶Table 18.7).

A basic laboratory workup is done and additional tests added depending on each particular situation (▶Table 18.8). As a general guideline, laboratory tests should be performed every 8 hours during the acute phase.

Escharotomy

This is the only urgent surgical treatment and is indicated in deep circumferential burns. There should be a low threshold to perform an escharotomy because the consequences of not doing so may be devastating. Because eschar tissue is insensitive, escharotomies may be performed in an emergency room without anesthesia with a scalpel, although using an electric cautery allows for improved hemostasis. The incision must run along the entire eschar and traverse its full depth up to unaffected underlying tissue (commonly subcutaneous).

Thoracoabdominal escharotomies are the only justifiable surgical therapy in prehospital care when ventilation is compromised. Thoracic escharotomy follows the anterior axillary lines to meet at the subcostal level (▶Fig. 18.9), whereas abdominal escharotomy can be performed drawing a quadrant pattern (▶Fig. 18.10). Neck escharotomy should follow the sternocleidomastoid muscle, avoiding the trachea and major blood vessels. Extremity escharotomies are done on the medial and lateral borders, avoiding superficial neurovascular structures, whereas on the dorsum of the hand they should follow intermetacarpal spaces, thus preserving the extensor tendons. Finger escharotomy must follow the dorsal and palmar skin juncture to preserve digital neurovascular bundles, with incisions ideally placed on the nondominant side (radial side on the thumb and fifth finger and cubital side on the others) (▶Fig. 18.11).

Topical Treatment

The goal of topical agents is to maximize epithelialization and reduce bacterial colonization. Since its introduction in 1968, the most widely accepted topical treatment is 1% silver sulfadiazine, applied every 12–24 hours as a thick layer (2 mm). This hydrophobic cream keeps the wound bed moist; is painless and easy to apply; has wide antimicrobial action that includes gram-positive cocci, gram-negative bacilli, and fungi; but penetrates the eschar poorly. It adheres to the wound bed forming a whitish layer (pseudoeschar) that sloughs as the burn reepithelializes; however, it might impair proper assessment of burn depth. Leukopenia is a common finding in the first few days after its use, but it reverses spontaneously without having to halt treatment. Allergic reactions are infrequent. Its use in pregnant or lactating women and newborns is not advisable due to its sulfamide content. Deep burns benefit from adding cerium nitrate at 2.2% to 1% silver sulfadizine, which increases its bacteriostatic potency, dries and hardens the

Table 18.7 Lund and Browder's Chart (numbers correspond to % TBSA)

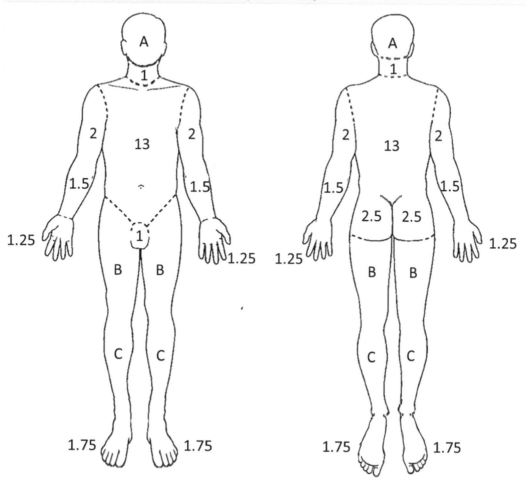

Age (years)	< 1	1-4	5-9	10-14	15	Adult
A (1/2 head)	9.5	8.5	6.5	5.5	4.5	3.5
B (1/2 thigh)	2.75	3.25	4	4.25	4.5	4.75
C (1/2 leg)	2.5	2.5	2.75	3	3.25	3.5

eschar, and allows for delay in the surgical treatment of unstable patients. Extensive descriptions of other topical treatments can be found in other texts. Finally, restrictive bandages must be avoided and the affected areas kept elevated.

Fluid Resuscitation

Resuscitation formulas should be considered only as an initial guideline, adjusting the perfusion according to hourly diuresis. Other variables to monitor

reanimation are clinical signs (level of consciousness, peripheral perfusion, heart rate, and blood pressure) and laboratory values (pH, base excess [BE], and lactic acid). Resuscitation should be assessed considering all variables and their trend over time rather than focusing on a particular single value.

During the first 24 hours, most adult patients are resuscitated effectively with 2-4 mL/kg/% TBSA burn although children requirements may approach 6 mL/kg/h. Half of the calculated volume should be administered during the first

Table 18.8 Workup on burn admission

Basic workup	Additional workup

• Blood: CBC (red series, white series, platelets), coagulation tests
• Biochemistry: Na⁺, K⁺, glucose, BUN, creatinine, liver enzymes, total serum proteins and albumin, CRP
• Acid–base balance
• Chest X-ray
• EKG
	• Inhalation injury: arterial blood gases with COHb
	• Other laboratory tests:
	  ∘ Pregnancy test
	  ∘ Toxic screening
	  ∘ Blood type
	• Other radiology tests:
	  ∘ Bone X-ray
	  ∘ CT scan

Abbreviations: BUN, blood urea nitrogen; CBC, complete blood count; COHb, carboxyhemoglobin; CRP, C-reactive protein; CT, computed tomography; EKG, electrocardiogram.

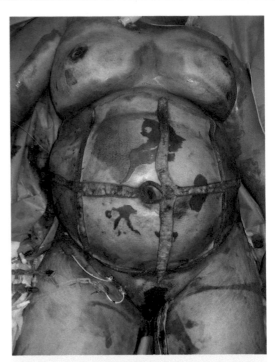

Fig. 18.10 Abdominal escharotomy.

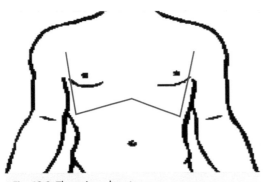

Fig. 18.9 Thoracic escharotomy.

8 hours and the other half in the remaining 16 hours, adjusting to endothelial permeability changes.

During the second 24 hours, with endothelial permeability restored, fluid resuscitation should be drastically reduced. The perfusion at a constant rate of about half of the volume given in the first 24 hours should be sufficient to maintain optimal diuresis. The addition of colloids in the form of fresh frozen plasma, dextran or human albumin improves resorption of edema increasing intravascular oncotic pressure (serum albumin level should be > 2.5 mg/dL). The premature use of colloids is generally discouraged for fear to worsening the hypovolemia and edema.

Certain conditions can cause volume requirements to be higher than conventional estimates. Examples include extensive third-degree burn, older patients, delayed resuscitation, associated trauma, smoke inhalation, and coincident alcohol intoxication.

When the volume given is insufficient to maintain diuresis or does so with volumes significantly higher than theoretical values, other strategies must be considered. The use of diuretics to force diuresis is not indicated, but earlier inclusion of colloids is a possibility because recent studies indicate that nonburned tissue's permeability begins to normalize 8–12 hours postburn. Refractory cases, particularly unstable patients with complex comorbidities, warrant invasive cardiovascular monitoring using a Swan–Ganz catheter or the less invasive Pulse Index Continuous Cardiac Output (PiCCO) monitor. PiCCO can provide information about the need for further resuscitation or vasoactive drugs; however, normal cardiac output values should never be the final goal, as it has been proven that this strategy favors hyperhydration. If the patient becomes oligoanuric, hemodialysis might be needed. Some authors recommend plasmapheresis or immediate burn debridement to reduce inflammatory response as a last resort.

Hypertonic crystalloid solutions, as Monafo first proposed, are an alternative to maintain diuresis with a reduced volume intake, risking hypernatremia and hyperosmolarity. Its proponents argue that

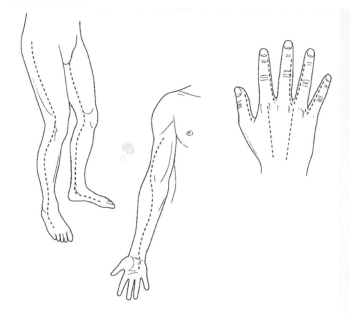

Fig. 18.11 Incisions for escharotomy in the extremities. (Reproduced from Bullocks et al, Plastic Surgery Emergencies Principles and Techniques, ©2008, Thieme Publishers, New York.)

it generates less edema but, in reality, what happens is cellular desiccation. This is precisely its limiting factor and urges caution. When serum Na^+ > 165 mEq/L, renal failure and cerebral edema occur.

Resuscitation finishes when diuresis is stable without the need for additional volume support, usually from the third day postburn. Patient monitoring during this period is based on fluid balance, patient weight, and daily laboratory results. The main hydroelectrolytic problems after resuscitation include the following:

1. *Volume overload (fluid creep):* A patient with a > 50% TBSA burn can experience a weight increase of up to 20% after resuscitation. Fluid overload causes cerebral edema, increased risk of compartment syndrome, and burn deepening as edema interferes with delivery of oxygen to tissues. At this point, treatment should provide basal fluid and electrolyte needs while favoring gradual edema resolution, with an advisable rate of 2–3% total body water loss per day until the initial weight is reached, around the 10th day. Of note, edema reabsorption may be deleterious in older patients with low cardiac output.

2. *High insensible losses of water through the burned surface:* This can be calculated by the following formula: Total insensible water loss (mL/h) = TBSA (m^2) × (25 + % TBSA burn).

3. *Low serum ions:* Dilutional low serum sodium (around Na^+ 130 mEq/L) tends to normalize with the hydric restriction applied during this phase. Ions such as K, Ca,P, and Mg tend to be low, and supplementation might be required.

Other Therapeutic Measures

In the absence of paralytic ileus, oral intake should be initiated as soon as possible to prevent villous atrophy and bacterial translocation. Insertion of a nasogastric tube should be considered in patients with extensive burn. Diet should be hyperproteic (1–2 g protein/kg/d) and hypercaloric (up to 150% of basal needs calculated using the Harris–Benedict formula), with a 3:1 ratio of carbohydrates to lipids. Total protein levels should be > 2.5 mg/dL. Administration of vitamins (A, C, D, E) and oligoelements (Zn, Se, Fe) supplements is advocated, whereas immunonutrition using glutamine, arginine, and omega-3 fatty acids still needs further evidence.

Additional metabolic stress caused by hypothermia, pain, and anxiety must be avoided. Medical strategies against stress response include anabolic drugs (growth hormone [GH], insulin, oxandrolone) and adrenergic blockers (propranolol). Nonsteroidal antiinflammatory drugs and glucocorticoids may impair wound healing.

Anemia, initially masked by hemoconcentration, soon becomes apparent and should be corrected with transfusion. Preventive measures against tetanus, stress ulcers, and deep vein thrombosis should be considered, whereas antibiotic prophylaxis is not encouraged.

Physical rehabilitation including elevation of affected areas to reduce edema and use of splints to prevent joint retraction, passive mobilization to reduce rigidity, and active mobilization against resistance to avoid muscle atrophy and osteoporosis should be started as soon as the patient's condition allows it.

Acute Surgical Management

Escharectomy

In 1970 Janzekovic proposed early escharectomy of deep burns and definitive coverage with skin grafts as opposed to waiting for spontaneous debridement and granulation tissue formation prior to grafting. The rationale behind early excision of burns is based on the reduction of inflammatory mediators and bacterial colonization of wounds. This practice has become the gold standard to treat burns with an expected spontaneous healing time of > 21 days, as it has been shown to reduce hospital stay, decrease mortality for extensive burns, and provide better functional and aesthetic results.

Remember   M!
The treatment of choice for deep burns is early debridement and definitive coverage with skin grafts.

Given that an early and accurate diagnosis is often difficult, especially in cases of partial-thickness burns with initially undefined depth areas, and the fact that clinical accuracy is as low as 66% and biopsy is of limited use (only valid for a region of the burn at a fixed time), multiple techniques have been proposed to analyze physical changes in burned skin, particularly those related to tissue perfusion. Among these, laser Doppler imagining has proven to have the maximal sensitivity and specificity.

Types of Escharectomy

Tangential debridement, the classical method originally described by Janzekovic, eliminates the eschar, layer by layer, until vital bleeding tissue is reached. It is carried out using specifically designed surgical knives, such as Watson's manual dermatome, or Goulian's knife for smaller areas.

Fascial debridement uses electrocautery to remove all the skin and subcutaneous fat down to but not including deep fascia. It is an aggressive technique that sacrifices viable tissue, exposes deeper structures, generates functional problems due to loss of superficial neurovascular structures, and causes significant corporal contour defects. Thus it is reserved for life-threatening burns like extensive third-degree and infected burns.

The hydrosurgery system (Versajet, Smith & Nephew) provides an interesting alternative, especially for delicate areas, such as the face, genitalia, and interdigital spaces.

There has been renewed interest in enzymatic debridement using bromelain (NexoBrid, MediWound), a proteolytic agent derived from pineapple that degrades only denatured dermal proteins in a 4-hour period (▶ Fig. 18.12). The process is painful and therefore is done under deep sedoanalgesia. Bromelain facilitates early diagnosis of burn depth, reduces the need for escharotomy for circumferential burns, and reduces blood loss when compared with surgical debridement.

Blood Loss and Hypothermia Management

Bleeding and hypothermia are the main limiting factors that put the patient's life at risk during surgery. Units of packed red blood cells, fresh plasma, and platelets must be readily available before surgery starts. Strategies to reduce bleeding include tourniquets, subcutaneous infiltration with diluted adrenaline solutions, fascial debridement, thorough hemostasis by applying solutions of oxygenated water or highly concentrated adrenaline, spraying the wound bed with thrombin or fibrinogen, placing compressive bandages, and limb elevation. Strategies to prevent heat loss include raising the room temperature to around 32°C, exposing only the areas that will be treated, using direct warming devices on the patient, and heating all intravenous fluids and anesthetic gases prior to their administration.

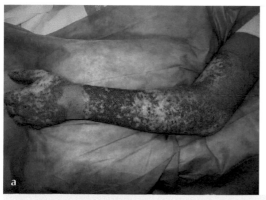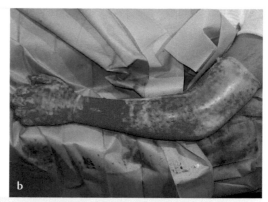

Fig. 18.12 (a) Flame second-degree burn of the upper extremity after enzymatic debridement with NexoBrid.
(b) Wound covered with Biobrane.

Definitive Wound Closure

Skin Substitutes

Split-thickness skin grafts (STSG) are the gold standard, provided that a healthy, well-vascularized wound bed is present. Laminar STSG are usually reserved to cover areas of particular functional or aesthetic value, whereas meshed STSG allow for better drainage and coverage of large surfaces when donor site availability is limited, though the final aesthetic and functional result may be worse. In extreme cases, maximum expansion is possible fragmenting the skin graft into small pieces as Chinese or Meek techniques.

Full-thickness skin grafts (FTSG) are rarely used in acute definitive coverage. Flaps are selected to cover poorly vascularized wounds or burns with exposed underlying structures.

Epidermal Substitutes

Cultured epidermal autografts (CEA) should be considered when donor sites are insufficient. They are obtained from a processed skin biopsy, and it takes 3–4 weeks to obtain 1 m². They are expensive, vulnerable to infection during the take phase, and, given the lack of a dermal component, provide unstable coverage due to weak fixation to the wound bed.

The ReCell system (Avita Medical) treats autologous skin enzymatically to obtain an epidermal cells suspension that is sprayed over the wound bed.

Dermal Substitutes (Dermal Matrices)

Dermal substitutes are membranes that adhere to the wound bed and become colonized by the host cells, working as a scaffold for a new dermis. Because they do not provide an epidermal layer, final coverage with a thin laminar STSG or a CEA is needed. Thinnest dermal matrices accept immediate epidermal graft. In other case, we must wait 3-4 weeks to allow its vascularization, although it can be accelerated using negative pressure wound therapy.

Some commercially available acellular biological dermal matrices include Integra (Integra LifeSciences), made of bovine collagen and glycosaminoglycan chondroitin-6-sulphate with an external silicone sheet; Matriderm (Skin and Health Care AG), a matrix of bovine collagen type I, III, and V and elastin; and Alloderm (LifeCell), a cryopreserved allogenic dermis. DermaGraft (Advance BioHealing) is an alloplastic dermal matrix made of polyglactin with allogenic neonatal fibroblasts.

Dermal substitutes can be used to cover areas with high functional or aesthetic value, as well as wounds with small areas of exposed structures, such as bones or tendons (▶Fig. 18.13). Dermal matrices are also a good option for revision burn surgery.

Temporary Wound Closure

Temporary dressings enable transient physiologic closure of wounds minimizing desiccation, risk of infection, local inflammatory reaction, and

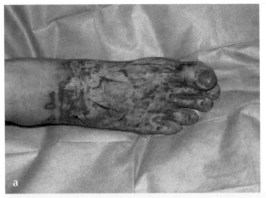
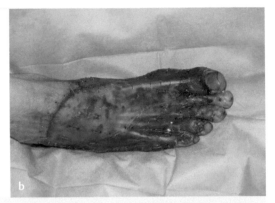

Fig. 18.13 (a) Third-degree burn on foot by sulfuric acid. (b) Definitive wound cover with a dermal substitute (Integra bilayer).

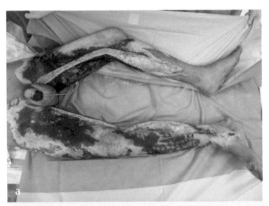
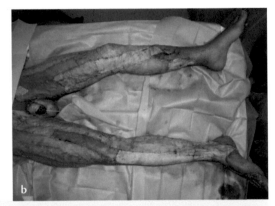

Fig. 18.14 (a) Flame third-degree burn on lower extremities. (b) After fascial debridement and coverage with skin homografts.

pain. They can be used to cover superficial burns and skin graft donor sites until spontaneous reepithelialization occurs, or as a bridge between debridement and definitive closure of deep burns.

Biological Temporal Substitutes

Cadaveric split-thickness skin homografts are the temporal substitute of choice (▶Fig. 18.14). Their cellular viability depends on the processing technique—whereas cell death occurs when they are preserved in glycerol or lyophilized, viable cells remain with cryopreservation or, better yet, refrigeration. Only homografts with viable cells become vascularized, acquiring a significant resistance to infection, greater than any other temporal substitute.

Homografts can be used to prepare the wound bed for definitive closure, providing growth factors, essential cytokines, and promoting angiogenesis. They might also work to test graft take in wound beds with uncertain viability. In Alexander's sandwich technique, homografts protect widely meshed autografts used to cover extensive burns.

Due to the burned patient's state of immunosuppression, homograft rejection does not occur until 1–2 weeks after application, although strategies are being studied to prolong homograft survival. Because of rejection, homografts require periodic replacement to avoid infection until definitive closure can be performed. Of note, part of their dermis may remain integrated in the wound, improving the quality of subsequent coverage. Disadvantages of homografts include their cost, the need for a tissue bank, and the possibility of disease transmission.

Other biological substitutes less commonly used are amniotic membranes and xenografts from porcine skin. Even though they may adhere to the wound bed they never vascularize.

Synthetic Temporal Substitutes

Biobrane (Dow B. Hickham) is constituted by a nylon layer impregnated with porcine collagen peptides and covered with a thin, perforated silicone sheet. It is a transparent occlusive dressing that allows wound monitoring by direct vision (▶Fig. 18.12b). It should be covered with a dry dressing (moisture interferes with its adherence to the wound bed) and never used on infected wounds. TransCyte (Advance Tissue Sciences) is composed of allogenic neonatal fibroblasts, which are then cultured over the nylon mesh of Biobrane. Suprathel (PolyMedics Innovations) consists of a porous layer of lactic acid polymers that is permeable to oxygen and water vapor and generates an acid antibacterial microenvironment favoring epithelialization. It adapts well to contours, and it degrades spontaneously by hydrolysis in approximately 4 weeks.

Surgical Strategy

Burns < 20% TBSA can be treated in a single surgical session. When depth is initially undefined, escharectomy should be delayed until the injury becomes fully demarcated, usually in 10-14 days. Conversely, when a diagnosis of a deep burn is made on initial assessment, early debridement and definitive wound closure should be performed as soon as possible. Burns > 20% TBSA will invariably require several surgeries until final closure is achieved and two surgical plans are possible.

One strategy follows the principle "debride first and cover later," that focuses on debridement to control the inflammatory response, the blood loss with escharectomy, and the risk of burn infection, using temporal substitutes until definitive coverage is possible. Complete debridement in one surgical session within the first 3 days is an aggressive approach with multiple logistical (operating room availability, qualified personnel on-call, available blood bank support) and medical problems (initial hemodynamic instability, unreliable early burn depth assessment, uncertain prognosis) that does not offer a clear reduction in mortality. In contrast, staged debridement is

a practice commonly adopted. It starts on the third day, when the patient is stable, debriding up to 20% TBSA every 2–3 days so that complete escharectomy is achieved within 7–10 days, before colonization of eschar by gram-negative bacteria occurs. The trunk and extremities are treated first, leaving the head, neck, and hands for the final surgical interventions because they represent smaller surfaces and more demanding surgery.

The other strategy focuses on definitive coverage and follows the principle "only debride what you can definitely cover," delaying future surgeries until donor sites become replenished. This strategy sets surgeries every 7–10 days, treating first the full-thickness burns and allowing demarcation of injuries of indeterminate depth. Problems with this approach are the prolongation of inflammatory response, higher risk of eschar infection, and increased blood loss during debridement as the wound increases its vascularization with time.

18.4 Electrical Injuries

18.4.1 Basic Science

Electrical current (EC) or electricity is a flow of charges initiated when two points with different electrical potential are joined by a conductor. Ohm's law defines EC in the following manner: $I = V/R$, where I represents intensity (flow of charges), R represents resistance (difficult current passage), and V represents voltage or electrical tension (electrical potential difference).

Electrical charges in movement collide with conductor molecules (opposition force), which increases their kinetic energy, that is, temperature. This phenomenon is known as Joule's effect, and the heat generated is described by the formula $Q = I^2 \times R \times t$, where t represents time.

Electrical lesions are classified according to whether EC has passed through the body (shock injuries) or not (flash injuries).

18.4.2 Electrical Flash Injuries

Flash injuries are caused by exposure to a voltaic arc phenomenon. When sufficient voltage is applied across an electrical insulator as the air, it turns into a conductor due to the ionization of its molecules. When the ionization reverts, the energy is emitted as thermal radiation (flash), burning exposed areas, typically face, neck, and hands. They are rarely full-thickness lesions unless ignition of clothes occurs. Furthermore, the arc phenomenon also causes extreme heating and dilation of the air due to the Joule's effect generating a shockwave that can lead to falls and associated traumatic lesions. In addition, flash injuries can show a carbonaceous aspect due to sublimated parts of the electrical panel traveling through the air and resting onto the exposed skin (traumatic tattoo).

18.4.3 Electric Shock Injuries

Electric shock (ES) or electrification entails the passage of electrical current through the organism. Electrocution refers to death by ES. In monopolar accidents the victim acts as a ground line (electric leak), whereas in bipolar accidents the victim becomes part of the circuit (short circuit).

The effects of EC can be categorized by the sensation, tetany, and heart fibrillation thresholds, which refer to the minimum intensity necessary to cause these effects (▶Table 18.9).

The EC produces both direct and indirect injuries.

Direct Injuries

1. *Thermal injury:* Resistance to current flow increases the temperature of the tissue (Joule's effect). When current flow ceases and tissues refresh, heat can be transferred to other adjacent tissues.
2. *Nonthermal injury:* Electricity causes membrane depolarization and activation of excitable muscle and nervous cells. Moreover, it causes denaturalization of macromolecules, such as proteins and nucleic acids, permeabilization of membranes with cellular edema (electroporation), and lysis.

Table 18.9 Clinical manifestations of different current intensities

Clinical effect	Current threshold (mA)
Tingling sensation	1–4
Let go	3–9
Tetany of skeletal muscle	16–20
Paralysis of respiratory muscles	20–50
Ventricular fibrillation	50–100

Indirect Injuries

1. *Thermal injury:* Indirect thermal injury is caused by accidental ignition of garments.
2. *Massive cellular death:* It results especially from muscle destruction, elevating compartment pressure (compartment syndrome), and releasing potentially harmful metabolites, such as potassium (cardiac arrhythmias) and myoglobin (obstruction of renal tubules).
3. *Vascular injury:* Low-flow and small-diameter vessels (< 4 mm) are the most affected. Injury to the intermediate layer may cause arterial bleeding, whereas injury to the intima causes thrombosis and ischemia of the corresponding angiosome. Cellular injury also stimulates the release of thromboxane A_2, promoting vasoconstriction. Both mechanisms may explain the progression of tissue necrosis after an ES.
4. *Associated trauma:* Falls are frequent after loss of consciousness or muscle imbalance, or due to explosive mechanisms linked to a voltaic arc. Tetany (sustained contraction) can cause dislocations and fractures.

Conditioning Factors

The main conditioning factors of injury are intensity and duration of EC. Higher-intensity currents reduce skin electrical resistance so that voltages > 600 V allow more current to flow to internal organs. Additionally, prolonging time of exposure lowers the intensity thresholds of sensation, tetany, and fibrillation (the heart fibrillation threshold falls especially when the duration of exposure exceeds the duration of a heartbeat). Because intensity and duration are rarely known, voltage is currently used to categorize the damaging potential of an EC, which is classified as high voltage (≥ 1,000 V) and low voltage (< 1,000 V).

The type of current is another conditioning factor. First, for the same duration, all three intensity thresholds are lower for alternating current (AC) than for direct current (DC). Secondly, whereas DC causes a single muscle contraction that throws the victim away from the electrical source, AC produces tetany that prolongs contact with the source, making it potentially more dangerous. Thirdly, whereas AC is more likely to cause arrhythmia, DC is more likely to cause asystole.

The path taken by an EC also determines which structures are affected, with the brain and heart being the most critical vital organs. Hand to hand pathways have a higher risk of fibrillation, whereas hand to foot pathways have a greater incidence of myocardial necrosis.

Tissue resistance increases with low water content, so heat production follows the order bone > fat > tendon > skin > muscle > mucous membranes > vessels > nerves. In addition, dry skin generates more heat than moist skin for the same reason. Resistance also increases when an EC traverses large paths with a small cross section so wrists and ankles habitually show the worst lesions.

Clinical Features

External Injuries

External injuries are generated by Joule's effect on the points of passage of the EC and may be absent in moist skin. Monopolar accidents commonly cause lesions in contact entry points (head or hands) and contact exit points (feet), whereas bipolar accidents are associated with injuries on both hands. Children may show mouth injuries when biting electric wires. Other possible patterns include a single wound (in AC the electricity enters and exits through the same point), one main lesion and several satellite secondary lesions (caused by magnetic fields that generate ancillary currents of erratic distribution), and symmetrical burns across flexures or "kissing burns" (EC jumps across flexures because its lower resistance due to its humidity).

Low voltage usually causes injuries of limited size that resemble third- or even fourth-degree burns. Conversely, high-voltage injuries have a greater potential for tissue damage and may show an explosive appearance.

Internal Injuries

Lesions caused by electricity typically show a discontinuous distribution ("patchy necrosis") and varying severity. External injuries have a poor correlation with the internal extent of damage (iceberg-like pattern) and are not good indicators of tissue injury.

> **Remember** **M!**
>
> Electrical shock injuries show a "patchy necrosis" pattern, and external injuries correlate poorly with internal injuries.

Skeletal muscle necrosis is characteristically located in deeper planes adjacent to the bone in discontinuity with cutaneous injuries. Clinically, it resembles a crush syndrome. Muscle necrosis causes massive release of K (which may alter the acid–base balance and also cause arrhythmias), cytolysis enzymes (e.g., aspartate transaminase, alanine transaminase, and CPK), and myoglobin (risk of renal failure due to tubule clogging). Destruction of muscle within the nonexpandable fascial envelope can cause a compartment syndrome, which is clinically characterized by the five P's: pain, paresthesia, paralysis, pallor, and pulselessness. Pain appears first and is disproportionate and exacerbated by passive extension of the affected muscle compartment. Paralysis and ischemic manifestations are late symptoms. The compartment is tense to the touch. The upper extremity assumes a typical posture characterized by a flexed elbow, pronated forearm, flexed wrist, and clawed hand (intrinsic minus posture with hyperextension of the metacarpophalangeal joint, flexion of the proximal and distal interphalangeal joints, and thumb adduction) (▶Fig. 18.15). In addition, muscle necrosis favors gaseous gangrene and sepsis.

Cardiac muscle necrosis is unlikely and clinically resembles cardiac contusion, altering the electrocardiographic (EKG) results and elevating CPK-MB. It can be mistaken with acute myocardial infarction, an otherwise extremely rare event in this scenario.

Electrical stimulation of skeletal muscle triggers involuntary contraction. Whereas affecting lower extremities can cause falls, in upper extremities it precludes the victim from releasing the electric source

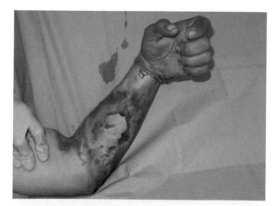

Fig. 18.15 High-voltage electrical injury. Compartment syndrome with the typical upper extremity position.

because flexors are more powerful than extensors, thus prolonging the duration of contact. Otherwise, muscle tetany can cause skeletal injuries (joint dislocation and fractures) and respiratory arrest (affecting diaphragmatic and thoracic muscles).

Electrical stimulation of the heart can cause asystole or arrhythmias. Ventricular fibrillation is the leading cause of sudden death following an ES. In survivors, the most commonly detected arrhythmias are atrial fibrillation and nonspecific repolarization disorders.

Nervous system lesions may occur as a consequence of direct electrical injury to neurons and myelin, or indirectly via vascular injury, compartment syndrome, and associated trauma. Clinical features can appear early or late, with the latter usually carrying a worse prognosis. Central nervous system affectation most frequently manifests as transient loss of consciousness with concomitant headache, confusion, and recent events amnesia. Cardiorespiratory arrest, focal neurological deficits, and seizures may also occur. Spinal cord disorders, both motor and sensitive, can develop and affect the lower extremities more frequently. Late onset is more commonly ischemic in nature and includes transverse myelitis, Guillain–Barré syndrome, and amyotrophic lateral sclerosis. Peripheral motor neuropathy is more prevalent than sensitive neuropathy, causing spasticity and weakness. Finally, sympathetic hyperactivity is the hallmark of autonomic injury, with visceral (intestinal, urinary, and sexual) and vascular dysfunction (vasospasm). Diverse neuropsychological manifestations might also be present.

Eye involvement typically manifests as late-onset cataracts, usually bilateral and years after injury. Their pathological mechanism is unknown.

Damage to visceras may occur directly due to current passage along them (especially hollow viscera) or indirectly secondary to vascular, neural or associated trauma injuries.

Pregnant patients require special consideration because cases of miscarriage and fetal injury have been described.

Lightning Injury

Lightning is an EC with millions of volts. A cloud-to-ground lightning is a voltaic arc that crosses the air and may enter the victim directly or indirectly. When it strikes directly over the victim, usually enters through head orifices (eyes, ears, and mouth). Conversely, when it first strikes the ground, the EC spreads out radially and enters the victim through the feet, whereas if it strikes a tree or any other nearby object, the EC enters the victim through the contact surface, such as hands.

Lightning injury rarely induces tissue necrosis because exposure time is minimal. Rhabdomyolysis is uncommon and skin lesions are typically superficial and small, punctate or linear in shape. The so-called Lichtenberg figure is a transient ramified erythema that quickly fades away, resembling an allergic rash. However, predominant clinical manifestations are heart and respiratory arrest, autonomous nervous system disorders, loss of consciousness, and vision and hearing damage. The associated shock wave may cause traumatic injuries from falls and barotrauma.

Treatment

Common problems during primary assessment include cardiorespiratory arrest, arrhythmias, multifactorial shock (hypovolemic due to burn and traumatic bleeding, cardiac due to arrhythmia and myocardial necrosis, and neurogenic due to spinal cord lesion), loss of consciousness, and other neurologic disorders. Resuscitation of a cardiorespiratory arrest should be aggressive and extended in time more than usual because there are high chances of success. Secondary assessment should rule out associated trauma, particularly in high-voltage injuries.

Victims of ES should be transferred to a burn unit immediately. Continuous EKG monitoring is mandatory during the first 48 hours in risk patients: loss of consciousness, those recovering from a cardiac arrest, initial abnormal EKG, high-voltage accidents, transthoracic current passage, and previous cardiovascular medical history. If the initial EKG is normal, late-onset arrhythmias are infrequent.

Because resuscitation formulas do not consider internal injuries, they usually underestimate the fluid requirements in electrical burns, which can reach up to 7 mL/kg/% TBSA. The goal is to obtain a urinary output of 1–1.5 mL/kg/h (75–100 mL/h) in adults until urine becomes clear to reduce the risk of tubular obstruction by myoglobin. Strategies to improve urine clearance include administration of mannitol and urine alkalinization.

Initial blood work should include markers of skeletal and cardiac muscle cytolysis (CPK, CPK-MB). Their levels correlate with the amount of muscle injury, risk of amputation, and length of hospitalization. They should be interpreted with caution because skeletal muscle cells can contain as much as 25% of CPK-MB fraction.

The development of compartment syndrome is a surgical emergency. Fasciotomies are indicated when absolute compartment pressure is > 30 mm Hg or when the difference between arterial diastolic pressure and compartment pressure is < 30 mm Hg. Nevertheless, in the presence of suggestive clinical findings it is better to proceed with surgery due to the devastating outcomes that a nontreated compartment syndrome can have. Fasciotomies should be performed in the operating room, under general anesthesia and limb tourniquet without exsanguination. Incisions are made through skin and deep fascia, making sure the affected compartment is adequately released (▶Fig. 18.16). Dressings should be used to prevent desiccation of exposed tissue while the wounds remain open.

Treatment of electrical injuries typically involves serial debridements before definitive closure, usually starting on the third day on a stabilized patient and repeated every 2–3 days until a viable wound bed is obtained. Urgent sessions might be needed in cases of severe systemic repercussion, such as refractory acidosis and renal failure. Amputations are frequently needed in high-voltage injuries.

Early assessment of the actual severity of the lesion is not easy. Imaging studies (CT scan, MRI and gammagram) are rarely required because they offer no more information than what is readily seen in the operating room, where failure of muscle to respond to electrocautery stimulation represents an ominous sign, even in the presence of active bleeding. Nerves, tendons, joints, and bones

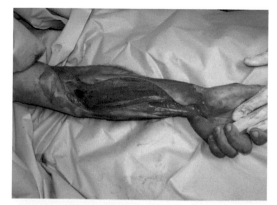

Fig. 18.16 Extensive fasciotomy for compartment syndrome decompression following an electrical injury to the upper extremity.

can be preserved by providing a well vascularized tissue cover. Once edema of the compartment has subsided around day 7–10, fasciotomy wounds may be closed primarily with presuturing devices, or alternatively, with skin grafts.

Rehabilitation plays a paramount role in the final treatment of ES lesions, though unfortunately sequelae are the rule. Long-term follow-up is necessary due to the possibility of late-onset ophthalmic and neurologic disorders.

18.5 Chemical Injuries

These are traumatic injuries caused by chemical agents affecting the hand and upper extremity more frequently. Most chemical products are composed of one or several active components mixed with excipients or additives that enhance their properties. They may come as solids, gases, or liquids. A large number and variety of chemical substances are available for domestic purposes (cleaners and disinfectants, fertilizers, insecticides), industrial applications, and even as chemical weapons.

18.5.1 Physiopathology of Injury

The severity of injury depends on the properties and quantity of the chemical agent, location and size of the lesion, the possibility of absorption, and the duration of chemical action.

Exposure to chemical agents usually implies contact through the skin and mucous membranes. Besides their local effect, chemical agents can produce systemic toxicity when an extensive area of skin surface is involved or when they are systemically absorbed by ingestion or inhalation. Importantly, the injurious effect of chemical agents is not limited to their exposure time. It only stops when all the reactants are consumed into their products or the chemical agent is neutralized.

> **Remember** M!
>
> Chemical agents continue to harm until the reactants are spontaneously consumed into their products or the chemical agent is neutralized.

Chemical agents damage tissues by interaction with proteins and other molecules. At least six different mechanisms have been described, with some agents involving more than one and others having an unknown mechanism:

- Oxidizing agents denature proteins by incorporating oxygen, chlorine, or sulfur atoms to their molecules. Examples: iodinated products, lye, oxygen, peroxides (hydrogen peroxide), potassium permanganate, and chromic acid.
- Reducing agents denature proteins by transferring electrons to them. Examples: hydrogen, nonmetal hydrides (hydrochloric acid), metal hydrides (aluminum and lithium hydrides), mercury products, nitric acid, and calcium hydroxide.
- Corrosive agents denature proteins by oxidation-reduction reactions and molecular breakdown (lysis). Alkaline corrosives tend to be more harmful than their acid counterparts. Examples: white phosphorus, carbolic acid, and alkaline agents (sodium and potassium hydroxides, lye).
- Desiccating agents extract water from tissues. Example: sulfuric acid.
- Protoplasm poisons block the use of certain ions essential for cell metabolism (hydrofluoric and oxalic acids) or create ester bonds with proteins, resulting in salts (formic and acetic acids).
- Vesicant agents typically cause blisters. They prevent cell division (mustards) or cell respiration (lewisite).

In addition, chemical agents may also produce thermal injury by releasing heat from an exothermal chemical reaction or by ignition of flammable products like alkali metals (ignite in contact with water) and white phosphorous (ignites in contact with oxygen).

18.5.2 Classification and Clinical Features

Chemical agents can be grouped according to pH in acids and bases. Strong acids (pH < 2) and strong bases (pH > 11.5) are those that are entirely dissociated in water. Acids work as proton donors causing *coagulative tissue necrosis*, whereas bases act as protons acceptors causing *liquefactive tissue necrosis* and *fat saponification*, a difference that explains the greater capacity of bases to damage deeper structures. Chemical agents can also be categorized as organic or inorganic according to their origin. As a general rule, organic agents cause cell membrane destruction, and inorganic agents rest primarily in the cellular interstitium.

Strong Bases

Sodium and potassium hydroxides are commonly used as household cleaning products and soaps and have corrosive effects, causing deep injuries with liquefactive necrosis. Eye injuries are particularly devastating (▶ Fig. 18.17).

Calcium hydroxide is a reducing agent constituting an integral part of cement. It typically affects the lower extremities, where it causes both a chemical and a thermal injury due to exothermal reaction.

Weak Bases

Sodium hypochlorite is a powerful oxidizing and corrosive agent, frequently used as a disinfectant (Dakin solution), a drinking water treatment agent, a textile bleaching agent, and in household cleaning products (lye).

Strong Acids

Usually presenting as colorless liquids, strong acids are widely used for industrial applications in metal purification and cleansing, and as laboratory intermediate reactants in the manufacturing process of fertilizers, pesticides, dyes, and plastic fibers.

Sulfuric acid is an inorganic acid with a powerful desiccant effect, which produces a strong exothermal reaction that leaves behind a typical blackish eschar. When in contact with hydrocarbons, it yields carbon, water vapor, and gases, such as carbon dioxide and sulfur dioxide, the latter being particularly toxic.

Hydrochloric acid (muriatic acid) is the least dangerous of strong acids. Its resultant eschar tends to be grayish, and inhalation of its fumes can lead to pulmonary edema.

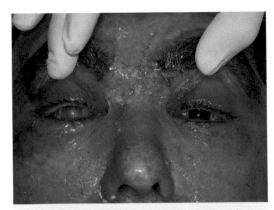

Fig. 18.17 Chemical burn on face and eyes by sodium hydroxide (strong alkali).

Hydrofluoric acid is a liposoluble inorganic acid. Although its protons act as a corrosive agent, the fluoride ion behaves as a protoplasm poison by three mechanisms: (1) binding cations, such as calcium and magnesium; (2) favoring the displacement of potassium to the extracellular space by blocking the Na^+/K^+-ATPase pump; and (3) causing a direct toxic effect on the myocardium, increasing its irritability and elongating the QT interval. Heart involvement (arrhythmias) is the leading cause of death following exposure. Local cutaneous injuries are very painful and usually appear with a whitish scar. In the fingertips, this acid may penetrate through the hyponychium and into the nail bed, causing osteolysis by decalcification of the distal phalanges.

Chromic acid is an oxidizing and corrosive agent that can easily penetrate cell membranes. Due to its local anesthetic effect the patient might underestimate the effect of injury. Burns > 10% TBSA are deadly due to multiple organ failure.

Nitric acid is a powerful oxidizing agent that leaves a yellowish eschar and when absorbed acts as a protoplasm poison by the formation of nitrates when it binds to proteins.

Oxalic acid is a reducing agent that forms insoluble precipitates with metal ions. In combination with calcium, it forms calcium oxalate, which may lead to hypocalcemia.

Weak Acids

Formic acid (methanoic acid) is the simplest organic acid with a single carbon atom. Though originally isolated from red ants, it is also present in bees and some species of nettles. It exhibits an irritating smell and acts as a protoplasm poison, forming ester bonds with proteins. It may cause multiple organ failure if systemically absorbed (▶Fig. 18.18).

Carbolic acid (phenic acid, phenol, hydroxybenzene) is a whitish agent with a strong, sweet smell, first used by Joseph Lister as a local disinfectant agent. In the health care sector, carbolic acid is used in the fabrication of acetylsalicylic acid, as a topical anesthetic, to infiltrate the amputation stumps of peripheral nerves, and as an exfoliating agent (chemical peeling). It is a powerful corrosive acid that initially forms a white covering of precipitate proteins onto the skin before sloughing. Skin absorption is almost as fast as inhalational absorption. It is cardiotoxic (arrhythmias),

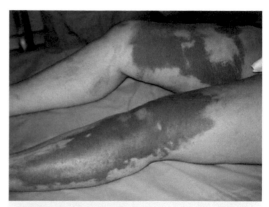

Fig. 18.18 Formic acid burn.

neurotoxic (painless injuries), and nephrotoxic. Burns affecting > 400 cm^2 are life threatening.

Alkali Metals

Remarkable examples are sodium, potassium, and lithium, which are always combined in nature. They function as reducing agents, oxidizing easily upon contact with oxygen and more so with water. In combination with water they yield the corresponding hydroxide and hydrogen, which produces a particularly explosive and exothermal chemical reaction.

White Phosphorus

Used as incendiary agent in weapons and pyrotechnics, and also in the manufacturing of disinfectants and pesticides, white phosphorus ignites spontaneously if temperature exceeds 34°C. Its oxidation generates phosphorus pentoxide and phosphoric acid, both highly corrosive agents that cause very painful injuries. The eschar is typically yellow and fluorescent. White phosphorus is readily absorbed due to its elevated lipid solubility, causing hypocalcemia, hyperphosphatemia, and cardiac arrhythmia. In the first 8 hours, patients may experience gastrointestinal symptoms, and after an indolent period of a few days, multiorgan failure and central nervous system dysfunction may result in death. Injuries > 10% TBSA are life threatening.

Vesicant Agents

Used as weapons, vesicant agents cause blisters in skin and mucous membranes, together with a strong burning sensation. Mustards owe their name to their smell. Sulfur mustard, commonly known as mustard gas, when absorbed, yields sulfonium, which impairs cellular division and function by alkylating nucleic acids and proteins. The basal cell layer of the epidermis, the most metabolically active, is particularly affected. The rupture of anchoring filaments with the basement membrane explains the formation of blisters, which concentrate in cutaneous flexures, conjunctiva, and the respiratory tract due to increased absorption in moist, warm areas. They form a few hours following exposure, may progress for up to 2 weeks, and heal considerably more slowly than a comparable thermal burn. In addition, melanogenesis is stimulated and the affected skin appears hyperpigmented.

Lewisite, a derivative of arsenic, is another oily liquid vesicant agent, which, unlike sulfur mustard, has increased local effect under conditions of low temperature and low humidity, and its systemic toxicity occurs more rapidly and is more severe. When absorbed it is hydrolyzed to hydrochloric acid and to chlorovinyldichloroarsine (lewisite oxide), both highly toxic. In alkaline solutions it can also form the trivalent form of arsenic, which blocks pyruvate dehydrogenase, among other effects.

18.5.3 Treatment

Prevention of rescue staff contamination, identification of the causative agent(s), assessment of systemic toxicity, and a formal ABCDE protocol are the initial priorities. All injuries caused by chemical agents should receive specialized emergency care.

The characteristics of the eschar may indicate the agent involved; however, depth of injury is not always readily evident on initial assessment, especially for alkalis. Although it has not been studied specifically, fluid resuscitation therapy should follow the same principles applied to other burns, and in cases where ophthalmic injury is suspected, specialist consultation should be sought.

Initial management requires urgent interruption of the chemical effect because the duration of contact is the major determinant of injury severity. Garments must be removed and blisters drained in order to eliminate possible agent reservoirs. Likewise, when the injury involves the fingertips, the nail of the affected digit should be removed to drain possible nail bed deposits. Solid agents (dry lime, cement, white phosphorus, alkali metals) must be brushed off the skin. Ultraviolet light might help identify fluorescent white phosphorus particles.

Irrigation of affected areas is of paramount importance because it both removes and dilutes the chemical agent and reduces the risk of thermal injury associated with exothermal reactions. Copious tap water at room temperature or normal saline should be used for at least 20 minutes for acids and 30 minutes for alkalis. Irrigation should be performed carefully from a safe distance and tilting the affected area so that fluid flows away from the patient and not to other areas of the body. Irrigation can stop when the pH of the rinsing fluid becomes neutral and the burning sensation disappears. Alkali metals (e.g., sodium, potassium, and lithium) should not be irrigated because they ignite in combination with water; instead, the area should be covered with petroleum jelly or mineral oil. Phenol must be made soluble with sponges soaked in 50% polyethylene prior to irrigation. White phosphorus, which ignites spontaneously at 34°C, requires water immersion or a wet gauze dressing to avoid oxygen exposure.

Diphoterine (Prevor) is a universal neutralizing agent with chelating and amphoteric properties, which blocks chemical reactions in tissues and is active against > 600 chemicals. Furthermore, it is hypertonic, which allows extraction of already impregnated chemicals. Generated wastes are not irritating or toxic, and its effectiveness is faster than simple washing with water.

The use of specific neutralization agents is controversial because they may trigger an exothermic reaction or add a chemical injury themselves. Importantly, irrigation of chemical injuries should never be delayed by the search for a neutralizing agent. Proposed specific agents include the following:

1. *White phosphorus:* Treatment involves both intralesional injection of superoxide dismutase and topical application of copper sulfate 0.5–5%, which turns black and helps to identify the extent of injury during debridement. Systemic absorption of copper sulfate may cause hepatic and renal damage.
2. *Chromic acid:* Topical application of sodium thiosulfate 5%, irrigation with dilute sodium hyposulfite, and immediate eschar excision are possible treatments suggested.
3. *Hydrofluoric acid:* Possible strategies include hemodialysis, ion-exchange resins to chelate fluoride ions, and administration of calcium to

counteract hypocalcemia. Calcium gluconate is used as a 3.5% gel for topical skin application, as a 10% solution for locally subcutaneous injections (0.5 mL/cm²), as an intra-arterial regional infusion, as 1% eyedrops, or as nebulization if inhaled. Local injections in acral parts, such as the fingertips, should be performed cautiously due to the risk of compartment syndrome. Hexafluorine (Prevor) is a specific neutralizer for hydrofluoric acid.

> **Remember** **M!**
>
> Never delay irrigation of a chemical injury to seek a specific neutralizer.

18.6 Cold Injuries

These are thermal lesions caused by exposure to cold. Humidity, wind, and altitude aggravate the injury. Predisposing factors are extreme age, dehydration, malnutrition, peripheral vascular disease, sensitive neuropathy, mental issues, and drug abuse (alcohol). The hands and feet account for 90% of reported injuries.

18.6.1 Physiopathology of Injury

Three phases are distinguished in cold injuries. During the *cooling phase*, mechanisms of heat preservation are activated, including peripheral vasoconstriction, which is interrupted by intermittent vasodilation to prevent irreversible ischemia, in a process called cold-induced vasodilation or hunting response. If temperature continues to fall, heat-generation mechanisms, such as shivering, are initiated. In small children, with little muscular mass, heat production by brown fat is fundamental. If core temperature falls < 30°C heat-generation mechanisms fail, and with temperatures < 28°C the hunting response disappears. Maximal peripheral vasoconstriction occurs at a tissue temperature of 15°C, with the affected area appearing cold, firm to the touch, and mildly edematous, with a pale or purple hue and weak peripheral pulses. When tissue temperature is < 10°C there is functional neural damage, and the initial pain and itching sensation are replaced by a complete loss of sensation. At this point the process is still reversible.

In the *freezing phase*, when tissue temperature drops to < − 2°C, ice crystals form and tissues become frozen. Crystals disrupt cell integrity and cause cellular death. Freezing also leads to microvascular occlusion with subsequent tissue anoxia. Additionally, when freezing is slow, crystals are first formed in the extracellular space, making it hypertonic and leading to cell dehydration. Nerves, endothelium, and cartilage are the most vulnerable to cold, whereas skin, fat, and connective tissue are the most resistant.

During the *rewarming/reperfusion phase*, cellular injury reminiscent of that seen in ischemia/reperfusion injury occurs, with platelet aggregation, microthrombosis, and extravasation of fluid and erythrocytes. The degree of endothelial damage is the main determinant of injury. Whereas in mild cases the affected part shows hyperemia, interstitial edema, and blistering, severe cases present with perivascular hemorrhage, hemorrhagic blisters, and tissue necrosis (gangrene).

18.6.2 Nonfreezing Cold Injuries

Frostnip is the mildest form of nonfreezing cold injury and occurs after limited exposure of acral areas to nonfreezing temperatures. There is no cell injury, and complete resolution is the rule upon withdrawal from cold.

Perniosis or chilblain occurs following prolonged exposure to nonfreezing temperatures, especially in high-humidity conditions. Acute chilblain presents as red-purple skin papules or plaques affecting symmetrically distal regions with associated edema, itching, and pain. Blisters and ulcers may appear in severe cases. Stopping cold exposure and applying topical hydrating creams allow the lesions to recede in about 3 weeks. Topical vasodilators (e.g., nifedipine) can help to accelerate resolution and reduce recurrence. Chronic chilblain occurs after repeated exposures and is characterized by persisting lesions, which can lead to scarring and atrophy.

Trench and immersion foot was described in soldiers exposed for long periods to wet and cold nonfreezing conditions in trenches and lifeboats. The condition is characterized by edema, blistering, and ulceration. Recovery is usually slow, lasting several months, and severe cases may require amputation.

18.6.3 Frostbite or Freezing Cold Injuries

Frostbite occurs predominantly in feet, followed by hands and face (nose and ears) and is frequently associated with systemic hypothermia and other traumatic injuries. These are the most severe cold injuries, and typical sequelae are amputations, peripheral neuropathy, and increased cold sensitivity.

18.6.4 Clinical Staging

Classically, a clinical staging system analogous to burn injuries has been used for cold injuries, with first-degree injuries showing hyperemia and edema without necrosis; second-degree showing hyperemia, serous blisters, and partial-thickness skin necrosis; third-degree showing numb, livid skin, hemorrhagic blisters, and total-thickness skin necrosis; and fourth-degree showing gray, purple, or spotted skin zones with necrosis affecting deep tissue layers. Nowadays, however, it is more useful to classify cold injuries as superficial (first and second degree) and deep (third and fourth degree).

The evolution of injury is slow, and final clinical staging can only be performed a few weeks after cold exposure. Technetium-99m triple-phase bone scans obtained 2 days postinjury provide the best prognostic information, predicting the level of amputation in 84% of cases. Case reports suggest magnetic resonance angiography is superior to Tc-99m bone scans.

18.6.5 Medical Treatment

The first aim is to stop the freezing process, protecting the victim from wind and humidity and replacing wet clothes with dry ones. Rubbing, mobilizing, and bearing weight on the affected area are strictly forbidden because they may cause further trauma.

Initial treatment for cold injuries must follow the ABCDE algorithm, always ruling out associated hypothermia and traumatic injuries. Fluid resuscitation is not necessary for the extent of cold injuries but to treat dehydration, which is frequent during hypothermia (cold diuresis mediated by antidiuretic hormone suppression) and among alpinists (high altitude increases its risk).

In stable patients, once hypothermia has been reverted, rewarming of the affected area is the next priority only if renewed exposure to cold can be excluded because this results in more severe injury. It must be made slowly in nonfreezing cold injuries and quickly in freezing cold injuries.

Frostbite injuries should be immersed for 30–45 minutes in water containing chlorhexidine or povidone iodine with a temperature of 37–39°C until distal tissue perfusion recovers and tissue

becomes pliable. Active motion during rewarming is advised. Reperfusion is a painful process that requires the use of narcotic analgesia. Following reperfusion, skin should be dried and blisters addressed, although there is no consensus as to their management, with some authors always debriding, others only debriding hemorrhagic ones, and others arguing for conservation if they are intact, with drainage only if movement is restricted. Topical aloe vera can be helpful due to its antiprostaglandin effect. Finally the affected extremity is loosely bandaged, immobilized in a functional position, and elevated

Ibuprofen 12 mg/kg/d during the first week, divided into two daily doses (maximum of 2,400 mg/d), should be given for its antiprostaglandin effect because it seems to reduce progression of injury. Prophylactic antibiotics are not initially required.

Other proposed strategies are vasodilators (calcium-channel blockers, pentoxifyline, iloprost) and thrombolytic agents (heparin, plasminogen). Hyperbaric oxygen and sympathectomy require further evidence to support their recommendation.

> **Remember M!**
> Cold injuries should be rewarmed only after hypothermia has been corrected and no new cold exposures can be ensured.

18.6.6 Surgical Treatment

Fasciotomies are sometimes necessary after rewarming. Because premature amputation increases morbidity, in the absence of local infection or sepsis, it is advisable to delay definitive surgical treatment until spontaneous mummification and necrotic tissues are fully demarcated, which occurs usually 2–3 months postinjury.

18.7 Key Points

- Burns are traumatic injuries that mainly affect the most vulnerable population groups living in the poorest social conditions.
- Fire/flames closely followed by scalds are the more frequent etiologic factors of thermal injuries.
- Thermal damage is heterogeneous in its spatial distribution and can change over time due to evolution of stasis and hyperemic zones.

- Burns involving > 20% TBSA extend systemically the inflammatory response and pose a vital risk to the victim. Associated inhalation injury is an independent factor that dramatically worsens the prognosis.
- Resuscitation formulas are only an initial guide.
- Early debridement and definitive wound closure with autologous skin grafts constitute the gold standard treatment of deep burns.
- Electrical shock injuries show a "patchy necrosis" pattern, and external injuries correlate poorly with internal injuries.
- Electrical flash injuries are thermal lesions.
- Chemical agents continue to harm until they are neutralized or their spontaneous consumption occurs. Irrigation of a chemical injury should never be delayed by trying to find a specific neutralizer.
- Cold injuries should be rewarmed only after hypothermia has been corrected and no new cold exposures can be ensured.

Recommended Readings

Aguilera-Sáez J, Binimelis MM, Collado JM, et al. Electrical burns in times of economic crisis: A new epidemiologic profile. Burns. 2016; 42(8):1861–1866

Almahameed A, Pinto DS. Pernio (chilblains). Curr Treat Options Cardiovasc Med. 2008; 10(2):128–135

American Burn Association. National Burn Repository. Report of data from 2005–2014. Version 11.0. 2015. http://www.ameriburn.org/2015NBRAnnualReport.pdf. Accessed June 6, 2016

Arnoldo BD, Hunt JL, Sterling JP, Purdue GF. Electrical injuries. In: Herndon DN, ed. Total Burn Care. 4th ed. London: Saunders Elsevier; 2012:433–439

Atiyeh BS, Costagliola M. Cultured epithelial autograft (CEA) in burn treatment: three decades later. Burns. 2007; 33(4):405–413

Bailey B, Gaudreault P, Thivierge RL. Cardiac monitoring of high-risk patients after an electrical injury: a prospective multicentre study. Emerg Med J. 2007; 24(5):348–352

Baldwin A, Xu J, Attinger D. How to cool a burn: a heat transfer point of view. J Burn Care Res. 2012; 33(2):176–187

Barajas-Nava LA, López-Alcalde J, Roqué i Figuls M, Solà I, Bonfill Cosp X. Antibiotic prophylaxis for preventing burn wound infection. Cochrane Database Syst Rev. 2013(6):CD008738

Barqouni L, Abu Shaaban N, Elessi K. Interventions for treating phosphorus burns. Cochrane Database Syst Rev. 2014(6):CD008805

Barret JP. Surgical approaches to the major burn. In: Barret J, Herndon D, eds. Principles and Practice of Burn Surgery. New York, NY: Marcel Dekker; 2005:249–256

Barret JP, Herndon DN. Modulation of inflammatory and catabolic responses in severely burned children by early burn wound excision in the first 24 hours. Arch Surg. 2003; 138(2):127–132

Baxter CR. Present concepts in the management of major electrical injury. Surg Clin North Am. 1970; 50(6):1401–1418

Baxter CR, Shires T. Physiological response to crystalloid resuscitation of severe burns. Ann NY Acad Sci. 1968; 150(3):874–894

Benichou G, Yamada Y, Yun S-H, Lin C, Fray M, Tocco G. Immune recognition and rejection of allogeneic skin grafts. Immunotherapy. 2011; 3(6):757–770

Benomran FA, Hassan AI, Masood SS. Accidental fatal inhalation of sulfuric acid fumes. J Forensic Leg Med. 2008; 15(1):56–58

Bier M, Chen W, Bodnar E, Lee RC. Biophysical injury mechanisms associated with lightning injury. Neuro Rehabilitation. 2005; 20(1):53–62

Blanchet B, Jullien V, Vinsonneau C, Tod M. Influence of burns on pharmacokinetics and pharmacodynamics of drugs used in the care of burn patients. Clin Pharmacokinet. 2008; 47(10):635–654

Brent J. Water-based solutions are the best decontaminating fluids for dermal corrosive exposures: a mini review. Clin Toxicol (Phila). 2013; 51(8):731–736

Cabanac M. Temperature regulation. Annu Rev Physiol. 1975; 37:415–439

Cartotto R. Fluid resuscitation of the thermally injured patient. Clin Plast Surg. 2009; 36(4):569–581

Cartotto RC, Peters WJ, Neligan PC, Douglas LG, Beeston J. Chemical burns. Can J Surg. 1996; 39(3):205–211

Carvajal HF, Parks DH. Optimal composition of burn resuscitation fluids. Crit Care Med. 1988; 16(7):695–700

Cauchy E, Marsigny B, Allamel G, Verhellen R, Chetaille E. The value of technetium 99 scintigraphy in the prognosis of amputation in severe frostbite injuries of the extremities: A retrospective study of 92 severe frostbite injuries. J Hand Surg Am. 2000; 25(5):969–978

Celebi A, Gulel O, Cicekcioglu H, Gokaslan S, Kututcularoglu G, Ulusoy V. Myocardial infarction after an electric shock: a rare complication. Cardiol J. 2009; 16(4):362–364

Chan TC, Williams SR, Clark RF. Formic acid skin burns resulting in systemic toxicity. Ann Emerg Med. 1995; 26(3):383–386

Cherington M, McDonough G, Olson S, Russon R, Yarnell PR. Lichtenberg figures and lightning: case reports and review of the literature. Cutis. 2007; 80(2):141–143

Choi IS. Carbon monoxide poisoning: systemic manifestations and complications. J Korean Med Sci. 2001; 16(3):253–261

Chung JY, Kowal-Vern A, Latenser BA, Lewis RW, II. Cement-related injuries: review of a series, the National Burn Repository, and the prevailing literature. J Burn Care Res. 2007; 28(6):827–834

Collado J, Barret J, Domínguez P. Protocol d'atenció inicial a pacients cremats. Hospital Universitari Vall d'Hebron Barcelona Spain. 2013. http://www.vhebron.net/documents/10165/13229994/vh_protocol_atencio_cremats_def2.pdf. Accessed June 10, 2016

Conner JC, Bebarta VS. Images in clinical medicine. White phosphorus dermal burns. N Engl J Med. 2007; 357(15):1530

Cotton BA, Guy JS, Morris JA, Jr, Abumrad NN. The cellular, metabolic, and systemic consequences of aggressive fluid resuscitation strategies. Shock. 2006; 26(2):115–121

Daanen HAM. Finger cold-induced vasodilation: a review. Eur J Appl Physiol. 2003; 89(5):411–426

Demling RH. The burn edema process: current concepts. J Burn Care Rehabil. 2005; 26(3):207–227

Pechura C, Rall D, eds. Dermatological effects of mustard agents and lewisite. In: Veterans at Risk: The Health Effects of Mustard Gas and Lewisite. Washington, DC: National Academies Press (US); 1993

Desai MH, Herndon DN, Broemeling L, Barrow RE, Nichols RJ, Jr, Rutan RL. Early burn wound excision significantly reduces blood loss. Ann Surg. 1990; 211(6):753–759, discussion 759–762

Despa F, Orgill DP, Neuwalder J, Lee RC. The relative thermal stability of tissue macromolecules and cellular structure in burn injury. Burns. 2005; 31(5):568–577

Devgan L, Bhat S, Aylward S, Spence RJ. Modalities for the assessment of burn wound depth. J Burns Wounds. 2006; 5:e2

Dirkmann D, Hanke AA, Görlinger K, Peters J. Hypothermia and acidosis synergistically impair coagulation in human whole blood. Anesth Analg. 2008; 106(6):1627–1632

Dries DJ, Endorf FW. Inhalation injury: epidemiology, pathology, treatment strategies. Scand J Trauma Resusc Emerg Med. 2013; 21:31

Duff K, McCaffrey RJ. Electrical injury and lightning injury: a review of their mechanisms and neuropsychological, psychiatric, and neurological sequelae. Neuropsychol Rev. 2001; 11(2):101–116

El-Helbawy RH, Ghareeb FM. Inhalation injury as a prognostic factor for mortality in burn patients. Ann Burns Fire Disasters. 2011; 24(2):82–88

Elena-Sorando E, Agulló-Domingo A, Juan-Garcia E, Amrouni B. Bilateral shoulder fractures secondary to accidental electrical injury. Ann Burns Fire Disasters. 2006; 19(1):41–43

Elijah IE, Sanford AP, Lee JO. Chemical burns. In: Herndon DN, ed. Total Burn Care. 4th ed. London: Saunders Elsevier; 2012:455–460

Evans EI, Purnell OJ, Robinett PW, Batchelor A, Martin M. Fluid and electrolyte requirements in severe burns. Ann Surg. 1952; 135(6):804–817

Farina JA, Rosique MJ, Rosique RG. Curbing inflammation in burn patients. Int J Inflam. 2013; 2013:715645

Fish RM, Geddes LA. Conduction of electrical current to and through the human body: a review. Eplasty. 2009; 9:e44

Flammiger A, Maibach H. Sulfuric acid burns (corrosion and acute irritation): evidence-based overview to management. Cutan Ocul Toxicol. 2006; 25(1):55–61

Fletcher JL, Cancio LC, Sinha I, Leung KP, Renz EM, Chan RK. Inability to determine tissue health is main indication of allograft use in intermediate extent burns. Burns. 2015; 41(8):1862–1867

Forjuoh SN. Burns in low- and middle-income countries: a review of available literature on descriptive epidemiology, risk factors, treatment, and prevention. Burns. 2006; 32(5):529–537

Fox CL, Jr. Silver sulfadiazine—a new topical therapy for Pseudomonas in burns. Therapy of Pseudomonas infection in burns. Arch Surg. 1968; 96(2):184–188

Franz MG, Steed DL, Robson MC. Optimizing healing of the acute wound by minimizing complications. Curr Probl Surg. 2007; 44(11):691–763

Fukuzaki S. Mechanisms of actions of sodium hypochlorite in cleaning and disinfection processes. Biocontrol Sci. 2006; 11(4):147–157

Gamliel Z, DeBiasse MA, Demling RH. Essential microminerals and their response to burn injury. J Burn Care Rehabil. 1996; 17(3):264–272

Goertz O, Hirsch T, Buschhaus B, et al. Intravital pathophysiologic comparison of frostbite and burn injury in a murine model. J Surg Res. 2011; 167(2):e395–e401

Gracia R, Shepherd G. Cyanide poisoning and its treatment. Pharmacotherapy. 2004; 24(10):1358–1365

Greenhalgh DG. Topical antimicrobial agents for burn wounds. Clin Plast Surg. 2009; 36(4):597–606

Greingor JL, Tosi JM, Ruhlmann S, Aussedat M. Acute carbon monoxide intoxication during pregnancy. One case report and review of the literature. Emerg Med J. 2001; 18(5):399

Guo Z, Sheng Z, Diao L, et al. Extensive wound excision in shock stage in patients with major burns. Chin Med J (Engl). 1995; 108(4):273–277

Gursul E, Bayata S, Aksit E, Ugurlu B. Development of ST elevation myocardial infarction and atrial fibrillation after an electrical injury. Case Rep Emerg Med. 2015; 2015:953102

Gurtner GC, Werner S, Barrandon Y, Longaker MT. Wound repair and regeneration. Nature. 2008; 453(7193):314–321

Guzman JA. Carbon monoxide poisoning. Crit Care Clin. 2012; 28(4):537–548

Haagsma JA, Graetz N, Bolliger I, et al. The global burden of injury: incidence, mortality, disability-adjusted life years and time trends from the Global Burden of Disease study 2013. Inj Prev. 2016; 22(1):3–18

Haberal M, Sakallioglu Abali AE, Karakayali H. Fluid management in major burn injuries. Indian J Plast Surg. 2010; 43(Suppl):S29–S36

Halim AS, Khoo TL, Mohd Yussof SJ. Biologic and synthetic skin substitutes: An overview. Indian J Plast Surg. 2010; 43(Suppl):S23–S28

Hamel J. A review of acute cyanide poisoning with a treatment update. Crit Care Nurse. 2011; 31(1):72–81, quiz 82

Handford C, Buxton P, Russell K, et al. Frostbite: a practical approach to hospital management. Extrem Physiol Med. 2014; 3:7

Heimbach D, Faucher L. Principles of burn surgery. In: Barret J, Herndon D, eds. Principles and Practice of Burn Surgery. New York, NY: Marcel Dekker; 2005:135–162

Herndon DN, Parks DH. Comparison of serial debridement and autografting and early massive excision with cadaver skin overlay in the treatment of large burns in children. J Trauma. 1986; 26(2):149–152

Hettiaratchy S, Dziewulski P. ABC of burns: pathophysiology and types of burns. BMJ. 2004; 328(7453):1427–1429

Hettiaratchy S, Papini R. Initial management of a major burn: II—Assessment and resuscitation. BMJ. 2004; 329(7457):101–103

Holm C, Mayr M, Tegeler J, et al. A clinical randomized study on the effects of invasive monitoring on burn shock resuscitation. Burns. 2004; 30(8):798–807

Hunt JL, McManus WF, Haney WP, Pruitt BA, Jr. Vascular lesions in acute electric injuries. J Trauma. 1974; 14(6):461–473

Hunt JL, Mason AD, Jr, Masterson TS, Pruitt BA, Jr. The pathophysiology of acute electric injuries. J Trauma. 1976; 16(5):335–340

Huzar TF, George T, Cross JM. Carbon monoxide and cyanide toxicity: etiology, pathophysiology and treatment in inhalation injury. Expert Rev Respir Med. 2013; 7(2):159–170

Imray C, Grieve A, Dhillon S; Caudwell Xtreme Everest Research Group. Cold damage to the extremities: frostbite and non-freezing cold injuries. Postgrad Med J. 2009; 85(1007):481–488

Imray CHE, Richards P, Greeves J, Castellani JW. Nonfreezing cold-induced injuries. J R Army Med Corps. 2011; 157(1):79–84

Jackson DM. The diagnosis of the depth of burning [in undetermined language]. Br J Surg. 1953; 40(164):588–596

Jandera V, Hudson DA, de Wet PM, Innes PM, Rode H. Cooling the burn wound: evaluation of different modalites. Burns. 2000; 26(3):265–270

Janzekovic Z. A new concept in the early excision and immediate grafting of burns. J Trauma. 1970; 10(12):1103–1108

Jelenko C, III. Chemicals that "burn". J Trauma. 1974; 14(1):65–72

Jeschke MG, Chinkes DL, Finnerty CC, et al. Pathophysiologic response to severe burn injury. Ann Surg. 2008; 248(3):387–401

Jeschke MG, Gauglitz GG, Kulp GA, et al. Long-term persistance of the pathophysiologic response to severe burn injury. PLoS One. 2011; 6(7):e21245

Jeschke MG, Mlcak RP, Finnerty CC, et al. Burn size determines the inflammatory and hypermetabolic response. Crit Care. 2007; 11(4):R90

Kao DS, Hijjawi J. Cold and chemical injury to the upper extremity. In: Neligan PC, ed. Plastic Surgery: Lower Extremity, Trunk and Burns. Vol 4. 3rd ed. Amsterdam, Netherlands: Elsevier; 2013:456–467

Keck M, Selig HF, Lumenta DB, Kamolz LP, Mittlböck M, Frey M. The use of Suprathel(®) in deep dermal burns: first results of a prospective study. Burns. 2012; 38(3):388–395

Kolios L, Striepling E, Kolios G, et al. The nitric acid burn trauma of the skin. J Plast Reconstr Aesthet Surg. 2010; 63(4):e358–e363

Kucheki M, Simi A. Phenol burn. Int J Occup Environ Med. 2010; 1(1):41–44

Kurmis R, Parker A, Greenwood J. The use of immunonutrition in burn injury care: where are we? J Burn Care Res. 2010; 31(5):677–691

Laloë V. Patterns of deliberate self-burning in various parts of the world. A review. Burns. 2004; 30(3):207–215

Lawson-Smith P, Jansen EC, Hyldegaard O. Cyanide intoxication as part of smoke inhalation–a review on diagnosis and treatment from the emergency perspective. Scand J Trauma Resusc Emerg Med. 2011; 19:14

Lee RC. Cell injury by electric forces. Ann N Y Acad Sci. 2005; 1066:85–91

Lee RC, Kolodney MS. Electrical injury mechanisms: dynamics of the thermal response. Plast Reconstr Surg. 1987; 80(5):663–671

Lee RC, Zhang D, Hannig J. Biophysical injury mechanisms in electrical shock trauma. Annu Rev Biomed Eng. 2000; 2:477–509

Lepock JR. How do cells respond to their thermal environment? Int J Hyperthermia. 2005; 21(8):681–687

Lewis T. Observations upon the reactions of the vessels of the human skin to cold. Heart. 1930; 15:177–208

Long WB, III, Edlich RF, Winters KL, Britt LD. Cold injuries. J Long Term Eff Med Implants. 2005; 15(1):67–78

Lumenta DB, Kamolz L-P, Frey M. Adult burn patients with more than 60% TBSA involved-Meek and other techniques to overcome restricted skin harvest availability—the Viennese Concept. J Burn Care Res. 2009; 30(2):231–242

Lund C, Browder N. The estimation of areas of burns. Surg Gynaecol Obs. 1944; 79:352–358

MacLennan L, Moiemen N. Management of cyanide toxicity in patients with burns. Burns. 2015; 41(1):18–24

Mandell SP, Gibran NS. Early Enteral Nutrition for Burn Injury. Adv Wound Care (New Rochelle). 2014; 3(1):64–70

Mann R, Gibran N, Engrav L, Heimbach D. Is immediate decompression of high voltage electrical injuries to the upper extremity always necessary? J Trauma. 1996; 40(4):584–587, discussion 587–589

Marques EG, Júnior GAP, Neto BFM, et al. Visceral injury in electrical shock trauma: proposed guideline for the management of abdominal electrocution and literature review. Int J Burns Trauma. 2014; 4(1):1–6

Marzella L, Jesudass RR, Manson PN, Myers RA, Bulkley GB. Morphologic characterization of acute injury to vascular endothelium of skin after frostbite. Plast Reconstr Surg. 1989; 83(1):67–76

Matey P, Allison KP, Sheehan TM, Gowar JP. Chromic acid burns: early aggressive excision is the best method to prevent systemic toxicity. J Burn Care Rehabil. 2000; 21(3):241–245

McBride JW, Labrosse KR, McCoy HG, Ahrenholz DH, Solem LD, Goldenberg IF. Is serum creatine kinase-MB in electrically injured patients predictive of myocardial injury? JAMA. 1986; 255(6):764–768

McQueen MM, Court-Brown CM. Compartment monitoring in tibial fractures. The pressure threshold for decompression. J Bone Joint Surg Br. 1996; 78(1):99–104

Meryman HT. Mechanics of freezing in living cells and tissues. Science. 1956; 124(3221):515–521

Miller BK, Goldstein MH, Monshizadeh R, Tabandeh H, Bhatti MT. Ocular manifestations of electrical injury: a case report and review of the literature. CLAO J. 2002; 28(4):224–227

Monafo WW. The treatment of burn shock by the intravenous and oral administration of hypertonic lactated saline solution. J Trauma. 1970; 10(7):575–586

Mosier MJ, Gibran NS. Surgical excision of the burn wound. Clin Plast Surg. 2009; 36(4):617–625

Neff LP, Allman JM, Holmes JH. The use of theraputic plasma exchange (TPE) in the setting of refractory burn shock. Burns. 2010; 36(3):372–378

Ng NYB, Abdullah A, Milner SM. A phosphorus burn. Eplasty. 2015; 15:ic15

Noordenbos J, Doré C, Hansbrough JF. Safety and efficacy of TransCyte for the treatment of partial-thickness burns. J Burn Care Rehabil. 1999; 20(4):275–281

Ong YS, Samuel M, Song C. Meta-analysis of early excision of burns. Burns. 2006; 32(2):145–150

Orgill DP, Piccolo N. Escharotomy and decompressive therapies in burns. J Burn Care Res. 2009; 30(5):759–768

Oscier C, Emerson B, Handy JM. New perspectives on airway management in acutely burned patients. Anaesthesia. 2014; 69(2):105–110

Paratz JD, Stockton K, Paratz ED, et al. Burn resuscitation—hourly urine output versus alternative endpoints: a systematic review. Shock. 2014; 42(4):295–306

Peck M, Pressman MA. The correlation between burn mortality rates from fire and flame and economic status of countries. Burns. 2013; 39(6):1054–1059

Peck MD. Epidemiology of burns throughout the world. Part I: Distribution and risk factors. Burns. 2011; 37(7):1087–1100

Peck MD. Epidemiology of burns throughout the World. Part II: Intentional burns in adults. Burns. 2012; 38(5):630–637

Pham C, Greenwood J, Cleland H, Woodruff P, Maddern G. Bioengineered skin substitutes for the management of burns: a systematic review. Burns. 2007; 33(8):946–957

Pontini A, Reho F, Giatsidis G, Bacci C, Azzena B, Tiengo C. Multidisciplinary care in severe pediatric electrical oral burn. Burns. 2015; 41(3):e41–e46

Pruitt BA, Jr. Fluid and electrolyte replacement in the burned patient. Surg Clin North Am. 1978; 58(6):1291–1312

Pruitt BA, Jr, Wolf SE. An historical perspective on advances in burn care over the past 100 years. Clin Plast Surg. 2009; 36(4):527–545

Raman SR, Jamil Z, Cosgrove J. Magnetic resonance angiography unmasks frostbite injury. Emerg Med J. 2011; 28(5):450

Reisner AD. Possible mechanisms for delayed neurological damage in lightning and electrical injury. Brain Inj. 2013; 27(5):565–569

Reiss E, Stirmann JA, Artz CP, Davis JH, Amspacher WH. Fluid and electrolyte balance in burns. J Am Med Assoc. 1953; 152(14):1309–1313

Rennekampff H-O, Schaller H-E, Wisser D, Tenenhaus M. Debridement of burn wounds with a water jet surgical tool. Burns. 2006; 32(1):64–69

Rhodes J, Clay C, Phillips M. The surface area of the hand and the palm for estimating percentage of total body surface area: results of a meta-analysis. Br J Dermatol. 2013; 169(1):76–84

Rice P. Sulphur mustard injuries of the skin. Pathophysiology and management. Toxicol Rev. 2003; 22(2):111–118

Ritenour AE, Morton MJ, McManus JG, Barillo DJ, Cancio LC. Lightning injury: a review. Burns. 2008; 34(5):585–594

Robinson EP, Chhabra AB. Hand chemical burns. J Hand Surg Am. 2015; 40(3):605–612, quiz 613

Robson MC, Murphy RC, Heggers JP. A new explanation for the progressive tissue loss in electrical injuries. Plast Reconstr Surg. 1984; 73(3):431–437

Rosenberg L, Krieger Y, Bogdanov-Berezovski A, Silberstein E, Shoham Y, Singer AJ. A novel rapid and selective enzymatic debridement agent for burn wound management: a multi-center RCT. Burns. 2014; 40(3):466–474

Rustin MH, Newton JA, Smith NP, Dowd PM. The treatment of chilblains with nifedipine: the results of a pilot study, a double-blind placebo-controlled randomized study and a long-term open trial. Br J Dermatol. 1989; 120(2):267–275

Sachs C, Lehnhardt M, Daigeler A, Goertz O. The triaging and treatment of cold-induced injuries. Dtsch Arztebl Int. 2015; 112(44):741–747

Shahi V, Wetter DA, Cappel JA, Davis MDP, Spittell PC. Vasospasm Is a Consistent Finding in Pernio (Chilblains) and a Possible Clue to Pathogenesis. Dermatology. 2015; 231(3):274–279

Shahrokhi S, Arno A, Jeschke MG. The use of dermal substitutes in burn surgery: acute phase. Wound Repair Regen. 2014; 22(1):14–22

Sharma N, Singh D, Sobti A, et al. Course and outcome of accidental sodium hydroxide ocular injury. Am J Ophthalmol. 2012; 154(4):740–749.e2

Sheridan R. Closure of the excised burn wound: autografts, semipermanent skin substitutes, and permanent skin substitutes. Clin Plast Surg. 2009; 36(4):643–651

Shin JY, Yi HS. Diagnostic accuracy of laser Doppler imaging in burn depth assessment: Systematic review and meta-analysis. Burns. 2016; 42(7):1369–1376

Singh V, Devgan L, Bhat S, Milner SM. The pathogenesis of burn wound conversion. Ann Plast Surg. 2007; 59(1):109–115

Soltani A, Karsidag S, Garner W. A ten-year experience with hemodialysis in burn patients at Los Angeles County + USC Medical Center. J Burn Care Res. 2009; 30(5):832–835

Sparić R, Malvasi A, Nejković L, Tinelli A. Electric shock in pregnancy: a review. J Matern Fetal Neonatal Med. 2016; 29(2):317–323

Tan H, Wasiak J, Paul E, Cleland H. Effective use of Biobrane as a temporary wound dressing prior to definitive split-skin graft in the treatment of severe burn: A retrospective analysis. Burns. 2015; 41(5):969–976

Tan J-Q, Zhang H-H, Lei Z-J, et al. The roles of autophagy and apoptosis in burn wound progression in rats. Burns. 2013; 39(8):1551–1556

Tarim A, Ezer A. Electrical burn is still a major risk factor for amputations. Burns. 2013; 39(2):354–357

Ulmer T. The clinical diagnosis of compartment syndrome of the lower leg: are clinical findings predictive of the disorder? J Orthop Trauma. 2002; 16(8):572–577

Ungley CC, Channell GD, Richards RL. The immersion foot syndrome. 1946. Wilderness Environ Med. 2003; 14(2):135–141, discussion 134

Venter THJ, Karpelowsky JS, Rode H. Cooling of the burn wound: the ideal temperature of the coolant. Burns. 2007; 33(7):917–922

Vivó C, Galeiras R, del Caz MDP. Initial evaluation and management of the critical burn patient. Med Intensiva. 2016; 40(1):49–59

Walker PF, Buehner MF, Wood LA, et al. Diagnosis and management of inhalation injury: an updated review. Crit Care. 2015; 19:351

Wang X, Zhang Y, Ni L, et al. A review of treatment strategies for hydrofluoric acid burns: current status and future prospects. Burns. 2014; 40(8):1447–1457

Warden GD. Fluid resuscitation and early management. In: Herndon DN, ed. Total Burn Care. 4th ed. London: Saunders Elsevier; 2012:115–124

Wibbenmeyer L, Liao J, Heard J, Kealey L, Kealey G, Oral R. Factors related to child maltreatment in children presenting with burn injuries. J Burn Care Res. 2014; 35(5):374–381

Williams FN, Branski LK, Jeschke MG, Herndon DN. What, how, and how much should patients with burns be fed? Surg Clin North Am. 2011; 91(3):609–629

Williams FN, Herndon DN, Jeschke MG. The hypermetabolic response to burn injury and interventions to modify this response. Clin Plast Surg. 2009; 36(4):583–596

Williams FN, Herndon DN, Suman OE, et al. Changes in cardiac physiology after severe burn injury. J Burn Care Res. 2011; 32(2):269–274

Wood FM, Giles N, Stevenson A, Rea S, Fear M. Characterisation of the cell suspension harvested from the dermal epidermal junction using a ReCell® kit. Burns. 2012; 38(1):44–51

Wood J, Walsh J, Genova R. Fasciotomy. 2015. http://emedicine.medscape.com/article/1894895-overview#a3. Accessed June 12, 2016

Woodson L. Anesthesia for acute burn injuries. In: Barret J, Herndon D, eds. Principles and Practice of Burn Surgery. New York, NY: Marcel Dekker; 2005:103–134

Xiang J, Sun Z, Huan JN. Intensive chromic acid burns and acute chromium poisoning with acute renal failure. Chin Med J (Engl). 2011; 124(13):2071–2073

Yarmolenko PS, Moon EJ, Landon C, et al. Thresholds for thermal damage to normal tissues: an update. Int J Hyperthermia. 2011; 27(4):320–343

Yoshimura CA, Mathieu L, Hall AH, Monteiro MGK, de Almeida DM. Seventy per cent hydrofluoric acid burns: delayed decontamination with hexafluorine® and treatment with calcium gluconate. J Burn Care Res. 2011; 32(4):e149–e154

Zack-Williams SDL, Ahmad Z, Moiemen NS. The clinical efficacy of Diphoterine® in the management of cutaneous chemical burns: a 2-year evaluation study. Ann Burns Fire Disasters. 2015; 28(1):9–12

Zhang ML, Chang ZD, Wang CY, Fang CH. Microskin grafting in the treatment of extensive burns: a preliminary report. J Trauma. 1988; 28(6):804–807

Zorrilla P, Marín A, Gómez LA, Salido JA. Shoelace technique for gradual closure of fasciotomy wounds. J Trauma. 2005; 59(6):1515–1517

19 Microsurgery

Diego Marré, Pablo Zancolli, Gustavo Pérez-Abadía, Héctor Roco

Abstract

Reconstructive surgery has the ability to offer a reliable and durable solution to patients suffering from conditions, wounds, or defects of increasing complexity. Surgeons can now use microsurgery to transfer tissues of varying compositions to restore anatomy and function with a high rate of success. Moreover, microsurgery allows replantation of amputated segments as well as the successful transplantation of allogeneic tissues. The principles of microsurgery as they relate to tissue handling and suturing have remained relatively unchanged for decades; however, significant improvements have been made in the manufacturing of instruments, sutures, and magnification, which, together with surgical experience and improvements in technique, have contributed to the remarkable rates of success, making microsurgery a safe and highly reproducible technique.

The route to becoming a proficient microsurgeon involves commitment, perseverance, and long sessions of laboratory training. After that, maintaining a reasonably steady flow of microsurgical cases during clinical practice is also important to maintain the skills. Despite experience and advances in technique and instruments, failure of a microsurgical anastomosis and subsequent flap loss are still possible; hence close postoperative monitoring is mandatory in order to promptly detect and treat a vascular complication. This chapter describes the fundamentals of microsurgery in relation to training and basic techniques as well as the main aspects of free flap failure.

Keywords: flap failure, free tissue transfer, ischemia, microsurgery, thrombosis

19.1 Introduction

Microsurgery literally means surgery under the microscope and the term *microvascular surgery* refers to the suturing of small blood vessels with the aid of magnification. In 1902, Alexis Carrel, a French surgeon, described the technique of triangulation for vascular anastomosis, and 10 years later he was awarded the Nobel Prize in Physiology or Medicine for his outstanding contributions on vascular sutures and the transplantation of organs and blood vessels. In 1921, Nylén was the first to use a monocular operating microscope for eardrum surgery, and soon after Holmgren would use a stereoscopic microscope for otolaryngological procedures. During the early and mid-1960s Jacobson and Katsumura reported the successful anastomosis of vessels of < 1.5 mm in diameter, while Buncke successfully replanted amputated digits and ears in rhesus monkeys and rabbits, respectively. In the clinical setting, in 1963, surgeons in China were able to replant a patient's hand amputated at the level of the wrist, and 1 year later Malt and McKhann reported two cases of arm replantation. Also in 1964, Nakayama et al used vascularized segments of intestines for esophageal reconstruction, which were attached by anastomosing vessels of 3–4 mm in diameter. Komatsu and Tamai in 1968 performed the first successful digit replantation, and then Cobbett in 1969 reported the first transfer of a hallux to the hand. During the early 1970s the world witnessed the first free flaps in the hands of Antia and Buch, who transferred a superficial epigastric artery skin flap to the face in 1971. McLean and Buncke reconstructed a scalp defect with an omentum free flap in 1972, and Daniel and Taylor, followed closely by O'Brien in 1973, independently reported the use of a free groin flap for lower extremity reconstruction. Microsurgery and free tissue transfer soon became the focus of attraction to numerous surgeons around the world and the technique began to expand rapidly. Although in the beginning microsurgery was performed in a selected number of places and the rates of success hardly reached 80%, today most tertiary units perform free flap surgery on a routine basis, with patency rates 95–98% due to a combination of careful preoperative planning, better instruments and surgical technique, and improved postoperative care. The fact that it is performed routinely and successfully in many institutions worldwide does not imply that microsurgery is a procedure to be taken lightly; rather, it is to be admired as the product of dedicated research, clinical work, and technical advances provided by the pioneering microsurgeons who paved the way to what we know and do today.

19.2 Training in Microsurgery

19.2.1 Preconditions in Microsurgery

Learning microsurgery requires both commitment and perseverance. In the authors' opinion, a 1-week laboratory course with neither cell phone interruptions nor clinical or social obligations is highly recommended to acquire the necessary basic skills. During such time, trainees are usually faced with a number of difficulties that, although irritating and frustrating at first, represent extremely valuable learning opportunities that will someday pay off when similar situations arise during clinical cases. Focusing on the technique and paying careful attention to the details are paramount during the process and should never be shadowed by the feeling of defeat when things go wrong.

Much has been said about the best way to prepare for a microsurgical procedure, which requires concentration, fine skills, and the right state of mind. Tobacco may affect concentration and performance for about 30 minutes and is therefore discouraged, whereas sticking to one's routine dose of coffee is highly recommended—tremor may be exacerbated not only by excess but also by the lack of it.

Time spent in the microsurgery laboratory is important and precious, but also limited. To make the most of it, regular breaks of 5–10 minutes every 60–90 minutes must be taken. During these breaks it is important to fully disconnect from the work being done so as to regain focus and concentration. Conversely, working restlessly for several hours will severely influence your judgment and ability to learn as well as significantly reduce your capacity to overcome difficulties in an intelligent and efficient manner.

> **Note**
>
> Trainees and surgeons wanting to become proficient in microsurgery should do as follows:
> - Dedicate a great amount of time to lab training.
> - Learn to deal with frustration and despair.
> - Not become discouraged by a poor result.
> - Not struggle under difficulties, but instead learn to identify, accept, and efficiently manage difficult situations.
> - Learn the anatomy of the working area, including vascular variations.

19.2.2 Posture

A correct and comfortable posture is an absolute requirement in microsurgery. Good positioning of the feet, body, and hands is important to avoid tremor and remain focused, whereas constant changes and movements usually result in loss of concentration and unnecessary delays, which eventually build up and undermine your surgical skills.

A good posture starts with the feet, which should be placed separate at an equal distance from the base of the stool, thus forming a three-point supporting base. Do not cross your legs or put them under the seat. Sit in the middle of the stool; the trunk should align in a way that allows the body to rest in space without effort. The seat must be set at a height that is just right for your eyes to meet the microscope's eyepieces without the need to flex, extend, or rotate the neck. The ulnar aspect of the elbows, forearms, and hands should rest flat on the table, making sure they are not bearing the weight of a forwardly inclined upper body. This position should allow you to work for a long time under the microscope without fatigue and employing little or no effort in maintaining a good posture. Furthermore, avoiding unnecessary muscle contraction greatly reduces the use of extrinsic hand musculature and helps to reduce tremor. Finally, the instruments should be held between the first three fingers, which will also enhance precision (▶Fig. 19.1).

19.2.3 Tremor

Tremor is the rhythmic, purposeless, trembling movement of the hand resulting from the

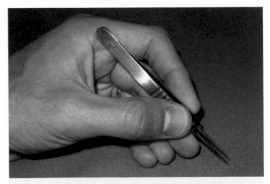

Fig. 19.1 Microinstruments are held using a three-digit grip with the instrument resting between the thumb, index, and middle fingers and the ulnar border of the hand lying flat on the working surface.

involuntary alternating contraction and relaxation of opposing skeletal muscle groups. There is a myth about surgeons with "steady hands"; everyone has a degree of tremor, although the author (GP-A) agrees that some trainees do show an "unusually stable" hand, which is explained by a higher capacity to control unwanted movement that allows them to perform better. As said earlier, there are a number of measures that help to reduce tremor, including consumption of the usual dose of coffee, a good body posture, proper hand positioning, and correct holding of instruments. After exercise, the resting activity of muscles increases, which is why strong exercises, particularly those involving the upper extremities, are discouraged during the 24 hours prior to a microsurgical procedure.

19.2.4 Nonliving Models

Nonliving models are an essential part of the microsurgical learning curve because they provide an excellent training opportunity allowing a steady transition on the route from inanimate models to living animals to living patients. Latex gloves, silicone tubes, leaves, petals, artificial vessels, chicken legs, and human vessels obtained from cadaveric dissections or discarded after a surgical operation have all been described and represent valid alternatives. Their use depends mainly on the preference and availability of each laboratory as well as the size of the suture—practicing with 11–0 or 12–0 nylon requires thin, delicate materials due to the small size and fragility of the needles.

In our microsurgery laboratory we have designed "Tavi," a modified stuffed toy with a piece of circular latex glove attached to a plastic ring on its the belly (▶Fig. 19.2). This model allows suturing in all directions, using both the dominant and the nondominant hand as well as direct visualization of the inner aspect of the suture line by flipping the latex piece. Three to 4 hours of practice on the glove during the first day in a regular 5-day microsurgery course is usually enough to master the use of 9–0, 10–0, and 11–0 nylon suture materials and learn the basics of microsuturing.

19.2.5 Living Models: The Rat's Groin

The rat is an excellent and relatively inexpensive model to start practicing on live, bleeding vessels. Bearing in mind that the goal is to obtain a patent anastomosis, only a living animal will allow the surgeon to contemplate the smooth and clear pulse of the artery at the end of the procedure.

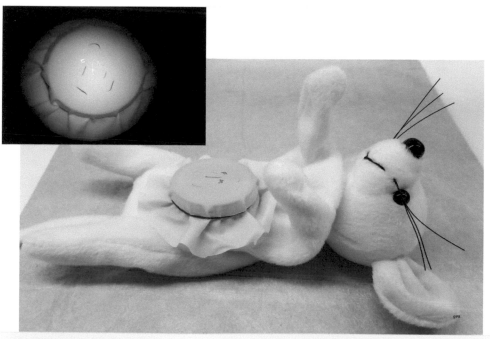

Fig. 19.2 The nonliving model, "Tavi."

Laboratory rats are easy to obtain, can tolerate prolonged anesthesia times, are clean and pathogen free, and in general very docile animals. Rats weighing around 350 g are ideal because their femoral vessels are approximately 1 mm in diameter (± 0.2 mm), a perfect size to work with.

The rat's groin represents an ideal area to practice microsurgery with several advantages over other regions, such as the neck (carotid artery and internal jugular vein) and the abdomen (aorta and vena cava). The femoral neurovascular structures are easy to access and expose through an incision running along the concavity between the abdomen and the leg. Bleeding in the area is easy to control and seldom life threatening for the animal. The common femoral vessels (artery and vein) are about 1.5 cm long, starting at the level of the inguinal ligament and running together within a common perivascular sheath, to end at the point where they divide into a superficial and deep branch. Of note, working with a rat's femoral vessels is more difficult than working with human vessels—their walls are thinner, and their diameter is smaller than most vessels used in clinical (adult) microsurgery, except for digital vessels. Practicing in smaller and thinner vessels is a good way to prepare for and face with confidence a clinical anastomosis.

Practicing with the carotid artery and internal jugular vein in the neck is an alternative to the femoral vessels; however, whereas surgical access is not difficult, their proximity to the trachea and heart increases the risk of a breathing problem or major bleeding that may result in the death of the animal. Using the abdominal vessels (aorta and vena cava) requires more advanced microsurgery skills. Despite their larger diameter, these vessels have important branches and are located deep in the retroperitoneal space, which makes their access more challenging, and bleeding is difficult to control. In this sense, it is advisable to progress to these areas once you feel fully comfortable with the femoral vessels.

19.2.6 Basic Techniques in Microsurgery

Microsurgery is a technique routinely used in reconstructive surgery and other surgical specialties. Although it has been around for almost 50 years, it is surprising how little the technique itself has evolved. The manufacturing of instruments and sutures has certainly improved over the years, but the surgical principles and actions involved in vessel/nerve suturing have stood the test of time and proven highly efficient and safe, as illustrated by the current > 95% overall success rates.

A basic microsurgery set comprises at least six elements: a needleholder, straight adventitia scissors, curved dissecting scissors, jeweller's forceps, dilator forceps, and microvascular clamps with their accompanying clamp application forceps (▶Fig. 19.3). Today, most units also include in their set of instruments the microvascular coupler system; a device used mainly for vein anastomoses with many advantages and similar

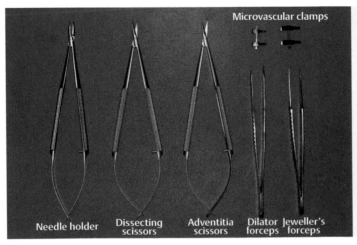

Fig. 19.3 Basic set of microsurgery instruments.

Microvascular clamps

Needle holder   Dissecting scissors   Adventitia scissors   Dilator forceps   Jeweller's forceps

patency rates when compared to the traditional hand-sewn anastomosis.

Vessel Preparation

The vessel ends need to be at a distance that allows anastomosis without tension and should rest flat on the surface so that no kinks or twists are seen once suturing is completed. During vessel preparation and throughout the whole procedure it is important to manipulate the vessels gently, always grabbing them by their adventitia and never their full thickness (▶Fig. 19.4). Clamps (single or double) are applied and the vessels' ends cut straight and cleanly with straight scissors and irrigated with heparinized lactated Ringer's solution (10 UI/mL) (▶Fig. 19.5a, b). The adventitia is then excised just enough to prevent it from getting into the line of anastomosis and is best done by pulling the tissue past the vessel end with forceps and cutting it flush with the vessel edge (▶Fig. 19.5c, d). Next, using dilator forceps, the vessels are carefully dilated. This allows better definition of the lumen and helps in preventing spasm by causing transient paralysis of the

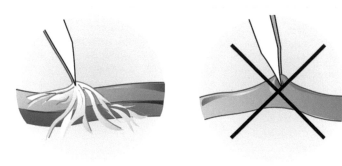

Fig. 19.4 The vessels should be grabbed by the adventitia and never full thickness. (Reproduced from Weerda, Reconstructive Facial Plastic Surgery: A Problem Solving Manual, ©2001, Thieme Publishers, New York.)

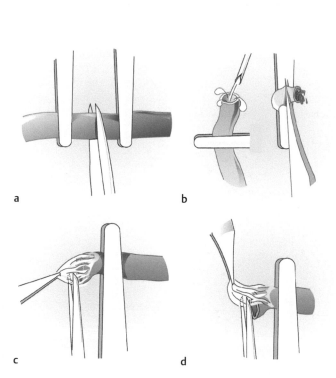

a

b

c

d

Fig. 19.5 Vessel preparation. **(a)** Once the clamps have been applied, a straight cut perpendicular to the axis of the vessel is made. **(b)** The vessels are flushed with heparinized solution or the blood remnants milked out. **(c, d)** Adventitia is trimmed from the vessel ends by gentle pulling and cutting flush with the vessel edge. (Reproduced from Weerda, Reconstructive Facial Plastic Surgery: A Problem Solving Manual, ©2001, Thieme Publishers, New York.)

smooth muscle of the vessel wall (▶Fig. 19.6). Remnants of blood or tissue inside the lumen are flushed with heparinized solution, and a background contrast material is finally placed under the vessels and clamps. The vessels are now ready for anastomosis.

End-to-End Anastomosis

Several techniques exist for end-to-end vessel anastomosis, including the triangulation technique, one way up technique, continuous technique, and spiral interrupted technique. This chapter describes the triangulation technique; however, it is important to note that irrespective of the technique used, some basic principles must be followed when performing a microvascular anastomosis:

- Stitches must be placed at a distance from the edge that is approximately twice the wall's thickness.
- The needle must pass perpendicularly through the whole thickness of the vessel wall, in one pass and avoiding repeated punctures (▶Fig. 19.7).
- Catching the back wall should be strictly avoided on every stitch and confirmed by direct visualization of the lumen.
- Tension of the knot should be sufficient to bring the edges together firmly but without tearing the wall.

- The number of stitches should be just enough to obtain a sealed anastomosis without undue trauma from unnecessary stitches.

All these measures are directed to minimize injury to the intima, which would otherwise expose the highly thrombogenic subendothelial collagen, likely resulting in thrombus formation at the anastomotic site. Likewise, at the end of the anastomosis the vessels' end should lie in perfect apposition or be slightly everted, but never inverted, because this exposes the thrombogenic external surface into the lumen. In addition, the lumen should be kept free of blood clots, tissue, and debris at all times throughout the procedure by repeated irrigation with heparinized solution.

The triangulation technique starts with two stay sutures, the most important ones placed at 120 degrees from each other on the front wall of the vessel (▶Fig. 19.8). This allows the back wall to fall away, which minimizes its risk of being caught while one is suturing the front. Next, depending on the diameter of the vessels, two or three stitches are placed between the two stay sutures, and this completes the front wall (▶Fig. 19.9). The vessel is then turned 180 degrees to address the back wall, which can be sutured in two ways. A stay stitch can be placed in the middle and two or three sutures placed on each side, or, alternatively, the wall can be sutured from one pole to the other.

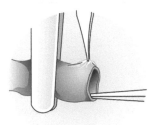

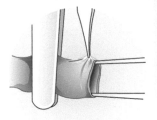

Fig. 19.6 Vessel dilation using dilator forceps. (Reproduced from Weerda, Reconstructive Facial Plastic Surgery: A Problem Solving Manual, ©2001, Thieme Publishers, New York.)

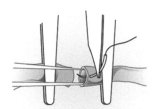

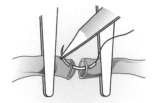

Fig. 19.7 Sutures are placed perpendicular to the vessel wall and full thickness. (Reproduced from Weerda, Reconstructive Facial Plastic Surgery: A Problem Solving Manual, ©2001, Thieme Publishers, New York.)

Once the artery and vein are finished, clamps are released, first the distal followed by the proximal one for the artery, and in the opposite way for the vein, and always releasing the vein first and artery second.

> ### Caution ⚠
>
> Remember to always release the vein first followed by the artery.

End-to-Side Anastomosis

An end-to-side anastomosis is mainly indicated in cases of severe vessel mismatch or when preservation of distal flow is needed (i.e., one vessel leg). Moreover, Godina advocated the use of this type of anastomosis under the observation that, after an arteriotomy, contraction of smooth muscle in the vessel wall tends to open up the space, thus reducing the risk of spasm. However, it is now widely known that the rates of success of an end-to-side anastomosis are no different, and as good as, those of end-to-end ones.

The procedure begins by performing an arteriotomy on the recipient vessel that matches the diameter of the donor vessel. Importantly, the adventitia must be completely removed from the site of the arteriotomy before making the cut. First, with the main vessel clamped proximally and distally, a stitch is placed and left long right in the middle of the proposed site. Next, two cuts are made at 45-degree angles in such a way that they meet exactly in the middle, thus creating an oval-shaped opening on the vessel wall (►Fig. 19.10). Alternatively, the arteriotomy can be performed using an arteriotomy set available from various manufacturers (ASSI; S&T), which eases the procedure and increases precision significantly. Next, key sutures are inserted at each extreme of the oval at 180 degrees from each other, followed by suturing of the front and back wall in either an interrupted or a continuous fashion (►Fig. 19.11). At this stage, it is critical to place the stitches radially in relation to the center of the arteriotomy and not perpendicular to the main vessel (►Fig. 19.12).

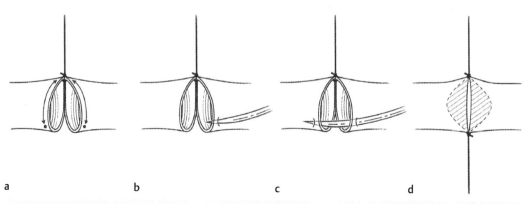

a   b   c   d

Fig. 19.8 (a-d) 120-degree suturing technique with back wall hanging down, which helps to prevent its being caught during suturing. (Reproduced with permission from Acland, Sabapathy, Practice Manual for Microvascular Surgery. 3rd edition, ©2008, Indian Society for Surgery of the Hand.)

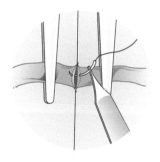
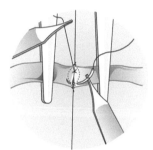

Fig. 19.9 Two or three stitches are placed between the two stay sutures to complete the front wall. (Reproduced from Weerda, Reconstructive Facial Plastic Surgery: A Problem Solving Manual, ©2001, Thieme Publishers, New York.)

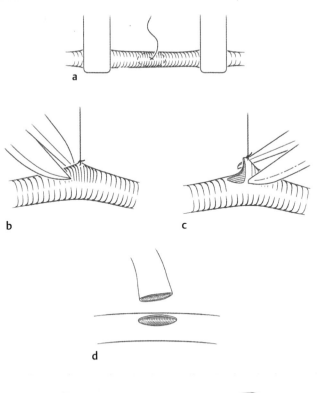

Fig. 19.10 (a–d) Arteriotomy for end-to-side anastomosis. (Reproduced with permission from Acland, Sabapathy, Practice Manual for Microvascular Surgery. 3rd edition, ©2008, Indian Society for Surgery of the Hand.)

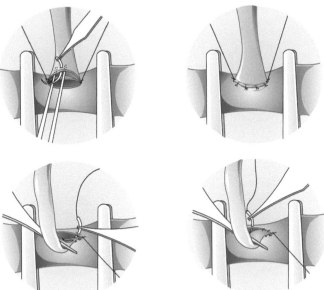

Fig. 19.11 End-to-side anastomosis. The procedure begins with one suture on each side, followed by suturing the front wall and finally the back wall. (Reproduced from Weerda, Reconstructive Facial Plastic Surgery: A Problem Solving Manual, ©2001, Thieme Publishers, New York.)

Microvascular Coupler System

Of the different devices developed for microsurgical anastomosis beyond the traditional hand-sewing method, the coupler system has been the most successful. Not surprisingly, this device has been incorporated into the routine practice of most units performing microsurgical reconstructions. The device consists of two rings, each containing six pins, attached to the end of a metallic piece with a turning handle on its back end (▶Fig. 19.13). The rings' diameter ranges from 1 to 4 mm, including half measures (e.g., 1.5, 2.5, and 3.5 mm), for a total of seven sizes to choose from. Following proper preparation, a "sizer" is placed right next to the vessels in order to select the diameter of the ring. Next each vessel end is passed through the corresponding ring, and the vessel wall is secured to the surrounding pins by gentle eversion and pushing using a specially designed forceps with an opening on its end that allows the passage of the pin. It is advisable to secure the longer or more mobile vessel first (usually the flap's pedicle) and then the shorter one to allow

more freedom of movement when working with the latter. Once both vessels have been "pinned" to their corresponding ring, the handle is turned and the rings are brought together. A hemostat is then used to gently squeeze the rings together, after which the system is released from the anastomotic site by continuous turning of the handle. In cases of size mismatch, the coupler system is able to accommodate a difference of up to 3:1 without the need of any additional maneuvers, always making sure that the selected ring size corresponds to the smaller vessel.

The coupler system works best in pliable vessels with a wall thickness of ≤ 0.5 mm. For this reason, this device has found its main application in

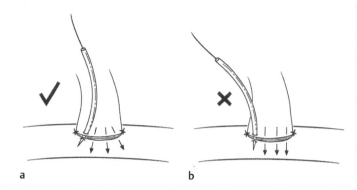

a b

Fig. 19.12 (a, b) During end-to-side anastomosis, stitches are placed radial to the center of the arteriotomy. (Reproduced with permission from Acland, Sabapathy, Practice Manual for Microvascular Surgery. 3rd edition, ©2008, Indian Society for Surgery of the Hand.)

Fig. 19.13 (a-c) The microvascular coupler system.

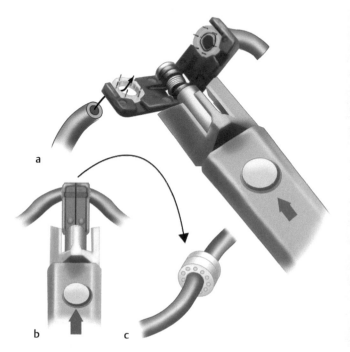

a

b c

venous anastomosis, where, compared to the traditional hand-sewn method, it is four to five times faster, has a shorter learning curve, and yields higher patency rates (e.g., close to 100%).

Size Mismatch and Patency Tests

A number of techniques have been described to deal with discrepancies in diameter between the donor and recipient vessels. For differences of up to 2:1, careful placement of the sutures farther apart on the larger vessel usually suffices (▶Fig. 19.14). Higher mismatches require additional maneuvers, such as the fish-mouth technique, beveling or tapering the larger vessel, and end-to-side anastomosis as described earlier. When beveling, an oblique cut of not more than 30 degrees is done at the edge of the smaller vessel, thus increasing the diameter of its opening (▶Fig. 19.15). Of note, for the anastomosis the beveled end should be placed parallel to the lumen of the other vessel. Tapering implies cutting the excess diameter obliquely and suturing it so that a narrower vessel end is obtained. This technique, however, does inflict more trauma to the vessel by the additional stitches and therefore should be done with utmost care.

The ultimate goal of a microsurgical anastomosis is to obtain a patent unrestricted flow. Different

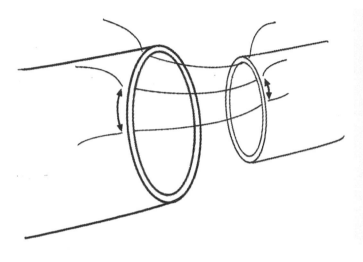

Fig. 19.14 Size mismatch up to 2:1 can be addressed by careful and proportioned placement of sutures. (Reproduced with permission from Acland, Sabapathy, Practice Manual for Microvascular Surgery. 3rd edition, ©2008, Indian Society for Surgery of the Hand.)

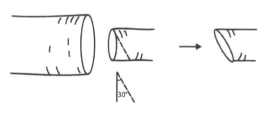

Not more than 30°

Fig. 19.15 Beveling of the small vessel end to overcome size mismatch. (Reproduced with permission from Acland, Sabapathy, Practice Manual for Microvascular Surgery. 3rd edition, ©2008, Indian Society for Surgery of the Hand.)

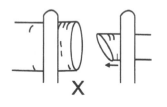

X

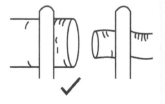

✓

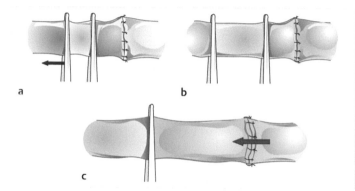

Fig. 19.16 (a-c) The milking test for patency check. (Reproduced from Weerda, Reconstructive Facial Plastic Surgery: A Problem Solving Manual, ©2001, Thieme Publishers, New York.)

methods to test patency are available, but these should be used judiciously because they imply vessel manipulation and therefore carry a risk of trauma. The least traumatic but least reliable is observation—a patent artery should be seen pulsating distal to the anastomotic site. However, in cases of clotting, a "pulse" may be mistakenly seen due to transmission of the longitudinal wave from the vessel pulsating proximal to the obstructed anastomosis. Besides, this method does not work for veins. In the uplift test, the vessel distal to the anastomosis is gently lifted and as it becomes stretched and occluded, alternating collapse and filling confirm the presence of pulsatile flow. Finally, highly reliable but traumatic is the milking test in which the vessel distal to the anastomosis is gently occluded with forceps and with another forceps blood is "milked" for several millimeters away from the anastomosis. Rapid refilling after releasing the proximal forces confirms patency. Unlike the previous two, this method can be used to assess venous patency (▶Fig. 19.16).

Practicing on a Living Model: End-to-End Anastomosis of the Rat's Femoral Artery

As Dr. Robert Acland used to say, "the secret of success is preparation." The procedure begins by making a 3–4 cm incision on the groin area, parallel to the inguinal ligament and reflecting the inguinal fat pad laterally while maintaining its attachment to the epigastric artery (▶Fig. 19.17a). The perivascular sheath is then incised with the dissecting (curved) microscissors parallel to the plane of the vessels (▶Fig. 19.17b, c) and the vessels completely freed by ligation or bipolar coagulation of their side branches. It is important to make sure that enough space is made for the vessel and clamp

to turn freely during the procedure. Next, a contrast background material is placed and a double clamp with a frame (Acland's clamp) brought into the field, and the vessels are prepared as explained earlier, including cutting, flushing, trimming of adventitia, and dilation. The front wall is addressed first, using 10–0 nylon suture, securing the two stay sutures to the suture-holding "cleat" on each side of the clamp, and placing two stitches in between to complete the anterior wall. The clamp is then flipped over to suture the back wall by placing the third stay stitch in the middle and two stitches on each side. Upon completion of the anastomosis, the stay sutures are cut and the clamp turned to its normal position and released, first distally and then proximally. The anastomotic site is covered with gauze, a sponge, or the inguinal fat pad, and gentle pressure is applied for 2 minutes. Finally, the vessel is carefully observed and patency tests performed to confirm permeability.

19.3 Basic Science of Free Flap Failure

The primary goal in any microsurgical tissue transfer is vessel permeability and flap survival. Whereas in the early days of microsurgery, patency rates barely reached 80%, today this figure rounds up to 95–98%. Furthermore, the indications for microsurgery have expanded to increasingly complicated cases and scenarios, most of which would have been judiciously denied the possibility of a microsurgical reconstruction in the past. Still, even in the most experienced hands, some flaps do fail. There are a number of biological, physical, and mechanical factors that can affect survival of a microsurgical transfer, which the (micro) surgeon must be aware of in order to anticipate what can go wrong and delineate a salvage plan when needed.

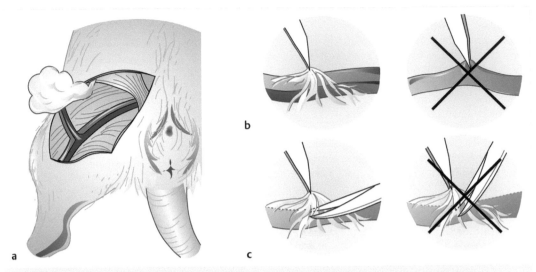

Fig. 19.17 Exposure of femoral vessels in the rat. (a) Isolation of the inguinal fat pad leaving it attached to its epigastric pedicle. (b) Vessels are grabbed by their adventitia and not full thickness. (c) The perivascular sheath is incised and dissected with the scissor's blades parallel to the plane of the vessels. (Reproduced from Weerda, Reconstructive Facial Plastic Surgery: A Problem Solving Manual, ©2001, Thieme Publishers, New York.)

19.3.1 The Endothelium and the Coagulation Cascade

The vascular endothelium is a highly dynamic and specialized layer of cells that serve a number of important functions locally and systemically. One of the main tasks of endothelial cells is to maintain blood flow by providing an antithrombotic surface that prevents the spontaneous formation of blood clots. Nevertheless, whenever the endothelial lining is disrupted and the subendothelial elements are exposed to the bloodstream, the coagulation cascade is activated. This chapter provides a summary of the main events and molecules involved in this process.

Endothelial cells express a number of factors with vasoconstrictive/vasodilating as well as prothrombotic/antithrombotic properties (▶Table 19.1). In the physiological state, the balance of these molecules, together with the negatively charged surface of endothelial cells, favors anticoagulation. However, when the intimal layer is injured, circulating platelets rapidly adhere to the exposed subendothelial collagen via links between von Willebrand factor (vWF) in the vessel wall and receptors in platelets' membranes. It is important to note that subendothelial collagen and the outermost layer of adventitia are the most powerful platelet attractants and thrombogenic

Table 19.1 Endothelial vasomotor and coagulation factors

Vasomotor factors		Coagulation factors	
Vasocon-strictive	Vasodilator	Prothrom-botic	Antithrom-botic
ACE	NO	vWF	PGI2
TXA$_2$	PGI2/PGE2	TXA$_2$	Thrombo-modulin
EDCF	EDHF	Thrombo-plastin	AT III
Leukot-rienes		Factor V	Proteins C
Free radicals		PAF	and S
Endothelin		PAI-1, PAI-2	tPA
			Heparin sulfate

Abbreviations: ACE, angiotensin-converting enzyme; AT III, antithrombin III; EDCF, endothelium-derived contracting factors; EDHF, endothelium-derived hyperpolarizing factor; NO, nitric oxide; PAF, platelet-activating factor; PAI-1, plasminogen activator inhibitor-1; PGE2, prostaglandin E2; PGI2, prostaglandin I2 (also known as prostacyclin); tPA, tissue plasminogen activator; TXA$_2$, thromboxane A$_2$; vWF, von Willebrand factor.

components of the vessel wall. After adhering to the injured site, platelets become activated and secrete arachidonic acid, which is converted to thromboxane A$_2$ (TXA$_2$) by cyclooxygenase (COX). TXA$_2$ is a potent vasoconstrictor and further stimulates platelet aggregation. Concomitantly, platelets also release vWF and fibrinogen from their alpha granules and adenosine diphosphate, calcium, and serotonin from their dense granules, all of which contribute to ongoing platelet aggregation. Coagulation leading to the formation of a fibrin clot has been traditionally represented as two pathways: intrinsic and extrinsic (▶Fig. 19.18). Although different in their mechanism of initiation, the end point is common for both, that is, the activation of prothrombin into thrombin, which in turn promotes the conversion of fibrinogen into fibrin. The intrinsic pathway is governed by normally circulating factors, whereas the extrinsic is initiated by the exposure of tissue factor (VII) on the injured endothelium. Finally, once the fibrin clot is formed, it is dissolved through a process called fibrinolysis, whereby plasminogen is converted to plasmin by several plasminogen activators, such as tissue plasminogen activator (tPA), released by endothelial cells. Plasmin is then responsible for the breakdown of fibrin and dissolution of the fibrin clot.

Upon completion of the anastomosis, injury caused by vessel division and suturing elicits a physiologic reparative/coagulative process, which results in the formation of a thin, nonobstructive layer of platelets and subsequent fibrin deposition. Careful handling of the vessels, precise apposition of their edges, and proper placement of sutures minimize exposure of collagen subendothelial prothrombotic agents, thus preventing coagulation and allowing the small platelet plug to disintegrate. During the next 72 hours, platelets are washed off and a pseudo-intima establishes at approximately 5 days. Finally a new endothelium forms 1–2 weeks after anastomosis.

Thrombosis can occur at any stage of a microsurgical transfer from completion of the microvascular anastomosis to several days later. In accordance with the physiology of vessel repair at the anastomotic site, most thrombotic events in free flap surgery occur during the first 72 hours, which is when platelets home to the anastomosis and, in the presence of a thrombogenic stimulus, may trigger coagulation. Arterial occlusion usually presents within the first 24 hours and is caused mainly by platelet aggregation and platelet plug formation, whereas venous thrombosis tends to develop later and results mainly from fibrin deposition. Although its benefit has not been fully demonstrated, it is common practice among the vast majority of microsurgeons to flush the vessels throughout the procedure with gentle jets of warm heparinized solution at a concentration of 10–100UI/mL to reduce the risk of thrombosis.

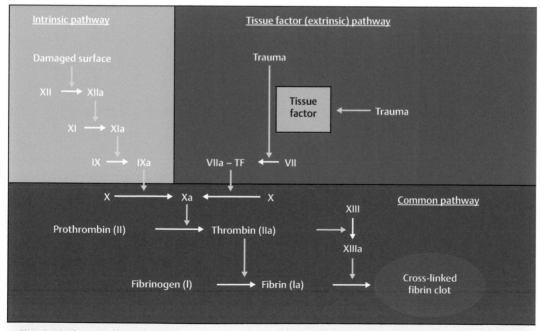

Fig. 19.18 The coagulation cascade.

19.4 Factors Influencing Flap Failure

19.4.1 Vessel Spasm

The exact mechanisms underlying vessel spasm have not been fully elucidated; however, several factors have been identified to contribute to it. Local factors include vessel trauma, presence of blood in the operative field, and tissue desiccation. Systemic factors, on the other hand, comprise low core temperature, hypotension, and sympathetic response to pain. It is therefore of paramount importance to keep these aspects in mind prior, during, and after any microsurgical procedure. Local factors are controlled mainly by a delicate and meticulous surgical technique, maintaining the (micro) surgical field clean of blood and tissue remnants and keeping the vessels and flap moist and warm. The management of systemic factors is usually done in consultation with the anesthetist and includes keeping the patient warm, under a suitable depth of anesthesia, and maintaining a stable hemodynamic state, especially regarding blood pressure. Despite the general tendency to avoid vasopressors and instead use fluids only to maintain an adequate systolic blood pressure, there is currently no robust evidence to support this practice because it has been demonstrated that use of vasoconstrictors in microsurgery does not correlate with a higher risk of flap failure. Adequate pain control during the postoperative period must also be contemplated.

There are a number of strategies that can be used to relieve spasm, of which patience is the most important, because spasm usually clears spontaneously after 5–10 minutes. Excessive manipulation in an effort to relieve the constricted vessel may result in further damage and spasm, which may at one point become irreversible; prolonged vasospasm has been shown to produce significant endothelial slough. Hence, as a first measure, the vessels should be left to rest covered with gauze soaked in warm solution containing lidocaine or papaverine. Lidocaine is one of the most commonly used topical antispasmodics and, although it is said to have its optimum effect at a concentration of 20%, in the clinical setting 2–4% formulations are generally used. Papaverine (30 mg/mL) is also used because it causes relaxation of smooth muscle on the vessel wall. Verapamil, a calcium channel blocker, has also been used topically for the same purpose. Mechanical strategies to relieve spasm include vessel dilation and stripping of adventitia. Vessel dilation alleviates spasm by eliciting temporary paralysis of the smooth muscle in the vessel wall, whereas removal of adventitia has a dual effect: vessel decompression and sympathetic denervation by dividing adrenergic nerve endings on the vessel wall. Both of these techniques should be used judiciously because excessive traction may cause injury to the vessel wall.

19.4.2 Surgical Technique

Surgical technique is the most important factor influencing success in microsurgical tissue transfer. In the words of Dr. Bernard O'Brien, one of the pioneers of microsurgery, no anticoagulation strategy can replace a meticulously executed microvascular anastomosis, a fact that highlights the importance of undertaking proper training before going into clinical practice.

During the anastomosis and throughout the whole microsurgical procedure, gentle handling of the vessels is mandatory. Grabbing the whole thickness of the vessel wall is forbidden because it is extremely traumatic and may result in endothelial disruption, platelet aggregation, and thrombus formation. Side branches should be ligated or cauterized using fine bipolar forceps at a low current setting and at a sufficient distance from its origin to avoid damage to the main vessel. Keeping the vessels warm and moist is also an important aspect to consider as cold desiccated vessels suffer endothelial sloughing with subsequent platelet aggregation. As stated earlier, the vessels should be cut cleanly with sharp straight microscissors and in one go. Irregular vessel ends may result in luminal exposure of endothelial flaps, which are highly thrombogenic. At times, due to radiotherapy or peripheral vascular disease, vessels may be of poor quality such that, once cut, the pressure of the scissors produces separation of the endothelium from the rest of the vessel wall. These vessels should be trimmed by placing one blade of the scissors inside and the other one outside the lumen so that the intima is pressed against the wall while cutting progressively around the circumference. In addition, while suturing, the needle should pass from inside to outside to avoid further separation of the different layers.

Clamp selection should consider the closing pressure of the clamp (measured in g/mm^2) and the diameter of the vessel (▶Fig. 19.19). There are five different clamp sizes, with two subcategories, A and V, for the first three. As a general

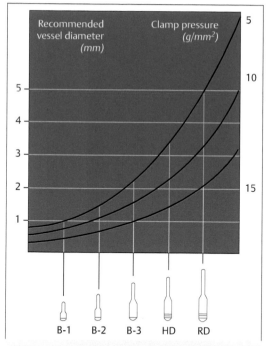

Fig. 19.19 Relationship between clamp size, recommended vessel diameter, and clamp pressure. (Adapted with permission from Acland, Sabapathy, Practice Manual for Microvascular Surgery. 3rd edition, ©2008, Indian Society for Surgery of the Hand.)

recommendation, the smaller clamp that effectively occludes the vessel should be used. Vessels can tolerate a clamp pressure of 20 g/mm² for 30 minutes without problems, whereas closing pressures over 30 g/mm² might cause significant damage to the vessel wall, especially veins.

The adventitia of vessels is highly thrombogenic, posing a high risk of failure if fibers get caught in the suture line and become exposed to the lumen. Although thorough trimming must be done to allow for a clean anastomosis, care should be taken to avoid excessive removal because this may result in endothelial damage, spasm, and an unnecessary waste of time.

Microsurgical needles are specially designed to cause the least possible trauma. Depending on vessel size, the vast majority of microvascular anastomoses are performed using nylon sutures between 8–0 and 11–0. Whereas the use of large sutures in small vessels results in significant trauma, suturing large vessels with thin sutures necessitates placement of a higher number of stitches, which is both time consuming and traumatic. Straight, full-thickness,

"one-shot" stitches should be placed because these are significantly less traumatic and achieve more precise vessel apposition than partial-thickness sutures, which may expose subendothelial collagen or cause inversion of the edges. Furthermore, taking an identical bite on both sides prevents overlap and exposure of intimal flaps at the anastomotic site. In addition, all efforts must be made to avoid undue tension at the site of anastomosis because this can otherwise result in medial discontinuity with subsequent formation of aneurysms at the suture line.

Not infrequently, anastomotic leaks are seen after releasing the clamps. It is important to identify the origin because it may come from a gap in the anastomosis, a tearing of the wall, or a side branch. Irrespective of the origin, leaks should be repaired rapidly and effectively, ideally without reclamping given that static blood within the anastomotic line is highly thrombogenic (remember Virchow's triad: blood stasis, intimal injury, and hypercoagulability). A large leak that suddenly stops is highly suggestive of thrombotic occlusion.

19.4.3 Mechanical Factors

Despite a finely executed microvascular anastomosis and reestablishment of a streamlined and unrestricted flow, flap survival may be hampered by mechanical factors, including pedicle twisting, kinking, compression, and hematomas. To prevent pedicle twisting, donor and recipient vessels must rest in their natural position prior to anastomosis, and the final position of the flap must be anticipated. In some cases, excessively long pedicles may suffer sharp bends (kinking) resulting in blood flow obstruction. When possible, this should be anticipated before suturing and the vessels cut to an adequate length; alternatively, the vessels may be fixed to the surrounding tissues at the desired position using microsutures, Surgicel (Ethicon) or Tisseel (Baxter Healthcare).

Tight wound closure and hematomas may compress the underlying pedicle, which underscores the need for correct preoperative planning of flap dimensions and meticulous hemostasis.

19.4.4 Local and Systemic Factors

Given the remarkable technical improvements in microsurgery, it is hard to establish absolute contraindications to a microsurgical repair other than the surgeon's judgment, a lack of tissues/ vessels, and the patient's inability to sustain a long surgery or postoperative recovery. In consequence, microvascular tissue transfers are being currently performed with a high degree of safety and success in increasingly complex situations. Notwithstanding, there are a number of local and systemic factors associated with increased rates of flap failure and wound healing problems that should be thoroughly investigated, anticipated, and managed during the preoperative planning to avoid unwanted surprises in the operating room and minimize postoperative complications.

Radiotherapy

The effects of radiation on wound healing are reviewed in Chapter 2. From a (micro) surgical perspective, damage from radiotherapy and scarring from previous ablative surgeries often precludes the use of local flaps for reconstruction, establishing the indication for regional or distant tissue transfer. Although some studies have reported an increased risk of flap failure, major complications, and reoperation rates in patients with preoperative radiotherapy, others have found no difference in flap survival. However, microsurgical reconstruction of irradiated defects may be complicated by poor quality of recipient vessels and a higher rate of wound healing problems. Finding suitable vessels in a previously operated and irradiated neck, for example, can be quite challenging. Likewise, irradiated internal mammary vessels in breast reconstruction may be surrounded by scar tissue, making their dissection sometimes difficult. Additionally, irradiated vessels are at times more friable and prone to intimal dissection during manipulation and suturing. In this regard, Guelinckx et al elaborated some important measures for suturing irradiated vessels (▶Table 19.2). When radiotherapy is administered after reconstruction there is a risk of flap shrinkage and induration, which may affect the functional and aesthetic outcome of the reconstruction. Hence it is preferable, when possible, to delay reconstruction at least until the initial inflammatory insult from radiotherapy has subsided. In all, whenever an oncologic reconstruction is planned, the issue of radiotherapy must be investigated as to doses, fractioning, and, most importantly, time elapsed since the last session. In situations in which postreconstruction radiotherapy is planned, close communication with the oncologic surgeon and radiotherapy oncologist is paramount to ensure both adequate delivery of radiation and a good reconstructive outcome.

Table 19.2 Measures to reduce trauma when suturing irradiated vessels

Suturing irradiated vessels
• Minimize recipient vessel injury by performing a limited dissection.
• Avoid use of electrocoagulation for arterial side branches.
• Minimize trauma by using small needles and sutures (e.g., 10–0 nylon sutures swaged on 70-mm needles).
• In the damaged vessel, pass the needle from inside to outside to prevent intramural dissection.
• Reduce clamping time.
• Rinse vessels with heparinized solution frequently throughout the procedure.

Source: Adapted from Guelinckx PJ, Boeckx WD, Fossion E, Gruwez JA. Scanning electron microscopy of irradiated recipient blood vessels in head and neck free flaps. Plast Reconstr Surg 1984;74:217–226.

Trauma

Microsurgical tissue transfer represents a reliable alternative for the reconstruction of traumatic defects. Not infrequently, the extent of trauma precludes closure with local tissues, either because they are lacking or unusable. Distant tissue, in turn, can provide a healthy, well-vascularized coverage for complex wounds, such as those presenting with bone or joint exposure, achieving good functional results and reduced rates of infection. The issue with microsurgical reconstruction of a traumatic wound has to do mainly with the quality of recipient vessels because they might be severely injured. In some cases, vascular reconstruction may be needed prior to bone and soft tissue repair to ensure adequate blood supply to the distal limb. Traumatized vessels are highly thrombogenic and should not be used as recipient, and it is often necessary to dissect proximally to find a suitable spot on which to connect the flap, because the extent of vessel damage may reach way beyond the actual wound. Angiographic studies, Doppler, and, ultimately, direct visualization of pulsatile flow are useful methods to assess vessel viability in a traumatized extremity. Flaps with long pedicles or vein grafts should be used in cases where there is considerable distance between the wound and recipient vessels. In addition, in critically perfused limbs, end-to-side anastomosis should be performed to preserve distal flow. Finally, although vascular anastomoses proximal to the site of injury are preferred, use of the distal stump is also acceptable as long as it is performed outside the zone of injury and after confirming adequate retrograde flow.

Smoking

While the use of tobacco has a proven negative effect on wound healing, there is no evidence to support that it affects free flap survival. Despite the fact that cigarette smoking produces a thrombogenic and vasoconstricted state, large series comparing outcomes between smokers and nonsmokers have failed to find elevated rates of flap failure in the former. There is, though, a higher risk of wound healing complications. Interestingly, smoking has shown to have a significant impact on replantation outcomes, which could be due to the digital vessels being more sensitive to the effects of nicotine and having stronger vasomotor control. In any case, cigarette-smoking cessation should be strongly encouraged both before and after any microsurgical procedure.

Medical Comorbidities

A complete review of the whole spectrum of comorbidities that can affect flap survival is beyond the scope of this chapter. Herein we will focus on two common conditions, namely diabetes and peripheral vascular disease. Diabetes is known to produce microangiopathy and is associated with atherosclerosis. Although free tissue transfer is a valuable tool for limb salvage in diabetics, the presence of diabetes has been identified as predictive of flap failure; therefore the indication for microsurgical reconstruction in these patients should be carefully assessed, balancing the risks and benefits of a complex reconstruction versus simpler methods or amputation. Peripheral vascular disease may pose difficulties to microsurgical reconstruction, with some cases needing vascular bypass surgery or endovascular revascularization prior to flap transfer. Vessels showing significant calcification and/or presence of obstructive atherosclerotic plaques precludes their use as either donors or recipients, thus limiting the alternatives. A careful preoperative assessment is therefore mandatory in patients at risk or with a previous history of vascular disease, and should include a through medical history and imaging by means of color Doppler ultrasonography, angiography, computed tomographic angiography, or magnetic resonance angiography. Consultation with a vascular specialist should be considered in cases of severe occlusion.

Hypercoagulability

Although it does not occur very often, there are cases in which thrombosis and flap failure occur without a readily identifiable cause. These patients should be thoroughly investigated for a potential hypercoagulability disease before embarking on a new microsurgical venture. Better yet, coagulation problems should be identified and managed during the preoperative planning, referring the patient to a hematology specialist if required. Prothrombotic states may be related to inherited and acquired conditions. Inherited thrombophilias include factor V Leiden, protein C and S deficiencies, and mutated antithrombin and prothrombin. Unfortunately, many of these patients are unaware of their condition preoperatively, and the disease reveals itself by "inexplicable" repeated thrombosis during the intra- or postoperative period. Acquired thrombophilias are associated with a number of factors that are commonly found in patients undergoing a microsurgical reconstruction, such as trauma, chronic inflammation, cancer, and infection. Use of hormonal contraceptives may also increase the risk of thrombosis, especially if combined with obesity and cigarette smoking. Whether it is due to an inherited or acquired condition, it is important to identify and treat thrombophilias prior to reconstruction. Conversely, in cases where the condition is unmasked by a failed microsurgical transfer, subsequent reconstructions should carefully balance the risks and benefits of performing a second free flap, and nonmicrosurgical options should be considered.

19.4.5 Ischemia–reperfusion Injury

Given the inherent nature of microsurgical tissue transfers, all free flaps must inevitably undergo a period of *primary ischemia*, which goes from pedicle division at the donor site until completion of anastomoses at the recipient site. Ischemic periods after this are called *secondary ischemia* and may be caused by intraoperative or postoperative thrombosis, pedicle compression, twists, and so forth. Interruption of blood supply to the tissues produces an important insult at the endothelial and cellular levels and should therefore be kept to the minimum possible. ►Table 19.3 summarizes the critical times of ischemia for different tissues.

The damage from ischemia is directly proportional to its duration. During primary ischemia, cells change their metabolism from aerobic to anaerobic. Under these circumstances, endothelial cells undergo molecular and structural changes that in turn initiate and drive a series of pathophysiological responses at the endothelium–cell interface. Proinflammatory cytokines as well as proinflammatory complement cleavage products are released, increasing endothelium permeability. The extravasation of fluid to the interstitial space produces edema and capillary narrowing, mainly by mechanical compression; this reduction in capillary caliber is further accentuated by failure to synthesize vasodilators and inability to degrade vasoconstrictors. In addition, due to the impaired blood flow, cellular waste products are not washed away, leading to their intra- and extracellular accumulation. Leucocytes are sequestered within the flap, and generation of oxygen free radicals begins. Sustained ischemia also leads to adenosine triphosphate depletion. Furthermore, prolonged ischemia leads to intracellular accumulation of H^+ and subsequent intracellular acidosis. In order to reestablish normal pH, exchange mechanisms are activated, which, in the absence of energy, leads to elevation of cytosolic Ca^{2+}. Excessive uptake of cytosolic Ca^{2+} by the mitochondria impairs adenosine triphosphate synthesis and results in cell death. Once microvascular anastomoses are completed and clamps released, reestablishment of blood flow not only provides nutrients and oxygen but also inflammatory cells, which are driven by the cytokines released during the ischemic period. Thus, an important number of neutrophils and platelets are attracted to the flap's microcirculation, where they become activated, migrate to the interstitial space, and release oxygen-free radicals. Restoration of blood flow also causes more edema, all of which

adds further damage to the already affected tissue. If the ischemic period is kept within the tissues' acceptable time frames, the flap will survive the insult. Conversely, prolonged ischemia will produce significant damage, and the flap will not be perfused after clamp release. The *no-reflow phenomenon* describes the situation where the flap is not perfused despite having patent arterial and venous anastomoses.

19.5 Free Flap Monitoring and Salvage

As mentioned earlier, despite the high rates of success in microsurgical tissue transfer, flap failure remains a concern, even among experienced surgeons. Adequate postoperative monitoring forms an integral part of the whole microsurgical process because early identification and treatment of a vascular complication have been shown to have a direct impact on flap survival. In 1975, Creech and Miller described the ideal monitoring device as quick and easy to perform, harmless to the patient and flap, accurate, inexpensive, able to be performed repeatedly without injury, and applicable to all kinds of flaps. Different methods have been described over the last 4 decades with none of them satisfactorily fulfilling all these characteristics. Furthermore, there is no evidence to support the use of one method over another.

19.5.1 Flap Monitoring

Clinical Monitoring

Clinical observation remains the most common technique and the gold standard to which the rest of monitoring methods should be compared. The four pillars of clinical monitoring are color, temperature, capillary refill, and turgor (►Table 19.4).

Table 19.4 Clinical findings of failing flaps

	Arterial	Venous
Color	Pale, mottled	Bluish-purple or cyanotic discoloration
Capillary refill	Slow (> 3 s) or absent	Fast (< 1 s)
Turgor	Decreased	Swollen
Temperature	Cold	Cold. Might be warm in initial stages

Table 19.3 Critical times of ischemia

Tissue	Critical times of ischemia (hours)	
	Warm	Cold
Skin and subcutaneous tissue	4–6	≤ 10
Bone	< 3	24
Muscle	< 2	8

In addition, handheld Doppler is routinely used in a number of reconstructive units. This device is very useful to assess pulsation of a perforator marked on the skin paddle as well flow through the pedicle, in which case it is very important to make sure that a signal *distal* to the anastomosis is being recorded. A strong, pulsating signal indicates arterial flow, whereas a smooth, continuous sound is characteristically venous. When in doubt, an additional adjunct is assessment of dermal bleeding by pinprick or gently scratching the flap's surface with a 24-gauge needle. Slow or absent bleeding is suggestive of arterial occlusion, whereas the presence of quick, dark bleeding indicates venous obstruction. Although the frequency of evaluation may vary among institutions, half-hourly checks during the first 24 hours and hourly over the next 24 hours is a reasonable scheme, consistent with the fact that most failures occur in the early postoperative period (first 48 hours). After that, 4-hourly checks should be performed until discharge. Buried flaps pose a significant challenge because they cannot be clinically monitored, and they have salvage rates close to 0% because their failure only becomes evident days after by indirect signs like swelling, dehiscence, fistulas, and infection. Strategies such as including a small monitoring paddle allow clinical monitoring of buried flaps.

Implantable Doppler Probe

The Cook-Swartz Doppler Probe (Cook Medical) consists of a 20-MHz ultrasonic probe implanted on a silicone cuff, which is wrapped around the vein distal to the anastomosis and secured with microclips, sutures, or fibrin sealant. The electrode is connected to a wire that exits the wound and is connected to a monitor that continuously records the audible venous signal. It is placed around the vein because this enables it to detect both an arterial and a venous obstruction. Once continuous monitoring is no longer required, the electrode is removed by pulling the wire with a recommended force of 50 g. This method is especially useful for buried flaps and has shown salvage rates between 61 and 94% after reexploration. The Flow Coupler device (Synovis) employs a similar concept where the probe is connected to one of the rings used for the anastomosis, which proceeds exactly the same as explained earlier.

Color Duplex Ultrasound

This noninvasive monitoring technique is used mainly for buried flaps in head and neck reconstruction. The system accurately records flow velocity and direction, allowing evaluation of donor and recipient vessels. However, because it is usually performed only once daily, it needs to be combined with other methods.

Microdialysis

This invasive monitoring technique consists of a double-lumen microdialysis catheter placed in the flap. As fluid passes through a semipermeable membrane in the catheter, the presence of certain metabolites like lactate, glucose, glycerol, and pyruvate is analyzed to assess the flap's metabolic state. An increase in glycerol concentration indicates cell membrane injury and is seen in both arterial and venous failure, whereas an elevated lactate:pyruvate ratio and low glucose are indicative of anaerobic metabolism from ischemia secondary to arterial obstruction. This method is able to detect vascular complications before clinical signs appear and is useful for monitoring buried flaps as well. Its downsides include its high cost and learning curve.

Near Infrared Spectroscopy

Near infrared spectroscopy (NIRS) measures hemoglobin content and oxygenation in small-diameter vessels (arterioles, venules, and capillaries), thus providing information on the status of microcirculation. Its depth of penetration of 20 mm makes it a suitable method for monitoring virtually any flap with a skin paddle to attach the probe to. This method is relatively inexpensive, harmless, highly reproducible, and reliable, which make it one of the best candidates for free flap monitoring currently available. Different studies have shown that NIRS is able to detect vascular complications before clinical signs appear. Furthermore, as opposed to simple pulse oximetry, NIRS is not affected by factors such as blood pressure changes, supplemental oxygenation, and perforator size and number. Salvage rates of 94–100% have been reported with the combination of NIRS and clinical monitoring.

Laser Doppler Flowmetry

Laser Doppler flowmetry is a continuous, noninvasive monitoring method in which the flap is illuminated with a laser light, and the light scattered in tissues is sent back, collected, and correlated with the average velocity of the cells moving within the tissue, thus yielding information on blood flow. The trend, rather than absolute values of flow, is evaluated. The main disadvantage of this technique is that its depth of tissue penetration is only 8 mm. Similar flap salvage rates have been reported with this versus clinical monitoring alone.

19.5.2 Flap Salvage

Once a diagnosis of flap compromise is made, a series of measures should be put in motion to reverse the situation as quickly and effectively as possible. Depending on the cause of failure, some flaps might be revised in the operating room, whereas others may be successfully managed at the bedside. Nonetheless, unnecessary delays must be avoided and, when in doubt, the take-back threshold should be low.

Bedside Strategies of Salvage

Whenever a flap is being monitored, either as a routine checkup or in response to a call from the ward,

it is good to have a mental checklist of the possible variables that might affect flap viability (▶ Table 19.5).

When the cause of obstruction is accumulation of underlying fluid/blood or tight closure, suture release and careful drainage and aspiration are very useful and highly effective measures that will improve the flap's characteristics immediately. Likewise, limb elevation or postural changes might also be effective, especially in cases of insufficient venous drainage. Open wounds from stitch removal should be adequately dressed and monitored to prevent infection, and closure (or grafting) is performed a few days later once postoperative edema has partially subsided and the flap has become adapted to the new situation. If the problem remains unchanged or a significant improvement is not observed, prompt take-back to the operating theater is indicated.

Surgical Strategies of Salvage

For cases undergoing urgent flap revision in the operating room, it is important to have an action plan considering both the clinical signs of failure and any clues the surgeon might have from the first surgery that could potentially explain and help correct the situation. For instance, in a case of venous insufficiency, the surgeon might have left a spare vein that would serve as a useful lifeboat.

Table 19.5 Flap monitoring checklist

Variable	Measure
Temperature	Ensure both patient and flap are warm. Cold patients/flaps are vasoconstricted and more prone to vessel spasm. Compare flap temperature with that of normal skin. A difference > 2°C is suggestive of vascular obstruction.
Doppler signal	Check for both arterial (pulsating) and venous (continuous) signals.
Tension	Tense wound closure is likely to compress the vascular pedicle, especially the vein. If this is the case, release sutures as necessary.
Hematoma	Look for signs of hematoma (rapid asymmetric bulging, bleeding, bruising, etc.). Release sutures and drain the accumulated fluid under sterile conditions. This is best done in the operating room.
Pain	Ensure proper management of postoperative pain. Release of catecholamines due to postoperative pain may produce vasoconstriction and contribute to vessel spasm.
Urine output	Fluid resuscitation should be kept within adequate limits. Aim for a urine output of 0.5–1 mL/kg/h. Underresuscitation increases blood viscosity and may lower blood pressure. Overresuscitation might produce flap edema and capillary compression.
Drain output	High output of fresh blood may indicate the presence of active bleeding and development of underlying hematoma. No output should raise suspicion of drain obstruction and risk of fluid/blood accumulation.
Position	Ensure the position of the flap is such that it facilitates venous drainage (as venous insufficiency is more common than arterial). This might need limb elevation or patient postural changes.
Anticoagulation	Check that a proper anticoagulation regime has been clearly charted in the patient's medications.

In other instances, it is hard to predict what the actual cause of failure is, and therefore the plan is "open and see." When performed in a timely manner, salvage rates of free flaps reach approximately 80%. The flap's pedicle and vascular anastomoses should be widely and clearly exposed and tested for patency. In the best of cases, the cause of obstruction will be pedicle compression, twisting, or kinking, all of which can be quickly resolved by repositioning. Immediate improvement should be observed. In cases in which no thrombosis or pedicle obstruction is found but blood inflow/drainage is still insufficient, techniques to improve arterial and/or venous flow by means of supercharging and/or turbocharging should be considered. In most instances, it is the venous drainage that needs to be boosted. Conversely, if thrombosis is noted, the affected anastomosis must be cut and the lumen of both donor and recipient vessels inspected because sometimes the thrombus extends beyond the suture line. Vessels should be trimmed to a healthy spot for reanastomosis. If the thrombus is confined to the anastomotic site, careful removal and vigorous flushing with a heparinized solution should be performed. However, if the thrombus extends beyond the suture line and into the pedicle, it may be an indicator of intraflap thrombosis. Again, irrigation with copious amounts of heparinized solution is performed, and once all clots have been removed anastomoses are redone. Fibrinolytics may also be used in a situation of massive pedicle thrombosis. An interpositional vein graft might be needed in cases where the recipient vessels fail and there are no nearby alternatives. Depending on the reconstructive need, vein grafts can be obtained from various sites, including the volar forearm, the long and short saphenous vein, and so forth. Even though vein grafts have a historical bad reputation for allegedly being associated with higher rates of thrombosis, this is no longer a reality because, when used primarily, they have been shown to achieve patency rates similar to those of normal anastomoses. What is true and should be considered though, is that, in the emergency situation of flap salvage, the scenario is far from ideal, and therefore a higher risk of failure should be expected—risk that is inherent to the procedure itself and not necessarily related to the use of a vein graft. Lastly a relatively aggressive anticoagulation protocol beyond routine prophylaxis should be indicated with close monitoring of bleeding and hematoma.

In cases in which the flap fails to become reperfused, an alternative reconstruction must be sought. Depending on availability, the cause of failure, and the patient's condition, a second free flap may be performed, although regional pedicled options should be considered as well. Likewise, the second reconstruction may be carried out immediately or in a delayed fashion, in which case the wound is dressed or covered temporarily with vacuum-assisted closure (VAC).

19.6 Postoperative Pharmacological Therapy in Microsurgery

The postoperative management of free flaps with regard to the use of antithrombotic therapy is extremely diverse and mostly based on personal experience rather than solid evidence. Given the wide array of factors that can affect the outcome in free flap surgery and the difficulty in designing randomized controlled trials, no formal guidelines exist as to type, doses, route of administration, and duration of antithrombotic medication following microsurgical tissue transfer or replantation. Protocols may vary from using one to three agents in combination to not using any medication at all.

As stated earlier, venous and arterial thrombi differ in their composition, with the former consisting mainly of fibrin and the latter of platelets, so in theory pharmacological strategies to prevent/treat each of them will be different as well. A potential target of pharmacological treatment that is currently being investigated is the administration of medications to reduce ischemia–reperfusion injury. Although this could be a promising solution for those complicated flaps that have been submitted to prolonged periods of primary and secondary ischemia, it does not address the main cause of failure, which is thrombosis at the anastomotic site. Furthermore, it should be noted that if no-reflow phenomenon has already ensued, the flap is most likely unsalvageable despite any pharmacological and surgical effort.

19.6.1 Heparin

Heparin is a naturally occurring glycosaminoglycan produced by mast cells and basophils. It acts by binding to and activating antithrombin III (AT III). Activated AT III then inactivates thrombin and factors IXa, Xa, XIa, and XIIa, which will ultimately prevent fibrin formation.

Heparin also decreases platelet adhesion. The effects of heparin are effectively reversed with protamine sulfate. One of the most feared complications related to the use of systemic unfractionated heparin is heparin-induced thrombocytopenia (HIT). Immune-related HIT (i.e., HIT-2) appears 5–14 days after administration and is a life- and limb-threatening complication because it is paradoxically associated with severe thrombotic events. Heparin and all heparin-related products should be stopped immediately and an alternative anticoagulant administered. Platelet transfusion is not indicated except for cases with active bleeding or patients undergoing procedures that carry a high risk of bleeding. While the use of intraoperative irrigation of microsurgical anastomoses is widespread, its systemic use is much less systematic. Although some surgeons give an intravenous bolus of 5,000 IU at the time of clamp release, others reserve it for cases of intraoperative and/or postoperative thrombosis, damaged vessels, and replantation of crushed/avulsed parts. Low-molecular-weight heparin (LMWH), such as dalteparin and enoxaparin, is a form of fractioned heparin that also acts by binding to AT III but in a way that it inhibits only factor Xa, without any effect on thrombin. LMWH cannot be monitored by partial thromboplastin time, but rather, by measuring anti-factor Xa activity, although this not often needed. Compared to unfractionated heparin, LMWH is administered fewer times a day and carries a smaller risk of both bleeding and HIT. Postoperative subcutaneous LMWH is more widely used in microsurgical cases.

19.6.2 Aspirin

Acetylsalicylic acid is a known antiaggregant that acts by irreversibly inhibiting platelet cyclooxygenase (COX-1). Inhibition of COX-1 blocks the production of TXA_2, a potent vasoconstrictor and proaggregant. Except for bleeding time, none of the other coagulation tests is altered by aspirin. It is important to note that, given its irreversible action, the effects of aspirin are reversed once platelet turnover occurs, which takes approximately 7–10 days. The usual adult dose is 80–325 mg by mouth daily, with which thromboxane but not prostacyclin (a vasodilator and platelet inhibitor) is blocked. Aspirin may be started 24 hours before or immediately after free flap surgery and continued for 2–4 weeks.

19.6.3 Dextran

Dextran is a complex polysaccharide clinically available in two forms depending on its molecular weight: dextran 40 (40,000 daltons) and de xtran 70 (70,000 daltons). Although dextran has been used mainly as a volume expander, it does a have a number of other medical applications. It acts as an antiplatelet/antithrombotic agent, mainly by increasing the negative electric charge of platelets, erythrocytes, and endothelial cells, which impairs platelet activation and fibrin plug formation. As a volume expander, dextran reduces blood viscosity, which also helps to reduce thrombus formation. Additionally, dextran acts by inactivating vWF and has been shown to have some fibrinolytic effect. Clinically, 10% dextran 40 is the most commonly used. An initial loading dose of 30–50 mL is administered upon completion of microvascular anastomoses, followed by 25–30 mL/h continuous infusion for 5 days, after which it is discontinued. Nowadays, most surgeons have abandoned the use of dextran in free flap surgery because of its potentially serious complications, including anaphylactic reactions, volume overload, pulmonary edema, renal failure, and hemorrhage. Furthermore, several reports have failed to show a significant improvement in flap survival with the use of dextran.

19.6.4 Thrombolytics

Although not routinely used in free tissue transfer, thrombolytics do have a role in the management of a failing flap or finger/limb replant. If a decision has been made to redo an anastomosis and thrombosis recurs after several attempts, then streptokinase, urokinase, or tissue tPA may be considered for thrombus breakdown and prevention of a new occlusion. All these agents act by activating plasminogen into plasmin, which then cleaves fibrin. Because streptokinase is produced by group Cβ-hemolytic streptococci, there is a risk of developing antibodies after a first administration, which can potentially reduce its action and induce a severe allergic reaction on a second administration. Urokinase and tPA, in turn, are human derived and therefore less immunogenic. Bleeding and hematoma, however, are complications common to all three. To reduce the chance of an allergic response and ameliorate the systemic bleeding risk, 100,000–250,000 IU of urokinase/streptokinase or 15 mg of tPA can be administered directly to the anastomosis through a side branch, making sure passage to the systemic circulation is avoided by, for example, leaving the flap to bleed through a nonanastomosed spare vein or by opening the venous anastomosis.

19.6.5 Antiglycoprotein IIb/IIIa

Glycoprotein (GP) IIb/IIIa is involved in platelet activation and subsequent aggregation. Tirofiban, abciximab, and eptifibatide, among others, act by inhibiting GP IIb/IIIa receptor on platelets' surface, thereby preventing their activation, and are most commonly used for acute coronary heart syndromes. In microsurgery, some experimental evidence using GP IIb/IIIa blockers alone or in combination with heparin and aspirin in animal models of thrombosed microvascular anastomosis showed good results; however, they are not routinely used in free tissue transfer.

19.6.6 Leeches

Several species of leeches are available for clinical use, with *Hirudo medicinalis* being by far the most common. In reconstructive surgery, leeches are mainly used to alleviate venous congestion of replanted fingers, although they can be used in pedicled and free flaps as well. After application, leeches start feeding on blood at the same time that they inject hirudin, a vasodilator and anticoagulant agent present in their saliva. Once the leech is fully fed, it falls off, but the surface continues to bleed for several hours due to the effect of hirudin. Patients on leech therapy may therefore necessitate blood transfusion. Leeches should be left to detach spontaneously and not be forcedly removed from the patient's skin because this can leave teeth behind and cause regurgitation, both of which can lead to infection. During leech treatment, it is important to administer antibiotic prophylaxis against *Aeromonas hydrophila*, for which a quinolone (e.g., ciprofloxacin) is usually prescribed.

19.7 Clinical Applications

19.7.1 Case 1

A 46-year-old man presented with a large scalp defect with exposed bone (▶Fig. 19.20a). An anterolateral thigh (ALT) flap was planned on the right side and elevated based on two perforators (▶Fig. 19.20b). The flap was connected to the superficial temporal artery and vein on the left side. Complete stable coverage was achieved (▶Fig. 19.20c).

19.7.2 Case 2

A 51-year-old woman suffered a complex traumatic injury to her left upper limb resulting in a large defect over the volar aspect of her forearm and wrist along with amputation of the ring and little finger (▶Fig. 19.21a). An ALT flap from the right thigh was harvested based on one perforator and connected to the radial artery and vein (▶Fig. 19.21b, c). One year after surgery the patient showed stable coverage of the wound, with good contour and excellent functional result with near full range of motion of the wrist and remaining digits (▶Fig. 19.21d-g).

19.7.3 Case 3

A 34-year-old man suffered a motor vehicle accident resulting in a complex lower limb injury (Gustilo type 3) with loss of soft tissues and exposed bone (▶Fig. 19.22a). After skeletal stabilization with an external fixator and serial

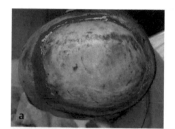
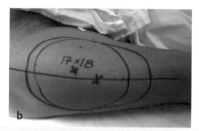
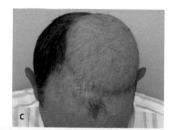

Fig. 19.20 Case 1. **(a)** Preoperative view of scalp defect. **(b)** Planned 17 × 18 cm right anterolateral thigh flap. **(c)** One year follow-up.

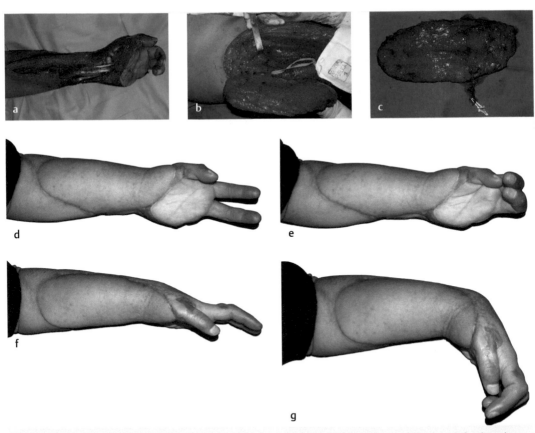

Fig. 19.21 Case 2. (a) Complex left forearm injury prior to reconstruction. (b) Right anterolateral thigh flap based on one perforator. (c) Flap disconnected and ready for transfer. (d-g) At 15-month follow-up showing stable coverage and excellent functional result.

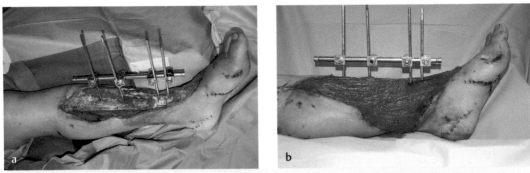

Fig. 19.22 Case 3. (a) Gustilo type 3 fracture after skeletal stabilization and serial debridements. (b) Soft tissue coverage with a free latissimus dorsi muscle flap.

debridements, the wound was resurfaced with a free latissimus dorsi muscle flap (▶ Fig. 19.22b), based on the thoracodorsal vessels, which were connected to the posterior tibial artery and vein. The flap was then covered with a split-thickness skin graft.

19.8 Conclusions

Acquisition of proficiency in microsurgery requires a high level of commitment and training. While the technical procedure itself (e.g., microsurgical anastomosis) may be seen as difficult at the beginning, with time and practice it becomes less challenging. However, microsurgery and free tissue transfer are far from being just about joining vessels and nerves under a microscope, but entail a whole process that includes wound and patient assessment, careful preoperative planning, meticulous execution, and thorough postoperative care. These aspects necessarily require a team that is coordinated by the lead reconstructive surgeon and includes surgical trainees, nurses, anesthetists, intensivists, and radiologists. Moreover, close communication with colleagues involved in the management of the patient, such as orthopaedic, head and neck, and general surgeons; medical and radiotherapy oncologists; pathologists; and rehabilitation physiotherapists, is paramount to ensure a successful microsurgical reconstruction.

19.9 Key Points

- Acquiring the basic skills in a dedicated microsurgery course prior to commencing clinical microsurgical work is highly recommended.
- Tremor is involuntary movement, and all surgeons have some degree of tremor. Correct positioning, adequate handling of instruments, a right state of mind, and control of regular habits (smoking, coffee, and exercise) all help to reduce it.
- Correct placement of stitches and gentle manipulation of vessels are critical to achieve a patent anastomosis.
- For venous anastomosis, the coupler system achieves similar or better rates of patency and is faster than the hand-sewn technique.
- Surgical technique is the main determinant of a successful microsurgical anastomosis and free tissue transfer. Other factors influencing the outcome include vasospasm, trauma, previous radiotherapy, hypercoagulability states, peripheral vascular disease, and diabetes. Nicotine has a significant impact on digital vessels following replantation.
- Topical 2% lidocaine and papaverine are the most commonly used agents to prevent/treat vasospasm intraoperatively.

- No reflow phenomenon is the end stage of ischemia/reperfusion injury and refers to the absence of flap perfusion despite a patent anastomosis.
- Clinical observation remains the gold standard in free flap monitoring. NIRS represents a reliable and inexpensive alternativ e of monitoring for flaps with a skin paddle big enough to accommodate the probe.
- Heparin is the most widely used anticoagulant; nevertheless, practice varies among institutions as to time of administration.
- Fibrinolytic therapy is not used routinely in free flap surgery; however, it does have a role in cases of flap revision and anastomotic thrombosis.
- Leeches feed on blood and inject hirudin, which is an anticoagulant. Complications associated with the use of leeches include bleeding necessitating transfusion, and infection. During leech treatment, ciprofloxacin is given as antibiotic prophylaxis against *Aeromonas hydrophila*.

Recommended Readings

Abdelrahman M, Sivarajah A, Thiemermann C. Beneficial effects of PPAR-gamma ligands in ischemia-reperfusion injury, inflammation and shock. Cardiovasc Res. 2005; 65(4):772–781

Acland RD, Raja Sabapathy S. Practice Manual for Microvascular Surgery. 3rd ed. Maharashtra, India: Indian Society for Surgery of the Hand; 2008

Antia NH, Buch VI. Transfer of an abdominal dermo-fat graft by direct anastomosis of blood vessels. Br J Plast Surg. 1971; 24(1):15–19

Ardehali B, Morritt AN, Jain A. Systematic review: anastomotic microvascular device. J Plast Reconstr Aesthet Surg. 2014; 67(6):752–755

Benatar MJ, Dassonville O, Chamorey E, et al. Impact of preoperative radiotherapy on head and neck free flap reconstruction: a report on 429 cases. J Plast Reconstr Aesthet Surg. 2013; 66(4):478–482

Bengtson BP, Schusterman MA, Baldwin BJ, et al. Influence of prior radiotherapy on the development of postoperative complications and success of free tissue transfers in head and neck cancer reconstruction. Am J Surg. 1993; 166(4):326–330

Bill TJ, Foresman PA, Rodeheaver GT, Drake DB. Fibrin sealant: a novel method of fixation for an implantable ultrasonic microDoppler probe. J Reconstr Microsurg. 2001; 17(4):257–262

Bui DT, Cordeiro PG, Hu QY, Disa JJ, Pusic A, Mehrara BJ. Free flap reexploration: indications, treatment, and outcomes in 1193 free flaps. Plast Reconstr Surg. 2007; 119(7):2092–2100

Buncke HJ, Jr, Schulz WP. Experimental digital amputation and reimplantation. Plast Reconstr Surg. 1965; 36:62–70

Buncke HJ, Jr, Schulz WP. Total ear reimplantation in the rabbit utilising microminiature vascular anastomoses. Br J Plast Surg. 1966; 19(1):15–22

Carrel A. The operative technique of vascular anastomoses and the transplantation of viscera. Med Lyon. 1902; 98:859

Chan WY, Matteucci P, Southern SJ. Validation of microsurgical models in microsurgery training and competence: a review. Microsurgery. 2007; 27(5):494–499

Chang LD, Buncke G, Slezak S, Buncke HJ. Cigarette smoking, plastic surgery, and microsurgery. J Reconstr Microsurg. 1996; 12(7):467–474

Chung TL, Pumplin DW, Holton LH, III, Taylor JA, Rodriguez ED, Silverman RP. Prevention of microsurgical anastomotic thrombosis using aspirin, heparin, and the glycoprotein IIb/IIIa inhibitor tirofiban. Plast Reconstr Surg. 2007; 120(5):1281–1288

Cobbett JR. Free digital transfer. Report of a case of transfer of a great toe to replace an amputated thumb. J Bone Joint Surg Br. 1969; 51(4):677–679

Colwell AS, Wright L, Karanas Y. Near-infrared spectroscopy measures tissue oxygenation in free flaps for breast reconstruction. Plast Reconstr Surg. 2008; 121(5):344e–345e

Creech B, Miller S. Evaluation of circulation in skin flaps. In: Grabb WC, Myers MB, eds. Skin Flaps. Boston, MA: Little, Brown; 1975:21-38

Daniel RK, Taylor GI. Distant transfer of an island flap by microvascular anastomoses. A clinical technique. Plast Reconstr Surg. 1973; 52(2):111–117

Disa JJ, Cordeiro PG, Hidalgo DA. Efficacy of conventional monitoring techniques in free tissue transfer: an 11-year experience in 750 consecutive cases. Plast Reconstr Surg. 1999; 104(1):97–101

Edsander-Nord A, Röjdmark J, Wickman M. Metabolism in pedicled and free TRAM flaps: a comparison using the microdialysis technique. Plast Reconstr Surg. 2002; 109(2):664–673

Few JW, Corral CJ, Fine NA, Dumanian GA. Monitoring buried head and neck free flaps with high-resolution color-duplex ultrasound. Plast Reconstr Surg. 2001; 108(3):709–712

Froemel D, Fitzsimons SJ, Frank J, Sauerbier M, Meurer A, Barker JH. A review of thrombosis and antithrombotic therapy in microvascular surgery. Eur Surg Res. 2013; 50(1):32–43

Furnas H, Rosen JM. Monitoring in microvascular surgery. Ann Plast Surg. 1991; 26(3):265–272

Gallico GG III. Replantation and revascularization of the upper extremity. In: McCarthy JG, May JW, Littler JW, eds. Plastic Surgery. Vol 7. Philadelphia, PA: WB Saunders; 1990:4355–4383

Godina M. Preferential use of end-to-side arterial anastomoses in free flap transfers. Plast Reconstr Surg. 1979; 64(5):673–682

Goodman JC, Valadka AB, Gopinath SP, Uzura M, Robertson CS. Extracellular lactate and glucose alterations in the brain after head injury measured by microdialysis. Crit Care Med. 1999; 27(9):1965–1973

Guelinckx PJ, Boeckx WD, Fossion E, Gruwez JA. Scanning electron microscopy of irradiated recipient blood vessels in head and neck free flaps. Plast Reconstr Surg. 1984; 74(2):217–226

Hallock GGA. A "True" false-negative misadventure in free flap monitoring using laser Doppler flowmetry. Plast Reconstr Surg. 2002; 110(6):1609–1611

Harris L, Goldstein D, Hofer S, Gilbert R. Impact of vasopressors on outcomes in head and neck free tissue transfer. Microsurgery. 2012; 32(1):15–19

Herle P, Shukla L, Morrison WA, Shayan R. Preoperative radiation and free flap outcomes for head and neck reconstruction: a systematic review and meta-analysis. ANZ J Surg. 2015; 85(3):121–127

Herrera FA, Lee CK, Kryger G, et al. Microsurgery in the hypercoagulable patient: review of the literature. J Reconstr Microsurg. 2012; 28(5):305–312

Hsu H, Chang CH, Lee CY, et al. A comparison between combined open bypass revascularization and free tissue transfer versus endovascular revascularization and free tissue transfer for lower limb preservation. Microsurgery. 2015; 35(7):518–527

Ilie VG, Ilie VI, Dobreanu C, Ghetu N, Luchian S, Pieptu D. Training of microsurgical skills on nonliving models. Microsurgery. 2008; 28(7):571–577

Jacobson JH, Miller DB, Suarez E. Microvascular surgery: a new horizon in coronary artery surgery. Circulation. 1960; 22:767

Jacobson JH, II, Katsumura T. Small vein reconstruction. J Cardiovasc Surg (Torino). 1965; 6:157–159

Jayaprasad K, Mathew J, Thankappan K, et al. Safety and efficacy of low molecular weight dextran (dextran 40) in head and neck free flap reconstruction. J Reconstr Microsurg. 2013; 29(7):443–448

Jones BM. Monitors for the cutaneous microcirculation. Plast Reconstr Surg. 1984; 73(5):843–850

Kaye JJ. A reliable, inexpensive temperature monitor for microsurgery. Orthop Rev. 1987; 16(9):630–632

Keller A. Noninvasive tissue oximetry for flap monitoring: an initial study. J Reconstr Microsurg. 2007; 23(4):189–197

Khouri RK, Shaw WW. Monitoring of free flaps with surface-temperature recordings: is it reliable? Plast Reconstr Surg. 1992; 89(3):495–499, discussion 500–502

Komatsu S, Tamai S. Successful replantation of a completely cut-off thumb: Case report. Plast Reconstr Surg. 1968; 42:374–377

Kroll SS, Schusterman MA, Reece GP, et al. Timing of pedicle thrombosis and flap loss after free-tissue transfer. Plast Reconstr Surg. 1996; 98(7):1230–1233

Kulkarni AR, Mehrara BJ, Pusic AL, et al. Venous thrombosis in handsewn versus coupled venous anastomoses in 857 Consecutive breast free flaps. J Reconstr Microsurg. 2016; 32(3):178–182

Lannon DA, Atkins JA, Butler PEM. Non-vital, prosthetic, and virtual reality models of microsurgical training. Microsurgery. 2001; 21(8):389–393

Laporta R, Longo B, Sorotos M, Pagnoni M, Santanelli Di Pompeo F. DIEP flap sentinel skin paddle positioning algorithm. Microsurgery. 2015; 35(2):91–100

Leonard AG, Brennen MD, Colville J. The use of continuous temperature monitoring in the post-operative management of microvascular cases. Br J Plast Surg. 1982; 35(3):337–342

Lin SJ, Nguyen MD, Chen C, et al. Tissue oximetry monitoring in microsurgical breast reconstruction decreases flap loss and improves rate of flap salvage. Plast Reconstr Surg. 2011; 127(3):1080–1085

Malt RA, McKhann C. Replantation of severed arms. JAMA. 1964; 189:716–722

McLean DH, Buncke HJ, Jr. Autotransplant of omentum to a large scalp defect, with microsurgical revascularization. Plast Reconstr Surg. 1972; 49(3):268–274

Mudry A. The history of the microscope for use in ear surgery. Am J Otol. 2000; 21(6):877–886

Murphy E, Cross HR, Steenbergen C. Na$^+$/H$^+$ and Na$^+$/Ca^{2+} exchange: their role in the rise in cytosolic free (Ca^{2+}) during ischemia and reperfusion. Eur Heart J. 1999 Suppl K:K18–K30

Nakatsuka T, Harii K, Asato H, et al. Analytic review of 2372 free flap transfers for head and neck reconstruction following cancer resection. J Reconstr Microsurg. 2003; 19(6):363–368, discussion 369

Nakayama K, Yamamoto K, Tamiya T, et al. Experience with free autografts of the bowel with a new venous anastomosis apparatus. Surgery. 1964; 55:796–802

Narasimhan K, Griffin JR, Thornton JF. Microsurgery. Selected Readings in Plastic Surgery. 2014; 11:1–63

Numata T, Iida Y, Shiba K, et al. Usefulness of color Doppler sonography for assessing hemodynamics of free flaps for head and neck reconstruction. Ann Plast Surg. 2002; 48(6):607–612

Nylén CO. The otomicroscope and microsurgery 1921–1971. Acta Otolaryngol. 1972; 73(6):453–454

Ozturk CN, Ozturk C, Ledinh W, et al. Variables affecting postoperative tissue perfusion monitoring in free flap breast reconstruction. Microsurgery. 2015; 35(2):123–128

O'Brien BM, MacLeod AM, Hayhurst JW, Morrison WA. Successful transfer of a large island flap from the groin to the foot by microvascular anastomoses. Plast Reconstr Surg. 1973; 52(3):271–278

Panchapakesan V, Addison P, Beausang E, Lipa JE, Gilbert RW, Neligan PC. Role of thrombolysis in free-flap salvage. J Reconstr Microsurg. 2003; 19(8):523–530

Repez A, Oroszy D, Arnez ZM. Continuous postoperative monitoring of cutaneous free flaps using near infrared spectroscopy. J Plast Reconstr Aesthet Surg. 2008; 61(1):71–77

Reus WF, III, Colen LB, Straker DJ. Tobacco smoking and complications in elective microsurgery. Plast Reconstr Surg. 1992; 89(3):490–494

Revenaugh PC, Waters HH, Scharpf J, Knott PD, Fritz MA. Suprastomal cutaneous monitoring paddle for free flap reconstruction of laryngopharyngectomy defects. JAMA Facial Plast Surg. 2013; 15(4):287–291

Riva FM, Chen YC, Tan NC, et al. The outcome of prostaglandin-E1 and dextran-40 compared to no antithrombotic therapy in head and neck free tissue transfer: analysis of 1,351 cases in a single center. Microsurgery. 2012; 32(5):339–343

Senchenkov A, Lemaine V, Tran NV. Management of perioperative microvascular thrombotic complications—the use of multiagent anticoagulation algorithm in 395 consecutive free flaps. J Plast Reconstr Aesthet Surg. 2015; 68(9):1293–1303

Seres L, Makula E, Morvay Z, Borbely L. Color Doppler ultrasound for monitoring free flaps in the head and neck region. J Craniofac Surg. 2002; 13(1):75–78

Setälä LP, Korvenoja EM, Härmä MA, Alhava EM, Uusaro AV, Tenhunen JJ. Glucose, lactate, and pyruvate response in an experimental model of microvascular flap ischemia and reperfusion: a microdialysis study. Microsurgery. 2004; 24(3):223–231

Setälä L, Papp A, Romppanen EL, Mustonen P, Berg L, Härmä M. Microdialysis detects postoperative perfusion failure in microvascular flaps. J Reconstr Microsurg. 2006; 22(2):87–96

Siemionow M, Arslan E. Ischemia/reperfusion injury: a review in relation to free tissue transfers. Microsurgery. 2004; 24(6):468–475

Smit JM, Acosta R, Zeebregts CJ, Liss AG, Anniko M, Hartman EH. Early reintervention of compromised free flaps improves success rate. Microsurgery. 2007; 27(7):612–616

Solomon GA, Yaremchuk MJ, Manson PN. Doppler ultrasound surface monitoring of both arterial and venous flow in clinical free tissue transfers. J Reconstr Microsurg. 1986; 3(1):39–41

Stone CA, Dubbins PA, Morris RJ. Use of colour duplex Doppler imaging in the postoperative assessment of buried free flaps. Microsurgery. 2001; 21(5):223–227

Suchon P, Al Frouh F, Henneuse A, et al. Risk factors for venous thromboembolism in women under combined oral contraceptive. The PILI Genetic RIsk Monitoring (PILGRIM) Study. Thromb Haemost. 2016; 115(1):135–142

Swartz WM, Jones NF, Cherup L, Klein A. Direct monitoring of microvascular anastomoses with the 20-MHz ultrasonic Doppler probe: an experimental and clinical study. Plast Reconstr Surg. 1988; 81(2):149–161

Swartz WM, Izquierdo R, Miller MJ. Implantable venous Doppler microvascular monitoring: laboratory investigation and clinical results. Plast Reconstr Surg. 1994; 93(1):152–163

Tan NC, Shih HS, Chen CC, Chen YC, Lin PY, Kuo YR. Distal skin paddle as a monitor for buried anterolateral thigh flap in pharyngoesophageal reconstruction. Oral Oncol. 2012; 48(3):249–252

Thankappan K. Microvascular free tissue transfer after prior radiotherapy in head and neck reconstruction—a review. Surg Oncol. 2010; 19(4):227–234

Udesen A, Løntoft E, Kristensen SR. Monitoring of free TRAM flaps with microdialysis. J Reconstr Microsurg. 2000; 16(2):101–106

Um GT, Chang J, Louie O, et al. Implantable Cook-Swartz Doppler probe versus Synovis Flow Coupler for the post-operative monitoring of free flap breast reconstruction. J Plast Reconstr Aesthet Surg. 2014; 67(7):960–966

van Adrichem LN, Hovius SE, van Strik R, van der Meulen JC. The acute effect of cigarette smoking on the microcirculation of a replanted digit. J Hand Surg Am. 1992; 17(2):230–234

Wang WZ, Baynosa RC, Zamboni WA. Update on ischemia-reperfusion injury for the plastic surgeon: 2011. Plast Reconstr Surg. 2011; 128(6):685e–692e

Wax MK. The role of the implantable Doppler probe in free flap surgery. Laryngoscope. 2014; 124 Suppl 1:S1–S12

Weinstein PR, Mehdorn HM, Szabo Z. Microsurgical anastomosis: vessel injury, regeneration, and repair. In: Serafin D, Buncke HJ Jr, eds. Microsurgical Composite Tissue Transplantation. St. Louis, MO: CV Mosby; 1979:111–144

Whitaker IS, Oboumarzouk O, Rozen WM, et al. The efficacy of medicinal leeches in plastic and reconstructive surgery: a systematic review of 277 reported clinical cases. Microsurgery. 2012; 32(3):240–250

Whitaker IS, Pratt GF, Rozen WM, et al. Near infrared spectroscopy for monitoring flap viability following breast reconstruction. J Reconstr Microsurg. 2012; 28(3):149–154

Whitaker IS, Rozen WM, Chubb D, et al. Postoperative monitoring of free flaps in autologous breast reconstruction: a multicenter comparison of 398 flaps using clinical monitoring, microdialysis, and the implantable Doppler probe. J Reconstr Microsurg. 2010; 26(6):409–416

Whitaker IS, Smit JM, Acosta R. A simple method of implantable Doppler cuff attachment: experience in 150 DIEP breast reconstructions. J Plast Reconstr Aesthet Surg. 2008; 61(10):1251–1252

Yano K, Hosokawa K, Nakai K, Kubo T, Hattori R. Monitoring by means of color Doppler sonography after buried free DIEP flap transfer. Plast Reconstr Surg. 2003; 112(4):1177

Yates YJ, Farias CL, Kazmier FR, Puckett CL, Concannon MJ. The effect of tirofiban on microvascular thrombosis: crush model. Plast Reconstr Surg. 2005; 116(1):205–208

Yuen JC, Feng Z. Monitoring free flaps using the laser Doppler flowmeter: five-year experience. Plast Reconstr Surg. 2000; 105(1):55–61

367

20 Facial Trauma

Nicolás Pereira, Patricio Andrades

Abstract

The face is one of the most commonly affected regions in a traumatized patient, occurring in approximately 10% of polytrauma cases. The craniofacial skeleton provides the framework for muscle attachment and defines facial dimensions, volumes, and contours; protects delicate structures (e.g., eyes, brain); and performs functional and structural roles in mastication and airway. In addition, the soft tissue component contains highly important aesthetic and functional elements, such as the ears, eyelids, nose, and lips. Maxillofacial injuries may include the soft tissues and the craniofacial skeleton, with each of these components needing proper assessment, accurate diagnosis, and timely and precise repair in order to optimize patient outcomes. Prior to maxillofacial evaluation, patients sustaining severe trauma should undergo more urgent interventions, namely airway management, bleeding control, and assessment of associated traumatic injuries. The main goals of facial fracture treatment include three-dimensional anatomical reduction, maximum immobilization at the fracture site, and the highest possible degree of freedom of movements that yields primary bone healing. Depending on the type of reduction and the degree of mobility of the fragments, treatment methods can be classified as *conservative* (e.g., interdental block, intermaxillary block, dental splints), with or without closed reduction, and *surgical*, comprising open reduction and internal fixation (rigid and semirigid). Finally, the rate of complications and sequelae are directly related to the complexity of the facial trauma and the difficulty of three-dimensional fracture reduction and fixation.

Keywords: facial lacerations, frontal fractures, mandibular fractures, maxillofacial buttresses, midface fractures, osteosynthesis, polytrauma

20.1 Introduction

Trauma is defined as the damage sustained by tissues and organs by the acute or chronic action of energy. Maxillofacial trauma involves both the soft tissues and the bony skeleton of the facial region and occurs in approximately 10% of multiple trauma patients.

Approximately 1.7 million head injuries occur annually in the United States. Alcohol is a contributing factor in almost 50% of head injuries. A review of the Maryland Shock Trauma Registry (1986–1994) reported that 11% of trauma patients (2,964 of 25,758) sustained maxillofacial fractures requiring subspecialty intervention.

Variables affecting type and severity of injury include the area of impact (the specific anatomical location that receives the energy), a resistant force (resultant movement of the head), and angulation of the impact, with more severe injury occurring with perpendicular delivery of energy than with tangential delivery.

20.2 Relevant Anatomy

The craniomaxillofacial skeleton is designed to protect vital soft structures, including the nervous system, eyes, and respiratory and digestive tracts. The head consists of the cranial vault and the maxillofacial skeleton with its vertical and horizontal buttresses (▶Table 20.1 and ▶Fig. 20.1). The buttresses are key elements that allow reconstruction of the facial skeleton and osteosynthesis fixation. Their proper reduction and stabilization guarantee optimal restoration of the volumes of the face. Bone healing after a fracture can occur through primary and secondary mechanisms:

- *Primary:* Without callus formation so that the process is shortened to one stage. For primary consolidation to ensue, a perfect reduction, good blood supply, rigid stabilization, and lack of micromovements are needed. Interfragmentary compression is important because the bone evolves according to the forces suffered and compression favors primary bone healing.

Table 20.1 Horizontal and vertical buttresses of the facial skeleton

Horizontal buttresses	Vertical buttresses
Superior orbital rim	Ascending process of maxilla
Inferior orbital rim	Lateral orbital ridge
Zygomatic arch	Zygomatomaxillary union
Maxillary alveolar ridge	Pterygomaxillary union
Mandibular body	Jaw ramus

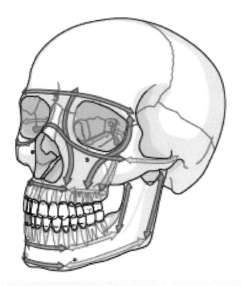

Fig. 20.1 Transversal, vertical, and sagittal buttresses of the facial skeleton.

- *Secondary:* Occurs with callus formation and is typically observed in fractures treated orthopaedically. It happens as a consequence of separation between fragments, a reduced vascular supply, poor stability, and lack of compression.

> **Remember** M!
>
> The aim of osteosynthesis is to achieve primary bone healing of the maxillofacial fracture.

20.3 Soft Tissue Trauma

20.3.1 Classification

- Abrasion: scraped area of skin.
- Laceration: jagged cut or tear.
- Avulsion: tearing resulting in an area of skin lifted off the underlying tissue.
- Crush: damage caused by compression; often results in greater tissue injury.
- Miscellaneous: gunshot wound (substantial soft tissue injury may warrant early intubation, soft tissue deficits are often minimal); bite (associated with polymicrobial infections: *Eikenella corrodens* and *Streptococcus viridans* in human bites, *Pasteurella canis* in canine bites, *Pasteurella multocida* in feline bites).

20.3.2 Initial Evaluation

A thorough and systematic assessment of the traumatized face is essential to make an accurate and complete diagnosis of the injury and provide appropriate treatment. Particular attention should be given to the mechanism of injury and characteristics of the wound. Patients with a significant mechanism of injury may have associated critical injuries, which mandates evaluation following Advanced Trauma Life Support (ATLS) guidelines. Careful attention is given to soft tissue injuries near specialized facial structures, such as the external auditory meatus, lacrimal apparatus, facial nerve, and parotid duct.

General Management

The risk of infection increases the longer the wounds remain open; therefore, closure should be performed as soon as the patient is stabilized. Of note, the rich vascularity of the head and neck makes it more resistant to infection than other areas of the body.

Bleeding

The rich vascularity of the head and neck region can lead to significant blood loss from lacerations, though rarely resulting in hypovolemic shock. Hemorrhage can usually be controlled with local pressure. Avoid blind clamping to prevent iatrogenic injury to specialized structures.

Irrigation and Debridement

Irrigation and removal of foreign bodies from wounds is essential before closure to reduce the risk of infection. In addition, debris that is not removed from the dermis can result in permanent (traumatic) tattooing. All devitalized tissue should be removed by sharp debridement. The surgeon needs to be conscious about the extent of debridement in functional and aesthetically important areas, such as the nose, periorbital region, lips, ears, and hair-bearing skin. Excessive removal of tissue in these zones may lead to severe disfigurement.

Repair

Local flaps should be avoided in the acute setting until the extent of the devitalized tissue has declared itself. Layered closure is preferred to reduce tension but may increase the risk of subsequent infection in a dirty wound.

- *Abrasions:* Partial-thickness wounds should be treated with antibiotic ointment while they are still fresh and moisturizing lotion once epithelialization occurs. Full-thickness tissue loss should be managed with dressing changes until the wound is stable and clean enough to be resurfaced with skin grafts or local flaps.
- *Lacerations/avulsions:* Closure of these wounds should ensure obliteration of dead space by layered closure, which may include tension-free approximation of skin, muscle, and fascia. Sutures should be placed carefully and at the appropriate tightness to prevent strangulation of tissues.
- *Bite wounds:* Bite wounds elsewhere in the body should be left open, whereas in the face they may be loosely approximated following aggressive irrigation and debridement. For commonly associated organisms, extended-spectrum β-lactam (amoxicillin/clavulanate) or fluoroquinolone antibiotics are appropriate. Administration of human rabies immunoglobulin and human diploid cell rabies vaccine should be considered depending on animal follow-up and the local epidemiological situation.

Medications

Prophylactic antibiotics may provide benefit in grossly contaminated wounds, immunocompromised patients, open fractures, wounds contaminated with oral secretions, and those presenting for delayed wound closure. In addition, tetanus prophylaxis should be considered in the presence of risk factors including time since injury (> 6 hours), depth of injury (> 1 cm), mechanism of injury (crush, burn, gunshot, puncture), presence of devitalized tissue, and contamination (grass, soil, saliva, retained foreign body). History of immunization and local epidemiological situation should also be considered.

> **Note**
>
> General management includes bleeding control, irrigation and debridement, structures repair, and medications.

Specific Management by Anatomical Zones

The sensory innervation and regional anesthetic blocks of the face and scalp are described in Chapter 5. The following section focuses on the technical aspects of wound closure in the different areas.

Scalp

Scalp lacerations usually bleed profusely. The scalp is richly vascularized, and the vessels running in the plane between the subcutaneous layer and the galea are attached to the latter, which prevents them from retracting upon sectioning. Layered closure should be performed approximating the galea with interrupted 2–0/3–0 absorbable sutures and epidermis with 4–0 nonabsorbable monofilament sutures or staples.

Forehead

Forehead lacerations may injure the frontal branch of the facial nerve or the frontalis muscle directly, which may cause brow ptosis. Layered closure should be performed, repairing the frontalis with interrupted 3–0/4–0 absorbable sutures and skin with interrupted 5–0/6–0 nonabsorbable monofilament sutures.

Eyebrow

The eyebrow is a unique structure that is difficult to replace. Therefore, it is important to preserve it as much as possible by performing minimal debridement and avoiding shaving. Wounds should be closed in a layered fashion using interrupted 5–0 absorbable sutures for the dermis and interrupted 6–0 nonabsorbable monofilament sutures for the epidermis.

Eyelid

The eyelid contains different structures that may be lacerated and need repair, including the tarsal plate, orbicularis muscle, and skin. Special evaluation is required for injury to the septum and levator palpebrae muscle—if left unrepaired, levator disruption may result in eyelid ptosis. Sutures adjacent to the cornea should be avoided to prevent abrasions. Eyelid lacerations should be closed using 6–0 absorbable sutures for the tarsus and orbicularis and 6–0 or 7–0 nylon for skin. Lacerations through the lid margin require careful closure to prevent lid notching and misalignment. The lid margin should be precisely approximated and the palpebral borders everted to prevent notching.

Lacrimal Apparatus

Tears drain into puncta located on the medial half of the upper and lower lids. Injuries to the lacrimal punctum are therefore associated with medial eyelid lacerations and occur most commonly on the lower eyelid. If a canalicular injury is suspected, it should be cannulated with a lacrimal probe to identify the site of laceration. Direct repair over a Silastic or polyethylene lacrimal stent is performed using 8–0 absorbable sutures, leaving the stent in place for 4 weeks. If cannulation is impossible dacryocystorhinostomy may be necessary.

Ear

Traumatic ear injuries are normally repaired in one layer by approximation of skin only using 5–0 or 6–0 nylon sutures with proper eversion to avoid unsightly grooves. Cartilage is not usually sutured as a separate layer as long as correct alignment and preservation of important landmarks are achieved with skin suturing. If cartilage needs to be sutured, 5–0 absorbable material is recommended.

Two of the most serious complications following injury to the auricle are hematoma and cartilage infection (e.g., chondritis). Hematomas may develop from bleeding from a laceration or as a consequence of blunt trauma in which the cartilage is detached from the overlying soft tissues and blood accumulates in the space. Hematomas can lead to cartilage resorption or reactive chondrogenesis, which results in a permanent thickened fibrotic deformity referred to as cauliflower ear deformity. Hematomas should therefore be drained as quickly as possible and compressed with a bolster dressing with or without through-and-through sutures. Cartilage infection may result in significant resorption and should be treated promptly. Unfortunately, chondritis is sometimes difficult to treat due to the reduced blood supply to the ear that prevents proper reach of antibiotics. Finally, in circumferential external auditory canal lacerations, a stent should be placed to prevent stenosis.

Nose

Nasal lacerations may comprise skin, cartilage, and mucosa. These need to be evaluated and repaired in a layered fashion if required. Skin and soft tissue are approximated using absorbable sutures for the deep dermis and nonabsorbable for the skin. If the cartilaginous framework is damaged, the pieces should be properly reduced and sutured separately from the skin using monofilament nonabsorbable suture. Finally, mucosal lacerations are approximated with 4–0 absorbable sutures. Patients with nasal injuries should undergo intranasal examination to rule out septal hematomas. Treatment involves incising the mucosa and nose packing to prevent reaccumulation. If overlooked, a septal hematoma can lead to septal perforation and saddle nose deformity.

Salivary Glands

Injury to the salivary glands can result in sialocele or cutaneous fistula if untreated. Lacerations through the cheek may injure the parotid (Stensen's) duct. If injury is suspected, the duct is located intraorally opposite the second maxillary molar and stented with a 24-gauge angiocatheter. Extravasation of saline after infusion indicates an injury, which should be repaired using microsurgical techniques. A direct repair over a Silastic stent may provide benefit. Submandibular gland lacerations should be marsupialized to the floor of the mouth.

Lip

The lips are an important aesthetic component of the face; therefore precise realignment of the structures involved is paramount. Full-thickness lacerations are repaired by approximating each layer separately, using 3–0/4–0 absorbable sutures for the mucosa and orbicularis muscle and 6–0/7–0 nylon for the skin and dry vermillion. The skin–vermillion border (white roll) must be exactly approximated to obtain the best cosmetic result. Discrepancies as little as 1 mm are noticeable at conversational distance.

> **Note**
>
> Align the lip injury at the level of the white roll to avoid obvious irregularities.

Nerves

Nerves at risk in any facial laceration are mainly branches of the trigeminal and facial nerves and should always be assessed prior to the administration of anesthesia. Facial nerve stumps can be identified with the aid of a nerve stimulator up to 72 hours after injury, after which the distal end may no longer be responsive, making stump identification more difficult. Also, it is important to note that facial nerve lacerations medial to the lateral canthus or the oral commissure may be too small to repair

Postoperative Care and Complications

Routine wound care of facial lacerations is indicated to prevent desiccation. Antibiotic ointment is applied until wounds are epithelialized, after which moisturizing lotion is recommended. Sutures are removed at 5–7 days for the face and neck and 2–3 weeks for the scalp.

As with any wound, head and neck lacerations may be complicated by hypertrophic scarring, hyperpigmentation, scar contracture, and alopecia. Sun exposure is the main cause of hyperpigmentation and should be avoided for up to 1 year after wounding, with the use of protective clothing and sunscreen. Scar contracture may lead to deformation of the normal anatomy and produce important functional deficits. Scar release and reconstruction with z-plasties or other procedures are usually performed once the scars have matured. Alopecia can be associated with excessive use of cautery and traumatic tissue handling, which should be minimized during wound repair.

20.4 Maxillofacial Trauma

20.4.1 Classification

1. Depending on the type of fracture:
   - Closed/open.
   - Simple/comminuted.
   - Displaced/nondisplaced.
   - Stable/unstable.
2. According to the parts involved and their location:
   - Soft tissue trauma (see previous section).
   - Trauma of the facial skeleton.
     - Upper third (fronto-orbital fractures).
     - Middle third (nasoorbitoethmoidal [NOE], zygomaticomaxillary fractures).
     - Lower third (mandibular fractures).

20.4.2 Clinical Evaluation

Initial Evaluation

Initial assessment of the patient with facial trauma should follow the ABCDE principles and ATLS guidelines. The following are the most important issues related to maxillofacial trauma:

- *Airway management:* Patients with severe maxillofacial trauma are at risk of upper airway obstruction due to clots, teeth, bone fragments, edema (floor of mouth, pharynx, and larynx), hyoid retroposition (in mandibular fractures), and aspiration of fluids (saliva, gastric content). Establishing an artificial airway is mandatory in cases of clear obstruction, inability to clear secretions, or unconsciousness, and is most commonly obtained by endotracheal intubation. This and other maneuvers aimed at maintaining a patent airway should be done with care in patients with cervical spine injury or skull base fracture because manipulation may further aggravate these injuries.
- *Bleeding control:* Massive hemorrhage from maxillofacial trauma is uncommon and may be seen in cases of massive scalp injuries, penetrating soft tissue injuries, and midface fractures. In most cases, bleeding can be effectively controlled by compression and hemostasis in the operating room. Middle third fractures may bleed copiously from less accessible sources, including the ophthalmic, maxillary, and ascending pharyngeal arteries. The sequence of treatment in these cases is anterior and posterior nasal packing, intermaxillary fixation, selective angiography and embolization, and ligation of external carotid and superficial temporal arteries.
- *Associated traumatic injuries:* Patients with maxillofacial trauma often have other injuries, such as serious cervical spine injury in 2–4%; encephalocranial trauma in 50%, including intracranial injury in 5–10% and skull base fracture in 25%; eye injury in 25–29%; and blindness in 2–6%. In these cases ophthalmologic evaluation and intervention are paramount.

Finally it should be noted that more serious and life-threatening aspects of the traumatized patient, such as establishing a patent airway, ensuring adequate ventilation, controlling bleeding, and surgical management of the thoracic, abdominal, and neurosurgical trauma, take priority over treatment of the maxillofacial trauma.

Maxillofacial Evaluation

- *Anamnesis:* The mechanism and time since injury can give an idea of the magnitude of the trauma and injuries. Among the patient's history, it is important to consider associated pathologies and comorbidities, alcoholism, allergies, medications, previous facial fractures, visual disturbances, denture condition, malocclusion, and previous treatments. In addition, the awake patient may report localized pain, hypoesthesia, malocclusion, and diplopia.
- *Physical examination:* The traumatized face should be systematically and rigorously examined so as not to overlook any potential injuries. Assessment should include inspection and palpation together with ophthalmic, auditory, nasal, and oral examinations.

  - *Inspection:* should include pictures prior to trauma and documentation of any soft tissue injuries, facial asymmetry, contour deformities, localized swelling and bruising.
  - Palpation: must be done in a systematic and orderly fashion, in a cephalocaudal direction examining bilateral bony prominences, fracture irregularities, localized pain, pathological mobility, bone crepitus, and hypoesthesia, which is indicative of nerve damage associated with the fracture.
  - *Ophthalmic examination:* should include visual acuity, visual field, ocular motility, pupil response, and fundus as well as documentation of any eyelid, conjunctival, and corneal injuries or lacerations. Raccoon eyes (periorbital ecchymosis) are indicative of skull base fractures.
  - *Auditory examination:* should include the ear canal and periauricular region, which can give clues about underlying fractures. Discharge of cerebrospinal fluid (CSF), hemotympanum, and Battle's sign (mastoid ecchymosis) are suggestive of skull base fractures. Otorrhea may also be present in condylar fractures.

  - *Nasal examination:* facial trauma involving the nose can present with epistaxis from a nasal fracture or CSF rhinorrhea, which is observed in cases of cribriform plate fracture in NOE fractures. Anterior speculoscopy must be done to rule out septal hematoma and CSF rhinorrhea.
  - *Oral examination:* should include assessment of edema, loose/displaced/fractured/ missing teeth, bleeding from gingival lacerations or other lesions, dental occlusion, caries, and mouth opening in patients that have sustained maxillofacial trauma.

> **Remember** **M!**
>
> Before maxillofacial evaluation, it is important to establish a patent airway, control bleeding, and rule out associated traumatic injuries.

Diagnostic Imaging

For an accurate and definitive diagnosis, patients with abnormal findings on physical examination should undergo maxillofacial computed tomography (CT) with axial and coronal sections and plain radiography depending on the injuries. CT is the gold standard imaging study for the upper and middle thirds and plain radiography is not necessary for the assessment of middle third fractures when CT is available, unlike what happens with mandibular fractures, in which orthopantomography is useful. In addition, two-dimensional CT is more accurate in evaluating orbital floor and medial orbital wall fractures, whereas three-dimensional CT is better for examining complex Le Fort and palatal fractures. Ideally, both 2D and 3D should be used for assessment and planning.

20.4.3 Principles of Treatment

The following are general principles for treatment of maxillofacial trauma:
- Early and one-stage treatment of all soft and hard tissue injuries.
- Wide exposure of all fractures sites.
- Precise anatomical reductions of all fragments rebuilding the buttresses of the facial skeleton.
- Maximal preservation of bone vascularity and other noble structures involved.

- Rigid fixation capable of maintaining the reduced bone fragments in place while neutralizing functional loads during bone healing.
- Early return of function.

To fulfill these principles we must understand the biomechanical properties and differences that exist between the upper and middle versus the lower third of the face (▶Table 20.2).

Surgical Approaches

The approaches to the facial skeleton must allow adequate access to the traumatized segment without causing functional or aesthetic alterations. The first possible approach is the soft tissue injury (e.g., laceration, tissue loss) itself. In some cases, this allows correct visualization and manipulation of the underlying fracture, whereas in others the laceration may need to be judiciously extended or a separate incision may be required to gain full access to the site of injury. Each approach has advantages and disadvantages that must be analyzed for each case individually (▶Fig. 20.2).

Timing of Operative Intervention

Prevention or minimization of secondary injury is of primary importance. The initial management of head-injured patients should be similar to that of polytraumatized patients without head injury, focusing on hemorrhage control and restoration of perfusion. Maintaining cerebral perfusion pressure (CPP) > 70 mm Hg during the preoperative, perioperative, and postoperative periods is critical because brain injury increases

with inadequate resuscitation and with operative procedures that allow hypotension or low CPP. The treatment protocol will be based on each patient's clinical assessment and treatment needs.

Maxillofacial Osteosynthesis (Association for Osteosynthesis/ Association for the Study of Internal Fixation [AO/ASIF] System)

The ultimate goal of osteosynthesis is to allow fracture fixation and bone healing. The fixation may be external, which is based on orthopedic reduction without surgery (e.g., intermaxillary fixation wires) thus promoting secondary bone healing; or internal, in which the fracture is reduced and fixed through the utilization of devices like plates and screws, that are applied directly to the fracture, allowing primary consolidation. It is important for the surgeon involved in the management of maxillofacial trauma to be fully familiarized with the nomenclature and organization of the osteosynthesis material. All systems include screws, plates, drill, screwdriver, sweep, guide, and bending, cutting, and drilling instruments (all for osteosynthesis). The screws are measured by the diameter of the core (e.g., excluding the thread body) in millimeters, and this number denominates the available systems as 1.0, 1.3, 1.5, 2.0, and 2.4 mm. In general, 1.0 and 1.3 systems are for osteosynthesis of the skull and upper third; 1.3, 1.5, and 2.0 for the middle third; and 2.4 for the lower third.

The implants used in maxillofacial osteosynthesis are made of steel, titanium, or biodegradable components. Steel is very rigid and has the potential for corrosion, which is why it is no longer used in plates. Steel wire fails to provide complete immobilization because it produces stabilization in two planes only, without preventing rotation around its axis. Titanium is biocompatible, adapts easily to the bone, and shows remarkable resistance, making it the most widely used material today. Biodegradable implants do not require subsequent removal, which is a great advantage, especially in children and in osteosynthesis of the upper third and midface. However, a material that complies with adequate strength and absorption for areas with higher functional load is not yet available.

Depending on the interaction between the implant and the bone with regard to loading, osteosynthesis implants are classified as follows (▶Fig. 20.3):

Table 20.2 Biomechanics of craniomaxillofacial trauma

	Upper and middle third	Lower third
Structure	Buttresses defining cavities	It behaves as a long bone
Composition	Predominantly cortical bone	Cortical-cancellous bone
Muscles	Weak muscles are attached	Powerful muscles are attached
Functional load	Less	Higher
Fragment displacement	Due to the impact	Due to muscle pull
Other elements	Paranasal sinuses, teeth and nerves	Teeth, nerves, and senile atrophy

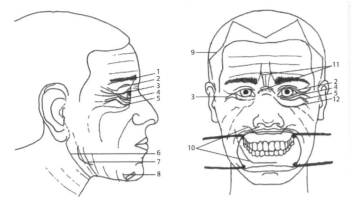

Fig. 20.2 Anatomical approaches. 1, Eyebrow incision; 2, upper blepharoplasty incision; 3, transconjunctival incision; 4, lower blepharoplasty incision; 5, subciliar incision; 6, face-lift incision; 7, mandibular angle; 8, skin lacerations; 9, coronal incision; 10, intraoral approaches; 11, glabellar incisions; 12, low eyelid incision.

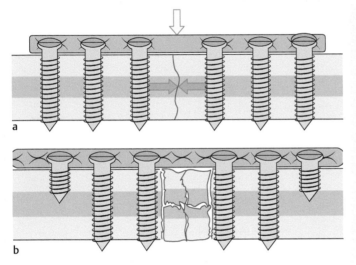

Fig. 20.3 (a) Load-sharing osteosynthesis. (b) Load-bearing osteosynthesis.

- *Load sharing:* The functional load is shared between the bone and plate. It is used in simple fractures allowing anatomical reduction.

- *Load bearing:* The entire load or functional effort is borne by the osteosynthesis plate. This type of osteosynthesis is used in complex comminuted fractures, when there is loss of fragments, and in the atrophic jaw. It requires thicker and more resistant plates, with bicortical screws of larger diameter.

Compression consists of pressing the bone fragments together to prevent interfragmentary mobility and promote primary bone healing and may be achieved with compression plates or lag screws (▶Fig. 20.4). Compression is not a requirement and is contraindicated in upper and middle third fixation. In addition, compression should not be used in situations in which a load-bearing osteosynthesis is being applied.

The sequence for open reduction and internal fixation of a maxillofacial fracture should follow these steps:

- Surgical approach and wide exposure of fracture site.
- Anatomical reduction of the fragments.
- Osteosynthesis system selection depending on the location and type of fracture.
- Plate selection and positioning. The plate should be selected according to the type of functional load that the implant will withstand. Plates should be positioned on the vertical and horizontal buttresses and be well adapted to the bone contour.
- Screw selection. Two to three screws are placed on either side of the fracture line, depending

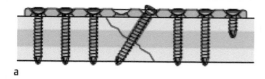

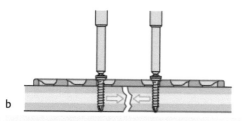

Fig. 20.4 (a) Compression with a lag screw and plate. (b) Compression with a low-contact dynamic compression plate.

on the functional load. Fixation in the upper and middle thirds should use screws that are 2–6 mm long, whereas fixation in the lower third should use screws that are 6–12 mm long. Monocortical screws can be used throughout the facial skeleton except in load bearing osteosynthesis (jaw pressure zone).

20.4.4 Facial Fractures

Frontal Sinus Fractures

Clinical Presentation

The frontal bone is a thick bone; in order to become fractured it requires two to three times the energy needed to produce a maxillary bone fracture. In addition, due to the high-energy impact, frontal sinus fractures are frequently associated with other craniomaxillofacial and body injuries.

The paired frontal sinuses are contained within the frontal bone and drain into the corresponding middle meatus in the nasal cavity through the nasofrontal ducts.

Indications for treatment of frontal sinus fracture include cosmetic issues derived from the loss of frontal contour in anterior table fractures, posterior table fractures, and nasofrontal duct obstruction that impairs normal drainage. Symptoms and signs of these fractures include bone depression, bruising, supraorbital anesthesia, crepitus, and CSF rhinorrhea.

Imaging

Plain X-rays may show fracture lines and air–fluid levels allowing diagnosis of major injuries but lack enough detail for treatment planning. CT scan allows a more accurate anatomical diagnosis of the fracture but still cannot clearly identify the drainage orifices and ducts.

Classification and Treatment

Frontal sinus fractures are classified as anterior, posterior, or inferior wall fractures (▶Fig. 20.5). In addition, for each of these locations fractures may be nondisplaced or displaced.

- *Anterior wall fractures:* Treatment is required only in those presenting with > 2–3 mm displacement, due to the cosmetic defect that results from the loss of convex frontal contour (▶Fig. 20.6).
- *Posterior wall fractures:* Management of posterior wall fractures with associated intracranial injury always require an extensive surgical approach and craniotomy. Sinus cranialization should be performed by removing the posterior wall, stripping off the mucosa and obliterating the drain ducts (▶Fig. 20.7).
- *Inferior wall fractures:* These are the most difficult to diagnose and treat. Overall if sinus drainage is good, the outcome after appropriate reduction is satisfactory. Complications such as sinusitis, mucoceles, osteomeningeal gap, meningitis, and intracranial and orbital abscesses, might develop if sinus drainage is inadequate.

Nasal and Nasoseptal Fractures

Clinical Presentation

Nasal bone fractures are the most common maxillofacial fracture. Depending on the magnitude, direction, and location of forces, the nasal bones, ascending process of the maxilla, and nasal septum can be affected. Symptoms and signs of nasal fractures include pain, airway obstruction, epistaxis, irregularities, nasal deviation, and depressions. It is very important to always perform a speculoscopy to rule out anterior nasal septum hematoma and assess previous or posttraumatic deviations.

Posttraumatic deformity of the nose is common after treatment and reported in up to 50% of patients. It can be minimized by accurate diagnosis

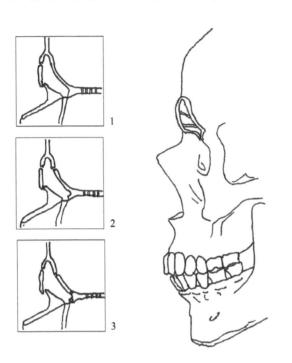

Fig. 20.5 Classification of frontal sinus fractures depending on the involvement of 1, anterior table; 2, posterior table; 3, nasal frontal duct. Fractures are either nondisplaced or displaced for each location.

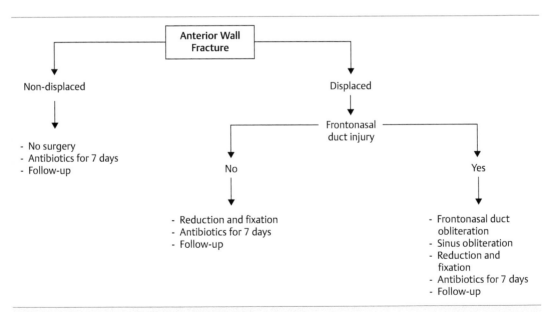

Fig. 20.6 Frontal sinus anterior wall fractures treatment algorithm.

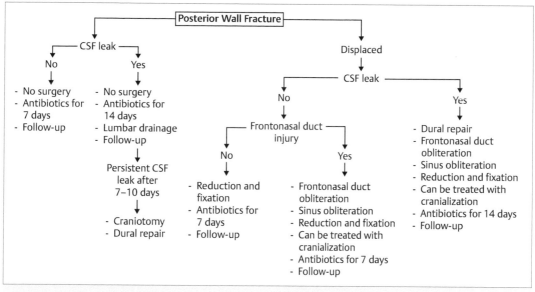

Fig. 20.7 Frontal sinus posterior wall fractures treatment algorithm.

and reduction following thorough external and internal nasal examination. Likewise, septal fractures are frequently undiagnosed and untreated, resulting in late deformity.

Imaging

Waters projection and radiography of the nasal bones are useful in diagnosis and have an important role in documenting injuries for medicolegal issues; however, they do not help in making treatment decisions. Definitive diagnosis of nasal and septal fractures is obtained with CT scan.

Classification and Treatment

Nasal trauma is classified as follows (▶ Fig. 20.8):
I. Nasal contusion.
II. Nasal bone fracture with mild or without displacement.
III. Nasal bone fracture with moderate to severe displacement.
IV. Complicated or extended nasal bone fracture.

Only 50% of nasal fractures require treatment, and 15% have acute septal injuries. Closed reduction of nasal bones can be deferred up to 2 weeks after trauma to allow the initial swelling to resolve, and it must be performed by a trained surgeon because posttraumatic nasal deformities may be as high as 15–45%. Septal hematomas should be drained through a retrocolumellar incision followed by anterior nasal packing. Septal fractures should be treated during the same procedure through an open or closed approach. Of note, this injury further increases the risk of having some deformity after treatment.

Closed nasal reduction and submucosal endoscopically assisted septoplasty for the treatment of nasoseptal fractures is an innovation that reduces the rates of secondary rhinoseptoplasty compared to those reported in the literature with traditional techniques.

Note

Always perform a speculoscopy to rule out anterior nasal septum hematoma.

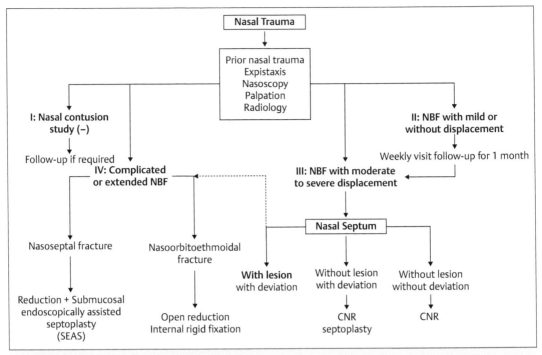

Fig. 20.8 Nasal trauma treatment algorithm. The dotted line depicts the treatment of nasoseptal fractures with SEAS. NBF, nasal bone fracture; CNR, closed nasal reduction; SEAS, submucosal endoscopically assisted septoplasty.

Nasoorbitoethmoidal Fractures

Clinical Presentation

NOE fractures are central face fractures involving the ethmoid bone (perpendicular plate, lamina papyracea, and cribriform plate), nasal bones, and ascending maxillary processes. This is the area of the face with the least resistance to fracture forces. Clinically, NOE fractures typically present with telecanthus, which is an increase in the distance between the medial canthi (intercanthal distance), and a flattened nose (saddle nose deformity). They may also exhibit similar findings to medial orbital wall and nasal fractures as well as periorbital edema or ecchymosis, step-offs at orbital rims, and subconjunctival hemorrhage.

Imaging

CT is diagnostic. Axial and coronal images are required for complete evaluation, and 3D CT can be very helpful. Aspects to assess with imaging of NOE fractures include degree of comminution in the region of the medial canthi, extent of orbital involvement, degree of posterior nasal displacement, and possible frontal sinus involvement.

Classification and Treatment

Markowitz et al classified NOE fractures in three different types depending on the involvement of the segment of bone on which the canthal ligament inserts (▶Fig. 20.9).

- Type I: single central fragment bearing the canthal ligament.
- Type II: comminuted central segment with medial canthal ligament still attached to a bone fragment.
- Type III: comminuted central segment with detachment of the medial canthal tendon from the bone.

Treatment of NOE fractures involves open reduction and internal fixation using a coronal approach. The most important step in the repair of NOE fractures is accurate positioning of the canthal ligament either by proper reduction and fixation of the ligament-bearing bone segment or by transnasal

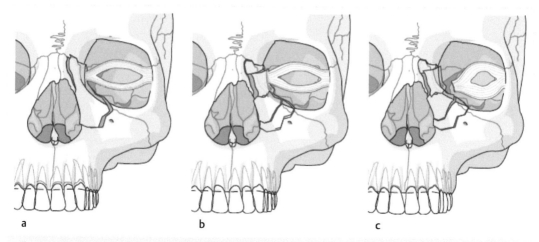

Fig. 20.9 Nasoorbitoethmoidal fractures. **(a)** Type I: single central fragment bearing the canthal ligament. **(b)** Type II: comminuted central segment with medial canthal ligament still attached to a bone fragment. **(c)** Type III: comminuted central segment with totally detached medial canthal ligament.

canthopexy. Bony structures are reduced and stabilized with low-profile miniplates. Cranial bone grafts are harvested to reconstruct nasal projection, and canthal tendons are reconstructed with transnasal wiring. Minimal hardware should be placed in the nasoorbital valley to reduce bulk. Finally, the management of NOE fractures also involves treatment of medial orbital wall and nasal septum fractures.

Orbital Fractures

Clinical Presentation

The bony orbit is formed by seven bones (zygomatic, sphenoid, frontal, ethmoid, lacrimal, palatal, and maxillary bone), which articulate to form a cone-shaped structure. The mechanism involved in orbital wall fractures is a force that produces a marked increase of the intraorbital pressure (bursting), which affects the weakest aspects, namely the floor and the medial orbital wall. Clinically, orbital fractures usually present with edema and periorbital ecchymosis, subconjunctival hemorrhage, enophthalmos or exophthalmos, diplopia, and infraorbital nerve paresthesia. In addition, patients may show limited eye excursion—whereas true entrapment is rare in adults and is usually a result of edema, in children entrapment of the recti must be ruled out and treated promptly. The following findings may be associated with specific locations:

- *Fractures of the anterior portion of the orbit:* orbital rim step-offs and infraorbital nerve injury
- *Fractures of the middle portion of the orbit:* alterations in the position of the eyeball (e.g., enophthalmos, hypophthalmos) and diplopia
- *Fractures of the posterior portion of the orbit:* when the fracture extends into the superior orbital fissure, nerves passing through this space may be damaged, namely, the oculomotor (III), trochlear (IV), abducens (VI), and ophthalmic division of the trigeminal nerve (V_1). Thus, patients with superior orbital fissure syndrome present with paralysis of extraocular movement, eyelid ptosis, mydriasis, and anesthesia/hypoesthesia of the eyelid, eyebrow, and forehead (CN VI). Orbital apex syndrome involves loss of visual acuity or blindness from optic nerve damage in addition to orbital fissure syndrome findings.

Imaging

A CT scan is the best study for orbital fracture evaluation. 3D reconstruction of the orbit and measurement of intraorbital volumes are recommended as well. Plain radiographs are of little use.

Classification and Treatment

Orbital fractures can be classified as follows:
- *Pure bursting:* Only the orbital walls are affected without involvement of the orbital rim.

- *Impure bursting:* The fracture is associated with adjacent facial bone fractures so the orbital rim is involved.

▶Table 20.3 lists the indications for treatment of orbital fractures. Treatment principles include reconstruction of the orbital rim and the orbital walls following reduction of herniated orbital content, and repair of soft tissue injuries. The orbital floor may be reconstructed with autologous (bone graft) or prosthetic (titanium mesh, polypropylene mesh, Medpor [Stryker]) material. After surgery, correct ocular motility should be confirmed by a forced duction test of the eye, which consists of grasping the inferior rectus muscle with forceps and smoothly rotating the eye upward as if the patient was looking up.

Zygomaticomaxillary Complex Fractures

Clinical Presentation

Zygomaticomaxillary complex (ZMC) fractures are the most frequent after nasal bone fractures. The zygomatic–maxillary complex has both aesthetic and functional features because the zygoma articulates with four bones: frontal (ZF), maxillary (ZM), sphenoid (ZS), and temporal (ZT). ZMC fractures usually disrupt most of these relationships, leading to malposition of the zygomatic bone in the anteroposterior, vertical, and horizontal dimensions. Symptoms and signs of ZMC fractures include bruises and periorbital edema, cheekbone flattening, zygomatic arch collapse, pain, upper vestibular ecchymosis, lower orbital rim and piriform aperture irregularities, lockjaw, infraorbital nerve hypoesthesia, subcutaneous emphysema, inferior displacement of the external canthus, altered pupil level, diplopia, and enophthalmos.

Table 20.3 Indications for surgery in orbital fractures

Clinical findings
Muscle entrapment in children
Persistent diplopia
Extraocular movement limitation
Enophthalmos > 2 mm
Hypoglobus > 2 mm
Difference > 2 mL between orbital volumes

Imaging

Waters, Hirtz, and oblique malar radiographic projections may help to establish proper diagnosis and even be of use for postoperative follow-up. A CT scan is diagnostic and should examine the degree of comminution (high- or low-energy), the presence of medial or lateral rotation of the zygoma, its anteroposterior projection, the position of the lateral orbital wall, and the need to reconstruct the orbital floor.

Classification and Treatment

There are many classifications for ZMC fractures, of which Knight and North's is the simplest, based on the presence of displacement.
- Nondisplaced (10%).
- Displaced (90%): arch (10%), body (80%: simple 60% and complex 20%).

The indication for surgery should be based on the aesthetic (visible deformity) and functional (eye or occlusal alterations) impact of the fracture. The surgical technique depends on the degree of instability of the zygomatic bone and may range from a semiclosed reduction using the Gillies maneuver to multiple approaches and osteosynthesis. The degree of instability is very difficult to establish and a matter of great controversy in the literature, with some saying that all zygomatic–maxillary fractures are unstable and they consequently operate on 100% of them, to others operating on only 15% of cases.

It is important to think of the zygoma as a chair with five supports, of which at least three should be correctly reduced and stabilized in order to achieve a good result (▶Fig. 20.10). Initial stabilization of the ZF suture with a malleable miniplate sets the vertical height and allows continued manipulation of the segment in the anteroposterior and horizontal dimensions. Following ZF, fixation of the ZM articulation should be performed. Additional fixation may be placed along the ZS articulation. Of note, the ZS articulation is the most important to assess for reduction.

Remember	M!
The zygoma has five contact points (ZF, ZM, ZS, ZT, and inferior orbital rim), and needs at least three properly reduced and stable supports for a good result. The zygomatic–sphenoid articulation is the most important to assess for reduction.	

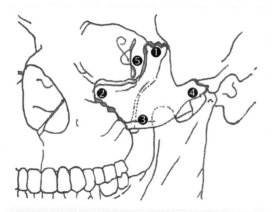

Fig. 20.10 Zygomatic bone articulations. 1, Frontal process; 2, infraorbital rim; 3, zygomaticomaxillary buttress; 4, zygomatic arch; 5, lateral orbital wall (zygomaticosphenoid).

Zygomatic Arch Fractures

Clinical Presentation

Fractures of the zygomatic arch entail an almost exclusively aesthetic concern, except in rare instances when the fracture segment impedes mandibular excursion by interfering with the coronoid process. These patients typically present with palpable deformity, contour deformity, and trismus.

Treatment

Uncomplicated fractures can be reduced using the Gillies approach through a temporal incision. Severely comminuted zygomatic arch fractures may require bone grafting or mandibular adaptation plates to restore aesthetic contour. Stabilization is generally unnecessary.

Maxillary Fractures

Clinical Presentation and Classification

The maxilla constitutes most of the midface skeleton and contains the maxillary sinus and dentition. Three major buttresses, the nasomaxillary, zygomatic, and pterygomaxillary, provide strength. Classically, three patterns of midface fractures, Le Fort I, II, and III, have been identified in reference to low-energy trauma (▶ Fig. 20.11). Today, however, due to the high-energy mechanisms

involved in trauma, these patterns are rarely found in isolation; instead combinations and varying degrees of comminution are more commonly seen.

- *Le Fort I:* This pattern describes a horizontal fracture through the upper alveolar line. Patients present with mobility of the whole dento-alveolar portion of the maxilla, an open bite due to molar contact, deviation of the maxilla from the midline, vestibulopalatal horseshoe-shaped bruising, significant edema of the upper lip, and mobility of the hard palate.
- *Le Fort II:* This pattern consists of a pyramidal fracture with extensive facial edema, raccoon eyes, nasal deformity and pathological mobility of the nasal bones, flattening and elongation of the middle third of the face, anterior open bite, infraorbital rim irregularities, pain, and mobility of the hard palate.
- *Le Fort III:* These fractures involve a complete separation of the facial skeleton from the skull base (craniofacial disjunction). Clinical findings are the same as for Le Fort II, plus significant facial edema that impedes eyelid separation to explore the eyeball, mobility of the entire face, hypertelorism, and airway obstruction by posterior displacement of the maxillary bone with the soft palate.

Imaging

Midface fractures are assessed and diagnosed by CT scan with axial and coronal sections, evaluating the following aspects:
- Degree of comminution.
- Presence of a sagittal fracture component.
- Fracture through the pterygoid plates.
- Level(s) of injury.

Treatment

The fundamentals of treatment in Le Fort I fractures are to achieve adequate reduction of the fractured segment and proper occlusion with intraoperative intermaxillary fixation and rigid internal fixation. Reduction can be achieved using Rowe forceps introduced through the mouth and nose (▶ Fig. 20.12).

In Le Fort II and III fractures, together with restoring occlusion, the external facial framework

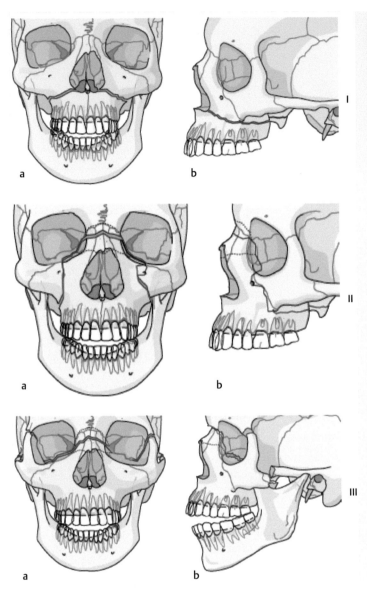

needs to be reconstructed in order to reestablish as much as possible the patient's facial dimensions and contours prior to the accident.

Dentoalveolar Fractures

Clinical Presentation

Dental trauma may occur as dislocation of the tooth, crown fracture, or root fracture, all of which may be associated with alveolar ridge fracture.

Imaging

The diagnosis is made by clinical and radiological examination (e.g., occlusal radiographs).

Classification and Treatment

Depending on the extent of injury and the layers affected, dental trauma can be classified as follows:
- Tooth dislocation, including contusion, subluxation and dislocation/intrusion or extrusion

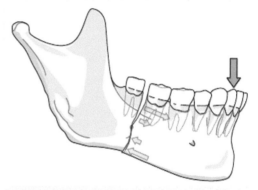

Fig. 20.13 Tension, neutral, and compression zones of a mandibular fracture.

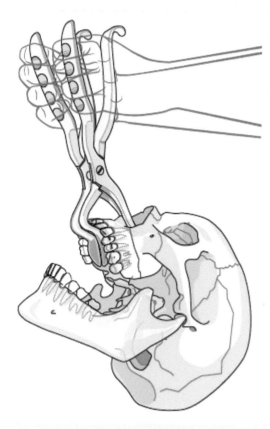

Fig. 20.12 Repositioning of Le Fort I fractures with Rowe's forceps.

- Crown fracture, which may affect enamel only, enamel and dentin, or pulp exposure
- Root fracture, which may occur at the cervical, central, and apical levels

Extrusions, dislocations, and subluxations require reposition of the tooth and stabilization to adjacent teeth. Intrusions generally require only observation for the tooth to erupt again.

Crown fractures involving enamel and dentin have a good prognosis and do not require intervention, whereas pulp exposure requires urgent treatment to maintain pulp viability.

Completely avulsed teeth should be replanted as soon as possible to optimize healing and restore the neurovascular supply. If the tooth cannot be replanted, it should be stored/transferred within its alveoli, in the oral vestibule, in saline or milk.

Limited fractures of the alveolar ridge require interdental fixation only, whereas extended lesions need internal fixation.

Mandibular Fractures

Clinical Presentation

From a mechanical and structural point of view, the mandible resembles a long bone in that it is composed of cortical and cancellous bone, it is mobile, it has powerful muscles attaching to it, and it withstands a high functional load. When a fracture occurs, the muscles will pull on the fragments, producing an area of tension on one side, a neutral zone at the midpoint (where the mental nerve runs), and an area of compression on the opposite side (▶ Fig. 20.13). Patients with mandibular fractures present with a variety of signs and symptoms, including pain, functional impairment, facial asymmetry, edema and bruising or hematoma at the fracture site, dental malocclusion, chin hypoesthesia, and preauricular condylar silence. Ipsilateral condyle fractures exhibit lateral deviation toward the fractured side, incomplete occlusion, and pain of the ipsilateral external auditory meatus, whereas fractures of both condyles result in an open bite.

Imaging

Plain radiographies including panoramic or orthopantomography allow good visualization of the jaw and are helpful in establishing a diagnosis; however, CT scan verification is always required.

Classification and Treatment

Mandibular fractures are classified according to several parameters:

- Presence of bone comminution: simple/complex
- Condition of teeth: fractures with teeth on both sides/one side/toothless
- Favorability for treatment: favorable (muscle forces draw the fragments together)/unfavorable (muscles distract the fragments apart). Depending on location and forces acting on the fractured segments, fractures may be vertically or horizontally favorable or unfavorable.
- Location: ▶Fig. 20.14 illustrates mandibular fracture classification according to location.

The use of antibiotics to prevent infection in mandibular fractures remains controversial. Maxillomandibulary fixation (also called intermaxillary fixation) is essential to maintain proper occlusion prior to fracture reduction and fixation and can be used intraoperatively or as definitive treatment alone. It is important to note that the compression area should be treated with strong bicortical screws and plates, whereas the area of tension requires thinner implants or simply the maintenance of the dental arch plates. In addition, the trauma system or universal 2.0 and 2.4 plates (with or without compression) are reserved for simple fractures with anatomical reductions, whereas the

reconstruction and unilock 2.4 systems are useful for complex fractures, with a high degree of comminution, loss of fragments, and atrophic jaws.

Finally, maintenance of proper oral hygiene and a soft diet during the postoperative period are essential to optimize outcomes.

> **Note**
>
> Load-sharing osteosynthesis is used in simple fractures allowing anatomical reduction.
>
> Load-bearing systems are used in complex fractures with significant comminution, fragment loss, and atrophic jaw.

Panfacial Fractures

Clinical Presentation

Panfacial fractures are those involving all three facial thirds, though some consider fractures of two-thirds as panfacial as well. These fractures are generated by high-energy mechanisms and are highly comminuted. The clinical findings in panfacial fractures vary depending on the different segments affected. They are usually severe and present with a mixture of symptoms and signs related to the specific areas, with significant soft tissue injury.

Treatment

Management of panfacial fractures requires careful planning on a case-by-case basis in a multidisciplinary environment. Treatment usually involves varied surgical approaches that allow correct visualization, anatomical reduction of the fragments, and stabilization with rigid internal fixation placed on vertical and horizontal buttresses. Bone grafts are normally required for reconstruction of multifragmented areas.

Anatomical reduction should follow an orderly and logical sequence: from cranial to caudal, from caudal to cephalic, or from outside in. Whatever the sequence, it is important that each maneuver constitutes the basis for the next one in order to restore facial diameters and volumes.

Anatomical reconstruction of the mandible should be performed initially to provide a stable

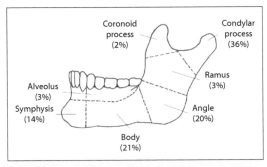

Fig. 20.14 Mandibular fractures classification depending on the anatomical location and frequency.

base from which to reconstruct the midface. If bilateral condyle fractures are present, at least one of them should be reconstructed to provide appropriate vertical height relationships for the midface. Next, anteroposterior dimensions of the zygomas should be reestablished to provide accurate facial projection. Reconstruction then proceeds inferiorly from the stable frontal process to the level of the maxilla. Fixation across the Le Fort I level is the last area to be stabilized. Because of the severity of these injuries, some degree of malreduction is inevitable; nevertheless, by reestablishing the major determinants of facial form early (mandibular base, vertical height, and anteroposterior projection), subtle malreductions may be tolerated at the Le Fort I level above the dentition.

20.5 Clinical Cases

Case 1: Nasal Bone Fracture

A 35-year-old man presented with a nasal fracture after a direct punch (▶Fig. 20.15a). The fracture is seen on X-ray (▶Fig. 20.15b) and confirmed on a CT scan where nasal deviation is observed corresponding to a type III nasal trauma: fracture with moderate displacement and septal deviation (▶Fig. 20.15c). Closed reduction and septoplasty was performed with excellent results at 6 months postoperative (▶Fig. 20.15d).

Case 2: Zygomaticomaxillary Complex (ZMC) Fracture

A 38-year-old man suffered direct trauma to his right cheek with a brick while working (▶Fig. 20.16a). A CT scan shows a complex zygomaticomaxillary fracture (▶Fig. 20.16b). Zygomatic–frontal and zygomatic–maxillary fixations were performed. ▶Fig. 20.16c shows three-dimensional reconstruction before and after surgery. An excellent result was obtained as shown in the 6 months postoperative picture (▶Fig. 20.16d).

20.6 Conclusions

The face is frequently affected in trauma. Nowadays, high-energy mechanisms account for a number of complicated injuries of one or more facial thirds. Regardless of the severity of the facial injury, it is important to always perform airway management and bleeding control and to rule out associated traumatic injuries, before maxillofacial evaluation. The diagnostic approach in these patients includes history of previous trauma, details of the accident and forces involved, clinical evaluation, and imaging. A precise diagnosis of facial fractures is essential for devising an adequate therapeutic plan, based on the best surgical approach that allows adequate visualization of the fracture, anatomical reduction, and rigid fixation when

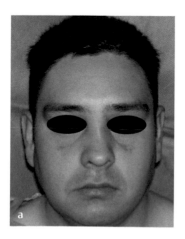
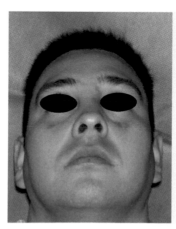

Fig. 20.15 Nasal bone fracture (see text for details).

(Continued)

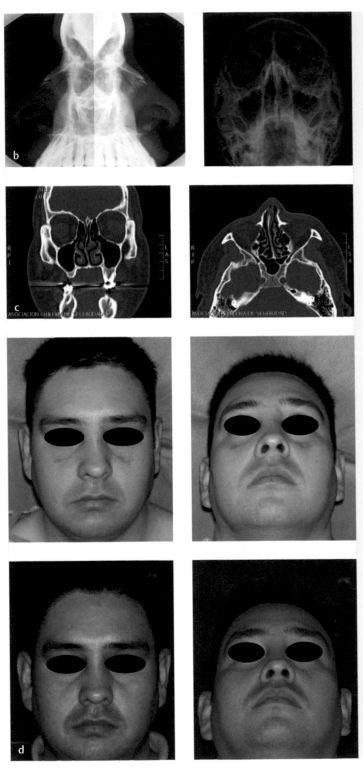

Fig. 20.15 *(Continued)* Nasal bone fracture (see text for details).

possible, in order to optimize patient recovery and obtain excellent functional and aesthetic results.

20.7 Key Points

- Before maxillofacial evaluation, it is important to perform airway management and bleeding control and rule out associated traumatic injuries.
- General management of maxillofacial trauma includes bleeding control, irrigation and debridement, repair of damaged structures, and postoperative medications.

- In lip wounds, exact alignment of the white roll is critical to avoid unsightly irregularities.
- The aim of osteosynthesis is to achieve primary bone healing of the maxillofacial fracture.
- In nasal trauma, always perform a speculoscopy to rule out anterior nasal septum hematoma.
- The zygoma has five contact points (ZF, ZM, ZS, ZT, and inferior orbital rim), and needs at least three properly reduced and stable supports for a good result. The ZS articulation is the most important to assess for reduction.

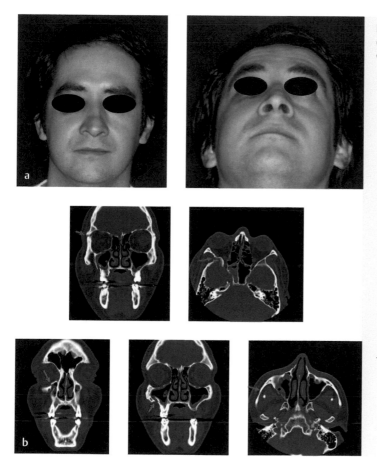

Fig. 20.16 Zygomaticomaxillary complex fracture (see text for details).

(Continued)

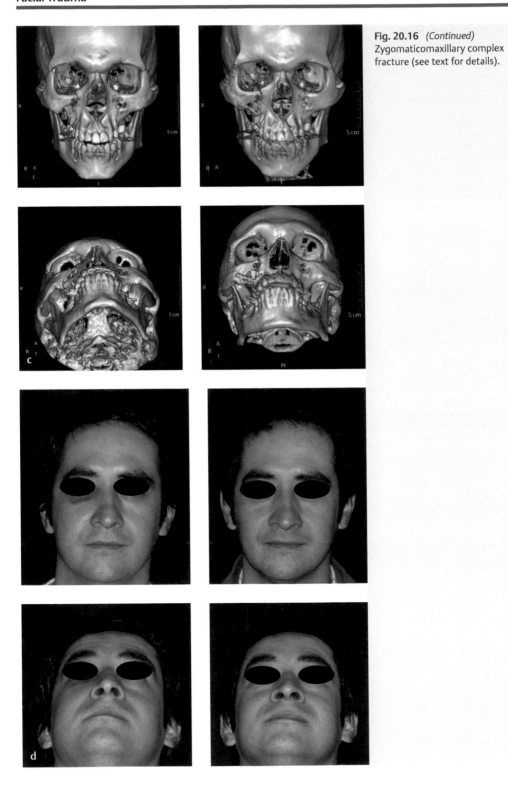

Fig. 20.16 *(Continued)* Zygomaticomaxillary complex fracture (see text for details).

Recommended Readings

American College of Surgeons. National Trauma Data Bank Annual Report 2012. http:// www.facs.org/trauma/ntdb/pdf/ntdb-annual-report-2012.pdf

Andrades P, Pereira N, Borel C, Rocha L, Hernández R, Villalobos R. A new approach to nasoseptal fractures: submucosal endoscopically assisted septoplasty and closed nasal reduction. J Craniomaxillofac Surg. 2016; 44(10):1635–1640

Antonyshyn O. Principles in management of facial injuries. In: Giorgiades G, Riefkohl R, Levin S, eds. Plastic, Maxillofacial and Reconstructive Surgery. Vol 33. Philadelphia, PA: Williams and Wilkins; 1997:339–350

Buck DW, II, Heyer K, Lewis VL, Jr. Reconstruction of the zygomatic arch using a mandibular adaption plate. J Craniofac Surg. 2009; 20(4):1193–1196

Ehrenfeld M, Manson PN, Prein J, eds. Principles of Internal Fixation in the Craniomaxillofacial Skeleton. New York, NY/Zurich: Thieme/AO; 2012

Ellis E, III. Sequencing treatment for naso-orbito-ethmoid fractures. J Oral Maxillofac Surg. 1993; 51(5):543–558

Ellis E, III, Kittidumkerng W. Analysis of treatment for isolated zygomaticomaxillary complex fractures. J Oral Maxillofac Surg. 1996; 54(4):386–400, discussion 400–401

Hale RG, Hayes DK, Orloff G, et al. Maxillofacial and neck trauma. In: Savitsky E, Eastridge B, eds. Combat Casualty Care: Lessons Learned from OEF and OIF. Falls Church, VA: Borden Institute; 2012: 225-277

Hollier L, Thornton J. Facial fractures I: upper two thirds. Select Read Plast Surg. 2002; 9(26):1–34

Jarrahy R, Vo V, Goenjian HA, et al. Diagnostic accuracy of maxillofacial trauma two-dimensional and three-dimensional computed tomographic scans: comparison of oral surgeons, head and neck surgeons, plastic surgeons, and neuroradiologists. Plast Reconstr Surg. 2011; 127(6):2432–2440

Kittle CP, Verrett AJ, Wu J, Mellus DE, Hale RG, Chan RK. Characterization of midface fractures incurred in recent wars. J Craniofac Surg. 2012; 23(6):1587–1591

Manson P. Facial fractures. In: Aston S, Beasley R, Thorne C, eds. Grabb and Smith Plastic Surgery. New York, NY: Lippincott-Raven; 1997:34

Marcus JR, Erdmann D, Rodriguez ED, eds. Essentials of Craniomaxillofacial Trauma. St Louis, MO: Quality Medical Publishing; 2012

Marik PE, Varon J, Trask T. Management of head trauma. Chest. 2002; 122(2):699–711

Markowitz BL, Manson PN, Sargent L, et al. Management of the medial canthal tendon in nasoethmoid orbital fractures: the importance of the central fragment in classification and treatment. Plast Reconstr Surg. 1991; 87(5):843–853

Nahum AM. The biomechanics of maxillofacial trauma. Clin Plast Surg. 1975; 2(1):59–64

North America AO. Review of surgical approaches to the cranial skeleton 2010. www.aona.org

Pereira N, Andrades P, Borel C, Rocha L, Hernández R, Villalobos R. Sub-mucosal endoscopically assisted septoplasty (SEAS) and closed nasal reduction. A comparative study versus traditional technique. Rev Cir Plast Iberolat. In press

Ridgway EB, Chen C, Colakoglu S, Gautam S, Lee BT. The incidence of lower eyelid malposition after facial fracture repair: a retrospective study and meta-analysis comparing subtarsal, subciliary, and transconjunctival incisions. Plast Reconstr Surg. 2009; 124(5):1578–1586

Rohrich RJ, Adams WP, Jr. Nasal fracture management: minimizing secondary nasal deformities. Plast Reconstr Surg. 2000; 106(2):266–273

Rohrich RJ, Hollier LH. Management of frontal sinus fractures. Changing concepts. Clin Plast Surg. 1992; 19(1):219–232

Thornton J, Hollier L. Facial fractures II: lower third. Select Read Plast Surg. 2002; 9(27):1–34

21 Hand Trauma

S. Raja Sabapathy, R. Raja Shanmugakrishnan

Abstract

Hand injuries are the most common injuries that occur in the workplace and often involve young people. Complications following even the "simple" injuries could lead to severe morbidity and lifelong disability to the individual. A systematic examination to assess injury to the tendons, nerves, bones, and blood vessels is important. All injured structures can be primarily repaired if the surgeon is confident of primary wound healing. Primary wound healing depends upon good debridement. When the injuries are associated with soft-tissue loss, skin cover with either grafts or flaps must be achieved as early as possible. In hand injury management, first time is the best time to get good results. Good management of hand injuries needs skilled surgeons experienced in the management of hand injuries, a supportive infrastructure, and supervised postoperative physiotherapy. If any of the required components of care are not available, it is better to refer the patient to the center where it would be available. With a better understanding of the healing of various structures of the hand and the advent of microsurgery, good outcomes are possible even in major injuries with loss of various tissue components. Microsurgery has made it possible to reattach even totally amputated hands and fingers. While amputated parts with no muscle like the fingers and thumb can stand long periods of ischemia, proximal amputations with large muscle component have to be revascularized within a few hours. Awareness of the possibility of replantation and indications will help surgeons to refer the patients to the replantation center. Accurate assessment of the injury, followed with appropriate care and physiotherapy can help get good functional outcomes even in major injuries.

Keywords: mangled hand, amputation, tendon injury, fracture, osteosynthesis, replantation, rehabililtation

21.1 Introduction

Hand is a commonly injured part of the body. Almost 40% of all injuries that happen in the workplace are to the hands affecting people in the most productive years of life. While in most parts of the body, wound healing is the end point, in the hand, restoring function is the end point. Proper assessment of the injury, with appropriate management provided at the right time, could result in a good outcome. Most patients would also need to undergo supervised rehabilitation protocols. If any one component of care is missed, it could result in severe morbidity to the individual. It could also result in an economic disaster with loss of employment and productivity, which the individual and the society could ill afford. Uniquely, the ultimate outcome depends upon the decisions made by the first doctor who examines the patient. So familiarity with the examination of an injured hand and the principles of its management is a must for a trauma surgeon.

> **Remember** **M!**
>
> - Forty percent of all injuries at the workplace are to the hands.
> - Ultimate outcome depends upon the initial diagnosis and appropriate primary care.

21.2 Relevant Anatomy

The structure and the capability of the hand distinguish the human being. In the hand, the second and the third rays act as stable rays, whereas the thumb and the ulnar two metacarpals possess movement. The position and mobility of the thumb are unique. The range of movement of carpometacarpal joint of the thumb is critical for hand function. Apart from the movement of the thumb, a length of at least up to the neck of the proximal phalanx is considered critical for function. Functional capability is drastically reduced with shorter thumb and a total loss of thumb equals 40% loss of function of the hand.

Every structure in the hand is well adapted for function. The palmar skin is thick, whereas the dorsal skin is thin and is loosely attached. So edema of the hand is more pronounced in the dorsum and it can pull up the metacarpophalangeal (MCP) joints into a nonphysiological position of hyperextension. The fibrous septa in the hand and fingers hold the volar skin tight and help in gripping.

The sensation of the fingertips can distinguish points with a gap of 3 to 4 mm. The neurovascular bundle in the fingers lies volar to the midlateral line, with the nerve lying volar to the artery. In the thumb, the digital nerves lie on either side of the flexor tendon (▶Fig. 21.1). The position of the nerves has to be kept in mind when performing digital blocks or exploring wounds. Digital nerves are identifiable and suturable structures almost to the level of the middle of the distal phalanx and as such must be repaired in cases of injury. Unrepaired digital nerves, apart from loss of sensation, can cause painful neuromas.

Important surface landmarks are useful in examining the hand. On the volar side, the distal wrist crease corresponds to the proximal limit of the flexor retinaculum, which extends distally for another 3 cm. The flexor retinaculum is attached to the pisiform and the hook of the hamate, which are both palpable on the ulnar side and to the tubercle of the scaphoid (a palpable landmark on the radial side) and the ridge of the trapezium. The distal palmar crease corresponds to the level of the MCP joints of the fingers and the proximal palmar crease in the base of the hand indicates the position of the carpometacarpal joint of the thumb. Any plasters crossing these lines will restrict the movement of the joints.

The hand is well supplied by radial and ulnar arteries, with the ulnar artery mainly contributing to the superficial palmar arch and the radial artery to the deep palmar arch. While the extensive anastomosis can compensate for injuries of a particular vessel, in major crush injuries it is advisable to repair blood vessels to get pulsatile blood flow into the hand,

which helps in wound healing, improved survival of local flaps, and planning secondary reconstruction.

The flexor tendons to the finger and the thumb reach the hand through the carpal tunnel. There is one flexor tendon for the thumb (flexor pollicis longus), whereas two for each finger (flexor digitorum profundus [FDP] and flexor digitorum superficialis [FDS]). The flexor tendons pass through an intricate system of fibro-osseous sheaths called pulleys. The FDS lies superficial to the FDP tendon up to the MCP joint level. At this level, the FDS tendon splits into two slips and through it the FDP becomes superficial to the FDS. The FDS is inserted at the middle phalanx and produces proximal interphalangeal (PIP) joint flexion. The FDP is inserted at the base of the distal phalanx and produces distal interphalangeal (DIP) joint flexion. Depending upon the relation of the flexor tendon to the pulley system and the surrounding anatomical structures, they are divided into five zones (▶Fig. 21.2). In zone 2, both the FDS and

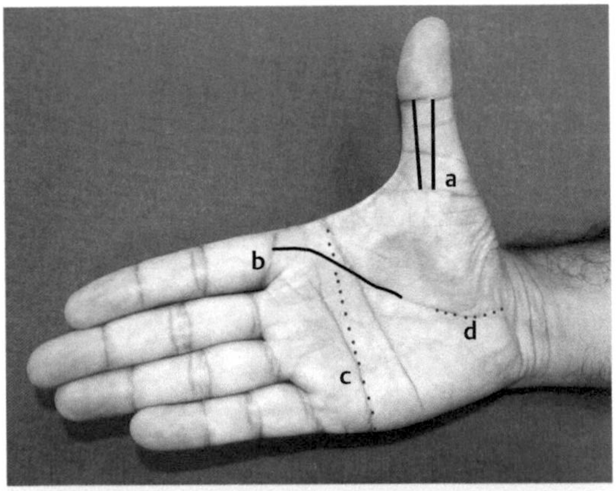

Fig. 21.1 Surface anatomy of the hand. (a) The line of digital nerves to the thumb. (b) The line of radial digital nerve to the index. (c) Dotted line shows the level of the metacarpophalangeal joints of the fingers. (d) Dotted line shows the carpometacarpal joint of the thumb. Plaster extending beyond these lines (c, d) blocks movement of the respective joints.

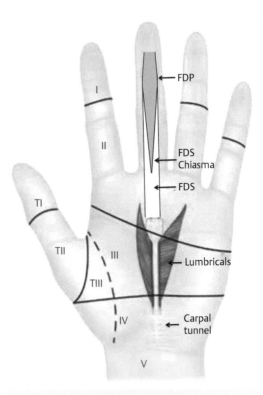

Fig. 21.2 Zones of the flexor tendon I to V (thumb TI-TV) in relation to important structures. FDP, flexor digitorum profundus; FDS, flexor digitorum superficialis.

FDP traverse in the narrow space of the pulley system. Repair of these tendons in this zone is considered a challenge, and hence the name of "no man's land." One has to be very precise in surgical technique to get a good result of flexor tendon repair at this level. At zone 4, all the flexor tendons are packed in a small space (carpal tunnel) along with the median nerve. An injury at this zone typically involves multiple structures. The pulleys prevent bowstringing of the tendons. There are five annular pulleys and three cruciate pulleys. A2 and A4 pulleys are considered important for function (▶Fig. 21.3).

Extensor tendon system is equally important. They are divided into nine zones. Odd numbers are used for regions overlying joints, whereas even numbers represent the regions between joints (▶Fig. 21.4). Distal to the MCP joint (zones 1–5), the extensor tendon is very flat and thin. Repairs of the tendon at these levels cannot be very strong; hence, they always require protection after repair, mostly in the form of a wire across the joint that the tendon is acting on.

21.3 Assessment of an Injured Hand

21.3.1 The Primary Survey

If the injured hand is not severely bleeding, the first few minutes of the patient examination must be spent on enquiring about the nature of the accident, the time of occurrence, handedness, occupation, and recreational demands of the individual. Comorbidities, if any, must be noted. Each factor has an important bearing on the management. If the hand has been injured in a roller injury or subjected to prolonged

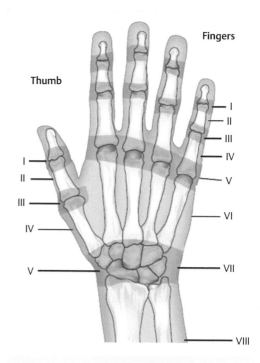

Fig. 21.4 The zones of extensor tendons.

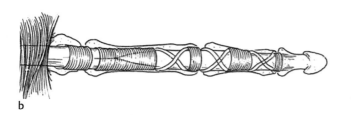

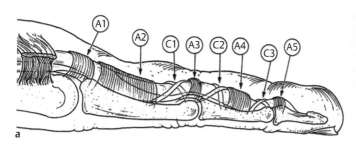

Fig. 21.3 (a, b) The pulley system in the fingers. A, annular pulleys; C, cruciate pulleys.

compression, the damage will be more than what is initially obvious. Time of occurrence of the injury will have a bearing on the decision to replant or revascularize the distal part. Surgical procedures are chosen depending on the work of the individual and the demands the hand will be put to. All major injured patients must go through the advanced trauma life support (ATLS) protocol so that an associated injury is not missed. Prophylactic antibiotics and tetanus prophylaxis must be administered. Hand injuries attract attention and if this protocol is not followed, it might lead to missed injuries and a poor outcome.

The opportunity must also be taken to provide a reassuring attitude because most hand-injured patients are concerned about the functional outcome.

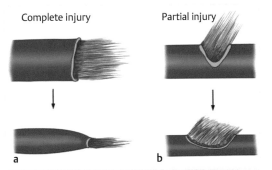

Complete injury   Partial injury

a   b

Fig. 21.5 (a) In the event of complete division of a vessel, the muscular walls contract and occlude the bleeding. (b) In the event of a partial division, the same mechanism opens up the rent and maintains it open, resulting in severe bleeding.

21.3.2 Controlling Bleeding

If the patient arrives with significant bleeding, the best way to control the bleeding is to apply a sterile dressing over the injured area and apply direct pressure over the bleeding surface with a compression dressing and elevate the injured part above the level of the heart. Bleeding will stop in most instances with this step in a few minutes. If significant bleeding persists, a partial injury to the vessel should be suspected. Whereas in a complete injury the contractile mechanism of the vessel wall helps control the bleeding, in a partially injured vessel it stretches the tear, making it wider (▶Fig. 21.5). In such cases, it is safer to inflate a tourniquet proximal to the level of injury. The tourniquet should be inflated beyond the systolic pressure and the time of application must be noted. Patients with an unanesthetized arm can tolerate a tourniquet for about 20 minutes, which would be adequate to seek the needed help. Even in such instances, a well-applied direct pressure will help control bleeding. The one measure that should not be done is to blindly plunge in hemostats to catch the bleeders. Important structures like nerves and tendons go along major vessels in the hand and this step has the risk of injuring them, making direct repair impossible (▶Fig. 21.6).

21.4 Identification of the Injured Structures

Good outcomes in hand injury management are achieved when the wound heals primarily and the injured structures are primarily repaired. The

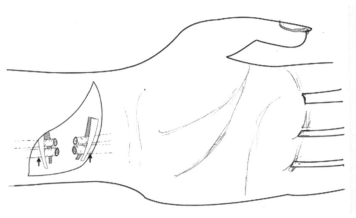

Fig. 21.6 Blind plunging of the artery forceps to control bleeding from the ulnar side wound can include the ulnar nerve as well.

hand is packed with functional tissues and therefore multiple structures may be damaged and it is quite easy to miss nerve or tendon injuries. The safe axiom is to consider all structures beneath the skin wound to be injured unless proved otherwise.

21.4.1 Vascular Supply

Vascularity of the hand and fingers is assessed by feeling the pulse and checking the color of the fingertips as well as capillary refill, which should be less than 3 seconds. If the fingertip is pale or congested, a vascular injury must be suspected. If the pulses are not felt in the injured limb although it is present on the other side or when a pulse oximeter does not pick up signals, a vascular injury is suspected. The absent pulse must not be attributed to vascular spasm or shock. In closed injuries, a hand-held Doppler can be run along the course of the main vessels. An abrupt drop in signals denotes the possible site of vascular injury and merits early exploration. Rarely do we resort to angiograms in upper limb injury.

Compartment syndrome is a situation of vascular compromise to tissues in a tight osseofibrous compartment. Bleeding inside a closed compartment, vascular injury, and muscle injury all could cause a reduction in the arteriovenous gradient preventing circulation in the muscles. Whenever the compartment pressure increases over 40 mm of Hg, circulation to the muscles is compromised. It may occur even in the presence of a palpable pulse in a major vessel. Whenever there is pain out of proportion to the injury accompanied by swelling and firmness over the compartment, compromised circulation should be thought of. Pain, pallor, paralysis, and pulselessness are the common findings, but the diagnosis of compartment syndrome should be done in the stage of pain itself. *Pain and increased resistance on passive stretch* of the fingers is the key to diagnose compartment syndrome. Because of the increased resistance component, this test could be used even in an unconscious patient. When present, it is an indication for careful frequent monitoring and if there is no improvement in a couple of hours, urgent decompression of the compartment should be done. Compartment pressures can be measured, but the person should be experienced in the technique to avoid false results. Time must not be wasted in doing an angiogram to diagnose compartment syndrome.

21.4.2 Tendons

The fingers have a normal resting cascade due to the tension of the musculotendinous units and any deviation from the norm in the presence of good joints could be due to tendon injury. On the flexor side, this is seen as inability of the fingers to maintain the cascade, whereas on the extensor side it is reflected by drop of the finger. When the extensor injury is close to the DIP joint, it causes mallet finger and at PIP joint it leads to boutonniere deformity. The patient is requested to actively go through the range of movements of the joints. While loss of movement occurs in complete injuries, even 10% of intact tendon will allow the patient to go through the full range of movement. Partial tendon injury should be suspected if there is pain on resisted movement of the fingers. In injuries in the palm and fingers, triggering of the finger could denote a partial injury with the injury site being caught at the rent in the pulley. In injuries to extensor tendons on the dorsum of the hand, finger extension might still be possible even with complete division of the tendon due to the presence of juncturae tendinae. The size of the wound has no bearing on the structures injured. Wounds due to knife or glass pieces are notorious for causing extensive injuries (▶ Fig. 21.7).

21.4.3 Nerves

Missing nerve injuries is the commonest cause of litigation in hand injuries. The nerves are suturable structures to the level of the middle of the pulp of the fingertip and hence injured nerves should be repaired. In the acute stage, the patient may not be aware of the loss of sensation. To diagnose a nerve injury, we need to systematically examine the muscles supplied by the nerve and distal sensation. While testing sensation in the emergency room, instead of asking the patient whether the patient feels the stimulus, we need to compare it with the uninjured side and ask the patient whether there is a difference between the two sides. If there is a difference, a nerve injury is suspected and the wound should be explored. In proximal injuries, sensation in the area of autonomous zones is checked (▶ Fig. 21.8). These are the minimum areas of overlap of sensory innervation between the three major nerves in the hand. The commonly used classification of nerve injuries is

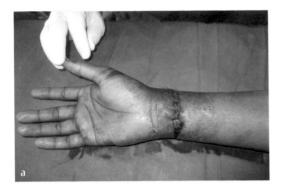

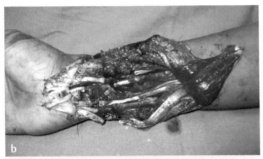

Fig. 21.7 (a) Coarsely sutured wound at another center, caused by a sharp knife, without recognizing the possibility of the injuries to critical structures. (b) Secondary exploration reveals the complete division of all flexors, median, and ulnar nerves and radial and ulnar arteries.

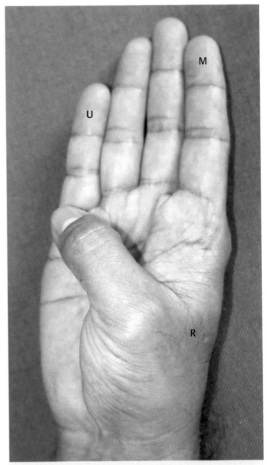

Fig. 21.8 Autonomous zone of sensation for testing nerves of the hand. U, ulnar nerve; M, median nerve; R, radial nerve.

given in ▶Table 21.1. Edema following closed compression injuries and electrical burns could cause compression of the median nerve in carpal tunnel. Hypoesthesia of the tips of the radial three fingers should raise suspicion of carpal tunnel compression, which if undetected could result in permanent sensory loss and intrinsic muscle paralysis.

21.4.4 Bone and Joint Injuries

Whereas it is easy to clinically identify fractures of shafts of the hand bones by deformity and local tenderness, assessment of the type of fracture and joint injuries requires good radiology. Good anteroposterior and lateral view radiographs are commonly ordered. When interphalangeal joint injuries are suspected, a perfect lateral view is important. If not specified in the request form, overlapping of the fingers will result in missing intra-articular fractures and subluxation of joints. An oblique X-ray is also taken

if an injury is suspected around the MCP joints. Two types of displacement, namely anteroposterior and rotational, can occur at the fracture site. Rotational displacement leads to scissoring of fingers, where the injured finger overlaps its neighbor. Ten degrees of rotation at the base of the metacarpal would result in 2 cm of overlap at the fingertip level (▶Fig. 21.9). Furthermore, the more proximal the fracture site, the greater the deformity.

If carpal injuries are suspected, a posteroanterior and lateral view radiographs are obtained. In suspected scaphoid fracture, in addition, an ulnar deviated posteroanterior view radiograph is also done. In the acute stage, if the plain radiographs are not conclusive, radiographs may be repeated

Table 21.1 Classification of nerve injury

Sunderland	Seddon	Injury
I	Neurapraxia	Conduction block resolves spontaneously
II	Axonotmesis	Axonal rupture without interruption of the basal lamina tubes
III		Rupture of both axons and basal lamina tubes, some scarring
IV		Complete scar block
V	Neurotmesis	Complete transection
VI (Mackinnon)		Combination of I through V and normal fascicles

Table 21.2 Indications for replantation

Definite indications
Thumb amputations
Multiple finger amputations
Any amputation in a child
Amputation at the level of the palm, wrist, or forearm
Single digit amputation distal to the FDS insertion

Relative indications
Ring finger avulsion injury
Single finger injury proximal to FDS insertion
Crush and avulsion amputations proximal to wrist

Abbreviation: FDP, flexor digitorum profundus; FDS, flexor digitorum superficialis.

after 2 weeks and the patient immobilized with a plaster or splint until then. If radiographs show scaphoid nonunion, magnetic resonance imaging is done to reveal the presence of the avascular segment.

21.4.5 Replantation Surgery and Indications

The advent of microsurgery has made reattachment of amputated parts possible. The goal of replantation surgery is to get good functional outcome rather than mere survival of the part. The definitive indications and relative indications are given in ▶Table 21.2. Whereas these recommendations serve as general guidelines, centers doing high-volume replantation have extended the indications. Hence, it is very prudent to discuss replantation referrals with the concerned units. The best way to transport the amputated part is to place the amputated part inside a plastic bag and tightly seal it with a knot. The plastic bag is put into a container with ice cubes all around. Direct contact with the ice or placing the amputated part in any fluid medium is not recommended. The proximal stump is given a compression bandage.

Replantations done distal to the wrist are called minor replantation and those done proximal

to the wrist are called major replantation. The words minor and major do not reflect the technical complexity involved in the procedure, but are more related to the risk of significant complications. Complications of replantation are directly related to the ischemia time and the quantum of ischemic muscle mass in the amputated part. In minor replantations, the amount of muscle mass is less and therefore able to withstand ischemia for a longer period of time. Parts like the thumb and fingers, which do not have muscles, can be replanted after long periods of ischemia provided they have been stored properly. For more proximal amputations, revascularization must occur faster and an above-elbow amputation must be revascularized within 6 hours even when the part has been properly stored during transport. Major replantations with longer ischemia time have the risk of causing reperfusion problems, with significant morbidity and even mortality. When properly executed, replantation offers the best form of reconstruction after amputation.

Note

- Spend the first few minutes in gathering details of the accident and looking for associated injuries.
- Never plunge in a hemostat to control bleeding. Use direct pressure and elevation of the hand.
- Size of the skin wound may be deceptively small with injury to many critical structures underneath; examine systematically.
- When there is an amputation, consult the microsurgery center about the possibility of replantation.

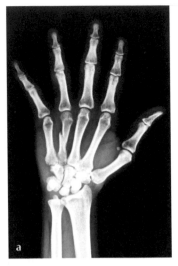
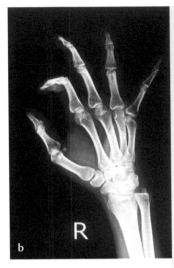

Fig. 21.9 (a) Radiograph showing healed fracture of the shaft of ring finger metacarpal. (b) On full extension, the fingers appear to be in good position. (c, d) On flexion, there is severe overlap (scissoring) of the fingers due to rotational malalignment at the fracture site.

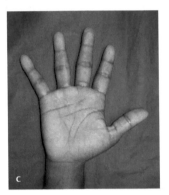
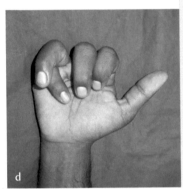

21.5 Management of Hand Injuries

21.5.1 Basic Principles

The goal of hand injury management is to achieve primary healing of the wound with early restoration of function. It is a basic principle that unless the skin wound heals primarily, we cannot expect the deeper structures to heal primarily. Common causes of poor wound healing are infection and poor judgment of the magnitude of skin injury. The injured hand has to be operated by a surgeon who is experienced to deal with the repair of the injured structures. First time is the best time to get good results. If the required skills and infrastructure are inadequate, the patient must be transferred to a center where they are available. Good anesthesia, tourniquet, and magnification are essential in hand injury management. Most hand injuries can be managed under regional anesthesia.

21.5.2 Management of Soft-Tissue Injury

Debridement

The important step in the management of open hand injuries is debridement of the wound. Quality of debridement determines whether the wound gets infected or not. Two types of debridement are described: serial debridement and radical debridement. During serial debridement, all the contaminants and obvious nonviable tissues are removed. This is followed by a second look under anesthesia 24 to 48 hours later. The procedure is repeated until one is sure that the wound is fit for closure or soft-tissue cover. In radical debridement, the emphasis is not on what is removed, but on what is left behind at the completion of the procedure. At the end of radical debridement, one must be sure that all that is left behind is viable and the wound is free of contaminants. This is also referred to as wound excision.

Debridement is done under tourniquet and loupe magnification by an experienced surgeon. This is done systematically starting with the skin. The ragged skin edges are excised. Sometimes the wound may need extension to gain access to deeper structures. Then layer by layer, the damaged and contaminated tissues are excised. Dead muscle looks red, and good muscle appears pale under tourniquet. Devitalized muscle is excised. Noncritical hypovascular structures are excised. Critical longitudinal structures like nerves, tendons, and bone are meticulously debrided. There is a thin filmy layer of tissue over these structures and even when there is severe contamination, by going beneath this layer these critical structures could be retained. Bone pieces without any soft-tissue attachment are removed. Cortical bones without any soft-tissue attachment cannot act as bone graft. Intermuscular planes and joint cavities, if open, are the common sites of missed contaminants. After a thorough wound excision, the wound is well irrigated. The tourniquet is let down, and if areas of avascularity are still seen, they are further debrided after reinflating the tourniquet. In this way, we convert a contaminated wound into a surgically clean wound, fit for primary reconstruction of injured structures and immediate soft-tissue cover (▶Fig. 21.10).

One has to be more careful in penetrating injuries, especially human bite injuries. These injuries over the MCP joints often appear innocuous; however, the teeth penetrate the joint and its coverings in various levels inoculating the pathway with bacteria. When the finger is extended, the layers separate, producing a good anaerobic environment for infection to occur. The recommended treatment for penetrating injuries is to excise the tract.

Timing of Soft-Tissue Cover

Good debridement allows safe primary cover of the wound. It has been proved that early soft-tissue cover prevents secondary loss of tissue by exposure, desiccation, and infection. Bare tendons and nerves tolerate desiccation much worse than bare bone. Pioneering work of Godina and the work pursued in that direction by many authors have proved that early flap cover following radical debridement is safe, reduces infection, and helps achieve better outcomes. Whereas the question

of maximum waiting period is still debated, the authors feel that it is better to achieve definitive soft-tissue cover within 48 to 72 hours. Only in exceptional cases like major electrical burns are serial debridement resorted to. Till definitive cover is achieved, the wound is covered with moist dressings. Negative pressure wound therapy (NPWT or vacuum-assisted closure dressing) can be used in the interim period. NPWT is used less frequently in the upper limb when compared to the lower limb. It is the authors' opinion that the use of NPWT must not be pushed in the upper limb as a means to avoid a flap when a flap is indicated at the end of debridement.

Type of Skin Cover

All areas with the potential to granulate will take a skin graft. On the contrary, bone devoid of periosteum, tendons without paratenon, bare nerves, vessel, and nerve repair sites need flap cover. When the defect is small, local flaps can be used. In major crush injuries, distant flaps, either pedicled or free, need to be used, with free flaps having the advantage of being one stage, providing coverage of large defects and allowing early initiation of physical therapy postoperatively (▶Fig. 21.11). Pedicled flaps include regional ones such as the radial artery flap or posterior interosseous artery flap. Distant pedicled flaps like the groin flap have the drawbacks of being a multistage procedure; however, when well executed, it obviates much of the potential drawbacks. Groin flaps continue to be the workhorse in the management of hand injuries in many parts of the world. Finally, the ultimate functional outcome depends not so much upon the type of cover, but whether the wound gets infected or not, which in turn depends on the quality of debridement and the timing of soft-tissue cover.

21.5.3 Management of Hand Fractures and Joint Injuries

In the management of hand fractures, fracture union alone is not the end point; restoration of hand function is equally important. Even during fracture union, mobilization of the uninvolved joints is undertaken. Fracture union after hand fractures is not a problem, unless it is an open fracture with bone loss, soft-tissue loss, or there is infection at the fracture site. Hence, nonunions

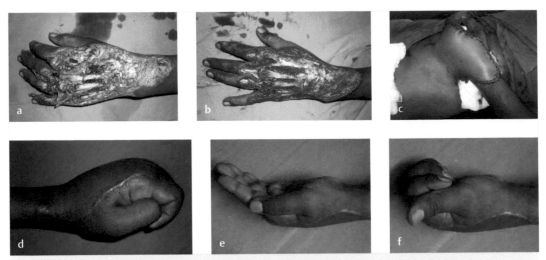

Fig. 21.10 (a) A major crush injury to the dorsum of the hand with composite tissue loss. (b) After radical debridement of the wound. (c) Primary pedicled abdominal flap cover to the wound. (d–f) The postoperative function without any reconstruction of the extensors. Extension achieved by relaxation of flexion.

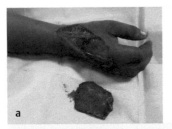
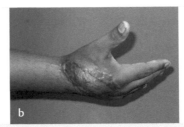
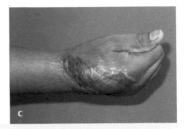

Fig. 21.11 (a) Defect over the dorsum of the hand. Damages to the extensor tendons have been repaired and the defect covered with a free muscle flap (shown in the picture). (b, c) Postoperative functional result.

are uncommon. Many of the hand fractures can be managed conservatively with good results. While performing operative fixation of the fractures, soft-tissue healing considerations take priority.

Fractures of the metacarpal can occur at the base, shaft, or the neck. Fracture of the base of the first metacarpal is called Bennett's fracture. It is an inherently unstable fracture because of the attachment of the abductor pollicis longus at the proximal fragment, which tends to displace this fragment proximally (▶Fig. 21.12). Hence, this fracture should always be fixed. A similar fracture of the fifth metacarpal is called "Baby Bennett" or "reverse Bennett" fracture where the extensor carpi ulnaris attachment acts as the displacement force needing fixation. Fractures of the base of other metacarpals can be managed conservatively. Definite indication for fixation in metacarpal fractures

is unstable rotational malalignment at the fracture site. The anteroposterior angular displacement can get molded and get better with time, but rotational malalignment never gets better with time and will require surgical correction. Fracture of the head of the fifth metacarpal is called boxer's fracture. Due to the good range of movement at the fifth carpometacarpal (CMC) joint, angulation up to about 45 degrees at the fifth metacarpal neck fracture is usually well tolerated, but angulation beyond that should be corrected surgically. The amount of angulation, which can be compensated, is less as we move radial to the middle and index due to the limited movement at their CMC joints, with the index tolerating a maximum of 20 degrees of angulation.

In the fingers, fractures of the proximal phalanges are the most common. Most proximal phalangeal fractures have a volar angular displacement

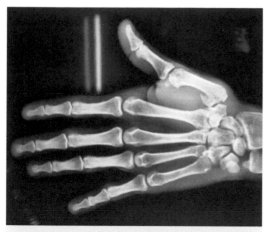

Fig. 21.12 Bennett's fracture dislocation showing the displacement of the larger fragment due to the pull of the attachment of abductor pollicis longus.

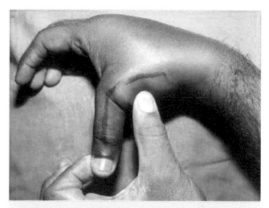

Fig. 21.13 Forced stress test showing the opening of the joint in a case of ulnar collateral ligament tear.

because of the flexion of the proximal fragment by the intrinsic muscle action. After closed reduction if the fractures are stable, simple immobilization with plaster is enough. On the contrary, all unstable phalangeal fractures, with gross displacement or angulation and fractures with rotational displacement, warrant surgical fixation. Intra-articular fractures need specialist attention.

Dorsal dislocation of the PIP joint is the commonest dislocation in the hand. It is easily reduced under digital block and treated by an extension block splint for 2 to 4 weeks. Volar dislocation at the PIP joint is *always* associated with central slip rupture and is treated by immobilization of the PIP joint by a K wire for 4 weeks, followed by gradual flexion exercises. When missed, it results in boutonniere deformity.

Dislocations of the MCP joint are classified as simple, when they can be managed by closed reduction, or complex when closed reduction is not possible. Complex dislocation, which is common in the MCP joint of the index finger, is irreducible due to the interposition of the volar plate and the flexors, with lumbricals and nerves getting looped around the neck. It needs operative intervention.

Ulnar collateral ligament (UCL) injury of the MCP joint of the thumb ("skier's thumb" or "gamekeeper's thumb") requires special mention as it is a commonly missed injury, which can be disabling if left untreated. If the injury is partial, it tends to heal well with rest and splinting. However, a complete avulsion of this ligament cannot heal because of the interposition of the adductor pollicis aponeurosis between the avulsed ligament and its original attachment site (e.g., Stener's lesion; ▶ Fig. 21.13). A stress test is performed by stressing the joint radially in full extension. Gradual opening of the joint without a firm end point is diagnostic of a complete tear. A stress view X-ray showing an opening up of more than 45 degrees is also diagnostic. All complete tears must be operated. The surgery involves fixing the avulsed ligament onto its anatomical location by periosteal sutures or interosseous sutures or by a suture anchor. The joint is immobilized for 4 weeks and then gradual movement of the joint and use of the hand can be initiated.

21.5.4 Tendon Injuries

Primary repair of flexor and extensor tendon injuries at all levels is the standard of care. Repair of tendons requires experience and a good infrastructure. If they are not available, it is better to refer to a center where they are available so that good primary repair can be carried out. First time is the best time to get good results. Results of repair of flexor tendons performed immediately or within 5 days from injury have not shown any difference in outcome. Whereas the definitive flexor tendon repair can wait, wound care cannot. The open wound must be debrided and the skin closed so as to prevent infection and achieve primary healing.

Numerous techniques are available for flexor tendon repair. Basically all have some form of core sutures and circumferential coaptation sutures, where increases in the number of strands in the core suture increase the strength of the repair. The author uses a four-strand suture with 4–0 nonabsorbable sutures and circumferential epitendinous suture with 6–0 polypropylene (▶Fig. 21.14). The circumferential suture not only makes the repair look tidy, but also adds strength to the repair site. Also, the technique of repair determines the feasibility of active range of movements during physiotherapy. Flexor tendon repair in zone 2 is usually challenging due to the presence of pulleys. Access is through cruciate pulleys, leaving A2 and A4 as uninjured as possible to prevent bowstringing during flexion. Adhesions and rupture are the two main complications after flexor tendon repair. Whereas adhesions are prevented by instituting rehabilitation protocols of active range of movement, rupture is avoided by a good technique during repair. Adhesions are diagnosed by the presence of more passive than active range of movement. Massage and therapy are the cornerstones of treatment and refractory cases undergo tenolysis usually done after

3 months. Rupture is diagnosed by the patient who usually refers a sudden pop at the repair site, followed by inability to flex the finger. Once rupture occurs, the treatment is immediate surgical exploration and tendon repair.

Extensor tendon repair, though considered easier than its flexor counterpart, shares the same level of complexity in obtaining good results. Extensor tendons are flat in most of their surface and the commonly used techniques of repair is shown in ▶Fig. 21.15. The extensor tendon (e.g., extensor digitorum communis) of each finger divides at the level of the proximal phalanx into a central slip and two lateral slips, which together with contributions from intrinsic muscles form the lateral bands. The central slip inserts at the base of the middle phalanx and the lateral bands join distally and insert at the base of the distal phalanx. Injuries at these insertion sites lead to specific deformities, namely mallet finger for the distal one and boutonniere deformity for the proximal one. Closed mallet injuries associated with an avulsion fracture of less than 25% of the articular surface of the distal phalanx can be

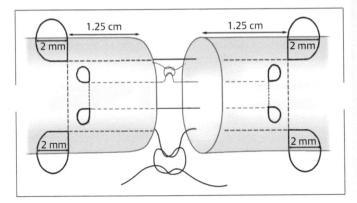

Fig. 21.14 Four-strand core suture repair of flexor tendons.

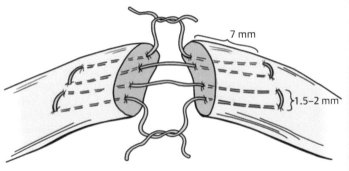

Fig. 21.15 Technique for suturing a flat tendon.

treated either conservatively or by surgery. Because conservative treatment requires continuous splitting for 6 weeks, we prefer to treat surgically by closed pinning of the DIP joint with a K wire. As mentioned earlier, division of the extensor insertion (central slip) at the middle phalanx leads to boutonniere deformity. In the acute phase, it can be diagnosed by the tendency of the finger to flex at the PIP joint and a tendency for extension at the DIP joint. Closed rupture of the central slip may be treated conservatively with 6 weeks of splinting of the PIP joint in extension while allowing movement at the DIP joint. Alternatively, the PIP joint can be fixed with a K-wire for 6 weeks. At all levels, supervised therapy is paramount to achieve a good outcome following repair. Loss of length or shortening of the extensor tendon or adhesions can cause severe loss of flexion of the fingers, which will be functionally disabling.

21.5.5 Nerve Injuries

Primary repair of injured nerves should be attempted whenever possible. When left unrepaired, the nerve ends retract and the changes occurring at the cut ends obscure the fascicular pattern, making their identification and correct matching difficult, particularly in mixed nerves. Both the vascular pattern on the surface of the nerves and the fascicular pattern at the cut ends are useful markers for the correct orientation and coaptation. In general, epineural repair with 8–0 to 10–0 nylon sutures is the recommended technique. Partial nerve injuries must be primarily repaired because secondary repair has the risk of injuring the uninjured fascicles and sometimes small grafts may be needed. When there is a nerve gap, suturing the nerves under tension is not recommended as tension reduces the intraneuronal blood supply and leads to fibrosis at the repair site. If the nerve ends cannot be securely held with a single 6–0 Prolene suture taken through the epineurium, then the use of nerve grafts should be considered. Techniques to bring the edges together and avoid grafts include flexion of the wrist joint up to 45 degrees, which is then gradually extended over 15 degrees every 3 weeks to neutral position. Another technique to avoid tension is mobilization of the nerves. Nerves have a good intraneuronal blood supply, making mobilization over long segments possible. The presence of branches, however, is the limiting factor in this method.

Most surgeons would hesitate to do primary nerve grafting. It could be done in cases where primary wound healing is highly likely and no further procedure on the tendons or bone will be required. If secondary nerve grafting is planned, then the cut ends are marked with sutures and their position recorded in the notes to avoid lengthy exploratory incisions. Sural nerve is the common donor nerve.

21.6 Clinical Cases

21.6.1 Case 1

A 21-year-old man sustained a major crush injury to his left hand in a road traffic accident. The dorsum of the hand had suffered abrasive injury with loss of skin and soft tissue around the wrist, division of extensor tendons, and loss of most of the carpal bones as well as the dorsal cortex of the distal part of the radius. The hand was attached only by volar soft tissues (▶Fig. 21.16a). On the volar side, apart from a partial injury to the median nerve, the flexor tendons and the vessels were intact. There was severe contamination.

The wound was radically debrided, which resulted in loss of most of the carpal bones (▶Fig. 21.16b). Bony stability was achieved by primary arthrodesis of the wrist with the wrist in about 20 degrees of dorsiflexion. The extensors to the fingers and the thumb were primarily repaired (▶Fig. 21.16c). Debridement resulted in loss of a few centimeters of extensor tendons, but the loss of the carpal bones and 20 degrees of dorsiflexion helped compensate for the loss of length. The raw area with exposed repaired extensor tendons and the implant was covered with a groin flap (▶Fig. 21.16d). The flap was divided after 3 weeks and the patient started supervised physical therapy. He had one procedure of flap thinning at 6 months. On follow-up at 1 year, the patient had full flexion and extension of the fingers and was able to resume his regular daily activities (▶Fig. 21.16e, f).

The learning points in this case study is that even though the wound at first sight may pose doubt about the possibility of salvage, through a combination of radical debridement, primary repair of the injured structures, and immediate flap cover, a very good outcome is possible to achieve. It also becomes apparent that primary reconstruction can be done with pedicle flaps as cover. In addition,

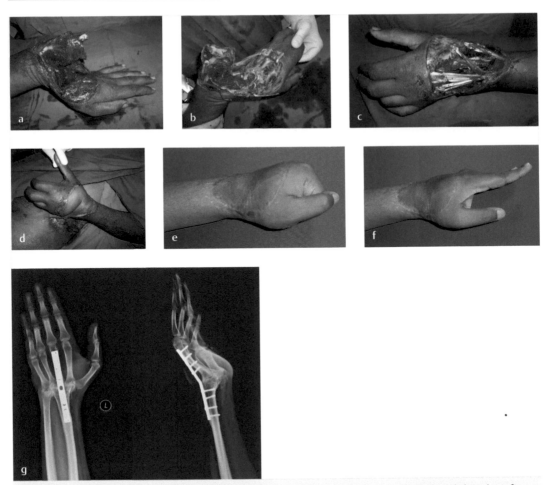

Fig. 21.16 (a) Major crush injury to the left hand in a road traffic accident with the hand hanging only by volar soft tissues. **(b)** Postdebridement picture. **(c)** Tendons were repaired after skeletal fixation. **(d)** The raw area being covered by a groin flap, the picture showing the flap prior to division. **(e, f)** Postoperative result showing good functional outcome. **(g)** Radiograph showing a well-united arthrodesis of the wrist.

more than the type of flap chosen, it is the radical debridement before flap coverage what determines whether the wound gets infected or not. Primary wound healing is fundamental to get a good outcome.

21.6.2 Case 2

A man sustained total amputation of his left forearm at the distal third while working in a saw mill (▶ Fig. 21.17a–c). The part was brought well preserved in a plastic bag kept in another bag containing ice within 2 hours of the accident. The part and the proximal segment were

debrided. Because it was a sharp injury, only a few centimeters of bone shortening was needed. Internal fixation of the fractures with plates and screws was done (▶ Fig. 21.17d). All tendons, the radial and ulnar arteries, two superficial veins and the venae comitantes, and the median and ulnar nerves were repaired. Total ischemia time was 5 hours. Replantation was successful and the patient underwent supervised physical therapy for 6 months. The patient developed good function, a 2-point discrimination of 10 mm and a DASH (disabilities of the arm, shoulder, and hand) score of 10. He is now back to his same job (▶ Fig. 21.17e, f).

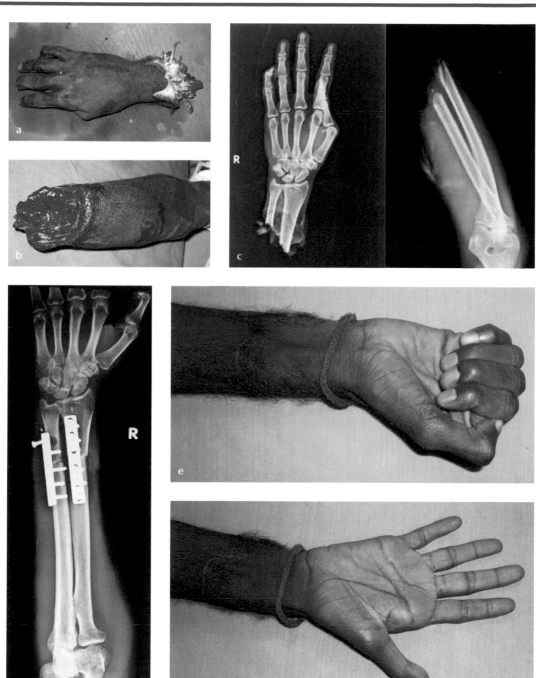

Fig. 21.17 (a–c) Total amputation of the right hand at the distal third of the forearm. **(d)** Radiograph showing bone union. **(e, f)** Functional outcome at 1 year.

The learning points in this case study are that immediate referral to the appropriate center is key to success. Even in a sharp injury, a few centimeters of bone shortening is advised. This is useful to perform quick fixation of bone ends, as well as to facilitate primary repair of nerves and tendons after debridement. Even in sharp injuries, most of the times the cut ends of the tendons and nerves need to be debrided, which inevitably conveys the shortening of these structures. Good and strong four-strand repair of the flexor tendons help start active mobilization protocol. Nerve repair helped re-innervate some intrinsic musculature. In such major replants, quick repair of all the structures is necessary. Because the ischemia time at arrival was only 2 hours and the part was well preserved, debridement, skeletal fixation, and nerve and tendon repairs were done first and the vessels were repaired last. Had the ischemia time been longer than 4 to 5 hours, a preliminary shunting of the vessels with a silicone catheter or the vessel repair technique is advisable.

Remember	M!

- First time is the best time to get good results.
- Debridement is the key to success to prevent infection and achieve primary healing.
- Achieve soft-tissue cover early.
- Minor rotational malalignments of fractures may lead to severe disability.
- Missed nerve injuries are the most common cause for litigation.
- Tendon repairs must be followed up with good rehabilitation protocols.

21.7 Conclusions

Hand injuries are just not medical problems; they could potentially become a source of great stress to the family. Forty percent of all injuries that occur in the workplace are to the hands and indirect costs of hand injury like lost wages and productivity and loss of employment are high. With proper treatment, the indirect costs come down and very often patients resume their previous job. To get good functional outcome, skilled and experienced surgeons and a supportive infrastructure are needed. Appropriate care rendered at the right time provides gratifying results.

21.8 Key Points

- Hand injury management needs special skills, a supportive infrastructure, and diligent follow-up.
- Indirect costs of hand injury like loss of wages, productivity, and employment can be reduced with good surgical care.
- It is paramount to achieve primary wound healing in all open injuries.
- Radical debridement with primary reconstruction yields the best results.
- Replantation when well executed offers the best form of reconstruction in total amputations.

Recommended Readings

Carlsen BT, Moran SL. Thumb trauma: Bennett fractures, Rolando fractures, and ulnar collateral ligament injuries. J Hand Surg Am. 2009; 34(5):945–952

Chandraprakasam T, Kumar RA. Acute compartment syndrome of forearm and hand. Indian J Plast Surg. 2011; 44(2):212–218

Freeland AE, Lindley SG. Malunions of the finger metacarpals and phalanges. Hand Clin. 2006; 22(3):341–355

Gelberman RH, Blasingame JP, Fronek A, Dimick MP. Forearm arterial injuries. J Hand Surg Am. 1979; 4(5):401–408

Gelberman RH, Garfin SR, Hergenroeder PT, Mubarak SJ, Menon J. Compartment syndromes of the forearm: diagnosis and treatment. Clin Orthop Relat Res. 1981(161):252–261

Giddins G. The Nonoperative Management of Hand Fractures in United Kingdom. Hand Clin. 2017; 33(3):473–487

Godina M. Early microsurgical reconstruction of complex trauma of the extremities. Plast Reconstr Surg. 1986; 78(3):285–292

Graham D, Bhardwaj P, Sabapathy SR. Secondary thumb reconstruction in a mutilated hand. Hand Clin. 2016; 32(4):533–547

Kleinert HE, Verdan C. Report of the committee on tendon injuries. J Hand Surg Am. 1983; 8(5 Pt 2):794–798

Lister G, Scheker L. Emergency free flaps to the upper extremity. J Hand Surg Am. 1988; 13(1):22–28

Lister G. The Hand: Diagnosis and Indications. 2nd ed. New York, NY: Churchill Livingstone Inc.; 1984:16–17

Meals C, Meals R. Hand fractures: a review of current treatment strategies. J Hand Surg Am. 2013; 38(5):1021–1031, quiz 1031

Raja Sabapathy S. Management of complex tissue injuries and replantation across the world. Injury. 2006; 37(11):1057–1060

Sabapathy SR, Bhardwaj P. Tendon injuries. In: Sivananthan S, Sherry E, Warnke P, Miller MD, ed. Mercer's Text Book of Orthopaedics and Trauma. London: Hodder Arnold; 2012:1292–1301

Sabapathy SR, Bajantri B. Indications, selection, and use of distant pedicled flap for upper limb reconstruction. Hand Clin. 2014; 30(2):185–199, vi

Sabapathy SR, Bharadwaj P. Soft tissue Cover in Hand Injuries. Curr Orthop. 2008; 22:1–8

Sabapathy SR. Treatment of mutilating hand injuries: An International Perspective. Hand Clin. 2016; 32:435–602

Scheker LR, Ahmed O. Radical debridement, free flap coverage, and immediate reconstruction of the upper extremity. Hand Clin. 2007; 23(1):23–36

Tsiouri C, Hayton MJ, Baratz M. Injury to the ulnar collateral ligament of the thumb. Hand (NY). 2009; 4(1):12–18

Venkatramani H, Sabapathy SR. Collagen sheets as temporary wound cover in major open fractures before definitive flap cover. Plast Reconstr Surg. 2002; 110(6):1613–1614

Verdan CE. Primary repair of flexor tendons. J Bone Joint Surg Am. 1960; 42-A:647–657

Index

Note: Page numbers set **bold** or *italic* indicate headings or figures, respectively.